FIFTH EDITION

HEALTH POLICY AND POLITICS
A NURSE'S GUIDE

Edited by:

**Jeri A. Milstead,
PhD, RN, NEA-BC, FAAN**

Senior Nurse Consultant, Dublin, Ohio
Professor and Dean Emerita
University of Toledo (Ohio) College of Nursing

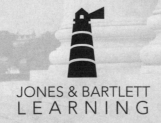

JONES & BARTLETT
LEARNING

World Headquarters
Jones & Bartlett Learning
5 Wall Street
Burlington, MA 01803
978-443-5000
info@jblearning.com
www.jblearning.com

06824-5

Production Credits

VP, Executive Publisher: David Cella
Executive Editor: Amanda Martin
Associate Managing Editor: Sara Bempkins
Production Editor: Sarah Bayle
Senior Marketing Manager: Jennifer Stiles
Art Development Editor: Joanna Lundeen
Art Development Assistant: Shannon Sheehan
VP, Manufacturing and Inventory Control:
   Therese Connell
Composition: Cenveo Publisher Services
Cover Design: Theresa Manley
Manager of Photo Research, Rights & Permissions:
   Lauren Miller
Cover Image: © Camrock/iStockphoto.com
Printing and Binding: Edwards Brothers Malloy
Cover Printing: Edwards Brothers Malloy

Library of Congress Cataloging-in-Publication Data
Health policy and politics (Milstead)
  Health policy and politics : a nurse's guide / [edited by] Jeri A. Milstead. — Fifth edition.
     p. ; cm.
  Includes bibliographical references and index.
  ISBN 978-1-284-04886-5 — ISBN 978-1-284-06824-5
  I. Milstead, Jeri A., editor. II. Title.
  [DNLM: 1. Legislation, Nursing—United States. 2. Health Policy—United States. 3. Politics—United States. WY 33 AA1]
  RT86.5
  362.17'30973—dc23
                              2014024733

6048

Printed in the United States of America
19 18 17 16 15   10 9 8 7 6 5 4 3 2

CONTENTS

Preface   ix
Acknowledgments   xv

**Chapter 1   Advanced Practice Registered Nurses and
    Public Policy, Naturally 1**
Jeri A. Milstead
Introduction   2
Why "Naturally"?   2
What Nurses Have to Offer Colleagues and Policymakers
    to Make Sustainable Change   12
Healthcare Reform in the Center of the Public Policy Process   17
Developing a More Sophisticated Political Role for Nurses   22
What Is Public Policy?   24
An Overview of the Policy Process   28
An Exciting Future   32
Conclusion   37
    Discussion Points   37
    Case Study: Pill Mills   40
    References   40

Chapter 2   Agenda Setting   45
Elizabeth Ann Furlong
Introduction   45
    *Case Study 1: A Nurse Practitioner–Initiated Bill in the Spring 2014
        Nebraska Unicameral Legislature*   46
    Case Study 2: The National Center for Nursing Research Amendment   48
Overview of Models and Dimensions   50
Summary Analysis of a National Policy Case Study   61
Theory Application to the Emerging State Case Study   62
    Discussion Points   65
    References   65

Chapter 3   Government Response: Legislation 69

Janice Kay Lanier

Introduction 70

Process, People, and Purse Strings 71

Playing the Game: Strategizing for Success 81

   Case Study: Workplace Safety 82

Conclusion 89

   Discussion Points 94

   References 96

Chapter 4   Government Regulation: Parallel and Powerful 99

Jacqueline M. Loversidge

Introduction 100

Regulation Versus Legislation 101

Health Professions Regulation and Licensing 103

The State Regulatory Process 113

   Case Study 1: Board of Pharmacy Regulation 118

The Federal Regulatory Process 120

Current Issues in Regulation and Licensure 131

The Future of Advanced Practice Nurse Regulation 135

Conclusion 140

   Discussion Points 141

   Case Study 2: Delegation of Medication Administration by APRNs ... 142

   Case Study 3: Changes in Regulations: The Weight of a Single Word ... 145

   References 147

Chapter 5   Policy Design 151

Patricia Smart

Introduction 151

The Policy Process 154

Review of Policy Research 154

The Design Issue 156

Policy Instruments (Government Tools) 157

Behavioral Dimensions 160

Using Tools as a Looking Glass 160

   Case Study 1: Comparative Analysis of Pregnancy Outcomes
      in Two Countries 162

Bringing Policy to the Classroom 165

   Case Study 2: Polypharmacy Problems 166

   Case Study 3: Teen Pregnancy in South Carolina 166

Conclusion. 167
    Discussion Points 168
    References 168

Chapter 6 Policy Implementation **171**
Marlene Wilken
Introduction 171
Implementation Research 173
Implementation: The Process 175
Conclusion. 180
Introduction to Case Studies 180
    Case Study 1: The Impact of Evidence-Based Practice on Patient Safety,
      Quality, and Cost 182
    Case Study 2: VHA Innovative Model 184
    Case Study 3: Nurse Managed Health Clinics 186
    References 187

Chapter 7 Program Evaluation. **189**
Ardith L. Sudduth
Introduction 190
Policy, Public Policy, and Social Programs. 192
Program Evaluation. 195
Theory and Ethics: Valuable Tools in Evaluation. 200
Program Evaluation Design Options 205
Evaluation Reports: Sharing the Findings. 207
Conclusion. 210
    Discussion Points 211
    Case Study 1: Evaluating Clinic Services 211
    Case Study 2: Clinic: For Episodic or Chronic Care? 212
    References 213
    Online Resources 216

Chapter 8 The Impact of Social Media and the Internet
  on Healthcare Decisions **219**
Elizabeth Barnhill and Troy Spicer
Introduction 220
Social Media: How They Have Changed Communication. 222
Social Media and Healthcare Information: A Mixed Blessing. 226
Beyond Informatics: Electronic Health Records. 232
Information, Legislation, and Health Care 236

The Future of Healthcare Policy in the Age of Social Media.................238
    Case Study 1: (In)secure Communication?...............................240
    Case Study 2: A Disconnect About Values/Beliefs..........................241
    Case Study 3: Ethics in a Clinical Setting................................242
    References...243

Chapter 9   Interprofessional Practice, Education, and Research.........247
Kimberly Ann Galt, J.D. Polk, Patrick DeLeon, and Jeri A. Milstead
Introduction 247
    References 251

Experiences and Perspectives on Interprofessional Education 251
Kimberly Ann Galt
Challenges Facing Interprofessional Education............................252
Overcoming the Challenges..253
    Case Study 1: Moving to a Common Core Interprofessional
        Patient Safety Curriculum.......................................254
Policy Implications..258
    References 259

The Evolving Interprofessional Universe 260
J.D. Polk
What Is Interprofessional Collaboration?..................................261
Core Attributes of Interprofessional Education............................261
    Case Study 2: An Adolescent with Diabetes: Typical Treatment Options?.......262
The "Team 4" Concept 264
    Case Study 3: Innovation and IPE in a Chilean Mine 267
The Future of IPE..269
    References and Bibliography...270

The Transformative Journey 270
Patrick DeLeon
Vision, Persistence, Patience 270
Perspectives on Being Involved 272
The Affordable Care Act..273
Final Reflections...281
    References 282
Conclusion..282

Chapter 10   Overview: The Economics and Finance of Health Care..... 283

Nancy Munn Short

Introduction 285

Economics: Opportunity Costs 286

Finance: Does More Spending Buy Us Better Health? 287

Economics: Health Insurance Market................................... 287

Finance: Health Insurance Exchanges.................................. 289

Finance: Healthcare Entitlement Programs............................. 291

Economics: Information Asymmetry 295

Finance: Comparative Effectiveness Research and QALYs................. 298

Finance: Bending the Healthcare Cost Curve Downward 299

   Discussion Points 302

   Case Study 1: Medicare Sustainable Growth Rate for
   *   Physician/Nurse Practitioner Payment* 303

   Case Study 2: Economic Value of BSN Education for RNs 304

   Case Study 3: Economic Impact of States Declining Medicaid Expansion 305

   References 306

   Online Resources 307

Chapter 11   Global Connections................................... 309

Jeri A. Milstead

Introduction 309

Global Issues 310

The Importance of Understanding the Cultural Context 313

The Nurse Shortage.. 315

Nurse Involvement in Policy Decisions................................. 316

   Case Study: The Resurgence of Polio.............................. 319

Conclusion.. 323

   Discussion Points 324

   References 324

Index 327

This is a contributed text for healthcare professionals who are interested in expanding the depth of their knowledge about the process of making public policy and in becoming more sophisticated in their involvement in public policy. The focus is on advanced practice registered nurses (APRNs), but the content, discussion points, and case studies can be used by all healthcare professionals including physicians, pharmacists, dentists, psychologists, those in allied health, and others. Chapters are written by contributors who have direct experience in real-world policymaking and political action. The scope of the content covers the whole process of making public policy. Components of the process are addressed within broad categories of agenda setting; government response; and program/policy design, implementation, and evaluation. The primary focus is at the federal and state levels, although the reader can adapt concepts to the global or local level.

Why a *Fifth Edition*?

The *First Edition* was a research-based text that covered the whole policy process. The *Second Edition* provided updated information. The book was well received and used in at least five countries.

The *Third Edition* found us in a different place. We live in a world of much uncertainty. The United States had lost its place as the benevolent, wise-for-our-age country where world leadership was a given. Other countries had lost confidence in our vision of economics, the environment, education, health care, and politics. We had been thrust into the world spotlight not because of our successes but because of our failures. The United States could no longer justify using so many environmental resources, could no longer justify rearing a generation (or more) of children who cannot read or compute and who are prone to unhealthy and violent behavior, and could no longer justify an economic system where the rich were getting richer and the poor were getting poorer and the middle class was beginning to diminish.

The *Third Edition* focused on practical examples and suggestions for actually becoming involved in the policy process. Both students and teachers were encouraged to use these activities to enhance their theoretical learning.

The *Fourth Edition* found us facing different challenges. The exponential growth of technology had affected not only our personal lives, but also our health system. Social media, genetics, and telehealth had become integral in our lives. Nurses accepted responsibility for making the health system more humane and ethical. We began to realize that leadership in policymaking and politics required commitment to becoming involved. Contributing authors had pursued other avenues of their roles that moved away from their original research, so they created case studies that tied policy concepts to real-world scenarios and developed discussion questions and activities for readers to use. The scenarios offered points to consider—there were no right or wrong answers. Posing different outcomes to each situation was intended to provide a safe place to try out solutions to some of the ideas presented and to help the reader become more flexible in thinking about options or choosing responses to very real circumstances.

The *Fifth Edition* builds on the prior editions and brings an exciting new dimension to readers in the form of a new chapter on interprofessional practice, education, and research. It was important that this chapter would not be written by nurses but by a physician, a psychologist, and a pharmacist who have had extensive experience in working with other professionals—in health care and other disciplines. As the 2010 Institute of Medicine (IOM) report noted, nurses can no longer afford to work in siloes; that is, we cannot ignore the power we can create when working together with our healthcare colleagues. This is not a new concept, but the IOM report gave substance and significance to a mandate to work with others. This new chapter offers examples of how our colleagues have been leaders in moving this idea forward.

Also in this edition, the chapter about nurses who are working in the policy arena has been retired—due to Nancy Sharp's personal retirement. We celebrate her future and acknowledge her wonderful past contribution. All of the contributing authors have updated and created new case studies and discussion points.

We hope readers will use this text to initiate discussions with their healthcare colleagues in related fields. We welcome your comments—let us know how this content has helped you in your practice.

Target Audience

This text is intended for several audiences:

- Nurses who work in advanced practice in clinical, education, administrative, research, or consultative settings can use this book as a guide for understanding the full range of the policy components that they did not learn in graduate school or may have forgotten. Components are brought to life through nursing research, real life cases, and theory. This book will help the nurse who is searching for knowledge of how leaders of today influence public policy toward better health care for the future. Nurses in leadership positions clearly articulate nursing's societal mission. Nurses, as the largest group of healthcare workers in the country, realize that the way to make a permanent impact on the delivery of health care is to be a part of the decision making that occurs at every step of the healthcare policy process.

- Doctoral and master's students in nursing can use this text for in-depth study of the full policy process. Works of scholars in each segment provide a solid foundation for examining each component. This book goes beyond the narrow elementary explanation of legislation and bridges the gap toward the understanding of a broader policy process in which multiple opportunities for involvement exist.

- Faculty in graduate programs and other current nurse leaders can use this book as a reference for their own policy activity. Faculty and other leaders should be mentors for those they teach and for other nurses throughout the profession. Because the whole policy process is so broad, these leaders can track their own experiences through the policy process by referring to the components described in this book.

- A wide variety of healthcare professionals who are interested in the area of healthcare policy will find this book useful in directing their thoughts and actions toward the complex issues of both healthcare policy and public policy. Physicians, pharmacists, psychologists, dentists, occupational and physical therapists, physicians' assistants, and others will discover parallels with their own practices as they examine case studies and other research. Nurses cannot change huge systems alone. Members of the healthcare team can use this book as a vehicle to educate themselves so that, together, everyone in the healthcare profession can influence policymakers.

- Those professionals who do not provide health care directly but who are involved in areas of the environment that produce actual and potential threats to personal and community health and safety will find this book a valuable resource regarding how a problem becomes known, who decides what to do about it, and what type of governmental response might result. Environmental scientists, public health officials, sociologists, political scientists, anthropologists, and other professionals involved with health problems in the public interest will benefit from the ideas generated in this book.

- Interest groups can use this book as a tool to consider opportunities to become involved in public policymaking. Interest groups can be extremely helpful in changing systems because their members' passion for their causes energizes them to act. Interest groups can become partners in the political activity of nurses by knowing how and when to use their influence to assist APRNs at junctures in the policy process.

- Corporate leaders can use this book to gain an understanding of the broad roles within which nurses function. Chief executive officers (CEOs) and other top business administrators must learn that nurses are articulate, assertive, and intelligent experts in health care who have a solid knowledge base and a political agenda. The wise CEO and colleagues will seek out APRNs for counsel and collaboration when moving policy ideas forward and make sure they are at the table when ideas are considered and decisions are made.

Using This Text

Each chapter in the text is freestanding; that is, chapters do not rely, or necessarily build, on one another. The sequence of the chapters is presented in a linear fashion, but readers will note immediately that the policy process is not linear. For example, readers of the policy implementation chapter will find reference to scholars and concepts featured in the agenda-setting and policy design chapters. Such is the nature of the public process of making decisions. The material covered is a small portion of the existing research, argument, and considered thought about policymaking and the broader political, economic, and social concepts and issues. Therefore, readers should use this book as a starting point for their own scholarly inquiry.

This book can be used to initiate discussions about issues of policy and nurses' opportunities and responsibilities throughout the process. The research studies that are presented should raise some questions about what should have happened or why something else did or did not happen. In this way, the book can serve as a guide through what some think of as a maze of activity with no direction but what is actually a rational, albeit chaotic, system.

The case studies and discussion points are ideal for planning a class or addressing an audience. Many ideas and concepts are presented, and I hope that they serve to stimulate the readers' own creative thoughts about how to engage others. Gone are the days of the "sage on stage"—the teacher who had all the answers and lectured to students who had no questions. Good teachers always have learned from students and vice versa. Today's teachers are interactive, technically savvy, curious and questioning, and capable of helping learners integrate large amounts of data and information. This text can serve as a guide and a beginning.

ACKNOWLEDGMENTS

Only a few nurses in the United States with master's degrees in nursing also hold earned doctorates in political science. When I discovered that several of these nurses had researched different components of the policy process, a contributed publication immediately came to mind. The authors realize that there is much more to public decision making than the process of writing laws, and that this knowledge affords them the opportunity and responsibility to contribute seriously to public policy. When I approached these nurses about contributing to this text, each agreed enthusiastically. Therefore, special thanks must go to Dr. Beth Furlong, Dr. Patricia Smart, Dr. Ardith Sudduth, and Dr. Marlene Wilken for their scholarly contributions.

I continue to thank Jones & Bartlett Learning (formerly Jones and Bartlett Publishers) for their encouragement and guidance in writing the *Fifth Edition* and for broadening the readership to include a wide range of healthcare professionals. Their confidence in all of the contributors has been consistent and unwavering. Amanda Martin, executive editor of the nursing division; Sara Bempkins, associate managing editor for nursing; and Rebecca Myrick, associate acquisitions editor for nursing, have kept the authors on track in meeting deadlines and in providing editorial assistance.

I also thank the readers of this text for their interest in the policy and political processes. For those of you who have integrated these components and concepts into your nursing careers, I applaud you. You will continue to contribute to the profession and to the broader society. For those readers who are struggling with how to incorporate one more piece of anything into your role as an advanced practice registered nurse, remember that you are advancing the cause of your own personal work, the profession, and healthcare delivery in this country and throughout the world every time you use the concepts in this text. Nurses are a powerful force and exercise their many talents to further good public policy, which, ultimately, must improve health care for patients, consumers, and families.

For the wide range of healthcare professionals (dentists, dietitians, pharmacists, physical and occupational therapists, physicians, physician's assistants, psychologists, and others) who may be reading this text for the first time, I encourage you to collaborate as colleagues in the 21st century definition of "team" and integrate policymaking into your practices. I hope the contents of this text have been helpful and will motivate you to implement the new healthcare paradigm.

Finally, I acknowledge my forever-cheering section—my four children, their spouses and significant others, and three grandchildren. They are always there for me and provide continuous support, encouragement, and unconditional love. I love you, Kerrin, Sunny, and George Biddle; Joan Milstead; Kevin Milstead and Gregg Peace; and Sara, Steve, and Matthew Lott. You are a fun bunch and you make me laugh. Special thanks, also, to the memory of my late fiancée, Ed Salser, who used to tease me by saying I never saw a committee meeting I didn't like, and to my late son-in-law, George A. Biddle, who read every word of the *Fourth Edition*.

Jeri A. Milstead

CHAPTER 1

Advanced Practice Registered Nurses and Public Policy, Naturally

Jeri A. Milstead

KEY TERMS

Advanced practice registered nurse (APRN): A registered nurse with a master's or doctoral degree in nursing who demonstrates expert knowledge, skills, and attitudes in the practice of nursing. An APRN is certified by a nationally recognized professional organization. Four types of APRNs are recognized by most nurse regulatory boards: nurse practitioner (NP), clinical nurse specialist (CNS), certified nurse midwife (CNM), and certified registered nurse anesthetist (CRNA).

Client/patient: The recipient of health care; *patient* carries a "sick" connotation whereas *client* may not. The terms will be used interchangeably throughout this chapter.

Healthcare providers (HCPs): Registered nurses, advanced practice registered nurses (APRNs), physicians, pharmacists, dentists, psychologists, occupational and physical therapists, and physician's assistants who are licensed by a state or territory to provide health care.

Nursing's agenda for health: Policy expectations of a vision for nursing practice that include prevention of illness, promotion of health, empowerment of individuals to assume responsibility for the state of their own health, expertise in the provision of direct nursing care, delegation and supervision of selected care to appropriate individuals, and the political influence to accomplish these goals.

Policy process: Bringing problems to government and obtaining a reply. The process includes agenda setting, design, government response, implementation, and evaluation.

Public policy: A program, law, regulation, or other legal mandate provided by governmental agents; also actual legal documents, such as opinions, directives, and briefs that record government decisions.

Introduction

This text originally was written to focus on the relevance of public policy to **advanced practice registered nurses (APRNs)**. The Institute of Medicine's report, *The Future of Nursing: Advancing Health, Leading Change* (Institute of Medicine [IOM], 2010), challenged nurses to work with other healthcare professionals in two ways: to learn from them and to help them learn from nurses. In this spirit of interprofessional cooperation and leadership, this text will incorporate a variety of **healthcare providers (HCPs)** into the discussion of public policy, case studies, discussion points, and reader activities. Although APRNs are the major focus, the astute reader will realize that the process is the same for all HCPs; the theories and scenarios that are presented have relevance to all providers. The authors hope that readers will recognize the spirit of respect and cooperation that is intended and begin to "gather at the table" together and to make decisions that truly integrate health care that benefits the **client/patient**.

Why "Naturally"?

The policy process is a broad range of decision points, strategies, activities, and outcomes that involve elected and appointed government officials and their staffs, bureaucratic agencies, private citizens, and interest groups. The process is dynamic, convoluted, and ongoing, not static, linear, or concise. The idea of "messy" may be uncomfortable to nurses who are known to expect action immediately, but the political arena requires patience, tact, diplomacy, and persistence. Knowledgeable nurses in advanced practice must demonstrate their commitment to action by being a part of relevant decisions that will ensure the delivery of quality health care by appropriate providers in a cost-effective manner. So why would anyone suggest that working at the policy level is "natural" to the nursing profession? This author proposes that involvement in policy decisions and the political process is an integral part of the role because of our history, practice, education, and professional organizations.

History

Florence Nightingale is regarded as the mother of nursing being a profession that requires education and practice. Although reared in an upper-class family, she viewed the service that nurses provided as worthy of respect, a standing generally not accorded to nurses at the time. She founded educational programs (known as nurse's training programs) and began the work of creating standards of care. She used her influence with her family's business and professional colleagues to obtain funding to send a cadre of trained nurses to the Crimea to care for soldiers during a war. The nurses focused on improving sanitary conditions and food in addition to attending to personal and medical care such as using clean dressings and linen. When she returned to England, she developed education programs that trained women in what became the principles of nursing. These schools raised the reputation of nurses and increased their credibility and visibility in the public's eye. Nightingale's political influence became legendary.

Over the years, other nurses have taken on health issues at various times and in various ways. Mary Mahoney was the first African American nurse in the United States (1879). She was a major advocate for equal opportunities for minorities. Nurses who exerted their considerable political influence in the early 20th century included Clara Barton, who founded the Red Cross; Margaret Sanger, whose leadership for Planned Parenthood resulted in arrest and conviction; and Lillian Wald, who worked diligently with the poor through neighborhood settlement houses, helped President Theodore Roosevelt create the Federal Children's Bureau, and suggested a national health insurance plan. Jessie Scott, DSc, RN, testified frequently before Congress in her position as director of nursing for the U.S. Public Health Service and was instrumental in passing the 1964 Nurse Training Act, legislation that provided funding for nurse education (especially graduate education) for many years. Faye Wattleton, RN, MS, was a forceful director of Planned Parenthood in the 1970s and 1980s during a time of great challenge to women's rights in general and, specifically, the right to determine the health of their own bodies. Ada Sue Hinshaw, PhD, RN, still is remembered today for her absolute persistence and her ability to gather a group of nurses in the late 1980s and 1990s who worked with federal legislators to create the National Center for Nursing Research that eventually became the National Institute for Nursing Research, one of the pillars of the National Institutes of Health. Mary Wakefield, PhD, RN, served as chief of staff for two U.S. senators before she became the current administrator of the Health Resources and Services Administration. There are many examples of nurses who have wielded political savvy and power to make significant changes to the profession. Our practice provides a firm basis for involvement in the process of making public policy.

Education

Public policy content pervades the nurse education programs of today in ways that would not have been considered in our early culture. The system of nursing education evolved from apprentice, hospital-based training to institutions of higher learning. Practice that once was found primarily in hospitals has moved into all facets of society—long-term care facilities, laboratories, clinics, industries, homes, and other situations. Specialization in nursing has moved from the early five major areas (medical, surgical, obstetric, pediatric, psychiatric) to include genetics, informatics, public policy, and a huge array of health- or medically related areas of expertise.

Today's nurse leaders are college-educated with doctoral, master's, baccalaureate, and associate's degrees. Baccalaureate programs are based on a liberal arts education of natural sciences (to understand the health and medical problems encountered), social sciences (recognizing that people live in families, groups, and communities), and the humanities (because nurses address the human condition) and provide a solid, broad education that forms the philosophical foundation from which nurses practice. Advanced education builds on education and experience and broadens the arena in which nurses work to a systems perspective. Nurses not only are well prepared to provide direct care to persons and families, but also act as change agents in the work environments in which they practice.

Nurses have developed theories to explain and predict phenomena that are met in the course of providing care. Nurses also incorporate theory from other disciplines such as psychology, anthropology, education, biomedical science, and information technology. Integration of all of this information reflects the extreme complexity of nursing care and its provision in an extremely complex healthcare system. Communication skills are integral to the education of nurses, who often must interpret complex medical situations and terms into common, understandable, pragmatic language. Nurse education programs have formalized a greater focus on communications than any other professional education program. From baccalaureate curricula through all upper levels of nurse education, full courses or major segments of courses on individual communications and group process are provided. Information and skills in these courses are integrated throughout programs and applied to practice in direct patient experiences known as *clinicals*. Communication skills are reinforced as requirements in advanced nurse education programs such as psychiatric nursing. Skills include active listening, reflection, clarification, assertiveness, role playing, and other techniques that build nurse competence levels. These same skills are used when talking with policymakers.

Complexity science "... fosters the health of individuals, families, communities, and our natural environment by helping people use concepts emerging from the new science of complexity" (Plexis Institute, 2009). Complexity science goes beyond systems theory; it acknowledges patterns in chaos, complex adaptive systems, and principles of self-organization and has great applicability to nursing (Curtin, 2010; Lindberg, Nash, & Lindberg, 2008). "The quantum concept of a matrix or field ... that connects everything together" (Curtin, 2011, p. 56) informs us that nurses are focused masses of energy who direct their behaviors and actions with patients in an intentional way toward accomplishing healthy states. The nurse–patient (or nurse–provider) relationship is not incidental or haphazard, but fully cognizant of purpose (Curtin, 2010; Husted, Scotto, & Wolf, 2015). Observing patterns in personal behavior can be useful in working with policymakers as they try to figure out the best or most cost-effective way to address public problems. Creative ways of examining problems and innovative solutions may not be comfortable to policymakers who have learned to be cautious and go slowly. Nurses and other professionals can help officials employ new ideas to reach their policy goals.

Quantum thinking also is crucial to the effectiveness of an organization in the 21st century (Porter-O'Grady & Malloch, 2014). Partnerships are valued over competition, and the old rules of business that rewarded power and ownership have given way to accountability and shared risk. Transforming the old systems into the new systems does not mean merely automating processes or restructuring the organizational chart. Transformation involves a radical, cross-functional, futuristic change in the way people think. Short-term planning is balanced with strategic planning, and vertical work relationships are replaced with networks and webs of people and knowledge. All workers at all levels share a commitment to the organization and an accountability to define and produce quality work. Rhoades, Covery, and Shepherdson (2011) are "convinced that positive, people-centered cultural values lead to higher performance" (p. 1). All workers share responsibility for self-governance, from which both the organization and the worker benefit (Porter-O'Grady, Hawkins, & Parker, 1997). Control is replaced by leadership. The new leader does not use policing techniques of supervision, but enables and empowers colleagues through vision, trust, and respect (Bennis & Nanus, 1985; Kouzes & Posner, 2007; Porter-O'Grady & Wilson, 2014). Encouragement, appreciation, and personal recognition are celebrated together in an effective organization (Kouzes & Posner, 1999). Building relationships is essential to the success of any current organizational model.

Policy content is understood as important to nurses and has become required by accreditation agencies for nurse education programs. Content essential at the undergraduate level includes "policy development ... legislation and regulatory processes ... social policy/public policy ... and political activism and professional organizations" (American Association of Colleges of Nursing [AACN], 2008a, p. 21). Content at the master's level for all students, regardless of their specialty or functional area, includes "policy, organization, and finance of health care" (AACN, 2008b, p. 6). Required content for doctoral students in advanced practice includes behaviors to "critically analyze ... demonstrate leadership ... inform policy makers ... educate others ... advocate for the profession" (AACN, 2006, p. 13).

Course syllabi include learning activities that involve students in various ways—from attending meetings of health-related or public policy–related boards to arranging time with legislators and their aides, attending sessions of regulatory boards and commissions, and testifying at hearings. Doctoral students, especially those in practice doctorates such as the Doctor of Nursing Practice (DNP), may conduct their final capstone projects around changing a law, regulation, or public policy. More action-oriented experiences are required at every level of education. Understanding the whole process of policymaking is essential for preparing nurses to become active with policymakers.

Nursing care is not just altruistic (although there is a noble component in the philosophy), but intentional action (or inaction) that focuses on a person or group with actual or potential health problems. The education of nurses puts them in the position of discovering and acknowledging health problems and health system problems that may demand intervention by public policymakers.

Practice

Nursing as a practice profession is based on theory and evidence. For many years that practice was interpreted as direct, hands-on care of individuals. Although this still is true, the profession has matured to the point where the provision of expert, direct care is not enough. Nurses of the third millennium stand tall in their multiple roles of provider of care, educator, administrator, consultant, researcher, political activist, and policymaker. The question of how much a nurse in advanced practice can or should take on may be raised. The Information/Knowledge Age continues to present new data exponentially. Nurses have added more and more tasks that seem important to a professional nurse and are essential for the provision of safe care to the client. Is political activism necessary? All health professionals are expected to do more with fewer resources. Realistically, how much can a specialist do?

The public policy process involves alerting government to issues and obtaining responses. Nurses spot healthcare problems that may need government intervention. Nurses work in areas of direct and indirect patient care. Their practice may be directed toward individual patients, families, groups, or communities. Nurses seek evidence through inquiry and research in order to provide appropriate interventions. Nursing education programs include courses and units on organizational development, general systems theory, and complexity science. Most nurses are employees (as are most physicians today) and must navigate the organizations in which they work. By being attuned to systems issues, nurses have developed the ability to direct questions and identify solutions. This ability is reflected in the relationships that nurses can develop with policymakers.

Major-General Irene Trowell-Harris, EdD, RN, USAF, retired, understood the political process when she was named director of the Department of Veterans Affairs Center for Women Veterans in 2001. She also was instrumental in establishing a nurse residency program for military nurses in the office of Senator Daniel K. Inouye (D-HI) in which one nurse from each of the four armed services was assigned (on a rolling basis) to that office for 1 year—a pragmatic and highly intense experience in the process of making public policy at the federal level.

Nurses have many personal stories that illustrate health problems and patients' responses to them. These stories can have a powerful effect when a nurse brings an issue to the attention of legislators and other policymakers. Anecdotes often make a problem more understandable at a personal level, and nurses are credible storytellers. Nurses also know how to bring research to legislators in ways that can be understood and can have a positive effect.

Nurses live in neighborhoods where health problems often surface and can often rally friends to the importance of a local issue. Nurses are constituents of electoral districts and can make contacts with policymakers in their districts. Nurses vote. It is not unusual for a nurse to become the point person for a policymaker who is seeking information about health-care issues. A nurse does not have to be knowledgeable about every health problem, but she or he has a vast network of colleagues and resources to tap into when a policymaker seeks facts. The practice of nursing prepares the practitioner to work in the policy arena.

Organizational Involvement

Over 20 years ago, a leader in organizational theory, Drucker (1995), addressed the need for more general-practitioner physicians rather than specialists. He redefined the generalist of that time as one who puts multiple specialties together rapidly. Nurses have benefitted from that thought. In Drucker's definition, the advanced practice registered nurse (APRN) must be a multidimensional generalist/specialist. This means that the APRN combines knowledge and skills from a variety of fields or subspecialties effectively to design the new paradigm of healthcare delivery. This also means that the APRN must demonstrate competence in the multiple roles in which he or she operates. To function effectively in the role of political activist, the APRN must realize the scope of the whole policy process, and the process is much broader than how a bill becomes a law.

Boards of nursing and other professional regulatory boards exert much influence in interpreting statutes that govern nursing. Scope of practice is defined by boards and, because each state and jurisdiction defines the practice of nursing differently, there is wide variation in how the scope of practice is conducted. A fear expressed by many boards is the interference with Federal Trade Commission (FTC) rules that restrict monopoly practices. The FTC recently published a policy paper addressing the regulation of APRNs with five key findings that policymakers must pay attention to. First, APRNs, after years of research, provide care that is safe and effective. Second, physicians' mandatory supervision of and collaboration with advanced nurse practice is not justified by any concern for patient health or safety. Third, supervision and collaborative agreements required by statute or regulation lead to greater cost, decreased quality of care, fewer innovative practices, and reduced access to services. Fourth, APRNs collaborate effectively with all healthcare professionals without inflexible rules and laws. Finally, APRN practice is "… good for competition and consumers" ("FTC Policy Paper," 2014, p. 11). APRNs must become knowledgeable about the regulatory process so that they can spot opportunities to contribute or intervene prior to final rulemaking ("The Regulatory Process," 1992).

Federal and state health-related agencies provide funding for nurse education, conduct surveys to compile nurse demographic data, and manage programs that address health issues. For example the U.S. Department of Health and Human Services (DHHS) is "the principle agency for protecting the health of all Americans and providing essential human services, especially for those who are least able to help themselves" (DHHS, n.d.). Check the DHHS website to discover the wide range of bureaus and departments included within DHHS.

Professional organizations can bring their influence to the policy process in ways that a single person may not. There are a myriad of organizations to which nurses belong, including specialty areas, education-related organizations, and leadership-related organizations. For example, the American Nurses Association, the National League for Nursing, and Sigma Theta Tau International state a commitment to advancing health and health care in this country and/or on a global scale, as noted in their mission statements and goals. These organizations are structured to offer nurses opportunities to develop personal leadership skills. Committees provide occasion to learn about the organization, the mission, and the outreach. Professional associations afford experiences to become knowledgeable about issues pertinent to the organization or the profession. These groups can expand a nurse's perspective toward a broader view of health and professional issues such as at the state, national, or global level. The change in viewpoint often encourages a member's foray into the process of public policy. Some nurses are experienced in their political activity. They have served as chairs of legislative committees for professional organizations, worked as campaign managers for elected officials, or presented testimony at congressional, state, or local hearings; a few have run for office. Political activism is a major expectation of most professional organizations.

Many organizations employ lobbyists who carry issues and concerns to policymakers. These sophisticated activists are skilled in the process of getting the attention of government and obtaining a response. Professional organizations provide information about many health issues. Specialty associations have their own agendas and are excellent resources from which to learn. Nurses also have an opportunity to voice their own opinions and provide information from their own practices through active participation in organizations. This give and take builds knowledge and confidence when nurses help legislators and others interpret issues.

Beverly Malone, PhD, RN, currently chief executive officer, National League for Nursing, was named by President Clinton as a member of the U.S. Delegation to the World Health Assembly (the governing board of the World Health Organization). Then from 2001 to 2006 she served as general secretary of the Royal College of Nursing, the most esteemed professional nurse's trade union in the world.

Joanne Disch, PhD, RN, served as chair of the board of directors for AARP. During her tenure, she was an example of how the knowledge and experience of a nurse has relevance in the broader community. Her influence illustrates the extensive effect that nurses have in addressing factors related to aging for a huge population of Americans. Her work with pharmaceutical manufacturers and her strong testimony to Congress in the early years of this century made possible several laws that addressed medication need, incompatibility, and cost for senior citizens. Through her recent term as president of the American Academy of Nursing she continued to demonstrate leadership and political shrewdness at the highest level.

Summary of Reasons

So nurses are uniquely prepared to be involved in the process of public policy through history, practice, education, and organizations. The nurses cited in this chapter are only a representative few of the leaders who have brought the profession to the position of respect and advocacy enjoyed today. Nurses can do much to improve the healthcare system through policy change. But they cannot do it alone any longer. Nurses and nursing care are at the center of issues of tremendous and long-lasting impact. Nurses cannot afford to limit their actions. It is natural for nurses to talk with bureaucrats, agency staff, legislators, and others in public service about what nurses do, what nurses and their patients need, and the extent of their cost-effectiveness and long-term impact on health care in this country. For too long, nurses only talked to each other. Each knew his or her value, and each told great stories; they "preached to the choir" of other nurses instead of sharing their wisdom with those who could help change the healthcare system for the better. We finally are listening to those who have espoused interprofessional collaboration, and we are realizing that, together with our colleagues in medicine, psychology, pharmacy, dentistry, allied health, and other professions, we can join forces and make a stronger presence in determining policy. In the end, the patient is the winner.

Today's nurses, especially those in advanced practice who have a solid foundation of focused education and experience, know how to market themselves and their talents and know how to harness their irritations and direct them toward positive resolution. Nurses are embracing the whole range of options available in the various parts of the policy process. Nurses are initiating opportunities to sustain ongoing, meaningful dialogues with those who represent the districts and states and those who administer public programs. Nurses are becoming indispensable to elected and appointed officials, and nurses are demonstrating leadership by becoming those officials and by participating with others in planning and decision making. Nurses are realizing that by working with colleagues in other health professions they often move an issue forward with more credibility and fewer barriers.

The advanced practice registered nurse of the third millennium is technically competent; uses critical thinking and decision models; possesses vision that is shared with colleagues, consumers, and policymakers; and functions in a vast array of roles. One of these roles is policy analyst. Policy and politics is a natural domain for nurses. We are on the brink of an opportunity for the full integration into practice of the impending major changes in the delivery of care in the United States. Nurses have prepared for these changes by initiating new nurse education programs, expanding the number of master's and doctoral programs, and focusing on issues important to patients such as the just and equitable delivery of health care. Nurses can bring a unique perspective to healthcare issues.

What Nurses Have to Offer Colleagues and Policymakers to Make Sustainable Change

Numbers

Nurses can bring numbers to the policy arena. Nurses comprise the largest group of healthcare workers in the world. According to a 2008 report of registered nurses, there are 3.1 million registered nurses in the United States, 84.8% of whom are working in nursing. Fifty percent hold bachelor's degrees in nursing; 13.2% have masters or doctoral degrees (DHHS, 2010). One-third of the RN workforce is near retirement age. Projections indicate that the long-standing nurse shortage is becoming worse now that baby boomers are retiring. This group of consumers grew up in a time of economic abundance and will expect an abundance of healthcare services when they leave the workforce. Nurse education programs recognize the opportunity to expand program enrollment but are faced with a dearth of qualified faculty and appropriate sites for direct care practice known as *clinical space*.

Technology

Nurses can bring their considerable knowledge of technology to the policy process. Nurse educators and administrators are using technology to enhance and supplement the learning process. Patient simulators are models that can mimic healthcare problems in a laboratory. These models are very sophisticated and expensive, and can be programmed to mirror a heart attack, congestive heart failure, or any number of health conditions and emergencies. For best effect, students work in teams with colleagues from nursing, medicine, physical therapy, and emergency medical technology; medical residents; and others. The lab approach can ease the need for direct experience with patients because of the focused approach and because a scenario can be analyzed and replayed for different outcomes. Boards of nursing are concerned about how much simulation is appropriate, but it is clear that simulation is an asset to learning. Another benefit of simulation is the experience of working with a team. Interprofessional education is fairly new in most educational programs, although the concept has been discussed for many years. The use of simulators is a natural way to implement the idea of interprofessional collaboration.

Online education also has become a major force in the United States. Whether described as distance learning, electronic education, or another similar term, most nursing education programs use at least some form of teaching that is not face-to-face (F2F) in a single classroom. Although correspondence courses were available in some educational institutions, the term "distance learning" was pioneered as television courses in the 1960s, in which a group of students met together at a location remote from the customary classroom and were taught by a faculty member in the primary classroom. Today's e-learning affords opportunities to learn in a flexible, anytime schedule that is not grounded in geography or time. Classes are held synchronously (all students together at one time) or asynchronously (each student may enter a virtual classroom at any time, not necessarily as a group) or a combination of both. The sophistication of software systems provides students and faculty with a wide range of presentations.

Telehealth, an outgrowth of e-learning and advanced diagnostic technology, allows patients and providers access to each other's domain without concerns about transportation, time lost from work, childcare during visits, and other major reasons why patients do not make or keep appointments. This sophisticated technology first was tested by military personnel and found to be an effective method for training and for practice. Currently phone applications are available that connect patients directly to providers who can monitor conditions, prescribe treatments and medications, and deliver educational information. Ethical issues, cost of equipment, the learning curve of the provider and patient, and laws and regulations are dictating how much telehealth the public will embrace.

Education

Nurses can bring the same creativity to solving public policy issues that they used in addressing educational issues. Although the profession has not solved the "entry" problem, there are efforts to move closer to requiring a bachelor of science in nursing (BSN) degree as the beginning point for professional nursing. Aiken and colleagues have reported over and over that hospitals with higher proportions of baccalaureate-prepared nurses demonstrate decreased patient morbidity and mortality (Aiken et al., 2003, 2011, 2014; Van den Heede et al., 2009; You et al., 2013; Wiltse-Nicely, Sloane, & Aiken, 2013). Aiken's research includes studies in the United States and in nine European countries. Over 90 nurse generalist and specialty organizations are on record as supporting the BSN as an entry point to professional nursing. Some states are moving legislation or regulation to require that graduates of hospital diploma and associate degree programs obtain a BSN within 10 years of graduation in order to be relicensed as registered nurses (RNs). Although the National Council of State Boards of Nursing has stated it is not ready to support legislation or regulation that requires a BSN to practice as a registered nurse, the marketplace is moving in a different direction. There is a mounting wave of healthcare agencies that are limiting new hires to those with at least BSNs and have developed policies that require RNs with associate's degrees or diplomas to complete a BSN within 5 years of employment. Academic institutions have expanded or created RN-to-BSN programs in response to the demand.

Accelerated nurse education programs, recalling similar programs during World War II, have been developed at the bachelor's and master's degree levels. These programs were created to accept applicants with college degrees in fields other than nursing and provide the student with an opportunity to graduate with a degree in nursing in an abbreviated time period; graduates are eligible to sit for the National Council Licensure Examination (NCLEX-RN) to become registered nurses. These popular programs provide new avenues that address the nurse shortage.

A new education model at the master's level, the clinical nurse leader (CNL), was created by the American Association of Colleges of Nursing (AACN), the national organization of deans and directors of baccalaureate and higher-degree nurse programs (AACN, 2008c). During meetings of leaders of the AACN, the American Organization of Nurse Executives, and other employers of nurses, the AACN asked: Are educational institutions providing appropriate professionals for the workforce? The answer was that the nurses of today and the future should be educated to manage a population of patients/clients (such as a group of diabetics or those with congestive heart failure) both in a hospital setting and after discharge and should be able to make changes at a microsystem (i.e., unit) level. The CNL master's-level program was proposed in 2003 to address those recommendations. As of 2014, 38 states conducted CNL programs whose graduates can sit for a national certification exam that provides credibility to employers. In 2014 there were more than 3,000 certified CNLs (AACN, 2014a).

At about the same time as the CNL program was initiated, much work had been accomplished in moving APRNs toward doctoral education as an entry point. Rationale included granting a degree appropriate to the knowledge base and credit hours required in master's-level APRN programs and placing the advanced practitioner on a level with other health professionals. Note that a physician (MD), dentist (DDS), physical therapist (DPT), occupational therapist (OTD), and audiologist (AuD) require a practice doctorate. In 2004, AACN members voted to establish a practice doctoral degree, Doctor of Nursing Practice (DNP), and to require that all advanced nursing practice move from the master's level to the DNP by 2015 (AACN, 2014b). The DNP is an expert in patient care and designs, administers, and evaluates the delivery of complex health care in new organizational arrangements and at the systems level. Areas of concentration are offered in direct care, informatics, executive administration, and health policy. Although some nurse educators still express concern over the impact of the DNP on APRN practice (Cronenwett et al., 2011), by 2013 more than 214 programs existed with 2,443 enrolled students and 14,699 graduates.

The CNL and DNP also reflect a change in how health care is provided. Certified CNLs work at the unit micro level (not the health systems macro level) and provide direct care to groups of patients, which includes teaching with the goal of self-management of their own health problems. Patients learn to notice early indicators of changes in their conditions so that they may seek help before serious symptoms arise, with the goal being to keep patients as healthy as possible and to reduce hospital readmissions. The DNP provides care at the macro systems level; that is, this provider is alert to problems in the healthcare organization and can seek solutions through policy changes. DNPs develop relationships within and outside the healthcare network in order to facilitate transformation.

Positive Relationships

Nurses will bring their positive relationships with other stakeholders with whom they have common issues. Nurses will lead the movement of interprofessional practice, education, and research to the policy arena. Perhaps the greatest potential for change in the education of nurses will be the effect of the report from the Institute of Medicine (IOM) of the National

Academies, *The Future of Nursing: Leading Change, Advancing Health* (IOM, 2010). Under the aegis of and funded by the Robert Wood Johnson Foundation (RWJF), the report recognizes that nurses (the largest health-care workforce in the United States) must be an integral part of a healthcare team. The report provided four key messages (IOM, 2010, pp. 1–3):

1. Nurses should practice to the full extent of their education and training.
2. Nurses should achieve higher levels of education and training through an improved education system that promotes seamless academic progression.
3. Nurses should be full partners with physicians and other healthcare professionals in redesigning health care in the United States.
4. Effective workforce planning and policymaking require better data collection and an improved information infrastructure.

How the messages are being received by the intended audiences—"policy makers; national, state, and local government leaders; payers; and health care researchers, executives, and professionals—including nurses and others—as well as ... licensing bodies, educational institutions, philanthropic organizations, and consumer advocacy organizations" (IOM, 2010, p. 4)—is having a seismic impact on nursing education, practice, administration, and research. Removing barriers to practice, expanding leadership opportunities, doubling the number of nurses with doctorates, and greatly increasing bachelor's degrees to 80 percent of the workforce will require money, commitment, energy, and creativity. Removing barriers to practice also will require a change in laws and, especially, regulations to allow nurses and other health professionals to practice at the top of their education and experience.

A consortium of professional organizations already is moving forward together to address common problems. The Josiah Macy Jr. Foundation (2014) developed recommendations that support working together in five areas: (1) engagement, (2) innovative models, (3) education reform, (4) revision of regulatory standards, and (5) realignment of resources. In 2009, leaders from six national organizations met to establish the Interprofessional Education Collaborative (IPEC, n.d.): the American Association of Colleges of Nursing (AACN), American Association of Osteopathic Colleges of Medicine (AAOCM), American Association of Colleges of Pharmacy, American Dental Education Association (ADEA), Association of American

Medical Colleges (AAMC), and Association of Schools and Programs of Public Health (ASPPH). In 2013 they expanded to include the CEO of the American Association of Colleges of Pharmacy (AACP). IPEC developed four core competencies for interprofessional collaborative practice: (1) values/ethics, (2) roles/responsibilities, (3) interprofessional communication, and (4) teams and teamwork. Geraldine "Polly" Bednash, PhD, RN, immediate past chief executive officer of the AACN, is the current chair of IPEC.

It is now up to nurses and our other professional colleagues to advance health care so that both patients and professionals will benefit. Nurses are not only reforming nurse education and practice, but also providing leadership in gathering other healthcare professionals (practitioners and educators) to begin paradigm-changing discussions to reform the entire system. The new system will focus on health care, prevention of disease/disability, and health promotion. Research will continue to produce breakthroughs in biomedical, behavioral science, and other relevant areas and will provide evidence for best practice. Research on outcomes of treatment will become essential.

The whole economic basis of capitalism—that is, the manufacturing system—had become rapidly outdated by the beginning of the 21st century. The new paradigm for organizations in this century began with a move to a perspective that was outside the usual way of thinking. What work is done, where it is done, how it is done, by whom it is done, and what it costs are important questions, and APRNs can provide creative answers. **Exhibit 1-1** compares the old paradigm of sick care and the new paradigm of health care.

Healthcare Reform in the Center of the Public Policy Process

There was talk for decades about reforming the U.S. healthcare system. In the 1990s, President Clinton established a group that made major recommendations, but the constant pressure of special interest groups, such as pharmaceutical and insurance companies that protected their own interests, delayed and ultimately derailed any serious attempt at overhauling this huge system. During the George W. Bush administration, defense was the number one issue on the agenda and health care was not a priority. President Obama declared early in his administration that a major priority would be health care for all, and in 2010 the Patient Protection and

Exhibit 1-1 Comparison of Old Sick Care Paradigm with New Healthcare Paradigm

Old Paradigm	New Paradigm
Hospital-based acute care	Short-term hospital stays, outpatient surgery, mobile/satellite clinics, telehealth/telemedicine
Physician in charge; nurses and others as subordinates	Team approach; collaborative; respect for all providers as full team members
Physician as primary decision maker	Relevant professionals and patient make treatment decisions
Traditional care "as we have always done it"	Evidence-based practice
Segmented care focused on separate body parts/systems	Seamless, coordinated, holistic care
Primary care physician and specialist separated	Patient-centered medical/health home
Paper records; some electronic health records (EHRs)	EHR systems that generate data used for change that can be retrieved for meaningful use (i.e., as evidence for change)
Fee-for-service	Mix of reimbursement packages
Hierarchical organizations	Value-based organizations
Positivist, linear thinking	Complexity science: quantum principles, patterns noted in chaos; networks are essential; interpersonal relationships are indispensable

Affordable Care Act (commonly known as the ACA) was established, a huge first for the United States.

Today's policymakers seem to be more divided than at any time in recent history; choices often are dichotomous or mutually exclusive and rulings follow a strict party line. Compromise can be perceived as losing power, and power seems to be revered over common sense or the common good. Splinter groups or loose arrangements of radical thinkers have appeared on the political scene and are challenging the traditional two- or three-party system. A long-time congressperson told this author that she has never seen this much bitterness and antagonism in her more than 30 years of elected office. Many citizens are becoming more and more angry over the inertia and lack of meaningful legislation and deep polarization on issues. Future elections will reflect the degree of dissatisfaction among voters. Nurses will have to be especially sensitive to the political positions of all policymakers when working in this arena. Communications techniques learned in basic baccalaureate and graduate programs will enable the nurse to transcend some of the pressures encountered in working through the political process. Physicians, psychologists, pharmacists, and other professionals will have to add communications content to their curricula in order to increase their effectiveness with policymakers.

The healthcare system in the United States is in the midst of huge changes. Many health problems are the result of lifestyles that do not support health. Obesity, hypertension, and cardiovascular illnesses are only three that are mentioned frequently. In order to promote a healthy population, we are in the early phases of a move toward prevention of illness and disability and promotion of healthy living. Many people know how to live a healthy life, but just as many do not actually engage in healthy practices. Healthcare professionals are changing the way they assess, diagnose, counsel, and treat patients.

People are living longer and are encountering many chronic problems. Who would have thought 5 years ago that cancer today is considered a chronic disease? Surgery has made great strides, especially as minimally invasive methods and robotics are perfected. Genetics and genomics have opened up a whole discipline that incorporates gene splicing and manipulation, genetic testing and counseling, and many other approaches to what have been considered irreversible or inevitable conditions. The use of prosthetics in many forms and for many body parts is maturing into a fast-growing business, especially with the recovery and return of military personnel from wars. Body parts grown in laboratories from stem cells taken from a recipient will reduce the probability of autorejection. Behavioral health experts (e.g., psychologists, psychiatrists, mental health nurses) must be integrated into the health team to help people address issues such as posttraumatic stress and other problems. Ethical questions are integral to policy arguments, especially as appropriations are examined with a critical eye toward costs.

Federal reform has mandated programs and policies that will demand action that is different from what is available today. The Patient Protection and Affordable Care Act of 2010 (ACA) is a federal law that is expected to transform how, where, and by whom health care is provided and how that care will be paid for. Whether or not the programs envisioned in the law will succeed (i.e., meet the needs of the populace and be politically acceptable) is being played out through federal and state legislatures, presidential influence, and judicial decisions. Bills were introduced in 2011 to seriously amend and terminate the law. Judicial decisions have been made and the courts will continue to weigh issues surrounding this program. Nurses and nurse organizations will be strong voices in the debates that will have lasting influence on health care in this country.

Hospitals are concerned with staffing the workforce with nurses and other healthcare providers. Staffing levels have become a huge issue, with two opposing camps: one supports actual numbers of nurses per patient or per unit and the other supports principles of staffing rather than actual numbers. The California Nurses Association (CNA), originally a state affiliate of the American Nurses Association, broke from the ANA mainly over staffing issues. The CNA (the group kept the name), under the umbrella of the National Nurses Organizing Committee (NNOC), became politically active in several states in its desire to establish legal, specific, numerical nurse-to-patient ratios. The ANA, in contrast, established "principles of staffing" that required including patient acuity, diagnosis, type of nursing unit, and other considerations rather than specific numbers. Buerhaus (2008, 2009) presented data and thoughtful discussion to support the need for nurses as the primary workforce in the United States. ANA brought together over 700 nurses whose work resulted in a document that assists nurses in constructing finance-based arguments that support safe staffing plans and that those plans use the knowledge of nurses in direct patient care (Lineweaver, 2013).

Most care providers recognize the problems inherent in offering care to the uninsured and underinsured. The disparity in care seen in low socioeconomic groups and vulnerable populations (e.g., children, the elderly) and groups with specific health concerns (e.g., diabetics, smokers) presents enormous challenges. Nurses have proffered solutions that have been taken seriously by major policy players. The Health Resources and Services Administration (an agency within the U.S. Bureau of Health Professions) has convened webinars since 2009 on major topics of quality improvement and reporting, health information technology (IT) diligence, health IT implementation/opportunities for workflow and budgeting, meaningful use, workforce and safety net providers, and health and quality programs and topics. Tactics and solutions gleaned from participants are used to develop strategies to address these major problems (Health Resources and Services Administration, 2010–2011).

For some policymakers, this seems as if nurses are trying to expand the scope of their practice. This opinion often comes about because policymakers do not know what nurses do or the actual dimensions of their roles. The nurse of today and the future is "not your mother's nurse," to paraphrase an old automobile commercial. Haas's (1964) early study of nurses clarified that their role had four dimensions: task, authority or power, deference or prestige, and affect or feelings. Each of those dimensions has changed drastically over the past 10 years. Nurses simply want to practice at the level of their education and within legal and professional definitions.

Expanding the historical boundaries of nursing takes skill in negotiation, diplomacy, assertiveness, expert communication, and leadership. Sometimes physician and nurse colleagues are threatened by these behaviors, and it takes persistence and certainty of purpose to proceed. Nurses must speak out as articulate, knowledgeable, caring professionals who contribute to the whole health agenda and who advocate for their patients and the community. All healthcare professions have expanded the boundaries of practice from their beginnings. Practice reflects societal needs and conditions; homeostasis is not an option if the provision of health care is to be relevant.

The American Academy of Nursing (AAN), a prestigious organization of approximately 2,000 select nurse leaders who work to change health care at the policy level, created a Raise the Voice campaign that "provides a platform to inform policymakers, the media, health providers and consumers about nurse-driven activities and solutions for an ailing health care system" (American Academy of Nursing, 2010, p. 1). This program, funded by a grant from the Robert Wood Johnson Foundation, cites "Edge Runners"—nurses who are leading the way to healthcare reform by creating models of care that "demonstrate significant clinical and financial outcomes" (p. 2). AAN members are committed to transforming the healthcare system from the "current hospital-based, acuity-oriented, physician-dependent paradigm towards a patient-centered, convenient, helpful, and affordable system" (p. 1).

A major influence in how health care is delivered is occurring as more and more people use online resources. Patients bring articles about diseases and conditions to their healthcare providers. Providers surf electronic databases in search of accurate information. The expansion of knowledge and the rapidity with which it can be disseminated has grown exponentially in ways that were not possible even 5 years ago. A unique resource, *The Nurse's Social Media Advantage* (Fraser, 2011), explains social media and, more importantly, discusses the necessity for nurses to understand how to use media resources in order to practice effectively in a fast-changing world.

Developing a More Sophisticated Political Role for Nurses

There has been a major shift in the roles that nurses assume. In addition to clinical experts, nurses are entrepreneurs, decision makers, and political activists. The nurse's role must be examined to determine if there is a power differential, what the unwritten rules are that acknowledge deference, and how both actors exhibit or control feelings. Many nurses realize that to control practice and move the profession of nursing forward as a major player in the healthcare arena, nurses have to be involved in the legal decisions about the health and welfare of the public, decisions that often are made in the governmental arena.

For many nurses, political activism used to mean letting someone else get involved. Today's nurse tunes in to bills that reflect a particular passion (e.g., driving and texting), disease entity (e.g., diabetes), or population (e.g., childhood obesity). Although this activity indicates a greater involvement in the political process, it still misses a broader comprehension of the whole policymaking process that provides many opportunities for nurse input before and after legislation occurs.

Nurses who are serious about political activity realize that the key to establishing contacts with legislators and agency directors is through ongoing relationships with elected and appointed officials and their staffs. By developing credibility with those active in the political process and demonstrating integrity and moral purpose as client advocates, nurses are becoming players in the complex process of policymaking.

Nurses have learned that by using nursing knowledge and skill they could gain the confidence of government actors. Communications skills that were learned in basic skills classes or in psychiatric nursing classes are critical in listening to the discussion of larger health issues and in being able to present **nursing's agenda for health**. Personal stories gained from professional nurses' experience anchor altruistic conversations with legislators and their staffs in an important emotional link toward policy design. Nurses' vast network of clinical experts produces nurses in direct care who provide persuasive, articulate arguments with people "on the Hill" (i.e., U. S. congressman and senators who work on Capitol Hill) during appropriations committee hearings and informal meetings.

Nurses participate in formal, short-term internship programs with elected officials and in bureaucratic agencies. Most of the programs were created by nurse organizations that were convinced of the importance of political involvement. The interns and fellows learn how to handle constituent concerns, how to write legislation, how to argue with opponents yet remain colleagues, and how to maneuver through the bureaucracy. They carry the message of the necessity of the political process to the larger profession, although the rank and file still are not active in this role.

As nurses move into advanced practice and advanced practice demands master's and doctoral degree preparation, the role of the nurse in the **policy process** has become clearer. Through the influence of nurses with their legislators, clinical nurse specialists, certified nurse midwives, certified registered nurse anesthetists, and certified nurse practitioners are named in several pieces of federal legislation as duly authorized providers of health care. The process has been slow; however, the deliberate way of including more nurse groups over time demonstrates that getting a foot in the door is an effective method of instituting change in the seemingly slow processes of government. Some groups of nurses do not understand the political implications of incrementalism (the process of making changes gradually) and want all nurse groups named as providers at one time. They do not understand that most legislators do not have any idea what registered nurses do. Those nurse lobbyists who worked directly with legislators and their staff in early efforts bore the brunt of discontent within the profession and worked diligently and purposefully to provide a unified front on Capitol Hill and to expand the definition of provider at every opportunity. The designation of advanced practice registered nurses as providers was an entry to federal reimbursement for some nursing services, a major move toward improved client and family access to health care. Advanced practice registered nurses became acutely aware of the critical importance of the role of political activist. Not only did APRNs need the basic knowledge, they understood the necessity of practicing the role, developing contacts, working with professional organizations, writing fact sheets, testifying at hearings, and maintaining the momentum and persistence to move an idea forward.

Although many nurses still focus their political efforts and skills on the legislative process, they understand the comprehensiveness of the policy process, the much broader process that precedes and follows legislation. For APRNs to integrate the policy role into the character of expert nurse they must recognize the many opportunities for action. APRNs cannot afford to do their own thing—that is, only provide direct patient care. They cannot ignore the political aspects of any issue. Nurses who have fought the battles for recognition as professionals, for acknowledgment of autonomy, and for formal acceptance of clinical expertise worthy of payment for services have enabled APRNs today to provide reimbursable, quality services to this nation's residents.

Today's nurses have a much clearer understanding of what constitutes nursing and how nurses must integrate political processes into their practices to further the decisions made by policymakers. Nurses continue to focus on the individual, family, community, and special populations in the provision of care to the sick and infirm and on the activities that surround health promotion and the prevention of disease and disability. Advanced practice nurses have a foundation in expert clinical practice and can translate that knowledge into understandable language for elected and appointed officials as the officials respond to problems that are beyond the scale or impact of individual healthcare providers. As nurses continue to refine the art and science of nursing, forces external to the profession compel the nursing community to consider another aspect—the business of nursing—that is paradoxical to the profession's long history of altruism.

What Is Public Policy?

So, what do the changes in education, practice, and organizations have to do with policymaking, especially in the public arena? A brief overview of the entire policy process will clarify what policy is and how influencing government policies has become crucial to the profession of nursing.

In this chapter, *policy* is an overarching term used to define both an entity and a process. The purpose of **public policy** is to direct problems to government and secure government's response; in contrast, politics is the use of influence to direct the responses toward goals. Although there has been much discussion about the boundaries and domain of government and the extent of difference between the public and private sectors, that debate is beyond the scope of this chapter.

The definition of public policy is important because it clarifies common misconceptions about what constitutes policy. In this text, the terms *public policy* and *policy* are interchangeable. The process of creating policy can be focused in many arenas most of which are interwoven. For example, environmental policy deals with health issues such as hazardous materials, particulate matter in the air or water, and safety standards in the workplace. Education policy is more than tangentially related to health—just ask school nurses. Regulations define who can administer medication to students; state laws dictate what type of sex education can be taught. Defense policy is related to health policy when developing, investigating, or testing biological and chemical weapons. Health policy directly addresses health problems and is the specific focus of this text.

Policy as an Entity

As an entity, policy is seen in many forms as the "standing decisions" of an organization (Eulau & Prewitt, 1973, p. 495). As formal documented directives of an organization, official government policies reflect the beliefs of the administration in power and provide direction for the philosophy and mission of government organizations. Specific policies usually serve as the "shoulds" and "thou shalts" of agencies. Some policies, known as position statements, report the opinions of organizations about issues that members believe are important. For example, state boards of nursing (government agencies created by legislatures to protect the public through the regulation of nursing practice) publish advisory opinions on what constitutes competent and safe nursing practice.

Agency policies can be broad and general, such as those that describe the relationship of an agency to other governmental groups. Procedure manuals in government hospitals that detail steps in performing certain nursing tasks are examples of the results of policy directives, but are not considered policies. Policies serve as guidelines for employee behavior within an institution. Although policies and procedures often are used interchangeably, policies are considered broader and reflect the values of the administration.

Laws are types of policy entities. As legal directives for public and private behavior, laws serve to define action that reflects the will of society—or at least a segment of society. Laws are made at the international, federal, state, and local levels and have the impact of primary place (i.e., are considered the principal source) in guiding conduct. Lawmaking usually is the purview of the legislative branch of government in the United States, although presidential vetoes, executive orders, and judicial interpretations of laws have the force of law.

Judicial interpretation is noted in three ways. First, courts may interpret the meaning of laws that are written broadly or with some vagueness, though laws often are deliberately written with language that addresses broad situations. Agencies that implement the laws then write regulations that are more specific and guide the implementation. However, courts may be asked to determine questions in which the law is unclear or controversial (Williams & Torrens, 1988). For example, the 1973 Rehabilitation Act prohibited discrimination against the handicapped by any program that received federal assistance. Although this may have seemed fair and reasonable at the outset, courts were asked to adjudicate questions of how much accommodation is "fair" (Wilson, 1989). Second, courts can determine how some laws are applied. Courts are idealized as being above the political activity that surrounds the legislature. Courts also are considered beyond the influence of politically active interest groups. The court system, especially the federal court system, has been called upon to resolve conflicts between levels of government (state and federal) and between laws enacted by the legislature and their interpretation by powerful interest groups. For example, courts may determine who is eligible or who is excluded from participation in a program. In this way, special interest groups that sue to be included in a program can receive "durable protection" from favorable court decisions (Feldstein, 1988, p. 32). Third, courts can declare the laws made by Congress or the states unconstitutional, thereby nullifying the statutes entirely (Litman & Robins, 1991). Courts also interpret the Constitution, sometimes by restricting what the government (not private enterprise) may do (Wilson, 1989).

Regulations are another type of policy initiative. Although they often are included in discussions of laws, regulations are different. Once a law is enacted by the legislative branch, the executive branch of government is charged with administrative responsibility for implementing the law. The executive branch consists of the president and all of the bureaucratic agencies, commissions, and departments that carry out the work for the public benefit. Agencies in the government formulate regulations that achieve the intent of the statute. On the whole, laws are written in general terms, and regulations are written more specifically to guide the interpretation, administration, and enforcement of the law. The Administrative Procedures Act (APA) was created to provide opportunity for citizen review and input throughout the process of developing regulations. The APA ensures a structure and process that is published and open, in the spirit of the founding fathers, so that the average constituent can participate in the process of public decision making.

All of these entities evolve over time and are accomplished through the efforts of a variety of actors or players. Although commonly used, the terms *position statement, resolution, goal, objective, program, procedure, law*, and *regulation* really are not interchangeable with the word *policy*. Rather, they are the formal expressions of policy decisions. For the purposes of understanding just what policy is, nurses must grasp policy as a process.

Policy as a Process

In viewing policy as a guide to government action, nurses can study the process of policymaking over time. Milio (1989) presents four major stages in which decisions are made that translate to government policies: (1) agenda setting, (2) legislation and regulation, (3) implementation, and (4) evaluation. Agenda setting is concerned with identifying a societal problem and bringing it to the attention of government. Legislation and regulation are formal responses to a problem. Implementation is the execution of policies or programs toward the achievement of goals. Evaluation is the appraisal of policy performance or program outcomes.

In each stage, formal and informal relationships are developed among actors both within and outside of government. Actors can be individuals, such as a legislator, a bureaucrat, or a citizen, but they also can be institutions, such as the presidency, the courts, political parties, or special-interest groups. A series of activities occurs that brings a problem to government, which results in direct action by the government to address the problem. Governmental responses are political; that is, the decisions about who gets what, when, and how are made within a framework of power and influence, negotiation, and bargaining (Lasswell, 1958).

One must recognize that the policy process is not necessarily sequential or logical. The definition of a problem, which usually occurs in the agenda-setting phase, may change during legislation. Program design may be altered significantly during implementation. Evaluation of a policy or program (often considered the last phase of the process) may propel onto the national agenda (often considered the first phase of the process) a problem that differs from the original. However, for the purpose of organizing one's thoughts and conceptualizing the policy process, the policy process is examined in this chapter from the linear perspective.

The opportunities for nurse input throughout the policy process are unlimited and certainly not confined narrowly to the legislative process. Nurses are articulate experts who can address both the rational shaping of policy and the emotional aspects of the process. Nurses cannot afford to limit their actions to monitoring bills; they must seize the initiative and use their considerable collective and individual influence to ensure the health, welfare, and protection of the public and healthcare professionals.

An Overview of the Policy Process

Advanced practice registered nurses should have an overview of the total process so that they do not get stuck on legislation. Many useful articles and books have been written about policy in general and even about specific policies, but few have addressed the scope of the policy process or defined the components. The elements of agenda setting (including problem definition), government response (legislation, regulation, or programs), and policy and program implementation and evaluation are distinct entities, but are connected as parts of a whole tapestry in the process of public decision making.

Agenda Setting

Getting a healthcare problem to the attention of government can be a tremendous first step in getting relief. The actual mechanism of defining a healthcare problem is a major political issue. APRNs have the capacity and opportunity to identify and frame problems from multiple sources.

The choice of a clinical problem on which to focus one's energy is a major decision. A nurse may be working in a specialized area and may see a need for more research or alternatives to existing treatment options; for example, those who work with patients and families with breast cancer already may have a passion for issues critical to this area. Other topics receiving attention include diabetes, obesity, AIDS, early detection and treatment of prostate cancer, child and parent abuse, cardiac problems in women, and empowering caregivers (Hash & Cramer, 2003; Pierce & Steiner, 2003).

Professional problems that are especially critical to nurses in advanced practice include reducing barriers to autonomy and reimbursement for nursing services. Workplace issues include advocacy for workplace safety and management strategies for training and redeploying nurses as work sites change. Related social problems that affect nurses include the increase of street violence and bioterrorism. A plethora of problems and "irritations" can arouse the passion of a nurse in advanced practice.

APRNs must come to understand the concepts of windows of opportunity, policy entrepreneurs, and political elites. *Sound bites* and *word bites* are tools used to gain the attention of viewers and readers and serve as a shortcut or an abbreviated version of a statement. Originally created as off-hand remarks, these oral and written snippets have become planned tactics. For example, a nurse who speaks at a press conference or who delivers a message to a politician should have a written message that includes bulleted sound or word bites that underscore the message and that emphasize the important points. These brief, focused points can serve as talking points for the media or a politician as they consider the message later. Another tactic that APRNs and their healthcare colleagues must develop is the *30-second elevator speech*. Any healthcare professional should have a brief, succinct explanation of the role of the professional, the problem to be addressed, or a proposed solution that can be shared verbally with a policymaker. Petitioners rarely are given much time to discuss issues, so a short, to-the-point statement may be the first, best opportunity to be heard.

Government Response

The government response to public problems often emanates from the legislative branch and usually comes in three forms: (1) laws, (2) rules and regulations, and (3) programs. Because only senators and representatives can introduce legislation (not even the president can bring a bill to the floor of either house), these elected officials command respect and attention. The work of legislation is not clear-cut or linear. Informal communication and influence are the coin of the realm when trying to construct a program or law from the often vague wishes of disparate groups. The committee structure of both houses is a powerful method of accomplishing the work of government. Conference committees are known as the "Third House of Congress" (*How Our Laws Are Made,* 1990) because of their power to force compromise and bring about new legislation. APRNs must appreciate the difference between the authorization and appropriations processes and seek influence in both arenas. Becoming involved directly with legislators and their staffs has been a training ground for many APRNs. Supporting or opposing passage of a bill often has served as the first contact with the political process for many nurses, but this often has been the stopping point for these nurses because they were unaware of other avenues of involvement, such as the follow-up process of regulations and rulemaking.

Lowi (1969) notes that administrative rulemaking is often an effort to bring about order in environments that are unstable and full of conflict. Some regulations codify precedent; others break new ground and address issues not previously explicated. An example of the latter is the Federal Trade Commission's (FTC's) Trade Regulation Rules. In 1964, the FTC, whose mission is to protect the consumer and enforce antitrust legislation, wrote regulations requiring health warnings on cigarette packages. The tobacco industry reacted so fiercely that Congress quickly passed a law that nullified the regulations and replaced them with less stringent ones (West, 1982). Decades passed before no-smoking rules actually were mandated in public places. Persistence and timing are integral to policymaking.

Programs are concrete manifestations of solutions to problems. Program design often is a joint effort of legislative intent, budgetary expediency, and political feasibility. There are many opportunities for nurses in advanced practice to become involved in the design phase of a program. Selecting an agency to administer the program, choosing the goals, and selecting the tools that will ensure eligibility and participation are all decisions in which the APRN should offer input.

Policy and Program Implementation

It is important that APRNs keep reminding their colleagues that the phases of the policy process are not linear and that policy activities are fluid and move within and among the phases in dynamic processes. The implementation phase includes those activities in which legislative mandates are carried out, most often through programmatic means. The implementation stage also includes a planning ingredient. Problems occur in program planning if technological expertise is not available. This is particularly important to nurses, who are experts in the delivery of health care in the broadest sense.

If government officials do not know qualified, appropriate experts, decisions about program planning and design often are determined by legislators, bureaucrats, or staff who know little or nothing about the problem or the solutions. As excellent problem solvers, APRNs have many opportunities to offer ideas and solutions. One strategy is to employ second-order change to reframe situations and recommend pragmatic alternatives to implementers (de Chesnay, 1983; Watzlawick, Weakland, & Fisch, 1974). Bowen (1982) uses probability theory to demonstrate how program success could be improved. She suggests putting several clearance points (instances where major decisions are made) together so that they could be negotiated as a package deal. She also advocates beginning the bargaining process with alternatives that have the greatest chance for success and using that success as a foundation for building more successes, a strategy she refers to as a "bandwagon approach" (p. 10). In the past, nurses have done the opposite: focused on failure and the perceived lack of nursing power. APRNs have begun to note successes in the political arena and are building a new level of success and esteem. The nurse in advanced practice today uses the strategies of packaging, success begets success, and persistence in a deliberate way so that nurses can increase their effective impact in the implementation of social programs. Another tactic useful to APRNs is a positive type of group process called appreciative inquiry (Hammond, 2013; Havens, Wood, & Lehman, 2006), in which participants focus on what has worked or what they want to happen in a situation rather than getting mired down in examples that have not worked in the past. Appreciative inquiry moves beyond the typical problem-solving model and can lead to positive organizational change.

Although nurses most often work toward positive impact, they have found that opposition to an unsound program can have a paradoxical positive effect. Although not in the public arena, an example of phenomenal success in the judicious use of opposition occurred when the professional body of nursing rose up as one against the American Medical Association's 1988 proposal to create a new type of low-level healthcare worker called a registered care technician. The power emerged as more than 40 nurse organizations stood together in opposition to an ill-conceived proposal that would have placed patients in jeopardy and created dead-end jobs.

Policy and Program Evaluation

For nurses who have worked beyond the nursing process through the process of clinical reasoning (Pesut & Herman, 1999), evaluation seems to be a logical component of the policy process. Evaluation is the systematic application of methods of social research to public policies and programs. Evaluation is conducted "to benefit the human condition to improve profit, to amass influence and power, or to achieve other goals" (Rossi & Freeman, 1995, p. 6). Evaluation research is a powerful tool for defending viable programs, for altering structures and processes to strengthen programs, and for providing rationale for program failure. Goggin, Bowman, Lester, and O'Toole (1990) propose that researchers investigate program implementation within an analytical framework rather than a descriptive one. They argue that a "third generation" of research established within a sound theory would strengthen the body of knowledge of the policy process. APRNs can contribute to both the theory and the method of evaluation.

Evaluation should be started early and continued throughout a program. An unconscionable example of a program that should have been stopped even before it was begun is the Tuskegee "experiment." From 1932 to 1972, a group of African Americans was used as a control group and denied antibiotic treatment for syphilis, even after treatment was known to be successful (Thomas & Quinn, 1991). Beyond evaluation research, this study clearly points out the moral and ethical concerns that are mandated when researchers work with human beings. Should a study or program be started at all? At what point should it be stopped? What is involved in "informed consent"? If a program involves experimental therapy, what are the methods for presenting subjects with relevant data so that participation preferences are clear (Bell, Raiffa, & Tversky, 1988)? These kinds of questions should be considered automatically by today's researchers, but it is the responsibility of APRNs as consumer agents to ask the questions if they have not been asked or if there is any doubt about the answers.

An Exciting Future

The multiple roles of the APRN—provider of direct care, researcher, consultant, educator, administrator, consumer advocate, and political activist—reflect the changing and expanding character of the professional nurse. Today is the future; action today sets the direction for what health care becomes for coming generations. As true professionals with a societal mandate and a comprehensive body of knowledge, nurses function as visionaries who are grounded in education, research, and experience. APRNs serve as the link between human responses to actual and potential health problems and the solutions that may be addressed in the government arena.

Full integration of the policy process becomes evident when professional nurses discern early the social implications of health problems, seize the opportunity to inform public officials with whom the nurses have credible relationships, provide objective data and subjective personal stories that help translate big problems down to a level of understanding, propose alternative solutions that acknowledge reality, and participate in the evaluation process to determine the effectiveness and efficiency of the outcomes.

Educating Our Political Selves

Nurses in advanced practice must be politically active. Basic content in undergraduate nursing programs must be reexamined in light of the needs of the profession. Educators must do more than plant the seeds of interest and excitement in baccalaureate students; they must model activism by talking about the bills they are supporting or opposing, by organizing students to assist in election campaigns, and by demanding not only that students write letters to officials, but also that they mail them and provide follow-up.

Educators can develop games in which students maneuver through a virtual bureaucracy to move a health problem onto the agenda. Brainstorming techniques can lead students to discover innovative alternative solutions. Baccalaureate students can analyze policy tools to discover how and when to use them. Teachers of research methods and processes can use political scenarios to point out how to phrase clinical questions so that legislators will pay attention. Program effectiveness can be studied in research and clinical courses. The theoretical components taught in class and followed by practical application through participation in political and legislative committees in professional organizations must serve as basic training for the registered nurse.

Graduate education must demand demonstrated knowledge and application of more extensive and sophisticated political processes. All graduate program faculty should serve as models for political activism. The atmosphere in master's and doctoral programs should heighten the awareness of students who are potential leaders.

Faculty can motivate students by displaying posters that announce political events and by including students in discussions of nursing issues framed in a policy context. Students who spot educators at rallies and other political and policy occasions are learning by example, so faculty should advertise their experiences as delegates to political and professional conventions. A few faculty can serve as mentors for students who need to move from informal to sustained, formal contact with policymakers and who have a policy track in their career trajectories. Both faculty and students should consider actual experience in government offices as a means of learning the nitty-gritty of how government functions and of demonstrating their own leadership capabilities.

If students hesitate and seem passive about involvement, educators must help these nurses determine where their passions are, which may help students focus on where they might start. Often the novice can be enticed by centering on a clinical problem. Every nurse cannot assume responsibility for all of the profession's problems or work on every healthcare issue. Issues can be at the practice level or the systems level (e.g., funding for nurse education or nurse-led research). Each nurse must choose the issue in which to invest energy, time, and other resources. Nurses can make a difference in the new healthcare system.

Strengthening Organized Nursing

The most productive and efficient way to act together is through a strong professional organization. As organizations in general have restructured and reengineered for more efficient operation, so will the professional associations. APRNs have a knowledge base that includes an understanding of how organizations develop and change. This theoretical knowledge must serve as a foundation for leadership in directing new organizational structures that are responsive to members and other important bodies. National leaders must talk with state and local leaders as new configurations are conceived. States must confer among themselves to share innovations and knowledge about what works and what does not.

Issues such as the role of collective bargaining units within the total organizational structure, the position of individual membership vis-à-vis state membership, the political role of a specialized interest group (nurses) in creating public policy, and the issue of international influence in nursing and health care require wisdom and leadership that APRNs must exert as the American Nurses Association addresses its place as a major voice of this country's nurses. The National League for Nursing (NLN) will exert leadership as many nurse education programs encourage graduates to continue their education and earn bachelor's degrees in nursing. Accrediting agencies (e.g., the Commission on Collegiate Nursing Education and the Accreditation Commission for Education in Nursing) must continue to be visionary and flexible in developing criteria and processes for accreditation. Boards of nursing must not become trapped in the slowness with which government bureaucracy can be mired, but must be bold and at the forefront of developing regulations that protect the public and allow nurses to work at their full capacity.

Issues inherent in multistate licensure are being debated today, and the outcome will reflect the extent to which nurses will use concepts of telehealth in their practices. Because APRNs already are eligible for Medicare reimbursement for telehealth services that are provided in specified rural areas (Burtt, 1997), these nurses are rich resources and must be included in reasoned discussions on this issue. State boards of nursing in every state and jurisdiction face issues of appropriate methods of recognizing advanced nursing practice, the role of the government agency in regulating nursing and other professions, and the analysis of educationally sound and legally defensible examinations for candidates.

Nurses who have been reluctant to become political cannot afford to ignore their obligations any longer. Each nurse counts, and collectively nursing is a major actor in the effort to ensure the country's healthy future. Nurses have expanded their conception of what nursing is and how it is practiced to include active political participation. A nurse must choose the governmental level on which to focus: federal, regional, state, or local. The process is similar at each level: Identify the problem and become part of the solution.

Advanced practice registered nurses understand the scope of service delivery, continuity of care, appropriate mix of caregivers, and expertise that can be provided by interprofessional teams. By being at the forefront of understanding, nurses have a moral and ethical mandate to lead the public policy process. Dynamic political action is as much a part of the advanced practice of nursing as is expert direct care.

Working with the Political System

By now, many APRNs have developed contacts with legislators, appointed officials, and their staffs. A group that offers nurse interaction is the Senate

Nursing Caucus (AACN, 2010). Established in March 2010, this group provides a forum for educating senators on issues important to nurses, as well as for hearing senators' concerns. Four senators established the caucus: Jeff Merkley (D-OR), Mike Johanns (R-NE), Barbara Mikulski (D-MD), and Olympia Snowe (R-ME). The Senate Nursing Caucus follows the lead of the Congressional Nursing Caucus in the U.S. House of Representatives, begun in 2003 by Representatives Lois Capps (D-CA) and Ed Whitfield (R-KY) (American Nurses Association, 2003). Members hold briefings on the nurse shortage, patient and nurse safety issues, preparedness for bioterrorism, and other relevant and pertinent issues and concerns.

APRNs must stay alert to issues and be assertive in bringing problems to the attention of policymakers. It is important to bring success stories to legislators and officials—they need to hear what good nurses do and how well they practice. Sharing positive information will keep the image of nurses in an affirmative and constructive picture. Legislators must run for office (and U.S. Representatives do this every 2 years), so media coverage with an APRN who is pursuing noteworthy accomplishments is usually welcomed eagerly.

Nurses absolutely must get their act together and work toward a unified voice on issues that affect the public health and the nursing profession. Whatever their differences in the past—anger from entry-into-practice arguments that have dragged on for over half a century; disparagement and animosity among those with varied levels of education; cerebral and pragmatic concerns about gaps between education and practice, practice and administration, or administration and education—nurses must put these kinds of divisive, emotional issues behind them if they expect to be taken seriously as professionals by elected and appointed public officials and policymakers. The 2010 IOM report is a wake-up call for nurses to work at their highest levels and to work with other health professionals.

Nurses cannot afford to stop arguing critical issues internally, but they must learn how to argue heatedly among themselves—and then go to lunch together. Nurses can learn lessons from television shows such as *Meet the Press, This Week, The O'Reilly Factor,* and *The McLaughlin Group* about how to challenge, contest, dispute, contend, and debate issues passionately, and then shake hands and respect the opponent's position. Passionate issues must not polarize the profession any longer and, more important, must not stand in the way of a unified voice to the public.

Conclusion

Nurses in advanced practice must have expert knowledge and skill in change, conflict resolution, assertiveness, communication, negotiation, and group process to function appropriately in the policy arena. Professional autonomy and collaborative interdependence are possible within a political system in which consumers can choose access to quality health care that is provided by competent practitioners at a reasonable cost. Nurses in advanced practice have a strong, persistent voice in designing such a healthcare system for today and for the future.

The policy process is much broader and more comprehensive than the legislative process. Although individual components can be identified for analytical study, the policy process is fluid, nonlinear, and dynamic. There are many opportunities for nurses in advanced practice to participate throughout the policy process. The question is not whether nurses should become involved in the political system, but to what extent. In the whole policy arena, nurses must be involved with every aspect. Knowing all of the components and issues that must be addressed in each phase, the nurse in advanced practice finds many opportunities for providing expert advice. APRNs can use the policy process, individual components, and models as a framework to analyze issues and participate in alternative solutions.

Nursing has a rich history. The professional nurse's values of altruism, respect, ethics, integrity, and accountability to consumers remain strong. In some ways, the evolution of nurse roles has come full circle, from the political influence recognized and exercised by Nightingale to the influence of current nurse leaders with elected and appointed public officials. The APRN of the 21st century practices with a solid political heritage and a mandate for consistent and powerful involvement in the entire policy process.

Discussion Points

1. Read Nightingale's *Notes on Nursing* (1859) and other historical sources from the mid-1800s and discuss how Nightingale's personal and family influence moved her agenda for the Crimea and for nursing education. How does this have implications for the future?

2. Discuss implications of the "BSN in 10" movement in relation to your own education. Research opportunities for BSNs and for APRNs. Dream about positions that might not be available today.

3. Compare the definitions of nursing according to Nightingale, Henderson, the ANA, and your own state nurse practice act. What are the differences in a legal definition versus a professional definition? What are the similarities? What did definitions include or not include that reflected the state of nursing at the time? Construct a definition of nursing for today and for 10 years from now.

4. Discuss the role of research in nursing. What has been the focus over the past century? What is the pattern of nursing research vis-à-vis topic, methodology, and relevance? To what extent do you think nursing research has had an impact on nursing care? Cite examples.

5. Trace the amount of federal funding for nursing research. Do not limit your search to federal health-related agencies; that is, investigate departments (commerce, environment, transportation, etc.), military services, and the Veterans Administration. What funding opportunities exist for nurse scientists?

6. Read books and articles about the changing paradigm in healthcare delivery systems. Discuss the change in nursing as an occupation and nursing as a profession. What does this mean in today's transformational paradigm?

7. Consider a thesis, graduate project, or dissertation on a specific topic (e.g., clinical problems, healthcare issues) using the policy process as a framework. Identify policies within public agencies and discuss how they were developed. Interview members of an agency policy committee to discover how policies are changed.

8. Have faculty and students bring to class official governmental policies. What governmental agency is responsible for developing the policy? For enforcing the policy? How has the policy changed over time? What are the consequences of not complying with the policy? What is needed to change the policy?

9. Identify nurses who are elected officials at the local, state, or national level. Interview these officials to determine how the nurses were elected, what their objectives are, and to what extent they use their nurse knowledge in their official capacities. Ask the officials if they

tapped into nurse groups during their campaigns. If so, what did the nurses contribute? If not, why?

10. Discuss the major components of the policy process and discuss the fluidity of the process. Point out how players move among the components in a nonlinear way.

11. Using Exhibit 1-1 as a framework, construct a healthcare organization in which access is provided and quality care is assured. What are the barriers to this type of paradigm?

12. Develop an assessment tool by which students can determine their own level of knowledge and involvement in the policy process. Reminder: Stretch your thinking beyond legislative activity.

13. Watch television programs in which participants discuss national and international issues, then analyze the patterns of verbal and nonverbal communication, pro-and-con arguments, and other methods of discussion. Discuss your analysis within the framework of gender differences in communication and utility in the political arena.

14. Construct a list of ways in which nurses can become more knowledgeable about the policy process. Choose at least three activities in which you will participate. Develop a tool for evaluating the activity and your knowledge and involvement.

15. Select at least one problem or irritation in a clinical area and brainstorm with other APRNs or graduate students on how to approach a solution. Discuss funding sources; be creative.

16. Attend a meeting of the state board of nursing, the district or state nurses association, or a professional convention. Identify issues discussed, resources used, communication techniques, and rules observed. Evaluate the usefulness of the session to your practice.

17. Discuss what skills (task, interpersonal, etc.) and attitudes are required for the nurse in the new paradigm. Who is best prepared to teach these skills, and what teaching techniques should be used? How will they be evaluated? Develop a worksheet to facilitate planning.

18. Discuss at least five strategies for helping nurses integrate these skills into their practices.

19. Convene a group of healthcare professionals and discuss common problems, potential solutions, and strategies to move forward.

CASE STUDY: PILL MILLS

APRNs have prescriptive authority including the ability to prescribe narcotics. In the past 10 years there have been only one or two instances in which APRNs have been sanctioned by the board of nursing for abusing prescriptive authority. Many legislators do not realize that APRNs have this authority. There has been a recent surge in "pill mills" (sites where prescriptions for large amounts of narcotics are provided without actual patient assessment). No nurses have been involved in writing these prescriptions.

Discussion Points

1. What can a nurse do to be invited to the table when a task force is convened by the governor or state health director?
2. What other healthcare professionals should be included in the discussion? What state agencies and regulatory boards could add value to the discussion?
3. Identify three issues that might derail a focus on the safety of the public during these discussions. What tactics can the nurse use to bring a discussion back to the issue of safety?
4. How can information about this issue be disseminated within the profession and to those outside the profession?

References

Aiken, L. H., Cimiotti, J. R., Sloane, D. M., Smith, H. L., Flynn, L., & Neff, D. F. (2011). Effects of nurse staffing on patient deaths in hospitals with differing nurse work environments. *Medical Care, 49*(12), 1047–1053.

Aiken, L. H., Clarke, S. R., Cheung, R. B., Sloane, D. M., & Silber, J. H. (2003). Educational levels of hospital nurses and surgical patient mortality. *Journal of the American Medical Association, 290*(12), 1617–1623.

Aiken, L. H., Sloane, D. M., Bruyneel, L., Van den Heede, K., Griffiths, P., Busse, R., et al. (2014). Nurse staffing and education and hospital mortality of European countries: A retrospective observational study. *The Lancet, 383*(9931), 1824–1830.

American Academy of Nursing. (2010). *Raise the voice*. Retrieved from http://www.aannet.org/raisethevoice

American Association of Colleges of Nursing. (2006). *Essentials of doctoral education for advanced nursing practice*. Washington, DC: Author.

American Association of Colleges of Nursing. (2008a). *Essentials of baccalaureate education for professional nursing practice*. Washington, DC: Author.

American Association of Colleges of Nursing. (2008b). *Essentials of master's education for advanced practice nursing*. Washington, DC: Author.

American Association of Colleges of Nursing. (2008c). Brief history of the CNL. Retrieved from http://www.aacn.nche.edu/cnl/about/history

American Association of Colleges of Nursing. (2010). Senate nursing caucus. Retrieved from http://www.aacn.nche.edu/government-affairs/senate-nursing-caucus

American Association of Colleges of Nursing. (2014a). CNL certification. Retrieved from http://www.aacn.nche.edu.leading initiatives/cnl-certification/pdf

American Association of Colleges of Nursing. (2014b). *DNP fact sheet: The doctor of nursing practice*. Retrieved from http://www.aacn.nche.edu/media/FactSheets/dnp.htm

American Nurses Association. (2003, March 19). *American Nurses Association commends Reps. Capps, Whitfield for forming congressional nursing caucus*. Retrieved from http://www.nursingworld.org/-pressrel/2003/pr0319.htm

Bell, D. E., Raiffa, H., & Tversky, A. (1988). *Decision making*. Cambridge, MA: Cambridge University Press.

Bennis, W., & Nanus, B. (1985). *Leaders*. New York: Harper and Row.

Bowen, E. (1982). The Pressman-Wildavsky paradox: Four addenda on why models based on probability theory can predict implementation success and suggest useful tactical advice for implementers. *Journal of Public Policy, 2*(1), 1–22.

Buerhaus, P. I., Staiger, D. O., & Auerbach, D. I. (2008). *The future of the nursing workforce in the United States: Data, trends, and implications*. Sudbury, MA: Jones & Bartlett Publishers

Buerhaus, P. I. (2009). Messages for thought leaders and health policy makers. *Nursing Economics, 2*(2), 125–127.

Burtt, K. (1997). Nurses use telehealth to address rural health care needs, prevent hospitalizations. *The American Nurse, 29*(6), 21.

Cronenwett, L., Dracup, K., Grey, M., McCauley, L., Meleis, A., & Salmon, M. (2011). The doctor of nursing practice: A national workforce perspective. *Nursing Outlook, 59*(1), 9–17.

Curtin, L. (2010). Quantum nursing. *American Nurse Today, 5*(9), 47–48.

Curtin, L. (2011). Quantum nursing II: Our field of influence. *American Nurse Today, 6*(1), 56.

de Chesnay, M. (1983). The creation and dissolution of paradoxes in nursing practice. *Topics in Clinical Nursing, 5*(3), 71–80.

Drucker, P. F. (1995, December). The age of social transformation. *The Atlantic*. Retrieved from http://www.theatlantic.com/past/docs/issues/95dec/chilearn/drucker.htm

Eulau, H., & Prewitt, K. (1973). *Labyrinths of democracy*. Indianapolis, IN: Bobbs-Merrill.

Feldstein, P. J. (1988). *The politics of health legislation*. Ann Arbor, MI: Health Administration Press.

Fraser, R. (2011). *The nurse's social media advantage*. Indianapolis, IN: Sigma Theta Tau International.

FTC policy paper examines competition and the regulation of APRNs. (2014). *The American Nurse, 46*(3), 11.

Goggin, M. L., Bowman, A. O., Lester, J. P., & O'Toole, L. J., Jr. (1990). *Implementation theory and practice: Toward a third generation*. New York: HarperCollins.

Haas, J. E. (1964). *Role conception and group consensus* (Research Monograph No. 17). Columbus, OH: The Ohio State University, Bureau of Business Research.

Hammond, S. A. (2013). *The thin book of appreciative inquiry*. Bend, OR: Thin Book.

Hash, K. M., & Cramer, E. P. (2003). Empowering gay and lesbian caregivers and uncovering their unique experiences through the use of qualitative methods. *Journal of Gay and Lesbian Social Services, 15*(1/2), 47–64.

Havens, D. S., Wood, S. O., & Lehman, J. (2006). Improving nursing practice and patient care. *Journal of Nursing Administration, 36*(16), 463–470.

How our laws are made. (1990). (House Document 101–139). Washington, DC: U.S. Government Printing Office.

Husted, G. L., Scotto, C., & Wolf, K. (2015). *Bioethical decision making in nursing and health care: A symphonological approach* (5th ed.). New York: Springer.

Institute of Medicine. (2010). *The future of nursing: Leading change, advancing health*. Washington, DC: National Academies Press.

Interprofessional Education Collaborative. (n.d.). *About IPEC*. Retrieved from http://www.ipecollaborative.org/About_IPEC.html

Josiah Macy Jr. Foundation. (2014). *Publications*. Retrieved from http://www.macyfoundation.org/publications/publications/aligning-interprofessional-education

Kouzes, J., & Posner, B. (1999). *Encouraging the heart: A leader's guide to rewarding and recognizing others*. San Francisco, CA: Jossey-Bass.

Kouzes, J., & Posner, B. (2007). *The leadership challenge* (4th ed.). San Francisco, CA: Jossey-Bass.

Lasswell, H. D. (1958). *Politics: Who gets what, when, how*. New York: Meridian.

Lindberg, C., Nash, S., & Lindberg, C. (2008). *On the edge: Nursing in the age of complexity*. Medford, NJ: Plexus Press.

Lineweaver, L. (2013). *Nurse staffing 101: A decision-making guide for the RN*. Washington, DC: American Nurses Publishing.

Litman, T. J., & Robins, L. S. (1991). *Health politics and policy* (2nd ed.). Albany, NY: Delmar.

Lowi, T. (1969). *The end of liberalism*. New York: Norton.

Milio, N. (1989). Developing nursing leadership in health policy. *Journal of Professional Nursing, 5*(6), 315.

Nightingale, F. (1859). *Notes on nursing*. Cambridge, England: Cambridge University Press.

Patient Protection and Affordable Care Act of 2010. (2010). Pub. L. No. 111-148, 124 Stat. 119.

Pesut, D., & Herman, J. (1999). *Clinical reasoning: The art and science of critical and creative thinking* (2nd ed.). Albany, NY: Delmar Learning.

Pierce, L., & Steiner, V. (2003). The male caregiving experience: Three case studies. *Stroke*, *34*(1), 315.

Plexus Institute. (2009, July). Making sense of complexity. Singapore: Civil Service College. Retrieved from http://c.ymcdn.com/sites/www.plexusinstitute.org/resource/collection/17978F03-1F91-4D5E-971C-651E9F9DC5FC/Cognitive_Edge_-_Making_Sense_of_Complexity_-_2009.pdf

Porter-O'Grady, T., Hawkins, M. A., & Parker, M. L. (1997). *Whole-systems shared governance: Architecture for integration.* Gaithersburg, MD: Aspen.

Porter-O'Grady, T., & Malloch, K. (2014). *Quantum leadership: Building better partnerships for sustainable health.* Burlington, MA: Jones and Bartlett Learning.

The regulatory process. (1992). *Capitol Update, 10*(23), 1.

Rhoades, A., Covery, S. R., & Shepherdson, N. (2011). *Building values: Creating an equitable culture that outperforms the competition.* San Francisco, CA: Jossey-Bass.

Rossi, P. H., & Freeman, H. E. (1995). *Evaluation: A systematic approach* (5th ed.). Beverly Hills, CA: Sage.

Thomas, S. B., & Quinn, S. C. (1991). The Tuskegee syphilis study, 1932 to 1972: Implications for HIV education and AIDS risk reduction education programs in the black community. *American Journal of Public Health, 8*(11), 1498–1505.

U.S. Department of Health and Human Services. (n.d.) *About HHS.* Retrieved from http://www.HHS.gov/about

U.S. Department of Health and Human Services, Health Resources and Services Administration. (2010). *The registered nurse population: Findings from the 2008 national survey sample of registered nurses.* Retrieved from http://bhpr.hrsa.gov/healthworkforce/rnsurveys/rnsurveyfinal.pdf

Van den Heede, K., Lesaffre, E., Diya, L., Vieugels, A., Clarke, S. P., Aiken, L. H., et al. (2009). The relationship between inpatient cardiac surgery mortality and nurse numbers and educational level: Analysis of administrative data. *International Journal of Nursing Studies*, *46*, 796–803.

Watzlawick, R., Weakland, C. E., & Fisch, R. (1974). *Change.* New York: W. W. Norton.

West, W. F. (1982, September/October). The politics of administrative rulemaking. *Public Administration Review*, 420–426.

Williams, S. J., & Torrens, P. R. (Eds.). (1988). *Introduction to health services* (3rd ed.). Albany, NY: Delmar.

Wilson, J. Q. (1989). *American government institutions and policies* (4th ed.). Lexington, MA: D. C. Heath.

Wiltse-Nicely, K. L., Sloane, D. M., & Aiken, L. H. (2013, June). Lower mortality for abdominal aorta aneurysm repair in high volume hospitals contingent on nurse staffing. *Health Systems Research, 48*(3), 972–991.

You, L.-M., Aiken, L. H., Sloane, D. M., Liu, K., He, G.-P., Hu, Y., et al. (2013). Higher percentage of baccalaureate nurses were strongly associated with relationships to better patient outcomes. *International Journal of Nursing Studies, 59*(2), 154–161.

CHAPTER 2

Agenda Setting

Elizabeth Ann Furlong

KEY TERMS

Contextual dimensions: Studying issues in the real world, in the circumstances or settings of what is happening at the time.
Iron triangle: Legislators or their committees, interest groups, and administrative agencies that work together on a policy issue that will benefit all parties.
Streams: Kingdon's concept of the interaction of public problems, policies, and politics that couple and uncouple throughout the process of agenda setting.
Window of opportunity: Limited time frame for action.

Introduction

This chapter will emphasize the agenda-setting aspect of policy by using exemplar case studies at both the state and national levels. Agenda setting is the process of moving a problem to the attention of government so that solutions can be considered. Advanced practice registered nurses (APRNs) and other healthcare professionals (HCPs) can apply the knowledge from these case studies to the many current concerns they face.

"At the end of my pilgrimage, I have come to the conclusion that among the sins of modern political science, the greatest of all has been the omission of passion" (Lowi, 1992, p. 6). This criticism does not apply to public policy researchers' scholarly interest in agenda setting, policy design, and alternative formulation, nor does it apply to certain policy communities who push for selected public policies. The passion of the former group, the researchers, is seen in their search and inquiry for a better understanding of public policy. The passion of the latter, policy communities, is reflected in their tenacity on policy design, in pushing to make sure that a policy is put into practice as it was intended.

APRNs and other HCPs, as well as policymakers and citizens, are interested in the best public policy to address society's concerns. In the past, political science researchers mostly studied the latter steps of policymaking—implementation and evaluation—to gain an understanding of public policy and knowledge that could be used by policymakers to create better public policy. Although all stages of the policy process have been studied, the need for more research on the earlier parts of policymaking—agenda setting, policy formulation, and policy design—has drawn more discussion (Bosso, 1992a; Ingraham, 1987; May, 1991). Research interest in these latter areas grew during the 1980s and 1990s and it continues into the second decade of the 21st century.

In this chapter, examples are presented of agenda setting at both the state and the federal levels. First, the state example is described. By reviewing this case study, APRNs and other HCPs can learn ways that issues get on the legislative state agenda. Following the description of the state agenda setting example, a classic national legislative exemplar is presented. Policy research and analysis of this national example was conducted by this author. Following that analysis, those same theories have been utilized for a beginning analysis of the emerging 2014 state case study.

CASE STUDY 1: A NURSE PRACTITIONER–INITIATED BILL IN THE SPRING 2014 NEBRASKA UNICAMERAL LEGISLATURE

One example of agenda setting in Spring 2014 was the introduction by Nebraska Nurse Practitioners (NNP), a state nursing association, of a bill into the Nebraska unicameral legislative session to eliminate the Integrated Practice Agreement (IPA) from the Nurse Practitioner Practice Act (Nebraska Legislature, 2014b). The public hearing for the bill was January 31, 2014; the sponsoring state senator's goal was for the bill to emerge from the seven-member Health and Human Services Committee with a near majority (S. Crawford, personal communication, January 2014).

Prior to this bill's introduction, the NNP had to undergo the Nebraska Credentialing Review (407) Program. This program had been created for evaluation of scope of practice of health professionals (i.e., was a healthcare provider changing their scope of practice, and/or was there a new provider with a new scope of practice?) (Nebraska Department of Health and Human Services, n.d.). For such a review, the particular group of healthcare providers, in this case the NNP, submitted extensive documentation to three review bodies—an ad hoc Technical Review Committee appointed by the director of the Division of Public Health, a second review by the State Board of Health, and a third review by the director of the Division of Public Health. These reviews represented input from the Department of Health and Human Services (DHHS) about what possibly could be concerns for Nebraskans in terms of either public health or safety. Another important aspect is that, although the recommendations at the three levels were advisory, they served as important data points for state senators when the latter considered and voted on legislation based on the three reports (D. Wesley, personal communication, June 2013). The NNP proposal received support at the first two levels; at the second level, the vote was 12–5 to remove the IPA from the current statute (Whitmire, 2013). There also were recommendations with this second vote to: (1) have practice requirements for the new graduate nurse practitioner (NP), and (2) have ongoing competency evaluations of all NPs. At the third level the director and chief medical director of the DHHS were strongly opposed to the NNP proposal (Ruggles, 2013).

Nurse practitioners in Nebraska set the agenda so they could: (1) decrease barriers to their full scope of practice, (2) provide more and needed access to health care (especially primary care and mental health care) in rural parts of the state, (3) meet the emerging primary healthcare needs with an increased Nebraska population

(continues)

now having health insurance because of the Affordable Care Act, and (4) decrease the exodus of NPs to contiguous states that do not have such IPA agreements (Sundermeier, 2013/2014). With passage of this bill in the 2014 unicameral, Nebraska would join 17 other states and the District of Columbia that facilitate NP practice in this way. This agenda-setting item is based on evidence-based practice studies and the promotion of all nurses working to their full potential as advocated by the Institute of Medicine (Institute of Medicine, 2010). Concurrent with introduction of this bill was another bill that attempted to modify Medicaid expansion; the bill did not pass in the 2013 session, so it was introduced again in 2014 (Nebraska Legislature, 2014a). Passage of the latter bill (LB887) would result in a further increase in the Nebraska population who will have access to primary care.

By introduction of a bill, NPs literally set the agenda. A variety of strategies were implemented to further the agenda. The author of this chapter serves as chair of the Nebraska Nurses Association's Legislative Advocacy and Representation Committee (LARC). This committee worked in unison and collaboratively with the NNP, its lobbyist, and the sponsoring senator to serve as the lead strategists and voices. Further, NPs used public media; for example, following the negative review from DHHS, one NP educated the public on data about NPs in the state's largest city's newspaper (Holmes, 2013). She noted several of the arguments or statements of support noted previously for why NPs want the IPA eliminated.

CASE STUDY 2: THE NATIONAL CENTER FOR NURSING RESEARCH AMENDMENT

Victor Hugo wrote, "Greater than the tread of mighty armies is an idea whose time has come" (Kingdon, 1995, p. 1). For nurses, one example of this was the initiation of legislation in 1983 that increased the funding base for nursing research. An amendment to the 1985 Health Research Extension Act, which created the National Center for Nursing Research (NCNR) on the campus of the National

Institutes of Health (NIH), is the focus of this chapter's national example of agenda setting.

Creation of the NCNR came about because a group of nurse leaders wanted to create a national institute of nursing within the NIH. In order to pass the legislation in 1985, a political compromise was made with congressional legislators to create a center instead of an institute. However, in 1993 the NCNR was changed to an institute, and today the agency continues as the National Institute of Nursing Research (NINR). Discussion in this chapter of the NCNR amendment focuses on the agenda setting and policy formulation that occurred from 1983 to 1985.

The Influence of National Nurse Groups

The creation of the National Center for Nursing Research on the campus of the National Institutes of Health was a policy victory for national nurse organizations. Despite this victory, APRNs and other HCPs still need a better understanding of agenda setting, policy formulation, and policy design as they work for other policy changes in the future. Although nurses' groups traditionally have not been considered strong political actors, these groups recognize the importance of political activity to bring about public policies that enhance patient care (Warner, 2003). In the last decade of the 20th century, nurse groups were just emerging as actors in policy networks; however, "a full cadre of nurse leaders who are knowledgeable and experienced in the public arena, who fully understand the design of public policy, and who are conversant with consumer, business and provider groups [did] not yet exist" (DeBack, 1990, p. 69).

In a study of national health organizations that play a key role in the health policymaking area (Laumann, Heinz, Nelson, & Salisbury, 1991), no nurse organizations were cited. Advanced practice registered nurses are well aware of this absence because state legislative and regulatory activity affects their professional practice on a daily basis. The scope and nature of nursing care and certain restrictions to providing that care are closely related to public policy. Raudonis and Griffith (1991) and Warner (2003) are three of the many nurse

(continues)

leaders who challenged nurses to be more knowledgeable about health policy. These leaders also urged nurses to become more empowered on health policy issues; if nurses were to become more involved in policymaking, public policy could better reflect the contributions of nurses to patient care, to the health of citizens, and to cost-effective quality solutions for the financial crisis of the healthcare system. Nagelkerk and Henry echoed this concern: "To date, few studies in nursing can be classified as policy research. Leaders in our field, therefore, have identified this type of undertaking as a priority" (1991, p. 20).

Research on the NCNR amendment is important because it studies political actors who are not generally studied (e.g., nurse interest groups), and so this research contributes to public policy scholars' knowledge of all actors in policy networks. Laumann et al. acknowledged that "we may even run a risk of misrepresenting the sorts of actors who come to be influential in policy deliberation" (1991, p. 67). The significance of policy research becomes obvious when the Schneider and Ingram model of social construction of target populations in policy design is applied to nurse interest groups (1993a). For example, how nurses were viewed by policymakers—the social construction of nurses as a target population—influenced not only the policy that nurses were interested in, but also passage of the total NIH reauthorization bill.

Dohler (1991) compared health policy actors in the United States, Great Britain, and Germany, and found that it is much easier to have new political actors in the United States because there are multiple ways to become involved. Dohler has written of the great increase in new actors since 1970. Baumgartner and Jones (1993) also described multiple paths of access to becoming involved.

Overview of Models and Dimensions

Several researchers have developed models of agenda setting and policy formulation (Baumgartner & Jones, 1993; Cobb & Elder, 1983; Kingdon, 1995), and several political scientists have developed theoretical modeling of policy design (Hedge & Mok, 1987). Ingraham is one of several authors who has noted the lack of one design, one theory, or one model in policy design (1987). Meanwhile, public policy scholars have pushed for more empirical study of agenda setting, alternative formulation, and policy design (Schneider & Ingram, 1993a).

Data analysis reveals the importance of the Schneider and Ingram model (1993a) of the social construction of target populations, and of the Kingdon model (1995) for an understanding of the agenda-setting process of this amendment to the NIH-reauthorizing legislative bill. Analysis of this legislation over the period of a decade also underscores the importance of the Dryzek (1983) definition of policy design. An analysis of the legislation supported the importance of studying the **contextual dimension** that has been advocated by Bobrow and Dryzek (1987), Bosso (1992a), DeLeon (1988-1989), Ingraham and White (1988-1989), May (1991), and Schneider and Ingram (1993b). The value of other models—institutional, representational communities and an institutional approach, and the congressional motivational model—is addressed as these models contribute to an understanding of this example. These findings will be discussed in more detail. For example, during the study of interest groups opposed to this legislation, this researcher noted two occurrences of **iron triangles** in the early 1980s where legislators and their staff and agency bureaucrats worked with interested parties to resolve issues.

Kingdon Model

One model that was explanatory for this research was the Kingdon model (1995), which explains how issues get on the political agenda and, once there, how alternative solutions are devised. The four important concepts are the three **streams** (policy, problem, and political) and the **window of opportunity**. A problem stream can be marked by systematic indicators of a problem, by a sudden crisis, by feedback that a program is not working as intended, and by the release of certain important reports. A practical application for APRNs and other HCPs is that they can be attentive to these indicators and maximize such opportunities to get an issue on the agenda. A policy stream relates to those policy actors and communities who attach their solutions (policies) to emerging problems. This concept also relates to the actual policy being promoted, and so APRNs and other HCPs can be attentive to identifying problems and framing their solutions to such concerns. The third stream of Kingdon's model is the political stream, which consists of the public mood, pressure group campaigns, election results, partisan or ideological distributions in Congress, and changes in administration. Other factors include committee jurisdictional boundaries and turf concerns among agencies and government branches. APRNs and other HCPs need to be constantly attentive to all of these political factors, which can integrate with the fourth concept, the "window of opportunity." This is when the previously discussed three streams integrate at a time that is favorable to solve a problem with one's preferred policy and with the least resistance. This window of opportunity is most often affected by the problem and political streams.

Interview data and a review of the literature showed many ways in which the Kingdon model explained the agenda setting for this bill. For example, for the problem stream, the following were variables: (1) the need for nursing research was recognized by many (e.g., Representative Madigan (R-IL), legislative staffers, and national nurse leaders); (2) there were data about the financial disparity in research funding for nurses; and (3) the timing of an Institute of Medicine (IOM) report (Cantelon, 2010) on this problem. For the political stream, these were the variables: (1) this policy would be valuable for Rep. Madigan's re-election, and (2) this was an important policy proposal for the Republican party to secure increased voting by women voters. For the policy stream, it was sound public policy. There was a window of opportunity, that is, the release of the IOM report in conjunction with the election cycle, the singular presence of many national nurse leaders who were policy and politically knowledgeable at this particular point in time, and a U.S. representative who initiated the idea for this bill; all came together quickly and at an opportune time. In summarizing these findings in relation to the Kingdon model, this example validated the importance of the political and problem streams. However, the NCNR amendment was passed without meeting the policy stream processes described by Kingdon, in that it did not go through a softening-up phase. This latter concept refers to several revisions being made to a particular policy as compromise and negotiations take place. As stated, the NCNR amendment was articulated once and moved forward; there was no tweaking or change in the language.

APRNs and other HCPs may be able to apply the Kingdon model to ongoing priority practice issues with which they are concerned. For example, APRNs and other HCPs can be attentive to the three streams (policy, problem, and political) and a window of opportunity in which to move forward their agenda. Specifically, for NPs, every year a legislative update is printed in *The Nurse Practitioner*, and this is one way to recognize the advances made in state policies in the areas of scope of practice, prescriptive authority, reimbursement practices, title protection, and emerging issues.

Although one of the exemplar case studies used in this chapter is that of the National Institute of Nursing Research getting on the political agenda and being passed as national legislation, APRNs and other HCPs also need to be aware that taking part in political activity in regulatory agencies could also be an ideal way to problem solve. In the early part of this century, nurse practitioners found increased difficulty in having mail-order pharmacies recognize and fill their prescriptions (Edmunds, 2003). Two nurse practitioners from New York and South Carolina addressed this problem stream by working with the Food and Drug Administration and the Federal Trade Commission. They recognized that working through regulatory agencies was the best initial solution for this problem (Edmunds, 2003).

Importance of Contextual Dimensions

Some authors, notably Bobrow and Dryzek (1987), Bosso (1992a), DeLeon (1988–1989), Ingraham and White (1988–1989), May (1991), and Schneider and Ingram (1993b), have emphasized the need to analyze the political context in which policies get on the agenda, alternatives are formulated, and policies are put into effect. Although neither a definitive nor an exhaustive list, five contextual dimensions are suggested by Bobrow and Dryzek (1987) for studying the success or failure of any designed policy: (1) complexity and uncertainty of the decision–system environment, (2) feedback potential, (3) control of design by an actor or group of actors, (4) stability of policy actors over time, and (5) stirring the audience into action. DeLeon writes that sometimes researchers, because of their unstructured environment, have chosen to study approaches and methodologies that may meet scientific rigor better, but in doing so come "dangerously close to rendering the policy sciences all-but-useless in the real-life political arenas" (1988–1989, p. 300).

DeLeon notes that it is difficult to impossible for researchers to "structure analytically the contextual environment in which their recommended analyses must operate" (1988–1989, p. 300). Whether analyzing the 1983 case study or the 2014 case study, APRNs and other HCPs must analyze the context in which they find themselves, apply theory, and evaluate the outcome later for theory application. Researchers and advocacy activists have to work in a world with great social complexity, extreme political competition, and limited resources. Of these writers, Bosso and May are especially strong in their advocacy of this contextual approach to the study of public policy. Bosso (1992b) echoes DeLeon's concern:

> In many ways, the healthiest trend is the admission, albeit a grudging one for many, that policymaking is not engineering and the study of policy formation cannot be a laboratory science. In policy making contexts do matter, people don't always act according to narrow self-interest, and decisions are made on the basis of incomplete or biased information. (p. 23)

For many healthcare professionals, this "messy" process is very uncomfortable.

Data from congressional documents, archival sources, and personal and telephone interviews showed the importance of the political context to all aspects of policy design—how the policy arrived on the agenda, how policy alternatives were formulated, the legislative process, implementation, and the redesign of the legislation 8 years later, resulting in new legislation within 2 years to accomplish the original goal (Bobrow & Dryzek, 1987; Bosso, 1992; DeLeon, 1988–1989; Ingraham & White, 1988–1989; May, 1991; Schneider & Ingram, 1993b).

Examples of Political Contextual Influence

First, partisan political conflict within Congress influenced the initial agenda setting of the amendment and the legislative process throughout the 2 years. Opposition to Rep. Waxman's (D-CA) NIH bill in the spring and summer of 1983 resulted in Rep. Madigan's initiating a substitute policy. An impetus to Rep. Madigan's bill was a perception that Rep. Waxman yielded too much power with NIH legislation. As noted by two congressional staffers, this was an example of partisan conflict. Another example of partisanship, noted by an interviewee, was that the appointment of Ada Sue Hinshaw, PhD, RN, as the first director of the NCNR was made easier because she was Republican. (The administration at the time was Republican.)

Second, a U.S. representative's concern with his re-election chances influenced the initial agenda setting because of the congressional perception that nurses were a target population that could help his re-election chances.

Several respondents noted that this was an important factor in the initial decision for this type of public policy.

A third contextual dimension was the bipartisan negotiation to enact policy. Such negotiations between Rep. Waxman and Rep. Madigan in early fall 1983 resulted in a firm resolve during the 97th and 98th Congresses to stay with the proposed NINR policy and during the 99th Congress to accept a compromise of an NCNR. Another example of bipartisan negotiation was the early committee work by Rep. Madigan, Rep. Broyhill (R-NC), and Rep. Shelby (D-AL) to forge a simple bipartisan four-line amendment. The bipartisan effort of these three representatives smoothed the way for passage of this amendment by the subcommittee. If there is bipartisan support for issues, there is a greater chance for passage of legislation. Legislators used this strategy early in the legislative process.

Fourth, interest group unity on the policy was a factor. Such unity by nurse groups was considered by many interviewees to be a crucial factor in the bill's passage, and this unity also was important in explaining why no other policy alternatives were pursued. Because the decision to support Rep. Madigan was officially made by the Tri-Council (the American Nurses Association, the National League of Nursing, the Association of Nurse Executives, and the American Association of Colleges of Nursing) in the summer of 1983, and although other policy alternatives were considered after that, the priority of presenting unity with Rep. Madigan was maintained by nurse organizations. Dohler (1991) reported on the importance of the unity of policy communities and concluded that the deregulation of two organizations, the Professional Standards Review Organization and the Health Systems Agencies, occurred because of the "weakened stability of the network segment" (p. 267). Dohler also determined that if there is not a stable, united policy community, programs falter. If there is such stability (as with the nurse community in this research), there is an increased chance of success.

Fifth, lack of interest group unity with a congressperson was seen as a negative factor. Such prior behavior by the American Association of Medical Colleges had disillusioned Rep. Madigan and increased his interest in initiating the NINR policy with the nurse providers' groups.

Sixth, partisan conflict between the White House and an interest group (nurses) that generally supported Democratic presidential and vice presidential candidates had an influence on this legislation's history. This campaign support by the American Nurses Association (ANA) for the Democratic candidates was evaluated as the reason for the 1984 Republican presidential veto of the NINR amendment and the NIH bill that had passed Congress. Interviewee data reported one congressperson's concern with how the ANA Political Action Committee (PAC) distributed its money—mainly to Democratic candidates. Research by Makinson (1992) a decade later on the 1990 election reflected that the ANA PAC gave 85 percent of its money to Democratic candidates.

Seventh, ideological and partisan conflicts over other issues within the larger NIH bill affected the bill's legislative history. Concerns about fetal tissue research and animal rights research caused much difficulty in the early 1980s, and concerns about immigration laws and immigrants with HIV infection raised concerns in the 1990s and affected compromises and passage of the bills. These issues, although not about the NINR amendment, had a major effect on the bill's legislative history. APRNs and other HCPs need to understand bills in their holistic context and the many pressures on a particular bill.

Eighth, concerns with the federal deficit influenced discussion of the bill and decision making. There was opposition to the creation of new federal entities because of the deficit concern, and President Reagan consistently used this argument as a reason not to create an NINR.

Ninth, legislation passed during a lame-duck presidential term was a factor. The NIH bill with the NCNR amendment was passed in 1985 when President Reagan was beginning his second term. Republican members of Congress did not feel as constrained to vote along party lines, and that was reflected in the 1985 legislative vote and the override vote. Thus, the timing of this vote in President Reagan's lame duck term helped the bill's passage. When the president vetoes legislation, another option for passage is for Congress to secure the necessary number of votes and override the president's decision. As will be explained in the thirteenth contextual variable, this was a significant political event for this nurse issue.

Tenth, the history of Congress with selected administrative agencies influenced the political context. Rep. Waxman's attempted control of the NIH was a factor in Rep. Madigan's initiation of NIH legislation during the summer of 1983. Data support the analysis that of all administrative agencies, the NIH consistently was regarded positively by members of Congress, and this was reflected in ample funding levels on a consistent basis. Contrary to this usual positive regard was the negative situation between Rep. Dingell (D-MI) and the NIH. Representative Dingell had "captured" letters sent by NIH officials to research scientists asking them to lobby their congresspeople for increased funding. Rep. Dingell reminded NIH officials that this activity violated law. Further, this situation led Rep. Dingell and other congressional members to ask: Who was and who should be in charge of the NIH?

Eleventh, the interaction of Congress, administrative agencies, and the Office of Management and Budget (OMB) also influenced the political context. The congressional funding pattern identified in the 10th factor changed somewhat in the early 1980s. National Institutes of Health officials became anxious when the OMB dictated that NIH make a last-minute revised budget to honor a 1980 promise to fund 5,000 new grants yearly. This mandated division of NIH's economic pie contributed to NIH officials not wanting new research entities on their campus that would further erode current programs and projects. A second similar budgetary crisis occurred at NIH in spring 1985 that, again, caused much consternation for NIH officials and research scientists.

Twelfth, the internal political dynamics of Congress also influenced this legislation. Rep. Waxman was a member of the congressional class of 1974, when the dynamic in Congress was a decentralization of power with a large congressional class. (A congressional class refers to that cohort of officials elected in a certain year.) The data revealed that Rep. Waxman was interested in gaining more power and control over the NIH. Although his committee had authorizing power over the NIH, it did not have the greater power of the Appropriations Committee that was responsible for funding. However, with his ability to authorize legislation, Rep. Waxman had leverage to gain more power. Waxman's attempt to micromanage the NIH resulted in Rep. Madigan's initiating substitute policy.

Thirteenth, interaction between the White House and Congress affected the legislation. For example, President Reagan publicly vetoed the legislation in 1984, although he could have done it quietly by not signing the bill. This was done to alert Congress to expect conflict the following year if the bill's provisions were kept the same. An example of the negative relationship between the White House and Congress related to the override vote in 1985. Data showed that members of Congress (and many of the president's party) felt betrayed over their work on this legislation and over what they thought their communication had been with the president about passing this policy and putting it into effect. This sense of betrayal spurred their work in securing the veto-override vote. Another example of the challenging relationship between the White House and Congress was the number of presidential vetoes by President Reagan of congressional legislation and the few veto-override votes. Since his inauguration, President Reagan had vetoed 41 legislative bills; this override of the NIH bill veto was the fifth successful override vote since 1981 (*Congressional Quarterly*, 1985). This override vote not only was a policy victory for nurses, but also was significant from a political science researcher's perspective.

Fourteenth, even international political relations were a consideration. During fall 1985, the Senate waited until the Geneva Summit was finished before beginning the veto-override vote. This was done to keep President Reagan from losing any credibility of leadership ability during the summit meeting because the Soviet leader would be aware of the veto-override vote.

Fifteenth, the skills and abilities of an interest group in furthering its intended policy had an influence on the context of legislation. Data revealed that in the early 1980s, many factors influenced the ability of nurse interest groups to promote this policy once it was on the agenda. These influences were: (1) the formation of the Tri-Council, (2) a special interest in public policy of the executive director of the National League for Nursing (NLN), (3) the anticipated need to reauthorize the Nurse Education Act, (4) many deans of nursing education programs who were policy-oriented, (5) a combination of people who saw the need, (6) much networking by nurses, (7) the presence of highly motivated people who were interested in furthering the nursing profession, (8) nurses appointed to positions within the White House, (9) more nurses working on Capitol Hill, and (10) the study conducted by Dr. Joanne Stevenson (personal communication, 1990) on nurse researchers' inability to obtain NIH grants. These 10 factors were obtained from interview data. Many of these influences demonstrate the increased numbers of nurses who were active in policy and politics in many dimensions and in many places: state and national governmental levels, professional associations, executive and legislative branches of the government, schools of nursing, and networking circles. Further, the research by Dr. Stevenson had shown that nurses had an increased opportunity of receiving NIH grants when they omitted their RN credential on their grants and only listed their PhDs (personal communication, 1983).

Sixteenth, the adage that "all politics is personal" influenced the legislation at various points. Data revealed the importance of personal relationships in getting the idea on the agenda, in gaining strategic information, in sharing needed information, and in making requests. For example, strategic networking at certain cocktail parties helped, as did carpooling with selected political actors. Savvy nurse leaders facilitated other nurses in meeting with legislators and legislative aides in these settings so nurses could lobby effectively. The importance of congressional staffers to the initiation and passage of legislation must be emphasized. Several interviewees spoke of the importance of certain staffers in their tenacity to ensure that the NCNR amendment was passed. Other staffers noted the importance of the professional education background and socialization of staffers in influencing the types of policy options that are initiated and pursued with vigor. Interview data attested to the tenacity of one Capitol Hill staffer during the conference committee.

Two of Bobrow and Dryzek's (1987) five contextual dimensions were in evidence and contributed to the success of this policy, both because the NCNR was passed as legislation in 1985 and because the NCNR became the National Institute of Nursing Research in 1993. The two criteria are related in this instance: the control of design by an actor or group of actors and the stability of policy actors over time. Once this policy was on the agenda and once nurses were united, the nurse interest groups were committed to the legislation. The nurse interest groups showed unity in working with Rep. Madigan and staying the course. Although other policy alternatives were discussed, they were never vigorously pursued by the nurse interest groups. Once the compromise for NCNR was made in 1985, the nurse interest groups found it acceptable because they knew they had a "foot in the door" and because they planned to accomplish their original design (an NINR) at a later date.

STABILITY OF POLICY ACTORS

The second dimension, stability of policy actors, also relates to the nurse interest groups. These groups of nurse leaders were stable for over a decade and kept tenaciously to their goal. Although the policy arrived on the formal agenda because of Rep. Madigan, a very unchanging group of nurse actors worked for over 10 years to see that the original policy design eventually was enacted (i.e., change from an NCNR to an NINR).

May (1991) writes that regardless of how one defines policy design, there is the "emphasis on matching content of a given policy to the political context in which the policy is formulated and implemented" (p. 188). This statement describes the contextual dimension of how this public policy arrived on the formal agenda. Rep. Madigan was going to introduce substitute legislation for Rep. Waxman's NIH bill. Rep. Madigan's NINR amendment was based on an appraisal of what policy content would best work in that political context.

Ingraham and White wrote: "Politics can influence both design process and design outcome in a number of ways. It can constrain problem definition and the range of alternative solutions available for consideration... . It can, in fact, eliminate the process of design altogether" (1988–1989, p. 316). Data indicate that this happened. Partisan and re-election politics influenced the design process, specifically the policy option that was chosen (the NINR proposal). That policy option moved quickly to the formal agenda, where it then moved forward in the legislative process. The politics of that option kept other alternative solutions from being seriously considered. Thus, the politics of this situation influenced the design process and the selection of the policy option and constrained the availability of other policy alternatives.

Schneider and Ingram Model

In addition to the political context emphasis, Schneider and Ingram (1991, 1993a, 1993b) specifically push for empirical research that studies the social construction of target populations (those groups affected by the policy). They propose that one can best understand agenda setting, alternative formulation, and implementation by knowing how elected officials perceive different target populations; in other words, by knowing the "social construction"—images, symbols, and traits—of such populations.

In their beginning work in this area, Schneider and Ingram proposed a theory in which there is a continuum of target populations categorized as the advantaged, contenders, dependents, and deviants. Their model suggests that there are pressures to initiate beneficial policy that helps those groups that are seen positively, whereas groups that are seen negatively will receive punitive policy. They argue that groups that are viewed positively are the "advantaged" and the "dependents" whereas the negatively perceived groups are the "contenders" and the "deviants." This is a beginning categorization, and they call for empirical research in this area. They admit that their theory needs three items:

Definitions of target populations and social constructions
An explanation of how social constructions influence public officials in choosing agendas and designs of policy
An explanation of how policy agendas and designs influence the political orientations and participation patterns of target populations

The Schneider and Ingram proposed theory, together with Kingdon's research, provide the best explanation for understanding the process of the NCNR legislation. Schneider and Ingram (1991, 1993a, 1993b) write that one can best understand agenda setting, alternative formulation, and implementation by knowing how elected officials see different target populations and by knowing the social construction, or images, symbols, and traits, of such populations. The data consistently revealed that this NCNR policy was initiated by Rep. Madigan because of the social construction of this target nurse population. Proposing public policy for this target population would help him pass his substitute NIH legislation. Nurses, as a target population, would be on the continuum of positively viewed groups. Although Schneider and Ingram acknowledge that theirs is an emerging theory that needs empirical testing to refine and define several of its phenomena, this author found it to be of explanatory value and extreme importance.

Mueller (1988) wrote: "Politicians must be convinced that they will gain from new policies—either through political success or through program effectiveness" (p. 443). The selection of nurses as a target population when congressional members, especially Republicans, needed the female vote contributed to a convincing argument for potential political success for them.

Summary Analysis of a National Policy Case Study

"No data are ever in themselves decisive. Factors beyond only the data help decide which policy is formulated or adopted by the people empowered to make the decision to form policy" (James, 1991, p. 14). James is referring to data in a problem stream as described by Kingdon. The accuracy of this quote was seen in this research because the Schneider and Ingram theory of the "social construction of target populations," together with the Kingdon model and the contextual dimension, explained the policy process.

The contextual dimension influenced all aspects of the policy, from agenda setting in 1983 through policy redesign in 1991, and later with the passage of the amended legislation in 1993 that accomplished the original 1983 goal. The importance of studying the political context was demonstrated by the 17 contextual dimensions that influenced this legislative policy process.

Of particular explanatory value in the early agenda-setting and policy-alternative formulation of this legislation were the Schneider and Ingram model and the Kingdon model. The particular amendment was pursued because of application of the "social construction of target populations"; that is, the target population of nurses was chosen because nurses would help Rep. Madigan's and other members of Congress's chances for re-election. With this model, the Kingdon theory adds to the further understanding of this legislation. Within Kingdon's model, neither the problem stream nor the policy stream was decisive for the process of this legislation; rather, it was the political stream. The factors of the political stream (re-election chances for Rep. Madigan and other congresspeople, partisan ideology in Congress, the public mood about gender issues, and turf concerns between government agencies) all strongly influenced the setting of this issue on the agenda. The hypotheses supported by this empirical research include that policy is more likely to be initiated for those target populations who are positively viewed by members of Congress; issues are more likely to reach the formal agenda when the political stream factors are related to positively viewed target populations; and the policy process is best understood in a contextual perspective.

Theory Application to the Emerging State Case Study

Although this chapter has emphasized this author's research of a national policy case study on agenda setting, the theories can also be applied to the emerging Nebraska 2014 case study. In the national case study, the goal of having a National Institute of Nursing Research was reached in 1993, having begun as a compromise bill initiating a National Center for Nursing Research. The agenda setting was initiated by a congressman. In contrast, in the state case study, NPs initiated and set the agenda (i.e., by seeking a state senator to introduce a bill, LB916). Nurse practitioners are knowledgeable about the problem, policy, and political streams; the window of opportunity; and the context of many variables within Nebraska and the nation that have had bearing on the progression of this bill. Variables include the 2010 IOM report, evidence-based research on the quality and safety of NP care, the 54,000 uninsured Nebraskans, the Affordable Care Act, whether the unicameral legislature passed a modified Medicaid Expansion bill during its session, the political conservatism of the state, and the structure of the unicameral as a short 60-day session in even-numbered years (J. Sundermeier, personal communication, December 2013). Specifically, the problem stream incorporates: (1) the factor that NPs in Nebraska do not meet the goal of the IOM report (i.e., are not working to their full scope of authority), and (2) that more Nebraskans, especially rural Nebraskans, could have enhanced access to health care if NPs have this full scope of authority. Nurse practitioners selected a policy stream proposal that was being furthered by the IOM report (i.e., work to one's full authority). Finally, NPs were aware of the political variables: (1) the modified Medicaid Expansion bill that did not pass in 2013 and that may or may not pass in spring 2014, with the resultant increase or nonincrease in the number of the newly insured population in the state; (2) the political conservatism of the state; (3) the short 60-day session (which means a prioritization of bills by the state senators); and (4) the push-back by the Nebraska Medical Association (NMA). As of late January 2014, the strategy of the NMA was to delay action on LB916 by seeking another study in addition to the thorough Nebraska Credentialing Review (407) Program that was undertaken for many months during 2013 (D. Wesley, personal communication, January 28, 2014). It is common to use a delaying tactic to proposed agenda setting instead of frontal opposition (D. Wesley, personal communication, January 28, 2014).

All of the variables listed in this state case study for the three streams have converged into a window of opportunity for NPs, who introduced the bill in January 2014. The Kingdon model, used here, continues to facilitate policy analysis with a range of policies (Kingdon, 2001; Lieberman, 2002). Further, the social construction theory used in the national case study was as relevant in 2014 in Nebraska with LB916 as it had been decades earlier. Schneider and Sidney (2009) continue with that analysis for policies. NPs in Nebraska struggle with the social construction perception of NPs versus physicians and hospital administrators and the amount of power each of these provider groups holds. For example, the Nebraska Hospital

Association took a neutral stance on the NP bill (D. Wesley, personal communication, January 28, 2014).

Besides taking the specific role of setting the agenda (i.e., introducing and shepherding a bill through a legislative body), there are other ways that APRNs and other healthcare providers were supportive of such agenda setting by their colleagues. For example, this writer serves in her third year as chair of the Legislative Advocacy and Representative Committee (LARC) of the Nebraska Nurses Association (NNA). Both LARC and the NNA were fully supportive of the NNP and followed the strategies of the NP plan. For example, verbal and written testimony were provided by LARC, representing the NNA, for the late January 2014 public hearing, and timely email messages were prepared by LARC and sent to all NNA members for appropriate advocacy with the respective Health and Human Services Committee senators who were considering this bill. Another way this writer furthered the agenda-setting goals of the NNP was by her membership in a League of Women Voters (LWV) chapter in a large midwestern city and education of LWV members on this bill. These LWV civic activists were encouraged, per their evaluation of the bill, to also advocate as citizen consumers.

LB916 passed the third and final vote (final reading) on April 17, 2014, with a 43–0 passage vote (six senators were either not present or abstained from voting). This was the last day of the unicameral session. On April 22, 2014, the governor vetoed the bill with rationale based on input from the physician director of the Nebraska Health and Human Services Department. Because April 17 was the last day of the legislature, it was not possible to have an override of the veto. The Nebraska Nurse Practitioner Association will reintroduce the bill in spring 2015.

Even though good ideas are presented to policymakers and the appropriate legislative process is followed, not all ideas take hold and not all solutions proposed come to fruition. In the case of the Nebraska unicameral, it is not atypical for an idea to move through as many as three bills within a 2-year legislative system; passage the first time around is unusual. Persistence and long-term planning are integral and critical to policymaking.

For APRN and HCP scholars, these case studies contribute to an understanding of agenda setting and policy design by having evaluated the importance of the Schneider and Ingram model, the Kingdon model, policy design, and the contextual dimension to policy initiation, development, implementation, and policy redesign in the creation of the National Institute for Nursing Research and in a state issue relating to full practice authority for NPs.

Discussion Points

1. How did the Kingdon model explain the NCNR getting on the political agenda?
2. How does the Kingdon model apply to the Nebraska case study?
3. How can APRNs and other HCPs become aware of factors in the problem stream to which Kingdon alluded? What problems are you concerned about in your specific profession?
4. What are examples of policy streams that APRNs and other HCPs could be advancing relative to their practice?
5. How can APRNs and other HCPs be involved in the political stream? How are you involved?
6. How can APRNs and other HCPs anticipate windows of opportunity? Given your profession, what will you specifically be observant for?
7. According to Schneider and Ingram, to which of the four target populations does your specific health provider group belong? Discuss the relevance to agenda setting.
8. What are ways that APRNs and other HCPs can network with congressional members and their staffers?
9. How can APRNs and other HCPs promote unity among themselves and with other healthcare providers?
10. How can all healthcare providers support one another and further some of the IOM goals?
11. What current contextual dimensions can promote APRN and other HCPs' practices?
12. How can APRNs and other HCPs best use the Kingdon model and the Schneider and Ingram model?
13. Given your specific health profession, what policy do you recognize that needs to be on the agenda at the local, state, or national level? What can you do to begin that process?

References

Baumgartner, F. R., & Jones, B. D. (1993). *Agendas and instability in American politics.* Chicago: University of Chicago Press.

Bobrow, D. B., & Dryzek, J. S. (1987). *Policy analysis by design.* Pittsburgh, PA: University of Pittsburgh Press.

Bosso, C. J. (1992a). Designing environmental policy. *Policy Currents, 2*(4), 1, 4–6.

Bosso, C. J. (1992b). *Policy formation: Current knowledge and practice.* Paper presented at the American Political Science Association meeting (pp. 1–30). Chicago, IL.

Cantelon, P. (2010). *National Institute of Nursing Research history book.* Washington, DC: NIH Publishers.

Cobb, R. W., & Elder, C. D. (1983). *Participation in America: The dynamics of agenda-building* (2nd ed.). Baltimore: Johns Hopkins University Press.

Congressional Quarterly. (1985, July 27). Washington, DC: U.S. Printing Office, p. 1493.

DeBack, V. (1990). Public policy—nursing needs health policy leaders. *Journal of Professional Nursing, 6*(2), 69.

DeLeon, P. (1988–1989). The contextual burdens of policy design. *Policy Studies Journal, 17*(2), 297–309.

Dohler, M. (1991). Policy networks, opportunity structures, and neo-conservative reform strategies in health policy. In B. Main & R. Mayntz (Eds.), *Policy networks: Empirical evidence and theoretical considerations* (pp. 235–296). Frankfurt, Germany: Campus Verlag.

Dryzek, J. S. (1983). Don't toss coins in garbage cans: A prologue to policy design. *Journal of Public Policy, 3*(4), 345–368.

Edmunds, M. (2003). Advocating for NPs: Go and do likewise. *The Nurse Practitioner, 28*(2), 56.

Hedge, D. M., & Mok, J. W. (1987). The nature of policy studies: A content analysis of policy journal articles. *Policy Studies Journal, 16*(1), 49–62.

Holmes, L. (2013, December 14). Give nurse practitioners more rein [in The Public Pulse Letters to the Editor]. *Omaha World Herald*, p. 4b.

Ingraham, P. W. (1987). Toward more systematic consideration of policy design. *Policy Studies Journal, 15*(4), 611–628.

Ingraham, P. W., & White, J. (1988–1989). The design of civil service reform: Lessons in politics and rationality. *Policy Studies Journal, 17*(2), 315–330.

Institute of Medicine. (2010). *The future of nursing: Leading change, advancing health.* Retrieved from http://www.iom.edu/Reports/2010/The-Future-of-Nursing-Leading-Change-Advancing-Health.aspx

James, P. (1991). Bravo to the nursing emphasis on policy research. *Reflections, 17*(1), 14–15.

Kingdon, J. W. (1995). *Agendas, alternatives, and public policies.* New York: Harper Collins College.

Kingdon, J. W. (2001). A model of agenda-setting, with applications. *Law Review, MSU-DCL,* (2), 331.

Laumann, E. O., Heinz, J. P., Nelson, R., & Salisbury, R. (1991). Organizations in political action: Representing interests in national policy making. In B. Marin & R. Mayntz (Eds.), *Policy networks: Empirical evidence and theoretical considerations* (pp. 63–96). Frankfurt, Germany: Campus Verlag.

Lieberman, J. M. (2002). Three streams and four policy entrepreneurs converge: A policy window opens. *Education and Urban Society, 34*, 438–450.

Lowi, T. J. (1992). The state in political science: How we become what we study. *American Political Science Review, 86*(1), 6.

Makinson, L. (1992). Political contributions from the health and insurance industries. *Health Affairs, 11*(4), 120–134.

May, P. J. (1991). Reconsidering policy design: Policies and publics. *Journal of Public Policy*, *11*(2), 187–206.

Mueller, K. J. (1988). Federal programs to expire: The case of health planning. *Public Administration Review*, *48*(3), 719–725.

Nagelkerk, J. M., & Henry, B. (1991). Leadership through policy research. *Journal of Nursing Administration*, *21*(5), 20–24.

Nebraska Department of Health and Human Services. (n.d.). *Credential review (407) program*. Retrieved from http://dhhs.ne.gov/pages/reg_admcr.aspx

Nebraska Legislature. (2014a). *LB887—Adopt the Wellness in Nebraska act*. Retrieved from http://nebraskalegislature.gov/bills/view_bill.php?DocumentID=21586

Nebraska Legislature. (2014b). *LB916—Eliminate integrated practice agreements and provide for transition-to-practice agreements for nurse practitioners*. Retrieved from http://nebraskalegislature.gov/bills/view_bill.php?DocumentID=21963

Raudonis, B. M., & Griffith, H. (1991). A model for integrating health services, research, and health care policy formation. *Nursing and Health Care*, *12*(1), 32–36.

Ruggles, R. (2013, December 11). A setback for key health players. *Omaha World Herald*, *149*(58), p. 1.

Schneider, A., & Ingram, H. (1991). *The social construction of target populations: Implications for citizenship and democracy*. Paper presented at the annual meeting of the American Political Science Association, Washington, DC.

Schneider, A. L., & Ingram, H. (1993a). How the social construction of target populations contributes to problems in policy design. *Policy Currents*, *3*(1), 1–4.

Schneider, A., & Ingram, H. (1993b). Social construction of target populations: Implications for politics and policy. *American Political Science Review*, *87*(2), 334–347.

Schneider, A., & Sidney, M. (2009). What is next for policy design and social construction theory? *The Policy Studies Journal*, *37*(1), 103–119.

Sundermeier, J. (2013/2014). Nebraska nurse practitioners move forward. *Nebraska Nurse*, *46*(4), 5.

Warner, J. R. (2003). A phenomenological approach to political competence: Stories of nurse activists. *Policy, Politics, and Nursing Practice*, *4*(2), 135–143.

Whitmire, T. (2013). Nebraska nurse practitioners. *Nebraska Nurse*, *46*, 9.

CHAPTER 3

Government Response: Legislation

Politics: Playing the Game

Janice Kay Lanier

"Politics Is the Art of Problem Solving."
— JONAH GOLDBERG, EDITOR-AT-LARGE, *NATIONAL REVIEW ONLINE*

KEY TERMS

Christmas tree bill: A term used to describe legislation that is moving speedily through the process when the legislative body is about to adjourn or take a prolonged break. Bills that have been enacted in one chamber are used as the vehicle (Christmas tree) for amendments from multiple bills that may have stalled during the process. Many tangentially related issues are tacked onto the moving bill with little or no formal committee consideration.

Congress: The legislative body charged with enacting laws at the federal level. At the state level, the name of the legislative body will vary. The term *Congress* is reserved for the federal entity.

Constituents: Residents of a geographic area who can vote for a candidate and whom the elected official represents.

Interest group: An organized group with a common cause that works to influence the outcome of laws, regulations, or programs.

Lame duck session: The weeks immediately following a November general election when an outgoing legislative body attempts to speed its priorities through the legislative process. Legislative activity can be particularly vigorous if control of the legislative or executive branch of government will change when the newly elected individuals take office in January.

Legislation: The bills considered by legislators that, if approved, become laws.

Legislator: An elected individual who serves in the legislature. These officials make decisions regarding bills and resolutions pending before the legislative body to which they have been elected.

Legislature: The legislative body made up of individuals authorized to enact laws.

Lobbyist: An individual who works to influence legislators and other governmental decision makers.

Political action committee (PAC): A formal organization that exists to engage in a process through which candidates for political office are endorsed and otherwise supported. It must adhere to state and/or federal laws in carrying out its activities.

Introduction

For many nurses and other healthcare professionals, "politics" is a dirty word; it is the seamy side of the policymaking process that they prefer to ignore. Unfortunately, participating in the political aspects of policymaking is not an optional exercise. In many respects, such participation is key to ensuring nurses have a place at the policy table. Before one can influence policy, one has to be in the room where policy is being debated and developed—policy is made by those who show up, not necessarily by people with special expertise, and the usual way into the room is through the door labeled "political participation and savvy." Even those who do see the need for political participation are somewhat naïve as to exactly what that participation entails and how to do it effectively. In part, politics means playing the political game by the rules—even distasteful rules—at least until nurses have sufficient presence and clout to be able to affect the rules themselves.

Some may believe involvement in policymaking is self-serving, concerned only with advancing selfish professional interests. Actually, the ultimate point of participating in policymaking is to improve patient outcomes. This chapter is intended to provide insight into the subtle rules governing political participation and set out the options available to nurses for finding their way through the political maze. In order to do that one must first have a basic understanding of the "rules of the game"—how laws are made and who is on the field of play.

Process, People, and Purse Strings

Process: Rules of the Game or How a Bill Really Becomes a Law

No one would presume to play a game of football without knowing the basic rules. Likewise, even simple board games, such as checkers or Monopoly, have rules one must follow to have a chance of winning. Lawmaking is no different. In many ways it is a game, admittedly with very high stakes, and there is a process that determines what must happen in order for an idea, concept, or concern to become part of the U.S. Code or state statutes.

Most students complete a government course in high school and promptly disregard much of the subject matter because it seemingly holds little relevance for them. Although diagrams depicting "How a Bill Becomes a Law" are important, they are also very rudimentary (see **Figure 3-1**). There is much more to the process than can be neatly depicted on a chart. It is also important to realize that although the process may seem straightforward, it can be circumvented when the will of the party in control determines it is expedient to do so. Parliamentary procedure maneuvers, filibusters, internal rule changes governing chamber proceedings, **lame duck sessions**, changes to committee appointments, and **Christmas tree bills** are all tactics or opportunities used to achieve one's legislative goals expeditiously. Whether or not these tactics engender good public policy has been the subject of much debate among political scientists; however, regardless of the debate, nurses must be aware of these options so as not to be the unwitting victims of a clever strategic move. Naïveté has no place in the policymaking arena.

INTRODUCTION

Bills are ideas that **legislators** have determined need to be enacted into law. The ideas can come from many sources: the legislator's own experiences; issues brought forward by **constituents**, special **interest groups**, or **lobbyists** on behalf of their clients; and not infrequently as a result of tragic events that trigger a public outcry for a new or amended law (e.g., school shootings that fan a debate over gun control). Once the concept is drafted into

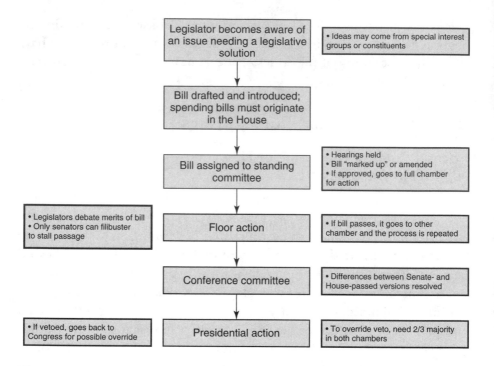

■ Figure 3-1   How a bill passes through Congress.

the proper bill format, it is introduced into the House or Senate, depending on the chamber to which the bill's chief sponsor belongs.[1] Each bill is numbered sequentially, and it retains this number throughout the process. Many bills are introduced during a legislative session, but few receive much attention in the form of committee consideration; fewer still actually become law.

COMMITTEE CONSIDERATION

Once introduced, a bill is referred to a standing committee for further consideration. These standing committees are generally subject-matter focused, so bills related to health care go to a health committee, finance issues to a banking committee, farm-related matters to an agriculture committee, and so on. Standing committees at the federal level tend to be permanent;

---

[1] All budget bills are initiated in the House, because our Founding Fathers designed this chamber to be most representative of the average citizens' interests and because of the importance of budgeting in regards to policymaking.

at the state level they can be configured differently over time depending on the vision of the leadership of the party in power at the beginning of each new legislative session. Subcommittees may be named to consider particular bills in greater detail. Bills are amended or marked up (voted on) in committee and subcommittee. These sessions are where testimony from affected parties is heard. Often the bill that emerges from committee bears little resemblance to the original proposal.

Committee hearings are important, but they often appear to be more chaotic than productive—at least to the average observer. That is because much of the real business of lawmaking is conducted behind the scenes in interested party meetings, but one must also participate in the defined committee processes to earn a place at the more informal behind-the-scenes tables.

Committee chairs are extremely influential, particularly with respect to the subject areas that are the focus of the committee's work. Chairs determine what bills will be heard and when, and they establish the procedural framework under which the committee operates. The chair's position on an issue can determine the fate of a bill from the outset. Because of the extent of their power and influence, committee chairs are able to raise large sums of money from special interest groups to support their re-election, and re-election is always an important consideration for lawmakers. House and Senate leadership (elected by their colleagues) determine who will be named as committee chairs. Certain committees are seen as more prestigious than others, so being named the chair of one of those committees is very important to an ambitious legislator. Not surprisingly, political considerations play a role in this entire process. Being aware of the dynamics that are the foundation of the overall committee process helps ensure more effective representation by those who want to influence the outcome of the committee's work.

FLOOR ACTION

If a bill is able to garner committee approval, it goes to the full chamber for a vote. The timing for scheduling a vote, as well as various attempts to amend the bill or delay the vote, are integral parts of the lawmaking process.[2] Much maneuvering occurs backstage, and the ability to influence

---

[2] Proponents of an issue are very aware of the potential vote count. If it appears the bill will not garner sufficient support, they will ask to have the bill pulled from the agenda so as to postpone the vote. As long as no action has been taken, the bill remains alive. If voted down it dies until the next session of the legislature convenes.

these less public interactions is as important as the words or concepts being debated. Again, people's relationships and politics determine the ultimate results. To be able to be effective in one's efforts to influence outcomes, one must be aware of these relationships and take them into account. Once a bill is approved in either the House or Senate, it must begin the process again in the other chamber.

CONFERENCE COMMITTEE

Seldom does a bill complete the journey through the second chamber without change, which means the originating chamber must agree to the new version of the bill. If it does not, the bill will be referred to a conference committee made up of representatives from the House and Senate who reconcile the differences and ask their respective chambers to support the conference committee report. If agreement cannot be reached, the bill dies.

CHIEF EXECUTIVE SIGNATURE

If there is agreement the bill goes to the chief executive (president or governor), who must sign the bill before it can become law. If the chief executive vetoes the bill, it will go back to the **legislature** for a potential veto override, which requires a two-thirds majority of both chambers.

All of this must happen within a single legislative cycle—2 years (a biennium). It is not surprising that it often takes several years for a particular legislative issue to finally become law, especially when powerful interest groups are on opposite sides of the proposal.

State legislatures typically follow the bicameral (two-chamber) structure of the federal government (see **Table 3-1**). The exception is Nebraska, which has a unicameral body. The number of legislators may vary from state to state as may the length of the term in office for the senators. Some states (but not the federal government) have adopted laws that limit the number of consecutive terms a legislator may serve in any one chamber. These term limits were adopted to deal with legislators who served multiple years in their respective chambers. Their re-election was seldom challenged, and voters became convinced that policymaking would be better served by changing the face of the lawmaker on a more regular basis. Not surprisingly, term limits have had unintended consequences, some of which have changed the dynamics within the legislature and affected policymaking in general. Relationship and leadership development, which take time, have

■ Table 3-1 Congressional Structure

Senate	House of Representatives
100 members, two from each state.	435 members based on a state's population. The number of representatives apportioned to each state changes every 10 years after national census data are obtained. Drawing and redrawing congressional district lines is a very political process that each state implements according to its own laws.
Six-year terms with one-third up for re-election every 2 years with no limit on the number of terms served.	Two-year terms with no limit on the number of terms served.
The vice president is the Senate leader but a president pro tempore is elected each session by the majority party.	The majority party elects the speaker of the House.

been short-circuited. Ambitious lawmakers frequently seek leadership positions without the foundations in place needed to be effective in these roles. Institutional memory has been lost, as has the depth of understanding of the complexity of the issues legislators must address. Finally, the interest in developing long-term solutions to challenging problems has been replaced with a more incremental immediate approach that focuses on short-term solutions rather than the underlying cause of the problems. These realities affect the strategies adopted by interest groups seeking a legislative solution to their problem or concerns.

Although there may be subtle differences between the state and federal lawmaking processes, the political dynamics that affect the ultimate outcome of any policymaking initiative are quite similar regardless of the venue.

People: Players in the Game

One might believe that the only players in the lawmaking game are the elected officials, the senators and representatives representing their respective states or districts. Although they are certainly integral to the process, there are many other individuals who are key to successfully achieving one's legislative goals. Those who take game playing seriously spend time learning the strengths and weaknesses of the people on the field or at the table with them. They study game film and read scouting reports and other resources to minimize surprises and help define their own strategies. That same attention to detail should apply in the policymaking game but it is often sadly neglected.

The majority of people cannot identify their federal, state, or local elected officials. Although many can name the President of the United States, few will be able to say with assurance who represents them in the halls of **Congress** and fewer still can name their state senators or representatives. Every nurse should know the identity of his or her U.S. senators and Congressional representative. It is equally or more important, however, for nurses to also know their state representative and senator because so much professional regulation occurs at the state level. Technology has made it easy to learn the identity of lawmakers at every level by simply going to federal or state government websites and entering zip code data. These sites also provide brief biographical information, photos, and other pertinent and helpful background material.

Why is this important? Politics is at heart a people process and, like other people-centered endeavors, the relationships among and between people determine outcomes. In order to have even the most basic conversation with elected officials, one must know who they are and what they care about.

LEGISLATIVE AIDES

In addition to knowing elected officials, one must also make an effort to know staff members—aides and others—who often control access to their bosses and influence how various issues are perceived and prioritized. At the federal level every legislator determines how his or her office will be staffed—usually using a chief of staff, legislative directors, press secretary, and legislative assistants (see **Table 3-2**). Federal lawmakers also maintain local or district offices with a small staff presence at each site. On the state level the number of aides can vary, but as state legislatures have become more than part-time endeavors, the use of aides has increased. Typically, state officials have at least one aide who is usually a generalist whereas federally the aides are more issue-focused.

Regardless of whether an aide is in Washington, D.C., or at statehouses across the country, elected officials rely on aides for the details and nuances associated with specific legislative initiatives. Aides delve more deeply into

■ Table 3-2   Staffing Patterns: Federal Level

Staff Member	Role Played
Chief of staff or administrative assistant	Oversight responsibilities
Legislative directors	Responsible for day-to-day legislative activities
Press secretary	Press releases and public relations
Legislative assistants (LAs)	Responsible for specific legislative issues. For example, the health LA might work on health issues as well as education and Social Security. LAs provide staff assistance to the congressperson at committee hearings and prepare the member's statements and witness questions. They may help draft bills by working in concert with the legislative council.
Committee staff	Support the work of congressional committees. Separate staffs are allocated to the majority and minority party with a larger number serving the majority party. Their focus is usually narrower than the legislator's personal staff and they are usually older and more experienced. They plan the committee agenda, coordinate schedules, gather and analyze data, draft committee reports, and so on.

the issue and work closely with other aides in developing strategies and alternative concepts that they then present to their legislators for consideration.

Although communicating with legislators is important, nurses should not underestimate the importance of aides and other staff members, who may provide the last word to a legislator regarding the issue or concern. Including aides and other staff members in communications and making special efforts to respectfully integrate them into the entire process is a tactic that is likely to yield positive results.

LOBBYISTS

Although nurses may not know the identity of specific lobbyists, it is important to understand the role lobbyists play in the policymaking process and how their influence affects the game of politics. No bill becomes law without lobbyists' input. Lobbying is the act of influencing—the art of persuading—a governmental entity to achieve a specific legislative or regulatory outcome. Although anyone can lobby, lobbyists are most often individuals who represent special interest groups and are looked to as the experts by lawmakers who need information and rationale for supporting or not supporting a particular issue.

The role of lobbyists has become even more critical as the complexity of **legislation** has increased; for example, the 1914 law creating the Federal Trade Commission was a total of 8 pages, the Social Security Act of 1935 totaled 28 pages, and the Financial Reform bill (conference version) of 2010 contained 2,319 pages (Brill, 2010). Legislators, often pressed for time and/ or newly elected to the legislature, rely on lobbyists' expertise to help them understand what they are voting for or against.

Some believe that, although the number of lobbyists in 2013 appears to indicate a decline (see **Table 3-3**), many individuals are actually working behind the scenes as "consultants" to avoid new and more stringent lobbyist reporting requirements. Congressional gridlock and a stagnant economy may be additional factors contributing to the decline. Lobbyists' overall influence has not waned, however (Auble, 2013).

Purse Strings: "Show Me the Money"

Game playing comes with a price in both athletic venues and legislative arenas. Not only are significant sums of money spent by special interest groups in support of their lobbying efforts, money also is critical to election

■ Table 3-3   Lobbying by the Numbers

Number of Lobbyists on Capitol Hill	Sample Lobbyist Numbers, 2013	Costs*
1998: 10,406	American Nurses Association: 8	1998: $1.45 billion
2007: 14,837	American Hospital Association: 75	2010: $3.55 billion
2013: 11,935	American Medical Association: 43	2013: $2.38 billion

*Costs include salaries and expenses lobbyists incur as part of their jobs. They could also include developing materials to support an initiative, or studies/surveys commissioned to support or refute a position.

Source: Data from The Senate Office of Public Records, Released October 18, 2013 (Center for Responsive Politics 2013c and Center for Responsive Politics 2013b).

On September 18, 1793, President George Washington laid the cornerstone for the U.S. Capitol. While the shovel, trowel, and marble gavel used for the ceremony are still displayed, repeated efforts to locate the cornerstone itself have been unsuccessful.

At times, policymaking seems as shrouded in mystery as the location of the Capitol's cornerstone. That's why you need an experienced partner (a.k.a. lobbyist) to help you unravel the mystery.

—A pitch for Capitol Tax Partners, a lobbying firm

and re-election campaigns. The role money plays in the policymaking process causes concern and discomfort for many nurses. It is where the notion of "politics" with all of its unfavorable connotations is on full display, and it is the reason many nurses (and others) consider political participation as something to avoid.

The amount of money that flows to and through the legislative process has raised serious questions as to whether the whole process is for sale to whoever has the deepest pockets. Unfortunately, winning an election or re-election, even at the local level, can be a very expensive proposition costing millions of dollars. In the 2012 election, the average cost of winning a U.S. House seat was $1.6 million; it was $10.35 million for a U.S. Senate seat (Center for Responsive Politics, 2013d). The total spending by political parties, candidates, and issue groups for the U.S. elections in 2012 was estimated to be nearly $6.3 billion, as compared with $86 million in Great Britain in 2010 (Zakaria, 2013). The spending trend is likely to continue

In its *Citizens United* ruling, the Supreme Court struck down the 2002 federal campaign finance law prohibiting unions and corporations from spending money directly advocating for or against candidates. The First Amendment was the basis for the Court's decision. The League of Women Voters has voiced its support of legislation that would require disclosure of the sources of the spending that is now legal and basically unlimited as long as the efforts are not coordinated with an individual's campaign.

due to the U.S. Supreme Court decision in *Citizens United v. Federal Election Commission* (2010) that basically allows unlimited spending by corporations and unions provided these efforts are not coordinated with an individual's campaign.

Not only has the amount of money flowing to campaigns increased dramatically, the source of those dollars (who has the deep pockets) also has changed and is expected to change even more in the future.[3] So-called "527 committees" are proliferating. These groups are not tied to any particular candidate or political party, but instead are funded by labor, big business, and superwealthy individuals (Center for Responsive Politics, 2013b). Other examples include American Crossroads GPS (the brainchild of Republican strategists Karl Rove and Ed Gillespie, both of whom held influential staff positions under former President George W. Bush), American Action Network, Republican Governors Association, and the Chamber of Commerce. These groups are based in Washington, D.C., and financed state political races across the country on behalf of Republican interests in 2012. Although these groups may appear to operate independently of each other, in actuality "coordination is as easy as walking across the hall" of their shared office space (Crowley, 2010, p. 31). On the Democratic side, organized labor, EMILY's List (Early Money Is Like Yeast), and the League of Conservation Voters continue to contribute millions to fund campaign messages (Crowley, 2010).

Experts have reported that "members of Congress spend three of every five workdays raising money" (Zakaria, 2013, p. E8), and that money usually is expected to yield a significant return on the donor's investment. The willingness of entities to invest the level of resources associated with influencing policy decisions is indicative of how important money is to the process. Members of special interest groups expect legislative success, and that success comes with a price. Nurses' willingness to pay that price remains an open question.

Although it may be distasteful, success in the halls of Congress and at statehouses is integral to the advancement of nurses' legislative agenda. That agenda includes measures intended to advance the profession itself, as well as societal values that are committed to better patient outcomes. Nurses

---

[3] Interestingly, women are underrepresented among campaign mega-donors, which has implications for the female-dominated nursing profession (Center for Responsive Politics, 2013e).

want their issues advanced successfully, and that expectation comes with a price tag that nurses must expect to pay.

Playing the Game: Strategizing for Success

Continuing the game-playing analogy, why are some teams more successful than others? If all the players know how to play the game, why are some consistent winners and others not? Why are the legislative agendas of some groups adopted seemingly with minimal opposition whereas others find it hard to get to the policy table? Much like athletic contests, the skill of the players, the expertise of the coaching staff, the financial investment of the team owners/supporters, and team chemistry all contribute to success on the field. Those same factors also determine success at the policymaking table.

Skill of the Players

Knowing the process and people, along with understanding how money affects the policymaking dynamics, is a start, but that alone will not ensure success. To move to the next level nurses and others must learn to think politically, to play politics, and to strategize with the political consequences and realities always at the forefront. In other words, they must apply their critical thinking skills in the policymaking context.

As political scientists have noted, politics underlies the process through which groups of people make decisions. It is the basis for the authoritative allocation of value. Simply put, politics is the effort and strategies used to shape a policy choice in all group relationships.

When one "plays politics," one is considered to be shrewd or prudent in practical matters, tactful, and diplomatic; playing politics is also seen as being contrived in a shrewd way, or being expedient. When one thinks like a politician it means he or she is looking beyond the issue itself and considering other forces and factors that affect what is likely to work and what has no chance of success. Deciding which of several policy options has the greatest benefit and the fewest costs in a world where re-election is a key consideration and media are a relentless presence means the best solution may not be the path ultimately chosen. The following scenario provides an example of what thinking politically might look like.

Clearly, success at the policy table involves more than the language of the proposal itself. Timing and the general political climate are key, unity is important, and quid pro quo is the reality in the statehouse halls. Politically

CASE STUDY: WORKPLACE SAFETY

Emergency department (ED) nurses have expressed concern about workplace safety, with many experiencing physical attacks on a routine basis. Many employers have been reluctant to report assaults to law enforcement because of the bad publicity it might engender. Nurses and others in psychiatric settings have similar concerns, as do nurses working in home health. Professional organizations representing these individuals, particularly ED nurses, formed a coalition to strategize about how to protect their members. Before the coalition had finished its work, the issue came to a head when an agitated family member assaulted a nurse, resulting in severe injuries to the nurse. Local media picked up the story and a state legislator, who is a member of the minority party and facing a difficult re-election, was surprised to learn that although teachers and law enforcement officials are part of a so-called "protected class," attacking healthcare workers was a misdemeanor rather than a felony offense. For protected workers the same assault carries the more stringent criminal designation that includes possible incarceration. The legislator decided to take on this issue, in part because he thought it might help his re-election efforts and because nurse organizations had supported his candidacy in the past. What factors must the politically savvy nurse consider if this issue is to move successfully from concept to legislation to law?

Thinking Like a Policymaker

Preliminary considerations	Issue: Problem identification	Is there a legislator to whom this issue may be of particular significance?
	Nurses are being assaulted in the workplace. Because the penalty for assaulting a healthcare worker is minimal, the law does not serve as an effective deterrent to such behavior. Is there another/better way to frame the problem?	Would that interested legislator be the best sponsor? Can s/he get majority party support? What is the level of commitment to the issue? How can the issue of sponsorship be finessed if a majority party cosponsor would increase the likelihood of success?

Looking at solutions through the eyes of the legislators	Possible solution: Make assaulting a nurse a felony offense Is there another solution or a compromise that would be more acceptable? How important are state budget considerations?	Would that solution be acceptable politically? Should all healthcare workers be included or nurses only? Would it mean more potential inmates in an already overcrowded prison system? Is that going to be costly to the state? If a patient is mentally ill does that change the dynamic?
Stakeholder identification and their influence on the overall issue	How politically connected are the stakeholders? How can their influence be minimized or maximized? What role would they be willing/able to play in supporting the legislator's re-election? How closely are they tied to those opposing the bill?	Stakeholders: Nurses; other healthcare workers who face the same dangers; trial lawyers; employers: hospitals, home health agencies concerned about what it means to their daily operations; mental health advocates concerned that the assaults occur because people are in stressful situations, which should not result in criminal charges. Others?
Values at play in this issue	What values/ideologies are paramount in the legislature? Is this proposal consistent with them? What are the majority party's priorities (e.g., health, economics, education)? How does this bill fit them?	Does the law really serve as a deterrent? Felony convictions could prevent someone from gainful employment in the future. Is that wise either socially or economically?
Resource analysis	What resources are available to support a legislative initiative? What contributions will nurse and other professional organizations be able/willing to make to the initiative?	How much money is needed to pass this initiative? How will the money be used? Will people be willing to testify? Is there administrative support to make the arrangements necessary to ensure coherent consistent advocacy?

(continues)

Power base and political considerations analysis	Who has the power? What is the political climate? How much time is left in the legislative session? Is the timing right for introducing the bill?	Is all the support coming from the minority party or is there bipartisan support? Is it an election year with legislators looking for an issue to champion that will resonate with the voters back home? Is this such an issue? Is the issue consistent with the governor and legislators' priorities?
Setting the stage	What groundwork needs to be laid before moving forward? What role will public opinion play, if any? What research should be brought forth and what does it say about the extent of the problem?	Is there a need to educate legislators on the issue? Do affected nurses live in the districts of key lawmakers? Would these nurses be willing to communicate with their senator/representative or testify? Are there personal stories that would resonate with legislators? Would a nurse's personal story be frowned upon by an employer who may not want the hospital's reputation seen as unsafe?

savvy nurses must be willing to take risks but should be smart when doing so (see **Exhibit 3-1**). In other words, they should enter the policy arena fully prepared for the challenges they will face.

Coaching Staff: Mentoring and Support

Given all the subtle factors that affect success on Capitol Hill or in state legislatures and the role money plays in the process, how can an individual hope to have sufficient knowledge or time to make a difference in the policymaking aspects of the profession? How can that nurse ever play the game effectively? Fortunately, the American Nurses Association (ANA) and its

Exhibit 3-1   Political Astuteness

- Issues always have at least two sides, and maybe more, that are reasonable depending upon one's point of view and experiences.
- Listen to what people are saying with an analytical ear. Critical thinking is not just for the practice setting. Apply theories and concepts about policymaking to the issues being considered. Use therapeutic communication techniques.
- Utilize a variety of sources; do not just rely on those that are consistent with your own ideology. Most sources have a bias, so broaden your reading and listening to get a more complete perspective and perhaps a bit closer to the truth. Always consider the source of the information provided.
- Connect with others who are involved in the policymaking side of the profession. Share what you learn with colleagues.

state constituent associations, as well as specialty nursing groups, can provide their members with the tools they need to be successful. The success of these organizations' efforts in the legislative arena depends in large part on their members' involvement with and understanding of the importance of an effective legislative presence on behalf of the profession in Washington, D.C., and in statehouses across the country. Many of these organizations offer opportunities for their members to come to Washington or to state capitals for lobby days that include briefings on both the issues and how to be effective spokespersons for the profession. These organizations know that it is the individual nurse, the so-called grassroots lobbyist, who has the most impact on the decisions made by elected officials. In fact, grassroots lobbying is seen by some as the most effective of all lobbying efforts (deVries & Vanderbilt, 1992).

Grassroots lobbyists are constituents who have the power to elect officials through their vote. When constituents have expertise and knowledge about a particular issue (such as nurses in healthcare policymaking), they are especially valuable resources for their elected officials. Although issues debated in Washington, D.C., are national in scope, members of Congress are still concerned about how the issue is perceived back home. The connections established by a nurse constituent with his or her lawmakers at the federal, state, and local levels may provide timely access and a listening ear at key points during the policymaking process.

Some professional organizations have established liaison or key person programs that match members with their elected officials, train them to be effective in the grassroots lobbying role, and provide periodic updates and information to help the nurses communicate in a timely manner with relevant messages targeted to the specific official. In turn, grassroots lobbyists establish ongoing connections with their elected officials that transcend specific legislative initiatives and communicate regularly with the sponsoring nursing organizations regarding what they learn through their interactions.

Coaching and mentoring nurses who are willing to engage in these kinds of supported liaison relationships will benefit both the individual nurse and the organizations doing the coaching. The nurse can markedly increase a legislator's understanding of nursing and the role nurses play in health care. With increased understanding, the legislator is more apt to be supportive of the profession's legislative agenda (see **Table 3-4**).

Investment: Time and Money

"A vision without resources is an hallucination." —Thomas Friedman

How much are nurses willing to pay to support the political activities of professional organizations? Are there sufficient resources available to make the vision of success a reality or is it destined to be a hallucination? What does that payment look like? Although the convergence of politics and money is not always pretty, ignoring the importance of financial contributions to moving a legislative agenda forward is naïve at best and will ultimately undermine efforts to advance the positive aspects of the nursing profession's agenda.

Some nurse organizations have established **political action committees (PACs)** that enable them to make contributions to political candidates and office holders who are supportive of nurses' legislative agenda. The money comes from the organization's members. An analysis of political contributions to federal candidates in 2013 showed contributions from nurse-related groups ranked far below those from other healthcare-related interest groups. For example, according to information compiled by the Center for Responsive Politics, based on reports from the Federal Elections Commission as of December 17, 2013, the highest amount contributed to federal candidates in 2013 by a healthcare PAC (the Cooperative of American Physicians) was $962,895. The American Hospital Association

■ Table 3-4 Communication Tips

Letters	■ Individually written letters are the most effective. Can send via U.S. mail, fax, or email. ■ Form letters/postcards have limited impact. ■ Timing is crucial. Send before the vote. Remember U.S. mail goes through a lot of security measures before delivery. ■ Send a typed message, no longer than two pages. ■ State purpose/position at the beginning and support it with clear, compelling rationale. ■ Include personal experiences. ■ Be polite. ■ Be respectful if expressing disappointment with a past vote. ■ Use your professional credentials. ■ Ask for a specific response.
Phone calls	■ Best if they come from the legislator's constituents. ■ Know what you want to say and say it respectfully and succinctly. ■ Identify self, including credentials. ■ Leave contact information and ask for a written response.
Social media	■ Do not discount social media as a mechanism for communicating. The messaging option on Facebook could result in rapid connection. ■ Identify yourself, your concerns, and your question professionally, regardless of the medium used
In-person meetings	■ Identify yourself, your work credentials, and your experience. ■ Avoid too much small talk but take advantage of shared personal experiences that might establish rapport. ■ Structure time to present the issue succinctly. ■ Do not assume the legislator has the level of expertise you do, so do not get too complex. ■ Provide a one-page summary of your key points. ■ Include the aide in the conversation. ■ Send a thank-you note afterwards.

spent $571,925. Both of these entities are designated as "heavy hitters" by the Center. The American Association of Nurse Anesthetists was the only nurse organization to appear on the list of top contributors ($460,250). With a contribution of $212,870, the American Nurses Association (ANA) did not make the list (Center for Responsive Politics, 2013a).

Given the contribution data, it should come as no surprise that organized nursing interests are at a disadvantage when trying to gain the ear of legislative decision makers. Were it not for other sources of power—numbers and the general trusted reputation of the nursing profession—trying to gain a seat at the policy table would be an elusive aspiration at best, at worst impossible.

Special interest groups may improve their chances for successful policymaking by endorsing candidates running for elective office. Candidates who want to demonstrate their appeal to the overall electorate prize these endorsements; this is particularly true for endorsements issued by nursing organizations such as the ANA on the federal level and state constituent associations of the ANA on the state level. This level of political activity occurs through the associations' PACs and must adhere to requirements set out in federal and state election laws.

Although money is a critical factor when considering the level of investment by the members of the nursing profession, membership in professional organizations is also symbolic of the extent of the commitment nurses have to the work of their representative organizations. Although nurses comprise the largest segment of the healthcare workforce, far too few invest in the profession by joining a professional organization. Approximately 6 percent of all nurses are members of any nurse organization (Haylock, 2012, p. 613). These low numbers significantly affect the amount of tangible and intangible resources available to associations for their work in the political arena. The strength of nurses is in their numbers, and that strength is enhanced when nurses support the work of their professional associations through their dues and volunteerism.

Team Chemistry: Getting Along with Each Other

Even with skilled players, strong support systems, and sufficient resources, a team will not succeed without that elusive quality: team chemistry. Divisiveness has long plagued the nursing profession and it remains an issue today. Disunity within the profession is a certain road to defeat and fuels the opposition's fire. Opponents are well aware of the potential impact a united nursing profession could have on health policy decisions and other important issues. Nurses' numbers alone are formidable. For that reason, competing interests subtly and purposefully poke at the hot spots that typically divide nurses (e.g., educational preparation, union vs. nonunion).

HEALTH POLICY AND POLITICS: A NURSE'S GUIDE; ED.
BY JERI A. MILSTEAD.
　　　　　　　　　5TH ED.　　　Cloth　　338 P.
SUDBURY: JONES & BARTLETT LEARNING, 2016

ED: UNIV. OF TOLEDO. TEXTBOOK--GRAD. W/ ONLINE
ACCESS.

　ISBN 1284048861　　　**Library PO#**　FIRM ORDERS

	List	99.95	USD
8395 NATIONAL UNIVERSITY LIBRAR	**Disc**	14.0%	
App. Date　9/23/15　SHHS　　8214-08	**Net**	85.96	USD

SUBJ: 1. NURSES--POL. ACTIVITY--U.S. 2. NURSING--
POL. ASPECTS--U.S.

CLASS RT86.5　　　　DEWEY# 362.1730973　LEVEL ADV-AC

YBP Library Services

HEALTH POLICY AND POLITICS: A NURSE'S GUIDE; ED.
BY JERI A. MILSTEAD.
　　　　　　　　　5TH ED.　　　Cloth　　338 P.
SUDBURY: JONES & BARTLETT LEARNING, 2016

ED: UNIV. OF TOLEDO. TEXTBOOK--GRAD. W/ ONLINE
ACCESS.

　ISBN 1284048861　　　**Library PO#**　FIRM ORDERS

	List	99.95	USD
8395 NATIONAL UNIVERSITY LIBRAR	**Disc**	14.0%	
App. Date　9/23/15　SHHS　　8214-08	**Net**	85.96	USD

SUBJ: 1. NURSES--POL. ACTIVITY--U.S. 2. NURSING--
POL. ASPECTS--U.S.

CLASS RT86.5　　　　DEWEY# 362.1730973　LEVEL ADV-AC

Nurses' tendency to align themselves within specialty practice groups and lobby or get involved only when an issue directly relevant to that particular group is being considered is encouraged without consideration of a broader perspective. Political astuteness would dictate that nurses recognize when they are being kept off balance by subversive divisive messages encouraged by those who benefit from nursing's disunity and ignore the discordant rhetoric. Further, all nurses should have a basic understanding or awareness of the legislative initiatives of specialty groups. They should actively support the initiatives of their colleagues or, at a minimum, refrain from opposing the cause publicly. Concerns should be shared privately and diligent efforts made to find a compromise position outside of the public eye.

Conclusion

Nurses with an understanding of how the policymaking process works can contribute to the political work of the organizations to which they belong and ultimately to the patients for whom they care. Such contributions are consistent with the obligations set forth in the profession's social policy statement and its code of ethics. *Nursing's Social Policy Statement* notes the connection between policymaking and the delivery of health care and the effect on the well-being of society. "Individual and inter-professional involvement is essential" (American Nurses Association [ANA], 2010b, p. 7). An essential feature of professional nursing is to "influence social and public policy to promote social justice" (p. 9). The *Code of Ethics for Nurses* (ANA, 2010a) repeatedly emphasizes the role nurses play in promoting, advocating, and striving to protect the health, safety, and rights of the patient, which extends to statehouses, boardrooms, and other arenas in which this advocacy can affect public policy. Finally, the *Future of Nursing* report issued by the Institute of Medicine in 2010 states that "nurses should be full partners with physicians and other healthcare professionals, in redesigning health care in the United States" (p. S-3). This role will be played out, in part, in the health policy context where nurses should participate in, and sometimes lead, decision making and be engaged in healthcare reform–related implementation efforts. To be ready to assume this responsibility, nurse education programs should include course content addressing leadership-related competencies for all nurses. These competencies include a firm grounding in politics and policymaking processes.

There is no substitute for visibility in the legislative arena. Showing up is what political activism is all about. "If you are not at the table, you are on the menu" is a sentiment frequently echoed in many policymaking venues. For too long nurses have been on the menu rather than active participants in shaping public policy around health care. Standing by watching the game and complaining about policy decisions will not change outcomes. Nurses must become convinced that they do have something valuable to contribute, that they have the ability and the time to do it, and that advocacy in the policy arena is not an option but a nonnegotiable professional responsibility.

Running for Elective Office: One Nurse's Experience

In 2008, after over 25 years of working in the state legislative arena as a lobbyist for nursing's interests, I became a candidate for the state House of Representatives. I had worked as a nurse in the clinical arena for many years and, after earning my Juris Doctor (JD), had practiced law as a healthcare attorney. I frequently spoke with nurses and nursing students about the importance of getting involved in the political process and often was asked why I didn't run myself. I had always managed to dismiss that possibility as far-fetched. Then healthcare reform became a major issue, along with education reform and the economy, and I soon became convinced that my background would appeal to voters who wanted change. Before proceeding, I had to make certain my family was on board, my employer would be supportive, and that I could put together a solid campaign team. If all those elements fell into place, I determined I would enter the race.

By the late fall of 2007, I had negotiated a satisfactory arrangement with my employer and was assured by my family that they were supportive as well. In addition, I found campaign managers who were excited to take on the Lanier campaign to put a nurse in the statehouse! Although the incumbent was not eligible for re-election due to term limits, the race was not going to be easy. I was running as a Democrat in a very Republican district, and I faced a challenge in the primary election, which meant the campaign needed to get busy fast for the early March vote.

A March election meant campaigning during the cruel winter months in Ohio. Climbing over snowdrifts to get signatures on candidate petitions, hammering campaign signs into frozen ground, and going door-to-door to meet voters in temperatures that would put Alaska to shame became routine. Was it fun? Not necessarily. But it was part of the job I signed on for when I said I wanted to be the candidate, so I did it almost without giving it a second thought.

In addition to the physical side, I also had to raise money to buy the signs, establish a credible Web presence, and print the campaign literature being distributed on my behalf. That meant making phone calls and sending what I called my "begging letter" to everyone I could think of who might support the effort financially. There was no how-to book that really addressed all the aspects of campaigning, so I was learning on the job each day, every day.

Nurses were my best supporters, and no one worked harder on our weekend "Nurses Make House Calls" initiatives. On the rainy, frigid-cold Election Day, nurses stood outside polling places with "Lanier" signs as one last reminder of whom to look for on the ballot. That night, as the election results came trickling in, we soon learned that we had been successful, so there were a few moments of celebration with friends, family, and supporters. What a fun night! Winning made it all worthwhile. The next day, however, the campaign for the general election started its 8-month marathon.

This time, the snow had turned to warm/hot days with more time for meeting voters and raising those elusive funds. By the time the November election day arrived, I had knocked on over 10,000 doors personally, and the total neared 16,000 when the efforts of volunteers were included. We had participated in numerous local parades and attended candidates' nights, festivals, and fundraisers. Many special interest groups had issued valued endorsements of my candidacy, whereas others disappointingly endorsed my opponent. I had answered countless questionnaires about my position on every issue imaginable. We had designed a series of direct mail pieces and other materials to give voters a reason to vote for me. I survived some hurtful negative encounters with people who were convinced that my party affiliation meant I was un-American, and I learned to ignore cruel blog comments that were focused on the superficial, rather than genuine issues. I shared a stage with presidential candidate Barack Obama and was introduced by then-Senator Hillary Clinton at a local rally. I attended a VIP briefing with a U.S. senator and was treated to some remarkably frank discussions about how to address some of the serious problems affecting the state and the nation.

Throughout the process, I learned how many people were struggling with the challenges posed by job losses and foreclosures. I talked with people who could not get the health care they needed because they had lost or never had adequate health insurance coverage. I watched as volunteers set up a health clinic designed to serve economically disadvantaged people, many of whom were working in minimum wage jobs. I visited local farms, preschools, and a school for children with autism.

Despite all the efforts by so many, I did not win the seat in the House I worked so hard to attain. [Editor's note: Ms. Lanier won nearly 40% of the total vote, a remarkable feat as a Democrat in a highly Republican district. She is to be celebrated for this effort.] Winning is lots more fun than losing, so the November election night party was subdued at best. In the end, all agreed that we ran a good campaign and had no regrets or "what ifs" to carry around. Although the loss was incredibly disappointing, I have no second thoughts about taking the chance. I have a whole new understanding of and appreciation for the political process and politics in general. I met people I would never have met otherwise, and my life is richer for having done it. My family, particularly my grandchildren, got to experience a political campaign first hand. They know what it feels like to distribute candy during a parade and to participate in a "lit drop" through many neighborhoods.

So what is it like to be a candidate for an elective position that was not featured in the local media, one that was more people-focused than media driven?

1. I found it to be one of the loneliest experiences of my life. Although I was constantly around people, I was really always on my own. Knocking on doors and never knowing what might be on the other side was disconcerting, but my nursing experience

prepared me well to deal with whatever arose. I probably had more information about people's health status than the local health department!

2. It was a very humbling experience with a huge learning curve. I learned how much I didn't know about the many issues facing people each day. I came to appreciate the unrealistic expectations we have for our elected officials. We elect people to state and federal legislatures expecting them to find solutions to all of the varied problems that challenge our cities, states, businesses, schools, industries, environment, and economy, and then do not give them the tools or time they need to be successful.

3. I realized once I received my first campaign contribution that it was no longer about my own personal ambitions, but it was bigger than that. I now owed something to others; my best effort was put forth to ensure their trust in me was not misplaced. When I got tired or discouraged, I thought about the $5 contributions I received from retired nurses who wanted to help me in some way, and that kept me moving ahead. I also learned, sadly, how those big contributions really do have an impact. Because a campaign, even so-called "down ticket" races, are expensive and few people (especially a nonincumbent) can raise the dollars needed or expected to be a credible candidate, when someone or some group hands you a check with multiple zeroes in the amount, it has an impact. That is a fact, like it or not.

4. You cannot do it alone. A good team is essential—campaign manager, treasurer, volunteer coordinator, media/public relations/ Web specialist, and a constituency willing to work for you. Being a candidate is a full-time job. It was a year out of my life in which I had to be on my best behavior at all times because you never knew who might be watching. My family members were also affected and had to be careful of what they said and did.

5. Hard work alone will not result in a victory. Timing and location (district demographics—the political index) are critical factors as well. No candidate should run unopposed, however, so candidates should be encouraged to come forward. Voters should

always have a genuine choice on Election Day. Sadly, the rigors of campaigning, including the personal scrutiny, discourage rather than encourage broad participation.

6. People actually thanked me for running, which really surprised me.

Government is only as good as the people who hold elective office. Cynicism and a lack of participation will eventually doom our form of government. Partisanship needs to take a backseat to collaboration in order to solve the very serious problems facing all of us. Nurses can be candidates or part of a campaign team or simply volunteers, but regardless of what they do, they should do something!

Discussion Points

1. Watch the HBO movie *Iron Jawed Angels*. What political considerations were at play in efforts to win voting rights for women?
   - To what extent have women today become complacent with respect to the importance of voting?
   - Describe the similarity of the fight waged by suffragettes and the one nurses have waged to gain recognition of advanced practice.
   - Discuss with colleagues how complacency imperils future professional advances for nursing.
2. There are many metaphors for the future role of advanced practice registered nurses in the healthcare system. Select one of the following metaphors and describe the political considerations that come into play with respect to the selected metaphor (adapted from Facing the Future, 2006).
   - The future role of advanced practice registered nurses is like a great roller coaster on a moonless night. It exists, twisting ahead of us in the dark, but we can only see the track that is just ahead. We are locked in our seats, and nothing we may know or do will change the course that is laid out before us; in other words, the future role is outside of our control.
   - The future role of advanced practice registered nurses is a huge game of dice. It is entirely random and subject only to chance.

Because everything is chance, all we can do is play the game, pray to the gods of fortune, and enjoy what luck comes our way; in other words, the future is totally random and we do not know how or if actions make a difference.

- The future role of advanced practice registered nurses is like a great ship on the ocean. We can travel freely upon it and there are many possible routes and destinations. There will always be some outside forces, such as currents, storms, and reefs, to be dealt with, but we still have the choice to sail our ship where we want it to go; in other words, we can choose whatever future we want if we are willing to work with a purpose and within the knowledge and constraints of outside forces.

- The future of advanced practice registered nurses is a blank sheet of paper. It is there for us to fill in with our actions and decisions in the present. If we choose the future we want and spend time within our professional lives trying to make it happen, it will probably materialize. If we leave it to the powers that be to decide upon and plan the future, we will have a very different kind of future—one dominated by traditional powerful forces. In other words, we have control over our future if we choose to act upon it.

3. Respond to the following statement in the context of the Patient Protection and Affordable Care Act.

> The suppliers of legislative benefits are legislators, and their primary goal is to be re-elected. Thus, legislators need to maximize their chances for re-election, which requires political support. Legislators are assumed to be rational and to make cost–benefit calculations when faced with demands for legislation. However, the legislator's cost–benefit calculations are not the cost–benefits to society of enacting particular legislation. Instead, the benefits are the additional political support the legislator would receive from supporting legislation and the lost political support they would incur as a result of their action. When the benefit to legislators (positive political support) exceeds their costs (negative political support) they will support the legislation. (Feldstein, 2006, p. 10)

- Consider how the cost–benefit analysis depicted in the statement affected the Affordable Care Act (ACA) that ultimately was enacted.

- Discuss how the cost–benefit analysis depicted in the statement did or did not affect decisions made by states about whether to expand Medicaid eligibility as allowed by the ACA.
- Discuss how the cost–benefit analysis depicted in the statement did or did not affect decisions made by states about whether to run a state-sponsored insurance exchange/marketplace or rely on the federal program.

4. Complete a legislative worksheet that requires use of the state and federal government websites to identify one's own elected officials, party affiliation, committee appointments, and other relevant background information.

References

American Nurses Association. (2010a). *Code of ethics for nurses.* Washington, DC: Author.

American Nurses Association. (2010b). *Nursing's social policy statement.* Washington, DC: Author.

Auble, D. (2013, March 20). *Lobbyists 2012: Out of the game or under the radar.* Washington, DC: Center for Responsive Politics.

Brill, S. (2010). On sale: Your government. *Time, 176*(2), 28–33.

Center for Responsive Politics. (2013a). *Health sector: PAC contributions to federal candidates.* Retrieved from http://www.opensecrets.org/pacs/sector.php?txt=H01&cycle=2012

Center for Responsive Politics. (2013b). *Influence & lobbying.* Retrieved from http://www.opensecrets.org/influence

Center for Responsive Politics. (2013c). *Lobbying database.* Retrieved from http://www.opensecrets.org/lobby

Center for Responsive Politics. (2013d). *OpenSecrets.org reports.* Retrieved from http://www.opensecrets.org/news/reports

Citizens United v. Federal Elections Commission. (2010). 130 S. Ct. 876.

Crowley, M. (2010). The new GOP money stampede. *Time, 176*(13), 30–35.

deVries, C. M., & Vanderbilt, M. (1992). *The grassroots lobbying handbook.* Washington, DC: American Nurses Association.

Facing the Future. (2006). *Lesson 38: Metaphors for the future.* Retrieved from http://www.facingthefuture.org/Curriculum/DownloadFreeCurriculum/tabid/114/Default.aspx

Feldstein, P. (2006). *The politics of health legislation: An economic perspective* (3rd ed., pp. 27–84). Chicago, IL: Health Administration Press, 10, 27–84.

Haylock, P. (2012). *Professional nursing associations: Meeting the needs of nurses and the profession.* In D. Mason, J. Leavitt, & M. Chaffee (Eds.), *Policy and politics in nursing and health care* (6th ed., pp. 609–617). St. Louis, MO: Elsevier Saunders.

Institute of Medicine. (2010). *Future of nursing report.* Washington, DC: The National Academies Press.

Zakaria, F. (2013, August 4). Washington is failing everyone except lobbyists. *Columbus Dispatch,* E8.

CHAPTER 4

Government Regulation: Parallel and Powerful

Jacqueline M. Loversidge

KEY TERMS

Administrative procedures act (APA): A state or federal law that establishes rulemaking procedures for state or federal agencies, respectively.

Board of nursing: A state government administrative agency charged with the power and duty to enforce the laws and regulations governing the practice of nursing in the interest of public protection.

Certification: A form of voluntary credentialing that denotes validation of competency in a specialty area, with permission to use a title.

Federal Register: A daily federal government publication that contains current executive orders, presidential proclamations, rules and regulations, proposed rules, notices, and sunshine act meetings.

Interstate compact: A legal agreement between states to recognize the license of another state and to allow for practice between states. The compact must be passed by the state legislature and implemented by the board of nursing in each state.

Licensure: A form of credentialing whereby permission is granted by a legal authority to perform an act that would, without such permission, be illegal, a trespass, a tort, or otherwise not allowable.

Multistate regulation: A provision that allows a professional to practice in more than one state based on a single license.

Mutual recognition: A method of multistate regulation in which boards of nursing voluntarily agree to enter into an interstate compact allowing the state to recognize and honor the license issued by the other state.

National Council of State Boards of Nursing (NCSBN): A not-for-profit, nongovernmental organization that provides a means by which boards of nursing may dialogue and act on matters of common interest relative to board of nursing missions, including development of licensing examinations.

Prescriptive authority: Legal authority to prescribe drugs and therapeutic devices, usually within a practice-specific formulary.

Professional self-regulation: Voluntary adherence to a set of moral, ethical, and professional standards, agreed to by a profession.

Public hearings: Meetings held by state or federal administrative agencies for the purpose of receiving testimony from witnesses who support or oppose regulations, or to receive expert testimony.

Recognition (official recognition): A form of credentialing that denotes a government authority has ratified or confirmed an individual's credentials.

Registration: A form of credentialing that denotes enrolling or recording the name of a qualified individual on an official agency or government roster.

Regulation: The act of governing or directing according to a rule or bringing under the control of a constituted authority, such as the state or federal government.

Regulations (rules): Orders or directives that provide detail or procedures to operationalize a law. They are issued by government agencies and have the force and effect of law.

Introduction

Regulation of the U.S. healthcare delivery system and practicing healthcare providers is extraordinarily complex. The vastness of the industry, the manner of healthcare financing, and the proliferation of laws and regulations that govern practice and reimbursement in the interest of public welfare contribute to that complexity.

This chapter focuses on major concepts associated with the regulation of healthcare professionals, with emphasis on advanced practice registered nurses (APRNs). An understanding of **licensure** and credentialing processes, and their impact on advanced practice nursing, is fundamental. Understanding how the healthcare system and individual providers are regulated empowers the APRN to advocate on behalf of the profession and consumers. Note that all healthcare professionals in every state are licensed within a defined scope of practice. Practice-specific boards or commissions (e.g., the Ohio Board of Nursing) or multiprofessional boards (e.g., Michigan's Department of Licensing and Regulatory Affairs) are government agencies that regulate each profession with the goal of protecting the public. Although the processes are similar, each professional is legally bound by the regulations in his or her own state.

Regulation Versus Legislation

The legislative and regulatory processes are parallel; both are public processes and are equally powerful. Together, legislation and regulations shape the way public policy is implemented. It is important for the APRN to understand both processes and how they are influenced. Major differences between the two processes are described here.

The legislative process is the first step in the production of laws and rules. Lawmakers in Congress, or in the state legislatures, introduce bills and conduct them through the lawmaking process. If they are passed by both houses, bills are signed into law by the president or governor. Once signed into law, implementation generally occurs in administrative agencies that are part of the executive branch of government.

Legislation (laws) and **regulations (rules)** are constructed differently. Note the terms *legislation* and *law* are synonymous, as are the terms *regulation* and *rule*; these synonyms are used interchangeably. Law is written using broad language to provide for flexibility and adaptability in application over time. The administrative agencies are charged, by the laws that govern them, with the responsibility to amplify those laws by writing regulations that describe, in detail, how the administrative agency will put the law into practice.

EXAMPLE: One provision in the nurse practice act (NPA) provides that a duty of the **board of nursing** is to develop criteria applicants must meet to be eligible to sit for licensure examinations, and for issuing and renewing licenses. The regulations amplifying that provision of law specify the criteria for eligibility, application procedures, the approved examination, renewal procedures, and fees.

Several details are worthy of note. First, the administrative agency's authority to write rules is specified by the law. Regulation must always tie directly to a section of law; an administrative agency is not permitted to promulgate rules that exceed its statutory authority. Second, both law and regulation have the same force and effect of law. From here forward the term *law* will be used instead of legislation, but *regulation* and *rule* will be used interchangeably. There are uses for which the word *rule* is preferable (e.g., rule-making authority).

The first step in establishing a new law or revising an existing law is the introduction of a bill by a legislator or group of legislators (sponsors) during a legislative session. The sponsor(s) may introduce legislation to address an issue or concern presented by constituents, or an administrative agency may seek a legislative sponsor to modify its practice act for a variety of reasons. If an administrative agency finds its regulations are inadequate to serve the needs of the public, it may seek statutory modification to add a section that allows additional rule-making authority in the law. Any bill introduced during a legislative session must pass in the session in which it is introduced, or else it "dies" and must be reintroduced in a subsequent session.

The regulatory process differs from the legislative process in a number of ways. Regulations can be promulgated at any time during the year by an administrative agency because rulemaking is not dependent on legislative session schedules. Some states require periodic review of regulations by the agency responsible for administering those regulations, in an effort to assure that regulations remain current and reflect changes in the environment. Some states revise regulations on a predictable schedule. Regulation promulgation, like lawmaking, is also a public process and requires disclosure of draft language, a period of time for public comment, and often a public hearing. Draft regulations may be amended by the issuing agency based on public input prior to publication of the final regulation. The administrative agency working on the regulation has discretion in determining what amendments, if any, are made. However, public comment may be very influential in determining the final outcome.

State governmental structures also have systems in place to assure checks and balances during the rule-making process. For example a body separate from the state agency, such as a Legislative Services Commission (LSC) may be charged with reviewing all administrative regulations to assure that: (1) the administrative agency does not exceed its statutory authority, and (2) proposed regulations do not encroach on other laws or regulations. The time frame for implementation of new or revised regulations varies according to the **administrative procedures act (APA)** of the state, but effective dates are generally within 30 to 90 days of publication of the final regulation.

Health Professions Regulation and Licensing

Definitions and Purpose of Regulation

Regulation, as defined in *Black's Law Dictionary*, means "the act or process of controlling by regulation or restriction" (Garner, 2009, p. 1398). Health professions regulation provides for ongoing monitoring and maintenance of an acceptable standard of practice for the professions, with the goal of protecting the interests of public welfare and safety.

Regulation is needed as a mechanism to protect the public because of the complexity of the healthcare system. Diversity in educational credentialing, proliferation of types of providers, lack of public information about healthcare provider competency, and the bundling of healthcare services make it difficult for the public to understand and evaluate options. Nursing requires independent decision making based on specialized knowledge, skills, and abilities. Nurses provide care at all points of service in a complex and rapidly evolving healthcare system. Laypersons cannot ordinarily judge the competency of a health professional, or whether the care delivered to them meets acceptable and prevailing standards of care. For these reasons, because of the potential risk for harm, and also because of the intimate nature of nursing care, states protect the public by establishing laws to regulate the professions (Russell, 2012).

The laws that credential and govern a profession are called *practice acts*. Practice acts vary by state, but all include the same basic elements: (1) creation of a board that serves as the decision-making body; (2) the definitions, standards, and scopes of practice; (3) the extent and limits of the board's power and authority and its composition; (4) standards for educational programs; (5) types of titles, licensure, and certification; (6) title protection; (7) licensure requirements; and (8) grounds for disciplinary action, including due process (remedies) for the licensee charged with violation of the practice act or regulations (Russell, 2012). The basis for mandatory continuing education and/or competency requirements for licensure or relicensure also are found in practice acts. The extent of the board's rule-making authority is also specified in the practice act.

A board of nursing's rule-making authority is found in the section that describes its power and authority; it is the rules, or regulations, that amplify the practice act and specify detail. Rules specify details related to provisions such as initial licensing requirements, standards of practice and delegation, requirements for the registered nurse (RN) and licensed practical nurse or licensed vocational nurse (LPN/LVN) educational programs, advanced practice registered nurse (APRN) standards and requirements for practice and prescribing, disciplinary procedures, and standards for continuing education. Some states regulate both continuing education and competence. Because continuing competence is a difficult outcome to measure, most states require mandatory continuing education instead. Regulations also define the methods the governing authority will use to enforce an existing law.

Regulations cannot be instituted by an administrative agency without the expressed intent of law. It cannot be presumed that silence of the law on an issue implies legislative intent. When there is no prior statutory authority or legislative precedent to address an issue, the legislative process must be initiated to allow the agency authority to promulgate new, specific regulations.

> EXAMPLE: An APRN petitions the board of nursing to clarify whether **prescriptive authority** for Schedule II controlled substances is within the scope of practice for the APRN. The board's staff refers the APRN to a provision in the statute that allows the APRN to "prescribe drugs and therapeutic devices" as long as the APRN's practice is in collaboration with a physician as required by law and rules, and is practicing in a way consistent with the nurse's education and certification. The staff conclude that "prescribe drugs and therapeutic devices" may include Schedule II controlled substances if permitted in the approved written protocols of the nurse and physician collaborator. No specific language is found in the law that authorizes the prescribing of Schedule II controlled substances. When the medical board receives the board of nursing's opinion, an attorney general's opinion is requested. The attorney general concludes that the board of nursing may not extend the scope of practice of the APRN through either opinion or regulation. The expressed will of the legislature in regard to the scope of practice for the APRN must be sought using the legislative process.

Subsequently, a legislative sponsor is sought to introduce a bill permitting APRNs to specifically prescribe Schedule II controlled substances. Note that not all state boards of nursing are granted statutory authority to express formal opinions; some must rely on the express language in the practice act and regulations, the official opinions of attorney general's office, or court decisions.

History of Health Professions Regulation

Physicians were the first healthcare professionals to gain legislative **recognition** for their practice. Most states had physician licensing laws in place by the early 1900s. Nursing followed; North Carolina was the first state to establish a regulatory board for nurses in 1903, and by the 1930s state licensing had been enacted by 40 states (Hartigan, 2011). Physician scopes of practice are very broad, and may include any act (or attempt) to diagnose or treat any individual with a physical injury or deformity. Some medical practice acts establish no scope of practice limits whatsoever. Herein lies the problem faced by APRNs and other nonphysician healthcare providers—how to define a scope of practice that delineates their roles, particularly those that may overlap with medicine's. The history of nursing regulation is characterized by efforts to accommodate this medical preemption (Safriet, 1992).

The early regulation of nurses was permissive (voluntary). Systems developed allowing nurses to register with a governing board, hence the title "registered nurse." In some states, nurses were registered by the medical board prior to establishment of a separate board of nursing. Registration is a minimally restrictive form of state regulation, and does not usually require entrance qualification (e.g., examination). Between the 1930s and 1950s, states enacted mandatory licensure laws, or nurse practice acts (NPAs), requiring that anyone practicing nursing obtain licensure with the state regulatory agency. These early NPAs defined nursing as a dependent practice, primarily involving the implementation of physician orders. In 1955, the American Nurses Association model definition was published, which laid the groundwork for NPA revisions to define independent functions for nurses, although the model reaffirmed that medical diagnosis and prescribing were prohibited (Hartigan, 2011).

Boards of nursing (BONs) began to establish licensure criteria, including board-approved courses of nursing education, and board-constructed licensure examinations. Board examinations could include multiple-choice or essay questions, performance examinations, or a combination; during that time, each BON set its own examination passing standard. BONs gained statutory authority to regulate schools of nursing and established requirements for structure, faculty, and curricula. Because interstate mobility was becoming more common, states developed *reciprocity* agreements with other states; these reciprocity agreements no longer exist today. The **National Council of State Boards of Nursing (NCSBN)** Nurse Licensure Compact has made interstate mobility, new technologies, and telehealth more feasible, but not all states participate, and this complex process should not be confused with the obsolete two-state reciprocal arrangements (Hartigan, 2011; National Council of State Boards of Nursing [NCSBN], 2014b).

By the 1940s the need for a standardized licensure exam became apparent. The State Board Test Pool Examination (SBTPE) was established by the National League for Nursing (NLN) in 1944. The SBTPE assured examination standardization and relieved state BONs of the burdens associated with writing and administering the examination. Over the years, questions about potential for conflict of interest were raised. Although individual BONs set their own passing standards, authority for the creation and control of the examination had been absorbed by a professional association. Concurrently, BON leaders created a forum in which they could meet and discuss matters of common interest, but that forum was structured as a council of the American Nurses Association (ANA). This created conflict between BONs' prescribed governmental duty to establish licensure standards and professional associations' rights and responsibilities to remain independent of governmental influence. To address these issues, the NCSBN was formed in 1978 with the assistance of a Kellogg Foundation grant. The NCSBN governance and voting body consist of representation from BONs; it is autonomous, and represents the states' interests rather than those of organized nursing (Hartigan, 2011). The NCSBN is not a governmental agency but serves as a forum for discussion and advice to BONs.

History of Advanced Practice Registered Nurse Regulation

The 1960s set the stage for the expansion of nursing practice and regulation of APRNs. The birth of the federal entitlement programs, Medicare and Medicaid, increased the number of individuals with access to government-subsidized health care. With a shortage of primary care physicians predicted, the first formal nurse practitioner programs were opened (Safriet, 1992).

Idaho became the first state to legally recognize diagnosis and treatment as part of the scope of practice for the APRN in 1971. The regulation of APRNs was accomplished through joint agreements between the state boards of nursing and medicine, and was specific for each "permissible" act of diagnosis and treatment. The model of regulation established in Idaho set a precedent for subsequent state regulation of APRNs to include some form of joint nursing and medical board oversight. The joint regulation model was designed to compensate for the broad definition of the practice of medicine, and was based on the determination that advanced practice nursing was a "delegated medical practice," necessitating some degree of medical board oversight. The struggle to define APRN scope of practice and determine whether medical board oversight is necessary continues in many states.

Since 1971, every state has developed some form of legal recognition of the APRN. Both the ANA and the NCSBN have proposed model rules and regulations for the governing of advanced practice nursing. However, practice acts are a product of individual states' political forces, so titles, definitions, criteria for entrance into practice, scopes of practice, reimbursement policies, and models of regulation are unique to each state.

Since 1988, *The Nurse Practitioner* has published a summary of annual survey data from each state's board of nursing and nursing organizations relative to the legislative status of advanced practice nursing. Significant advances have been made by many states, particularly with regard to APRN practice independent of direct physician supervision. Currently, 18 states report that nurse practitioners (NPs) are regulated solely by a board of nursing and have both independent scope of practice and prescriptive authority; these 18 states report no requirement for physician collaboration, delegation, or supervision, with Nevada and Rhode Island appearing as the newest additions. In the remaining 32 states, APRNs are regulated either by the board of nursing alone with the addition of medical board oversight or jointly by the board of nursing and medical board. In jointly regulated states APRNs generally find their licensure "home" with the board of nursing. In either model, medical board oversight may include requirements for physician collaboration, consultation, and delegation or supervision circumscribing the nurse practitioner's authority to practice, prescribe, or both (Phillips, 2014). All states have allowed some form of prescriptive authority for more than 20 years (Pearson, 2002).

Methods of Professional Credentialing

Health professions regulation is facilitated through a variety of credentialing methods. The method is determined by the state government and is based on at least two variables: (1) the potential for harm to the public if safe and acceptable standards of practice are not met, and (2) the degree of autonomy and accountability for decision making that is considered standard practice for a particular profession. The least restrictive form of regulation to accomplish the goal of public protection should be selected (Gross, 1984; Pew Health Professions Commission, 1994). Four credentialing methods are used in the United States; each credentials and regulates the individual provider. Credentialing methods are described in the following sections, moving from the most restrictive to the least restrictive method.

LICENSURE

A license is "a permission ... revocable, to commit some act that would otherwise be unlawful" (Garner, 2009, p. 1002). The licentiate is "one who has obtained a license or authoritative permission to exercise some function, esp. to practice a profession" (Garner, 2009, p. 1005). Licensure is the most restrictive method of credentialing and requires anyone who practices within the defined scope of practice to obtain the legal authority to do so from the appropriate administrative state agency.

Licensure implies competency assessment at the point of entry into the profession. Applicants for licensure must pass an initial licensing examination, and then comply with continuing education requirements or undergo competency assessment by the legal authority charged with assuring that acceptable standards of practice are met. Because competency is unique to the individual professional it is difficult to measure; most licensing agencies require mandatory continuing education in lieu of continued competency assessment for license renewal. Licensees are also held to practice act provisions and relevant regulations. Licensure offers the public the greatest level of protection by restricting use of the title and the scope of practice to the licensed professional who has met these rigorous criteria. Unlicensed persons cannot call themselves by the title identified in the law, and they cannot lawfully perform any portion of the scope of practice.

The administrative agency holds the licensee accountable for practicing according to the legal, ethical, and professional standards of care defined in law and regulations. A licensee holds a greater public responsibility than a nonlicensed citizen. Disciplinary action, through an administrative disciplinary procedure, may be taken against licensees who have violated provisions of law or rule. State administrative practice acts (APAs) assure that licensees subject to disciplinary action are provided due process. However, the fact that a license is revocable means that the legal authority (BON) may divest the licensee of the license if it is deemed that the license holder has violated law or regulations, and that it is in the best interest of the public to rescind a license. Health professions are largely regulated by licensure because of the high risk of potential for harm to the public if unqualified or unsafe practitioners are permitted to practice.

REGISTRATION

Registration is the "act of recording or enrolling" (Garner, 2009, p. 1397). Registration provides for a review of credentials to determine compliance with the criteria for entry into the profession, and permits the individual to use the title "registered." Registration serves as title protection, but does not preclude individuals who are not registered from practicing within the scope of practice, so long as they do not use the title or hold themselves out to be a "registered" professional.

Registration does not necessarily imply that prior competency assessment has been conducted. Some state laws may have provisions for removing incompetent or unethical providers from the registry, or "marking" the registry when a complaint is lodged against a provider. However, removing the person from the registry may not necessarily protect the public, because the individual is permitted to practice without use of the title. A registration exemplar is the states' Nurse Aide Registry, which tracks individuals who have met criteria to be certified for employment in long-term care settings; this registry was required by the Omnibus Budget Reconciliation Act of 1987.

CERTIFICATION

A certificate is "a document certifying the bearer's status or authorization to act in a specified way" (Garner, 2009, p. 255). In nursing, **certification** is generally thought of as the voluntary process that requires completion of requisite education, competency assessment, and practice hours. This type of certification in nursing is granted by proprietary professional or specialty nursing organizations and attests that the individual has achieved a level of competence in nursing practice beyond entry-level licensure. Certification, like registration, is a means of title protection. Certification awarded by proprietary organizations does not have the force and effect of law.

However, the term *certification* may also be used by state government agencies as a regulated credential; states may offer a "certificate of authority" or an otherwise-titled certificate to practice within a prescribed scope of practice. In this case, certification is required by law for practice in the specific role. For example, an APRN may need to hold a certificate as a nurse practitioner (NP) from a proprietary organization to qualify for a certificate of authority from a state board of nursing to practice as an NP in that state. Most states have enacted regulations requiring nationally recognized specialty nursing certification for an APRN to be eligible to practice in the advanced role.

In addition, states may offer certification to otherwise unlicensed assistive personnel, such as dialysis technicians or medication technicians. Astute consumers may ask whether a provider is certified, as a means of assessing competency to practice. Employers also use certification as a means of determining eligibility for certain positions or as a requirement for internal promotion.

RECOGNITION

Recognition is "confirmation that an act done by another person was authorized ... the formal admission that a person, entity, or thing has a particular status" (Garner, 2009, p. 1385). Official recognition is used by several boards of nursing as a method of regulating APRNs, and implies the board has validated and accepted the APRN's credentials for the specialty area of practice. Criteria for recognition are defined in the practice act and may include requirements for certification.

PROFESSIONAL SELF-REGULATION

Self-regulation occurs within a profession when its members establish standards, values, ethical frameworks, and safe practice guidelines exceeding the minimum standards defined by law. This voluntary process plays a significant role in the regulation of the profession, equal to legal regulation in many ways. Professional standards of practice and codes of ethics exemplify **professional self-regulation**. National professional organizations set standards of practice for specialty practice. By means of the certification process, these organizations determine who may use the specialty titles within their purview. Continuing education requirements and documentation of practice competency or re-examination are usually required for periodic recertification. Standards are periodically reviewed and revised by committees of the membership to assure current practice is reflected.

Although professional organizations develop standards of practice, they have no legal authority to require compliance by certificate holders; only legal regulation provides a mechanism for translating standards of practice into enforceable regulatory language, for monitoring the actions of licensees, and for taking action against licensees if regulations are violated. Administrative agencies regulating professions generally recognize prevailing professional standards of practice when making decisions about what constitutes safe and competent care. Legal regulation and professional self-regulation are two sides of the same coin, working together to fulfill the profession's contract with society.

Regulation of Advanced Practice Registered Nurses

The evolution of APRN practice across the United States has been inconsistent because the U.S. Constitution gives states the right to establish laws governing professions and occupations. As a result, titles, scopes of practice, and regulatory standards are unique to each state. To bring some uniformity to the regulation of advanced nursing practice, the NCSBN, at the behest of its board of nursing membership, convened the Advanced Practice Task Force in 2000. The NCSBN joined with the American Association of Colleges of Nursing (AACN) to facilitate a consensus-building process to develop the Consensus Model for Regulation: Licensure, Accreditation, Certification, and Education (LACE). This report is the outcome of the work of the APRN Consensus Work Group and the NCSBN APRN Advisory Committee. It defines APRN practice, titling, and education requirements; describes an APRN regulatory model and new APRN roles/population foci; and offers strategies for implementation (APRN Joint Dialogue Group, 2008). At the time of its publication, 40 nursing organizations endorsed the Consensus Model; only one was a state board of nursing. Although state boards of nursing are interested, most maintain a position of neutrality that is standard practice for government agencies in such matters and work through their legislatures to effect change.

National specialty nursing organizations and their affiliate certifying organizations play an important role in the professional regulation of

APRNs. Specialty certifying organizations are nongovernmental bodies that develop practice standards and examinations to measure the competency of nurses in an area of clinical expertise. Most boards of nursing require the APRN to hold a graduate degree in nursing and national certification in the specialty area relevant to their educational preparation. Boards of nursing promulgate regulations allowing acceptance of national certification examinations for purposes of state advanced practice certification, if predetermined criteria are met. A document published by the NCSBN (2002) serves as a guide for state boards of nursing in determining those criteria. It is imperative that criteria for evaluating the eligibility of national certification examinations as a part of the APRN application to practice be established in regulation, because boards of nursing may not abdicate regulatory authority by passively accepting examinations from independent bodies without having conducted a thorough evaluation of the examination's regulatory sufficiency and legal defensibility (NCSBN, 1993). The basis for regulatory sufficiency and legal defensibility of any licensure or certification examination includes: (1) the ability to measure entry-level practice, based on a practice analysis that defines job-related knowledge, skills, and abilities; and (2) development using psychometrically sound test construction principles.

The NCSBN developed *The Requirements for Accrediting Agencies and Criteria for APRN Certification Programs* in 1995. This document has since been updated, and serves as a guide for state boards of nursing in their review of advanced practice certification examinations' suitability for meeting regulatory standards. It also serves as a means to advance greater standardization in establishing certification criteria at the state level (NCSBN, 2009).

The criteria can be located on the NCSBN website at http://www.ncsbn .org.

National organizations that prepare certification examinations for APRNs include the following:

- American Academy of Nurse Practitioners
- American Association of Nurse Anesthetists Council on Certification
- American College of Nurse-Midwives Certification Council
- American Nurses Credentialing Center
- National Certification Board of Pediatric Nurse Practitioners
- National Certification Corporation for the Obstetric, Gynecologic, and Neonatal Nursing Specialties

The State Regulatory Process

The 10th Amendment of the U.S. Constitution specifies that all powers not specifically vested in the federal government are reserved for the states. One of these powers is the duty to protect its citizens (police powers). The power to regulate the professions is one way states exercise responsibility to protect the health, safety, and welfare of its citizens. State laws, specifically practice acts, create administrative agencies that implement practice acts and assume responsibility for regulation of the professions. These agencies are given referent authority by their governments to promulgate regulations and enforce both the law and regulations for which they are responsible. Administrative agencies have been called the "fourth branch" of government because of their significant power to execute and enforce the law.

Boards of Nursing

Each state legislature designates a board or similar authority to administer the practice act for the profession. Nurse practice acts vary by state, but all NPAs include the major provisions, or elements, discussed earlier in this chapter. Provisions included in NPAs focus on a central mission—protection of the public safety and welfare.

There are 60 boards of nursing (BONs) in the United States, including in the 50 states, U.S. territories, and the District of Columbia; each of these is known as a *jurisdiction*. Each BON is a member of the NCSBN. Some states have separate boards for licensing RNs and licensed practical nurses/licensed vocational nurses (LPNs/LVNs). As members of the NCSBN, BONs represent the interest of public safety with regard to the construction and administration of the National Council Licensure Examinations (NCLEXs), are allowed the privilege of using the examinations, and meet to discuss and act on matters of common interest (NCSBN, 2008).

Some states do not have a single board for RNs and/or LPNs/LVNs. Multiprofessional boards are found in several states. These types of boards have jurisdiction over a variety of licensed professionals such as physicians, nurses, dentists, and the like.

COMPOSITION OF THE BOARD OF NURSING

Boards of nursing are generally composed of licensed nurses and consumer members. In most states the governor appoints members, although in at least one state, North Carolina, elections are held to fill board vacancies.

Nurses who are interested in serving as board members may be helped to gain appointment to those positions by securing endorsements from their professional associations and support from their district legislators.

Some state laws designate board member representation from specific practice areas, from advanced practice nursing, and in the case of joint boards, representation from LPN/LVNs in addition to RNs/APRNs. In other states, criteria for appointment only require licensure in the profession and state residency. Information on vacancies can be obtained directly from the BON or from the governor's office. Knowing the composition of the board and its vacancy status allows professional organizations to politically influence representation on the board. Information related to serving on boards and commissions is found later in this chapter.

Board Meetings

All state government agencies must comply with open meeting or "sunshine" laws that permit the public to observe and/or participate in board meetings. Board meetings may vary in degree of formality. Public participation is usually permitted, but an open dialogue between board members and the public is not generally invited. The opportunity to address the board may be scheduled on the meeting agenda (e.g., during an open forum time). Board policies may require advance notification from individuals who wish to address the board during a meeting, so their name, topic, and the organization they represent (if applicable) can be identified on the agenda. Boards generally go into closed executive session for reasons specified in the state's APA (e.g., to obtain legal advice, conduct contract negotiations, and discuss disciplinary or personnel matters). Boards must comply with APA regulations regarding subject matter that may be discussed in executive session and report out of executive session when public session resumes. All voting is a matter of public record, and board action occurs only in open public session.

Most state APAs require the board to post public notice of meetings and make the agenda available, usually 30 days prior to the meeting. Sometimes the notice of meeting is published in major state newspapers or it may be posted on the board's website. Agendas are often updated immediately prior to the meeting date.

Board meeting participants include board members, board staff, and legal counsel for the board. Legal counsel advises the board on matters of law and jurisdiction. Some boards may have "staff" counsel, but many state boards receive advice only from an assigned representative of the state attorney general's office, known as an assistant attorney general (AAG). Staff and invited guests may present reports during the meeting, and individuals or organization representatives may provide testimony to the board on matters of interest.

Board members must take several factors into consideration when they vote. These include implications for the public welfare and safety, the legal defensibility of the outcome of the vote, and the potential statewide impact of the decision. First and foremost, the board must act only within its legal jurisdiction. Because all board actions are a matter of public record, BONs must make major actions taken during meetings available to the public. BONs may publish newsletters, which include action summaries, and may also include articles written by board members and staff that explain sections of law and rule. BON newsletters typically include disciplinary action taken against licensees, including nurses' names, license numbers, offense, and the specific disciplinary action (e.g., permanent revocation, suspension, practice restrictions, etc.). Some states mail newsletters to all licensees, or they may be available only on request. Many BONs make newsletters available to the public on their website.

Monitoring the Competency of Nurses: Discipline and Mandatory Reporting

The licensed nurse is accountable for knowing the laws and regulations governing nursing in the state of licensure and for adhering to legal, ethical, and professional standards of care. Some state regulations include standards of practice; other states may refer to professional or ethical standards established by professional associations. Employing agencies also define standards of practice through policies and procedures, but these are separate from, in addition to, and superseded by the state's NPA and regulations. When a nurse violates provisions of the NPA or regulations, the BON has authority to conduct an investigation and take possible action on the license. In the case of an APRN, the BON's authority includes the license or certificate to practice as an APRN and prescriptive authority.

Because the BON's most critical role is to assure the public safety, most NPAs include provisions for mandatory reporting that require employers to report violations of the NPA or regulations to the BON. Licensed nurses also have a moral and ethical duty to report unsafe and incompetent practice to the BON. The NPA defines acts of misconduct and provides a system for investigating complaints against licensees that assures due process for the license holder. Procedures for filing complaints, conducting investigations, and issuing sanctions for violations are enumerated in regulations. A nurse who holds a multistate license (i.e., a license that permits a nurse to practice in more than one state in accordance with a multistate compact agreement) is held accountable for knowing and abiding by the laws of the state of original licensure as well as the compact state in which the nurse practices. Multistate regulation is discussed in more detail later in this chapter. Nurses with multistate licenses should be aware that ignorance of the law in any state of licensure and/or practice does not excuse misconduct.

Most state NPAs and regulations are now available online, either directly from the BON website or linked from the board's website to a state law register website. The NCSBN also provides links to state boards of nursing (see http://www.ncsbn.org).

Instituting State Regulations

A state agency has the authority and duty to promulgate regulations amplifying its law, so long as rule-making authority has been granted in that law. Because law is created through an act of the legislature and is general in nature, rule-making authority allows state agencies to add the process details required for implementation of the law. The APA of each state specifies the process for promulgating and ratifying regulations, including requirements for public notification of proposed regulations and for providing an opportunity for public comment. State processes differ; some states designate government commissions or committees as the authorities for review and approval of regulations, whereas other states submit regulations to the general assembly or to committees of the legislature. Certain elements are common to the promulgation of regulations. These include: (1) public notice that a new regulation or modification of an existing regulation has been proposed, (2) opportunity to submit written comment or testimony, (3) opportunity to present oral testimony at a rules hearing, and (4) publication of the final regulation in a state register or bulletin. It is important that the APRN becomes familiar with all phases of rule promulgation, particularly the process for providing comment.

In some states, a fiscal impact statement is required. This statement provides an estimate of the costs that will be incurred as a result of the rule, both to the agency and to the public. In states where the rule promulgation process is overseen by a commission of legislators, the commission's role is to ensure that the regulatory agency filing the rule: (1) has the statutory authority to do so, (2) does not exceed the scope of its rule-making authority, and (3) does not draft rules that would conflict with its own law or that of any related discipline. For example, in the case of nursing, legislative commissions would cross-check other health professions' laws and regulations.

Monitoring State Regulations

Administrative agencies promulgate hundreds of regulations each year. Regulations that affect advanced nursing practice may be implemented by a variety of agencies. Knowing which agencies regulate health care, healthcare delivery systems, and professional practice, and monitoring legislation and regulations proposed by those agencies is important for safeguarding APRN practice.

Chief among the agencies APRNs should consider tracking are the health professions licensing boards, including medicine, pharmacy, and counselors and therapists. In addition, state regulations determining reimbursement for government programs should be monitored (e.g., Medicare and Medicaid). In this rapidly changing healthcare environment, conflicts related to scopes of practice, definitions of practice, right to reimbursement, and requirements for supervision and collaboration may occur.

Exhibit 4-1 provides some key questions to consider when analyzing a regulation for its impact on nursing practice.

It is critical for APRNs to be aware of regulations that mandate benefits or reimbursement policies and to lobby for inclusion of APRNs. Several states have instituted open-panel legislation, known as "any willing provider" and "freedom of choice" laws. These bills mandate that any provider who is authorized to provide the services covered in an insurance plan must be recognized and reimbursed by the plan. Insurance company and business lobbyists oppose this type of legislation. As managed care contracts are negotiated, APRNs must ensure that APRN services are given fair and equitable consideration. Other important areas include workers' compensation participation and reimbursement provisions, and liability insurance laws.

In summary, health professions licensing boards and state agencies that govern licensing and certification of healthcare facilities, administer public health services (e.g., public health, mental health, and alcohol and drug

Exhibit 4-1   Questions to Ask When Analyzing Regulations

1. Which agency promulgated the regulation?
2. What is the source of the agency's authority (the law that provides authority for the regulation to be promulgated)?
3. What is the intent or rationale of the regulation? Is it clearly stated by the promulgating agency?
4. Is the language in the regulation clear or ambiguous? Can the regulation be interpreted in different ways by different individuals? Discuss advantages of language that is clear versus ambiguous.
5. Are there definitions to clarify terms?
6. Are there important points that are not addressed? That is, are there omissions?
7. How does the regulation affect the practice of nursing? Does it constrain or limit the practice of nursing in any way?
8. Is there sufficient lead time to comply with the regulation?
9. What is the fiscal impact of the regulation?

CASE STUDY 1: BOARD OF PHARMACY REGULATION

Assume the board of pharmacy has drafted the following definition of the practice of pharmacy: The practice of pharmacy includes, but is not limited to, the interpretation, evaluation, and implementation of medical orders; the dispensing of prescription drug orders; initiating or modifying drug therapy in accordance with written guidelines or protocols previously established and approved by a practitioner authorized to independently prescribe drugs; and the provision of patient counseling as a primary healthcare provider of pharmacy care.

Discussion Points

1. Use the questions in Exhibit 4-1 to analyze the proposed regulation. Based on your analysis, do you consider this a "good" or "bad" regulation? What could you do to improve the regulation?

2. This definition requires that anyone responsible for "... initiating or modifying drug therapy in accordance with written guidelines or protocols ..." must be licensed as a pharmacist by the board of pharmacy. If this definition were to be included in the pharmacy practice act, how would this affect the practice of nursing, especially APRN practice?

3. The definition in this case study is an example of a scope of practice definition that could have significant overlap with the advanced practice of nursing and result in practice restrictions for APRNs. It may be that the authors of the definition had not considered the infringement on APRN practice. Develop talking points to initiate a conversation between the representatives of the nurse organization, pharmacy representatives, and the regulation's authors to negotiate a solution; the addition of an exemption for APRNs in the pharmacy practice act would suffice.

agencies), or govern reimbursement are agencies that may potentially promulgate regulations that could have implications for APRN practice.

Serving on Boards and Commissions

One way to actively participate in the regulatory process is to seek an appointment to the state BON or other health-related board or commission. Participation in the political process, especially during times of rapid change and reform, will ensure that APRNs have a voice in setting the public policy agenda.

Appointments to boards and commissions should be sought strategically. It is important to select an agency with a mission and purpose consistent with your interest and expertise. Because most board appointments are gubernatorial or political appointments, it is important for the APRN to obtain endorsements from legislators, influential community leaders, and his or her professional associations. Individuals seeking appointment are more likely to acquire endorsements if they have an established history of service to the professional community.

Letters of support should document the APRN's primary area of practice and contributions to professional and community service. Delineate involvement in local, state, and national organizations. A letter from the employer is recommended, as both an indication of the employer's willingness to support time away from work to fulfill the responsibilities of the position during the term of office and as an endorsement of professional merit; the letter should speak to both. A personal letter from the APRN seeking appointment should include the rationale for volunteering to serve on the particular board or commission, evidence of a good match between one's expertise and the role of that board or commission, and expression of a clear interest in serving the public. A résumé or curriculum vitae should be attached. Letters should emphasize desire to serve over self-interest; ideally, appointment decisions are based on a determination of the individual's potential contributions to the work of the board or commission. This kind of public service requires a substantial time commitment, so it is wise to speak to other members of the board or call the executive director/agency administrator to determine the extent of that commitment.

The Federal Regulatory Process

The federal government has become a central factor in health professions regulation. A number of forces have influenced this trend; however, one of the most significant was the advent of the Medicare and Medicaid programs. Federal initiatives that have grown from these programs include cost containment initiatives (prospective payment), consumer protection (combating fraud and abuse) (Jost, 1997; Roberts & Clyde, 1993), and the initiatives and programs written into the Affordable Care Act and Health Care and Education Reconciliation Act of 2010 (U.S. Department of Health and Human Services [DHHS], 2014).

A significant change occurred in July 2001 when the Centers for Medicare & Medicaid Services (CMS) was created to replace the former Health Care Financing Administration (HCFA). The reformed agency provides an increased emphasis on responsiveness to beneficiaries, providers, and quality improvement. Three business centers were established as part of the reform: Center for Beneficiary Choices, Center for Medicare Management, and Center for Medicaid and State Operations (Centers for Medicare & Medicaid Services, 2014). In 2003, President George W. Bush signed the Medicare Prescription Drug, Improvement, and Modernization Act (MMA) into law. The act created a prescription drug benefit for Medicare beneficiaries and established the Medicare Advantage program (O'Sullivan, Chaikind, Tilson, Boulanger, & Morgan, 2004), effectively providing seniors with prescription drug benefits and more choice in accessing health care.

The practice of APRNs has been influenced by the changes in Medicare reimbursement policy as it has continued to evolve. In 1998, Medicare reimbursement reform was enacted, allowing APRNs to be directly reimbursed for provision of Medicare Part B services that, until that time, had been provided only by physicians. In addition, the reform lifted the geographic location restrictions that had limited patient access to APRNs. More recent revisions to the required qualifications, coverage criteria, billing, and payment for Medicare services provided by APRNs are specific, depending on whether the APRN is a certified registered nurse anesthetist (CRNA), nurse practitioner (NP), certified nurse-midwife (CNM), or clinical nurse specialist (CNS). Reimbursement for APRNs has generally improved; for example, nurse practitioner services are now paid at 85% of the amount a physician is paid (DHHS, CMS, 2011). Because of their education, experience, and practice, APRNs in many states are working toward reimbursement at 100% of the amount paid to physicians.

Relationships between the state and federal regulatory systems are continuously evolving. Responsibilities once assumed by the federal government have been shifted down to the state level, including administration and management of the Medicaid and welfare programs. The perspective that states are better equipped to make decisions about how best to assist their citizens, coupled with a public sentiment that generally seeks to diminish federal bureaucracy and its accompanying tax burden, have been instrumental in shifting the placement of authority to the states. However, although states have primary authority over regulation of the health professions, federal policies continue to have a significant effect on healthcare workforce regulation. Policies related to reimbursement and quality control over the Medicare and Medicaid programs are promulgated by the U.S. Department of Health and Human Services (DHHS) and administered through its financing agency,

CMS. APRNs should familiarize themselves with other federal laws that have a regulatory impact on healthcare providers:

- Clinical Laboratory Improvement Amendments of 1988 (CLIA 88)
- Occupational Safety and Health Act of 1970 (OSHA)
- Mammography Quality Standards Act of 1987 and 1992 (MQSA 87 and 92)
- Omnibus Budget Reconciliation Act of 1987 and 1990 (OBRA 87 and 90)
- Americans with Disabilities Act of 1990 (ADA)
- North American Free Trade Agreement of 1993 (NAFTA, effective date January 1, 1994)
- Telecommunications Act of 1996
- Health Insurance Portability and Accountability Act of 1996 (HIPAA)
- Patient Protection and Affordable Care Act (ACA, effective date March 23, 2010)

The Veterans Health Administration, the Indian Health Service, and the uniformed armed services are regulated by the federal government. Large numbers of health professionals, many of whom are nurses/APRNs, are employed by these federal agencies and departments. Health professionals who are federally employed must be licensed in at least one state/jurisdiction. These individuals are subject to the laws of the state in which they are licensed, as well as the policies established by the federal system in which they are employed. However, the state of licensure need not correspond with the state in which the federal agency or department resides, because practice that occurs on federal property is not subject to state oversight.

The Supremacy Clause of the U.S. Constitution, Article VI, Paragraph 2, establishes that federal laws generally take precedence over state laws (Legal Information Institute, n.d.). State laws in conflict with federal laws cannot be enforced. At times, the courts may be asked to determine the constitutionality of a law or regulation to resolve jurisdictional disputes.

The Commerce Clause of the U.S. Constitution limits the ability of states to erect barriers to interstate trade (Gobis, 1997). Courts have determined that the provision of health care constitutes interstate trade under antitrust laws, and this sets the stage for the federal government to preempt state licensing laws regarding the practice of professions across state boundaries if future circumstances make this a desirable outcome for the nation.

The impact of technology on the delivery of health care, for example telehealth, allows providers to care for patients in remote environments and across the geopolitical boundaries defined by traditional state-by-state licensure. This raises the question as to whether the federal government would have an interest in interceding in the standardization of state licensing requirements to facilitate interstate commerce. If this occurred, the federal government would be in the position of usurping what is presently the state's authority. Licensing boards have an interest in avoiding federal intervention, and are beginning to identify ways to facilitate the practice of telehealth, while simultaneously preserving the power and right of the state to protect its citizens by regulating health professions at the state level. One approach to nursing regulation that addresses this conundrum is **multistate regulation**, which is discussed later in this chapter.

The most recent federal initiative is the Patient Protection and Affordable Care Act (ACA). The enactment of this law in 2010 represented progress toward comprehensive and far-reaching national healthcare system reform. The ACA represents the broadest revamping of health care since the Medicare and Medicaid programs were created in 1965. The provisions of this law, which is being implemented over a 5-year period (through 2015), include requirements for consumer protection, improvement of healthcare quality, lowering of healthcare costs, increased access to affordable care, and greater insurance company accountability (Commonwealth Fund, 2014; HealthCare.gov, 2010). Note that changes in the ACA have been evolving since its inception. That is the nature of the process of legislation and regulation; few laws are written perfectly, and many are altered during implementation.

The ACA also includes a number of provisions related to nursing, many of which are applicable or specific to the APRN. Among these are increased funding for a primary care workforce, grants for funding nurse-managed health centers through DHHS, and clarification of the funding of advanced practice nursing education to include accredited nurse-midwifery education. In addition, the Nurse Corps Loan Repayment Program, the Nurse Scholarship Program, and Faculty Loan Repayment Program have been expanded. Even more specifically applicable to APRNs are provisions related to the inclusion of nurse practitioners and clinical nurse specialists as accountable care organization (ACO) professionals. ACOs are legally formed structures composed of a group of providers and suppliers who are responsible for managing and coordinating care for Medicare fee-for-service beneficiaries. The law also authorizes DHHS to establish a grant program for states or designated entities to establish community-based interprofessional teams to support primary care practices, increases Medicare payments for primary care practitioners, and increases reimbursement rates for certified nurse-midwives. There are numerous other provisions in this law; a complete list of key provisions related to nursing may be found on the American Nurses Association website (http://www.nursingworld.org).

Promulgating Federal Regulations

The federal regulatory process is established by the federal Administrative Procedures Act. A notice of proposed rulemaking (NPRM) is published in the proposed regulation section of the *Federal Register*, which includes information for the public about the substance of the intended regulation. The notice also provides information about public participation in the regulatory process, including procedures for attending meetings or hearings, or providing comment. Once public comment has been received it is given careful consideration by the agency, and amendments to the draft regulations are made, if warranted. The agency issues final regulations by means of publication in the rules and regulations section of the *Federal Register*. The rules become effective 30 days after publication (see **Figure 4-1**).

Emergency Regulations

Provisions for promulgating emergency regulations are defined at both the state and federal levels. Emergency regulations are enacted if an agency determines that the public welfare is in jeopardy and the regulation will serve as an immediately enforceable remedy. Emergency regulations often take effect upon date of publication, are generally temporary, and are effective for a limited time period (usually 90 days), with an option to renew. Emergency regulations must be followed with permanent regulations that are promulgated in accordance with APA procedures.

Locating Information

The *Federal Register* is the federal government's bulletin board, or newspaper. It is published on the U.S. Government Printing Office website and updated daily, Monday through Friday, except for federal holidays. It contains executive orders and presidential proclamations, rules and

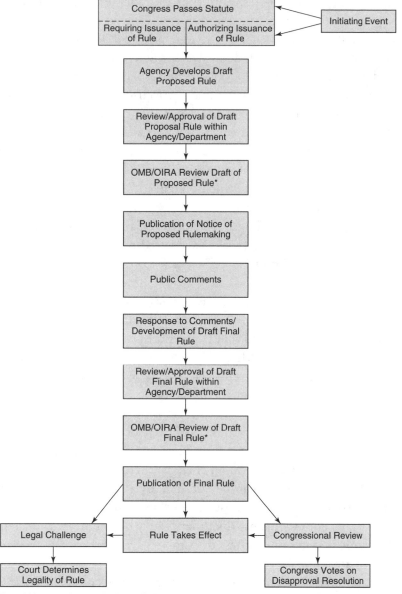

* The Office of Management and Budget's (OMB)/Office of Information and Regulatory Affairs (OIRA) reviews only significant rules, and does not review any rules submitted by independent regulatory agencies

■ Figure 4-1 The federal rulemaking process.

Source: Reproduced from Carey, M. P. (2013, June 17). *The federal rulemaking process: An overview*. Congressional Research Service Report RL32240. Retrieved from http://www.fas.org/sgp/crs/misc /RL32240.pdf

regulations, proposed rules, notices from federal agencies and organizations, sunshine act meetings, and corrections to previous copies of the *Federal Register*. Daily issues of the *Federal Register* also include a table of contents alphabetized by federal department. Daily issues may be downloaded in their entirety, or documents particular to a federal department of interest may be searched. Department-specific information begins with a heading including the name of the department, relevant information (e.g., the Code of Federal Regulations title), and a content synopsis. Deadlines for comments or effective dates are provided, as is contact information and other supplementary information. The *Federal Register* may be accessed online via the Government Printing Office (GPO) website at http://www.gpoaccess.gov/fr/index.html.

The Code of Federal Regulations (CFR) is the official compilation of all final regulations issued by the executive branch agencies of the federal government. The CFR consists of 50 titles representing broad subject areas. The CFR is updated annually on a staggered basis, and is available for download from the CFR website. The Electronic Code of Federal Regulations (e-CFR) is an unofficial, editorial compilation of the CFR material and *Federal Register* amendments that is produced by the National Archives and Records Administration Office of the *Federal Register* (OFR) and the GPO. The OFR updates the e-CFR daily. Titles may be browsed using a drop-down list. The Code of Federal Regulations is found online at the GPO website at http://www.gpoaccess.gov; the e-CFR is found at http://www.ecfr.gov.

Each state government publishes similar documents that identify proposed regulations, notices, final regulations, and emergency regulations. The publication is usually called the State Register or the State Bulletin, and the publication cycle can be obtained by accessing the state legislative printing office/website or the state legislative information system office/website. Hard copies of these documents may be available at local libraries; however, most states make these documents available on the state's government website.

State and federal agencies promulgate numerous regulations. It is in the APRN's best interest to belong to at least one professional nurse organization because most large organizations employ professional lobbyists who track legislation and report to their membership. Specialty organization newsletters and journals, legislative subscription and monitoring services, and bulletins summarizing proposed regulations are also resources that are helpful for monitoring legislation and regulations. Subscription services that track legislation and proposed agency regulation revisions provide summaries of the bill or regulation's substance and progress reports showing the status of the measure in its journey through the legislative or regulatory process. Both free and subscription legislative information services are available online.

In addition, numerous private services are available and can be found by searching the Internet. Several nursing and healthcare associations also feature relevant updates and information on current legislative and public policy issues (see **Exhibit 4-2**).

Providing Public Comment

There is a small window of opportunity for public input into the development of regulations. Most comment periods last 30 days from the date of publication of the proposed regulation, although sometimes an NPRM will provide for a longer comment period if the agency anticipates the issue has strong public interest or involves controversy. It is important that APRNs remain vigilant with regards to tracking comment period deadlines.

Public hearings are held by the agency proposing the regulation. Public agencies must comply with APA regulations regarding public hearings. Federal agencies are generally required to hold hearings when a numeric threshold is reached (i.e., a certain number of individuals or agency/organization representatives make requests to offer testimony). Written comments received by the agency are made a part of the permanent record and must be considered by the agency's board or commission members prior to publication of the final regulation. A final regulation can be challenged in the courts if the judge determines the agency did not comply with the APA or ignored public comments.

The *Federal Register* provides agency contact information on its website, making it reasonably easy for the public to provide comment on proposed regulations. Only written comments are included in the public record, although it is permissible to call the agency and provide comments orally if time is of the essence. Instructions for submitting electronic comments or written submissions by mail, hand delivery, or courier are generally included on the filing agency's *Federal Register* webpage. It is imperative to meet the deadline posted in the *Federal Register*; comments received after the comment period is closed can be legitimately disregarded by the agency.

Exhibit 4-2   Selected Websites of Interest

http://www.statenet.com Legislative and regulatory reporting services from all 50 states and Congress. A subscription service that provides comprehensive and timely information on legislation.

http://thomas.loc.gov Thomas Legislative Information System, sponsored by the U.S. Library of Congress. Summarizes bills and provides the full text of bills and the *Congressional Record*, information on the legislative process, and U.S. government Internet resources.

http://www.ahrq.gov Agency for Healthcare Research and Quality. Provides information on healthcare research, evidence reports, clinical practice guidelines, and consumer health information; part of the U.S. Department of Health and Human Services.

http://www.ctel.org Center for Telehealth and e-Health Law. Information on the latest findings in the regulation of telehealth and e-health, and state-by-state updates on telehealth legislation.

http://www.nursingworld.org American Nurses Association. Access to all ANA services and the *Online Journal of Issues in Nursing*, which is jointly prepared with Kent State University.

http://www.ncsbn.org National Council of State Boards of Nursing (NCSBN). Information on all NCSBN services and committee activities, access to state nurse practice acts, and information on the progress of multistate regulation.

http://www.hhs.gov U.S. Department of Health & Human Services. Access to all agencies within the department, including the Centers for Disease Control and Prevention (CDC), CMS, Health Resources and Services Administration (HRSA), and National Institutes of Health (NIH). Includes consumer and policy information.

http://www.hschange.com Center for Studying Health Systems Change. A Washington, D.C.–based research organization dedicated to studying the nation's healthcare systems and the impact on the public.

http://www.nurse.org State-by-state display of advanced practice nursing organizations, links to related sites that contain legislative and regulatory information, and NP Central (a comprehensive site for APRN continuing education offerings, salary information, and job opportunities).

http://www.nursingethicsnetwork.org Nursing Ethics Network. A nonprofit organization committed to the advancement of nursing ethics. Site contains ethics research findings and online inquiry.

http://www.aanp.org American Association of Nurse Practitioners. Comprehensive site for this NP membership organization featuring information on the latest trends and issues affecting APRN practice and regulation, advocacy, continuing education, and professional development.

http://www.cms.gov Centers for Medicare & Medicaid Services. Provides the latest legislative and regulatory information on reimbursement and HIPAA implementation.

http://www.hhs.gov/ocr/hipaa Office for Civil Rights. Fact sheets, sample forms, and frequently asked questions (FAQs) on HIPAA implementation, along with related links and educational materials.

http://www.iom.edu Institute of Medicine. Provides objective, evidence-based information helpful for advancing science and health policy. A leading and respected authority on health issues. Access to published reports.

When providing comment in writing, or written/oral testimony at a hearing, it is important for the APRN to:

- Be transparent about identity, background, and representation status; that is, the APRN should be clear about whether comments/testimony are representative of an organization's position or are representative of the individual APRN's position.
- Be specific regarding whether the position you are representing is in support of or opposition to the regulation. Give examples using brief scenarios or experiences when possible.
- Have credible evidence to back the position. Explain major points using common language; avoid nursing/medical jargon.
- Know the opposition's position and respond to these concerns.

- Convey a willingness to negotiate or compromise toward mutually acceptable resolutions.
- Demonstrate concern for the public good, rather than self-interest.
- Be brief and succinct. Limit remarks to one or two pages, or 5 minutes for oral testimony.

Regulatory agencies charged with public protection are more likely to address concerns that are focused on how the public may be harmed or benefited rather than concerns that give the impression of turf protection and professional jealousy. Demonstrate support for your position by asking colleagues who represent a variety of organizations, professions, and interests to submit comments; interprofessional solidarity projects a powerful message. In addition, if a significant number and variety of professionals and organizations form a coalition around a single issue, this demonstrates the degree of concern and a high level of commitment toward finding a solution. In this way, the volume and breadth of interest expressed in a proposed regulation can serve as the deciding factor in assisting an agency to assess support or nonsupport for the proposed regulation.

Strengths and Weaknesses of the Regulatory Process

The regulatory process is much more ordered than the legislative process, in that the state or federal APAs direct the respective processes. APA process guarantees opportunity for comment and public input. The regulatory process also includes built-in delays and time constraints that slow the process. On the other hand, administrative agencies are able to exert a great deal of control over the rule-drafting process. Agency staff generally draft proposed regulations; staff have an interest in assuring the final regulation has sufficient detail that it can be reasonably enforced. However, it is possible that agency staff, although skilled regulators, may not be knowledgeable about a regulation's impact from the practitioner point of view. If the agency did not invite stakeholders to assist with the original drafting of the regulation, then public input during the comment period is especially important.

In addition to enforcement, administrative agencies may have legislative authority to interpret regulations. Be aware that regulations may be misinterpreted by the agency staff or board members, resulting in the imposition of a new meaning that is not aligned with the original intent of the regulation.

New interpretations of existing laws and regulations may occur over time. These interpretations may be published as opinions, interpretive statements, and/or declaratory rulings of the board, attorney general opinions, or opinions of the court. Official opinions carry the force and effect of law even though they are not promulgated according to the APA. There is a fine line between the duty to interpret existing laws and regulations and establishing new regulations without complying with the APA or new laws without going through the formal legislative process. In some states, official interpretations of law or regulation are only permitted by the attorney general's office or the courts. BONs may be able to offer interpretive statements to facilitate licensee/consumer understanding of a section of a law or regulation, but nothing stronger or enforceable. The courts have been known to revoke board rulings that were made without statutory authority, or unofficial BON "opinions" that were not "properly filed" as rules. If this occurs, the BON unofficial opinion may be rescinded by court order and appropriate means to obtain enforcement authority must be sought. This may require legislation if a change in the practice act is required, or rulemaking if legislative intent for a new rule or rule amplification already exists in the practice act.

Current Issues in Regulation and Licensure

Regulation in a Transforming Healthcare Delivery System

Healthcare professionals are regulated based on a longstanding system of regulating the individual licensee. As new healthcare occupations and professions have developed, there has been increasing professional debate about scopes of practice. Overlapping scopes of practice have naturally emerged in nursing, medicine, pharmacy, social work, physical therapy, respiratory therapy, and other licensed health professions. The overlap may be appropriate when areas of educational preparation and competency are substantially equivalent in more than one profession, but restrictive practice acts have made overlap a source of debate. Questions have been raised as to whether a system regulating individual licensees by means of separate practice acts serves the interests of public protection, or whether the system has become a means to protect the professions and create monopolies for services (Gross, 1984; Pew Health Professions Commission, 1994).

In 1995, the Pew Health Professions Commission published a sweeping report that began to change thinking about existing regulatory systems. The report suggested that the current system, based on a century-old model, was out of sync with the nation's healthcare delivery systems and financing structures. The Pew Health Professions Commission suggested that major reform was needed, and asked states to review regulatory processes with the following questions in mind (Dower & Finocchio, 1995, p. 1):

- Does regulation promote effective health outcomes and protect the public from harm?
- Are regulatory bodies truly accountable to the public?
- Does regulation respect consumers' rights to choose their own healthcare providers from a range of safe options?
- Does regulation encourage a flexible, rational, and cost-effective healthcare system?
- Does regulation allow effective working relationships among healthcare providers?
- Does regulation promote equity among providers of equal skill?
- Does regulation facilitate professional and geographic mobility of competent providers?

Workforce regulation has a significant impact on healthcare cost and accessibility. Restrictive scopes of practice limit the ability of comparably prepared health professionals to provide care. Boundary disputes within and across the health professions create tension and are counterproductive to efforts to improve interprofessional collaboration. A workforce response to regulatory restrictions has been to increase the use of unlicensed assistive personnel (UAP), who are unregulated and less expensive, in both acute and primary care settings. In many employment settings, UAPs are used appropriately. However, when employers misunderstand the roles of these unlicensed individuals or expand their job descriptions in an effort to provide more and less costly care, there is a risk that UAPs may be asked to function in a way that approaches nursing practice without the education or license to do so. Potential dangers include unsafe patient care, when UAPs are asked to function beyond their capacity; liability for nurses who, because of their employment situations, feel forced to delegate more nursing tasks to UAPs than safe standards of delegation would dictate; and infringement on professional nursing practice by unlicensed workers.

The Pew Task Force on Health Care Workforce Regulation challenged state and federal governments to respond to the complex health professions education and regulation issues identified in the report. The task force made

10 recommendations to improve state regulatory systems' responsiveness to changes in the nation's healthcare system. Recommendations addressed the use of standardized and understandable language, standardization of entry-to-practice requirements, assurance of initial and continuing competence of healthcare practitioners, and the redesign of professional boards, including the creation of super-boards with a majority of consumer representatives. The report also called for better methods of assessing the achievement of objectives and improved disciplinary processes (Pew Health Professions Commission, 1995). Since the 1995 task force report, the Institute of Medicine (IOM) has issued a number of reports related to safety in health-care systems, known as the Quality Chasm Series. In its first report, *To Err Is Human*, the IOM called for licensing and certification bodies to pay greater attention to safety-related performance standards and expectations for health professionals (Kohn, Corrigan, & Donaldson, 2000).

A consensus report, focused singularly on nursing, was jointly issued by the Robert Wood Johnson Foundation (RWJF) and the IOM in October 2010. This report, *The Future of Nursing: Leading Change, Advancing Health*, provides four key messages to guide changes and remove barriers that prevent nurses from being able to function effectively in a rapidly evolving healthcare system. These are that nurses should be enabled to practice to the full extent of their education and training, should be able to access higher levels of education and training in an improved education system that allows for academic progression, should be full partners in the interprofessional redesign of the U.S. healthcare system, and finally that effective workforce planning and policymaking need better data collection and information infrastructures. Eight recommendations for fundamental change are found in the report, along with related actions for Congress, state legislatures, CMS, the Office of Personnel Management, and the Federal Trade Commission and Antitrust Division of the Department of Justice. These are: (1) remove scope-of-practice barriers, (2) expand opportunities for nurses to lead and diffuse collaborative improvement efforts, (3) implement nurse residency programs, (4) increase the proportion of nurses with a baccalaureate degree to 80 percent by 2020, (5) double the number of nurses with a doctorate by 2020, (6) ensure that nurses engage in lifelong learning, (7) prepare and enable nurses to lead change to advance health, and (8) build an infrastructure for the collection and analysis of interprofessional healthcare workforce data (Institute of Medicine, 2010).

The Josiah Macy Jr. Foundation, an organization dedicated to improving the health of the public through the advancement of health professions education, has been instrumental in providing direction for regulatory reform. In 2013, the foundation held a consensus conference with health professions education leaders to discuss a vision for a joint future of healthcare practice and education. Conference participants made recommendations for immediate action in five areas; one of these was to "revise professional regulatory standards and practices to permit and promote innovation in interprofessional education and collaborative practice" (Josiah Macy Jr. Foundation, 2013, p. 2).

The sum total of these reports and recommendations provides a body of evidence substantive enough to leverage for reform of health professions regulation that can serve the needs of the 21st century. APRNs have a window of opportunity and must be open to the notion that collaboration with other health professions is essential if new regulatory models are to emerge. Regulation determines who has access to the patient, who serves as gatekeeper in a managed care environment, who is reimbursed, and who has autonomy to practice. APRNs must be visible participants in the political process to shape a dynamic, evolving system that is responsive to the healthcare environment, authorizes APRNs to practice to the full extent of their education in a collaborative environment as equal team members, and ensures consumer choice and protection.

Multistate Regulation

State BONs have made progress facilitating interstate mobility for nurses. Cumbersome licensure processes across geopolitical boundaries make seamless transition difficult or impossible, particularly for APRNs. The Nurse Licensure Compact (NLC) model was adopted by the NCSBN delegate assembly in 1997 during the same timeframe the Consensus Model (LACE) was in development. The NLC is nursing's **mutual recognition** model of multistate licensure. States adopting the model voluntarily enter into an **interstate compact** to legally recognize the licensure policies and processes of a licensee's home state and permit practice in a remote state without obtaining an additional license (NCSBN, 1998). The NLC requires the licensee to comply with the NPA in each state. Nurses are subject to those NPA provisions and regulations, and therefore are accountable and subject to discipline in the state of practice, whether it is the original state of licensure or the remote compact state. To implement the mutual recognition model, the cooperating states' legislatures must enact the interstate compact provisions into law. APRNs have not been included in the compact agreements to date, so although the compact may apply to a nurse's RN license, it does not extend to cover advanced practice. Therefore, the APRN must apply for licensure in each state of practice.

A number of states moved quickly to enter the compact when it was instituted, but many states remain independent. As of July 2014, 24 states are participating as compact states and 3 states have NLC legislation pending (NCSBN, 2014). To promote APRN participation in multistate regulation and APRN competitive advantages in a global market, state NPAs would need to be revised to include the Uniform APRN Requirements. Alternatively, the NLC would need to be expanded to include APRNs.

The Future of Advanced Practice Nurse Regulation

Much of the discussion in this chapter has focused on ways regulatory systems affect APRNs. However, not all challenges associated with practice limitations and patient access are external to the profession; some dilemmas have been created from within. The lack of common APRN role definitions, growing numbers of advanced practice specializations, deliberations about credentials and scopes of practice, and inconsistency in educational standards and state regulations have contributed to public confusion and limited patient access to APRNs as care providers (NCSBN, 2010).

A number of forces within the profession are working independently to address these issues. These forces could coalesce to potentially remedy some of the challenges faced by APRNs. They are: (1) the development of an APRN Consensus Model that has been widely endorsed by nursing organizations; (2) individual states' progress toward Consensus Model implementation through legislation; (3) consolidation of APRN nursing organizations, in particular the two national nurse practitioner organizations; (4) advancing the future of postgraduate APRN education to a level equivalent with other healthcare providers, specifically the practice doctorate; and (5) directions in research on credentialing in nursing.

The NCSBN 2006 draft vision paper, *The Future Regulation of Advanced Practice Nursing*, was the subject of considerable debate among advanced practice nursing organizations and the American Association of Colleges of Nursing (AACN) (Nelson, 2006; NCSBN, 2006). The final report of the Consensus Work Group and the NCSBN Advisory Committee, the *Consensus Model for APRN Regulation: Licensure, Accreditation, Certification, and Education* (Consensus Model), referred to as LACE, was a major step in reaching a level of agreement between stakeholders in organized nursing (APRN Joint Dialogue Group, 2008). Note that the Consensus Model and LACE are not one and the same. The APRN Consensus Model is a stand-alone product of the NCSBN APRN Advisory Committee and the APRN Consensus Work Group, whereas LACE is a mechanism to engage interested stakeholders who are necessarily communicating about and implementing the Consensus Model. The Consensus Model provides detailed definitions for four APRN roles, the certified registered nurse anesthetist, certified nurse-midwife, clinical nurse specialist, and certified nurse practitioner. Realization of the Consensus Model is dependent on how quickly its recommendations, including the merged adult-gerontology foci for NP and CNS curricula, are embedded in educational programs to assure continued graduate eligibility to sit for national certification, and how quickly states are able to enact legislation actualizing recommendations in the NPA. The Consensus Model target date for full implementation is 2015; however, not all APRN groups are on the same timeline, so some variation in timing will occur. The NCSBN document *APRN Consensus Model Frequently-Asked Questions* clarifies questions APRNs may have about implications for their roles, titles, practice, grandfathering, specialization, population foci, and timelines (NCSBN, 2010). In 2008, the NCSBN revised the *Model Nursing Practice Act* and *Model Nursing Administrative Rules* to reflect the Consensus Model (NCSBN, 2011).

The status of implementation of the Consensus Model by each state is unique. The NCSBN has developed a grid to track states' status in adopting elements of the model. Elements tracked include titles, roles, license, education, certification, and whether practice and prescribing is independent for each of the four APRN titles. The grid assigns points to each element enacted; a color-coded map of the United States is periodically updated on the NCSBN website as APRN laws change. As of May 2014, the states that have achieved 100 percent implementation are Idaho, Montana, Nevada, New Mexico, North Dakota, Utah, Minnesota, and Vermont (NCSBN, 2014).

The voice of APRNs is stronger when it is unified and consistent. The American Academy of Nurse Practitioners and American College of Nurse

Practitioners (2012) have consolidated to better position a single organization, the American Association of Nurse Practitioners, to capitalize on growth in NP demand; direct NP legislative and policy agendas; achieve the goals and objectives of NPs; provide enhanced resources for education, research, and grant writing; increase public awareness; and work toward globalization.

Directions in the education of advanced practice nurses parallel changes in regulation. The national standard in health professions education is moving toward the clinical doctorate; pharmacy, physical therapy, and other health professions have advanced the level of graduate education required for entry accordingly. In 2004, the AACN Board of Directors endorsed a *Position Statement on the Practice Doctorate* in nursing, which calls for a change from masters-level educational preparation to the clinical doctorate for APRNs by 2015 (American Association of Colleges of Nursing, 2004). The AACN cites the need for change in graduate nursing education as a response to the increasing complexity of the nation's healthcare environment, and points to national calls to action from the IOM, the Joint Commission (an independent company that accredits healthcare organizations and programs), and the 2005 National Institutes of Health (NIH) report calling for the development of nonresearch (clinical) doctorates in nursing. As of May 2014, 235 DNP programs in the United States enrolled students and more than 100 others were under development (AACN, 2014a).

Finally, credentialing bodies play a crucial role in advancing the profession. Quality in credentialing speaks to the value of creating a system that aims to improve the performance and healthcare outcomes of its credential holders. In 2012, the American Nurses Credentialing Center (ANCC) announced the formation of an Institute of Medicine Standing Committee on Credentialing Research in Nursing. Among other activities, the committee discusses short- and long-term strategic planning, maintains surveillance of the credentialing field, and serves as a public venue of communication for relevant stakeholders. It is within the committee's purview to address the following topics: priorities for nursing credentialing research; relevant research methodologies, measures, and outcomes assessment related to the impact of credentialing in nursing on healthcare quality improvements; and strategic planning for advancing research in nursing credentialing. The ANCC is the primary sponsor of this activity (American Nurses Credentialing Center, 2012; Institute of Medicine, 2014).

Reimbursement

Significant breakthroughs are being made in reimbursement policy for APRNs, largely as a result of the formation of grassroots lobbying efforts and coalitions of APRN specialty nursing organizations. With the passage of federal legislation in 1997 allowing APRNs to bill Medicare directly for services, consumers' access to care provided by APRNs has improved. Managed care markets value efficiency and provider effectiveness. Understanding the concept of market value has motivated APRNs to become more skilled in costing out services and winning contracts in a competitive market.

Discrepancies in Medicare APRN reimbursement still exist, and the reimbursement structure for comparable services is arbitrary. Calls to achieve pay parity have suggested the CMS lead demonstrations of market-based, population-based, and performance-based initiatives to facilitate recognition of NPs as eligible providers (Naylor & Kurtzman, 2010).

Impact of the Nurse Shortage on Regulation and Licensure

Supply and demand projections substantiate that the shortage of nurses will continue well into the next decade. Factors driving the shortage include: (1) the fact that nurse education capacity is not growing rapidly enough to meet the projected demands, in part because of nurse faculty shortages; (2) the aging of the nurse workforce, resulting in a large cohort of retiring nurses; (3) a growth in the aging population, resulting in an increased number of individuals who will require complex care; and (4) insufficient staffing levels and stressful job environments, which are motivating nurses to leave the profession (AACN, 2014b). In December 2013, the U.S. Department of Health and Human Services announced $55.5 million in funding in FY 2014 to strengthen health professions education and increase the size of the healthcare workforce. The majority of funding, $45.4 million, was earmarked to support nursing workforce development. Areas targeted included: (1) increasing the number of nurse faculty, (2) improving diversity in nursing, (3) increasing traineeships in nurse anesthesia and supporting advanced practice nurse education, and (4) supporting the development of interprofessional collaborative practice models (DHHS, 2013). It is expected that nursing workforce issues will continue to fuel policy on work environment issues across the nation.

Although projections in job growth are expected, the nurse workforce able to fill vacant or new positions continues to decline. Several issues bear monitoring during this period. They include the following:

- *Comprehensive U.S. healthcare reform:* Provisions in the ACA will increase access for the nation's under- and uninsured, estimated at more than 50 million. It is also estimated that in more than 6,400 shortage areas in the United States, 66 million Americans are limited in access to primary care (American Nurses Association [ANA], 2011). The need for APRNs in a variety of settings, but particularly in primary care, will be enormous, but their usefulness is dependent on the lifting of practice restrictions in their state of licensure.

- *Delegation and supervision of unlicensed assistive personnel (UAP):* Utilization of UAPs will continue to be debated and expanded as the shortage of licensed nurses makes it difficult to meet the public's demands for care. Providing safe and effective care while delegating care tasks appropriately to a potentially growing cadre of UAPs will place additional responsibilities on the licensed nurse.

- *Mandatory overtime legislation:* The IOM report, *Keeping Patients Safe: Transforming the Work Environment of Nurses* (2003) presented a body of evidence associating the nurses' work environment and patient safety. Nurses commonly work extended hours; this work environment factor was found to be associated with diminished work performance, increased risk of errors, and potential patient harm. Employers have coerced nurses to remain on duty against their will by threatening termination, using the concept of patient abandonment as "cause." Employers follow coercion with threats of reporting the alleged patient abandonment to the licensing board. Disciplinary sections in NPAs typically read in such a way that the employers' threats are empty; most state boards do not consider refusal to work additional consecutive shifts as an incident that constitutes patient abandonment. Fourteen states have protected nurses from this kind of employer threat by enacting restrictions on the use of mandatory overtime in law, and two states have included provisions in regulation (ANA, 2014).

- *Staffing ratios:* In some states, nurses have organized to pass legislation implementing staffing ratios based on patient acuity. Staffing ratios have both positive and negative implications. Although staffing ratio regulations may require a facility to employ a certain minimum number of nurses, or staff units with a minimum number of nurses, employers may interpret the regulated minimum ratios as the maximum number of nurses that *must* be employed, and subsequently place a cap on hiring.

- *Foreign nurse recruitment:* Employers may seek to recruit foreign-educated nurses during acute nurse shortages. Deregulation of licensure and examination standards has historically been enacted during these periods. Few countries outside the United States have nurse education systems equivalent in academic breadth or rigor, or in clinical requirements. The nurse community must be vigilant to these attempts to lower the standards for licensure, which could lead to increased risk for patients and a change in public perception of the profession.
- *Proliferation of new nursing education programs:* Colleges, universities, and other legitimate, accredited public and private educational institutions are finding the business of nurse education is becoming more attractive. The number of qualified applicants for nursing programs far exceeds the number of available seats. However, proprietary organizations are also seeing nursing education as an opportunity for profit, and may not consider the infrastructure and support systems necessary to carry out a quality program. State BONs are challenged to strike a balance between the concept of an open marketplace and a desire to protect the stretched interests of existing programs that are struggling to maintain a cadre of qualified faculty and ensure clinical placements for their students.

Other trends and issues will surface over the next several years that may affect the regulation of nurses and APRNs. It will be increasingly important to stay abreast of legislative and regulatory initiatives, and to affiliate with professional organizations to preserve and protect professional standards.

Conclusion

The capacity to adapt is crucial in an era of rapid change. Healthcare reform is transforming healthcare delivery systems, but it is also providing momentum for fundamental changes in APRN practice and regulation. A window of opportunity has presented itself for politically astute APRNs to shape public policy by working with coalitions of nurses, other health professionals, and consumers to advocate for regulations that will allow the public greater access to affordable, quality health care. It is essential for APRNs to develop skills to capitalize on the chaos present in the healthcare and political environments and create opportunities to advance the profession.

Familiarity with the regulatory process will give APRNs the tools needed to navigate with confidence. Knowing how to access the status of critical issues involving scopes of practice, licensure issues, and reimbursement will allow the APRN to influence outcomes. Participation in specialty professional nurse organizations is especially advantageous. Participation builds a membership base, providing the foundation for strong coalition building and a power base from which to effect change in the political and regulatory arenas. Participation also presents members with access to a colleague network, legislative affairs information, and professional and educational opportunities. Although supporting the profession through participation is central, it is equally important to remember that each APRN has the ability to make a difference.

Discussion Points

1. Compare and contrast the legislative and regulatory processes.
2. Describe the major methods of credentialing. List the benefits and weaknesses of each method from the standpoint of public protection, and protection of the professional scope of practice.
3. Discuss the role of state BONs in regulating professional practice.
4. Compare the role of state BONs with the role of professional organizations in regulating professional practice.
5. Obtain a copy of a proposed or recently promulgated regulation. Using Exhibit 4-1, analyze the regulation for its impact on nursing practice.
6. Assume the BON has promulgated a regulation requiring all APRNs to have 20 contact hours of continuing education credit in pharmacotherapeutics each year to maintain prescriptive authority. Write a brief (no more than two pages) testimony supporting or opposing this proposed regulation.
7. Describe the federal government's role in the regulation of health professions. Do you believe the role will increase or decrease over time? Explain your rationale.
8. Discuss the pros and cons of multistate regulation. Based on your analysis, defend a position either for or against multistate regulation.
9. Prepare written testimony for a public hearing defending or opposing the need for a second license for APRNs.

10. Contrast the BON and the national or state nurses association vis-à-vis mission, membership, authority, functions, and source of funding.

11. Identify a proposed regulation. Discuss the current phase of the process, identify methods for offering comments, and submit written comments to the administrative agency.

12. Download at least one resource from one of the websites listed in Exhibit 4-2 and evaluate the credibility of the author (the "author" may be the organization), the most recent update, and the appropriateness of the data. Share the resources with colleagues.

13. Evaluate the APRN section of the nurse practice act in your state using the *NCSBN Model Nursing Practice Act* (March 2011).

14. Identify the states that have implemented nurse-staffing ratios. List some of the obstacles one of the states has encountered in the implementation phase.

CASE STUDY 2: DELEGATION OF MEDICATION ADMINISTRATION BY APRNs

The authority to administer medications in one state is restricted and specific. The NPA allows RNs to delegate medication administration to BON-certified medication aides in nursing homes and residential care facilities. Unlicensed persons may assist an individual with self-administration of certain medications, may give oral or apply topical medication in accordance with the laws and regulations of the Department of Disabilities, and may administer prescribed medication to a student if they are employed by a board of education or charter school and medication administration procedures are in accordance with law regulating boards of education. Dialysis technicians have limited delegated authority to administer only specific relevant medications. Physicians may delegate medication administration to physician assistants and medical assistants, in accordance with a section of the Medical Practice Act. However, with the exception of the special instances just identified, RNs and APRNs are not permitted to delegate medication administration to non-nurses, including medical assistants. This is problematic for APRNs, particularly NPs and CNSs who function in primary care settings.

Patients in primary care settings frequently need immunizations, TB skin tests, or routine medications. Because current law largely prohibits APRNs from delegating medication administration to unlicensed personnel, APRNs must interrupt the flow of patient care to administer the medication themselves and perform all associated tasks, unless there is another RN who is available to administer the medication. This prohibition is a significant barrier to productivity and efficiency.

APRNs and stakeholder nurse associations approached a legislator who has been a friend to nursing and is interested in improving healthcare delivery in the state. This member of the House of Representatives sought a colleague to cosponsor the bill who is a member of the Senate, and a member of the other party. A house bill, jointly sponsored by a representative and a senator, one a Democrat and one a Republican, is uniquely collaborative, and sends a message about the need for the measure.

The bill, as introduced, would allow certain APRNs to delegate medication administration to a trained, unlicensed person, such as a medical assistant, so long as certain conditions are met. These conditions include: (1) APRN assessment of the patient prior to administration to determine appropriateness; (2) the APRN has determined the unlicensed person has completed the requisite education, and has the knowledge, skills, and ability to administer the drug safely; and (3) delegation is in accordance with rules that are established by the BON. Additional safeguards include: (1) the drug must be within the formulary established by the BON for APRNs, is not a controlled substance, and is not to be administered intravenously; (2) the employer has given the APRN access to employment records documenting the unlicensed person's education, knowledge, ability, and skills with regards to medication administration; and (3) the APRN must be physically present at the location where the drug is administered by the unlicensed person. Language in the bill clarifies that the APRN delegating authority law would not affect or change

(continues)

the current law governing delegation authority in certain facilities, including nursing homes and residential care facilities. This legislation has, to date, received four hearings in the House Health Committee and has been reported out with sponsor amendments that would add ambulatory surgical facilities to the list of sites where an APRN cannot delegate medication administration and would move the rule authority language to the general rule authority of the nurse practice act. Although this second amendment is technical, it is beneficial to APRNs in that it will authorize the BON to promulgate rules without the advice and counsel of its multidisciplinary Committee on Prescriptive Governance.

One state nursing association and one APRN testified on behalf of nursing as proponents for the bill. The state medical association has remained neutral throughout the process.

Discussion Points

1. Identify ways to increase the likelihood for the legislation to pass in this General Assembly or the next.
2. Determine a complete list of possible stakeholders. In addition to state nurses' associations, what other associations or organizations might have an interest?
3. Discuss the position of neutrality on the part of the state medical association. Would you expect this? Why or why not? Could their position change? Why or why not? If so, what could you do in anticipation to assure passage of the bill?
4. Although a number of state nurses' associations have an interest in this bill, only one formally provided proponent testimony for the record. In addition, one adult NP, who represented herself as a single practitioner, provided testimony. What are the implications of limited proponent testimony? What does a small turnout, or silence, say to legislators? What might be done differently, or in addition, when the bill reaches the Senate?

CASE STUDY 3: CHANGES IN REGULATIONS: THE WEIGHT OF A SINGLE WORD

APRNs may find themselves in educator roles; schools of nursing often employ APRNs to teach advanced practice graduate students, or they may be asked to teach at the undergraduate level. APRNs engaged in teaching roles must have an understanding of the regulations affecting nursing education in addition to those affecting general and advanced nursing practice. This case focuses on changes in education rules in one state, although the process could easily be applied to changes in any regulations affecting nurses.

In most states, education regulations devote a section to the supervision of nurse students by qualified faculty and instructional personnel, and also speak to the leadership of the nurse education program by qualified administrators (e.g., chairs, deans, or directors). In one state, a long-standing regulation described procedures nurse education programs must follow to account for the occasional absence of the program administrator in the case of illness or other personal reason. The regulation stated that if the program administrator was absent for a period of 30 or more business days, a qualified interim administrator would need to be named and the BON notified. This regulation protected the integrity of nurse education programs by assuring continuity of program leadership.

During a comprehensive revision of the education regulation section, the rule in question was redrafted so that the period of time was extended from 30 days to 90 days, in an apparent effort to make the time frame more generous. However, additional language in the same rule was added so that the scope of the rule expanded from the coverage of short absences, lasting a month or more, to include the *vacating* of the position by the administrator (i.e., resignation). In addition, the word *interim* was deleted. In effect, a nurse education program would be required to replace the administrator within a 90-day period if the rule went into effect as drafted. This time frame is inadequate for conducting a search for a qualified person to fill the

(continues)

position; it is not uncommon for chair/dean searches to take a year or more.

A group of nurse education program leaders in the state discussed the impact of the draft rule. The BON held an open public hearing as a part of the rule-making process, and the group sent a representative to give both oral and written testimony. The BON heard the testimony, and as a result had a more complete understanding of the meaning of the rule change to nurse education programs. The BON revised the rule to include both absences and vacancies, and language was added to require the designation of a qualified registered nurse to replace the program administrator *or* to serve as an interim program administrator.

Discussion Points

Keeping in mind that it is imperative for nursing programs to comply with all board of nursing rules to maintain their approval status, consider the following questions:

1. If the draft language had not been changed, what would have been the effect on nursing programs if an administrator resigned unexpectedly?
2. What was the impact of removing the word *interim* in the first draft? What is the impact of the word *or* in the revised language? Discuss the importance of reading draft regulations for explicit detail.
3. Identify ways that APRNs can stay abreast of potential changes in relevant nursing or related regulations.
4. Discuss the value of involvement with nurse organizations as a means to have an impact on changes in regulations; that is, how might a regulatory agency weigh the testimony of an individual versus the testimony of an organization representative?

References

American Academy of Nurse Practitioners & American College of Nurse Practitioners. (2012, July 3). *Two national nurse practitioner organizations announce plans to consolidate.* Retrieved from http://www.aanp.org/28-press-room/2012-press-releases/996-plans-to-consolidate

American Association of Colleges of Nursing. (2004). *AACN position statement on the practice doctorate in nursing.* Retrieved from http://www.aacn.nche.edu/DNP/DNPPositionStatement.htm

American Association of Colleges of Nursing. (2014a). *DNP program schools.* Retrieved from http://www.aacn.nche.edu/dnp/program-schools

American Association of Colleges of Nursing. (2014b). *Nursing shortage fact sheet.* Retrieved from http://www.aacn.nche.edu/media-relations/NrsgShortageFS.pdf

American Nurses Association. (2011). *Advanced practice nursing: A new age in health care.* American Nurses Association Backgrounder. Retrieved from http://www.nursingworld.org/functionalmenucategories/mediaresources/mediabackgrounders/aprn-a-new-age-in-health-care.pdf

American Nurses Association. (2014). *Mandatory overtime.* Retrieved from http://www.nursingworld.org/MainMenuCategories/ThePracticeofProfessionalNursing/NurseStaffing/OvertimeIssues/Overtime.pdf

American Nurses Credentialing Center. (2012, September). *American Nurses Credentialing Center announces members of the IOM committee on credentialing research in nursing.* Retrieved from http://www.nursingworld.org/FunctionalMenuCategories/MediaResources/PressReleases/2012-PR/IOM-Committee-on-Credentialing-Research-in-Nursing.pdf

APRN Joint Dialogue Group. (2008). *Consensus model for APRN regulation: Licensure, accreditation, certification & education.* Retrieved from www.aacn.nche.edu/education-resources/APRNReport.pdf

Centers for Medicare & Medicaid Services. (2014). *History.* Retrieved from http://www.cms.gov/About-CMS/Agency-Information/History.Index.html

Commonwealth Fund. (2014). Affordable care act reforms. Retrieved from: http://www.commonwealthfund.org/topics/affordable-care-act-reforms

Dower, C., & Finocchio, L. (1995). Health care workforce regulation: Making the necessary changes for a transforming health care system. *State Health Workforce Reforms, 4,* 1–2.

Garner, B. A. (2009). *Black's law dictionary* (9th ed.). St Paul, MN: Thompson West.

Gobis, L. J. (1997). Licensing & liability: Crossing the borders with telemedicine. *Caring, 16*(7), 18–24.

Gross, S. (1984). *Of foxes and hen houses: Licensing and the health professions.* Westport, CT: Quorum.

Hartigan, C. (2011). APRN regulation: The licensure-certification interface. *AACN Advanced Critical Care, 22*(1), 50–65.

HealthCare.gov. (2010). *About the law: Patient protection and Affordable Healthcare Act.* Retrieved from http://www.healthcare.gov/law/about/Index.htm

Institute of Medicine (2003). *Keeping patients safe: Transforming the work environment of nurses.* Washington, DC: National Academies Press.

Institute of Medicine. (2010). *The future of nursing: Leading change, advancing health.* Retrieved from http://www.iom.edu/~/media/Files/Report%20Files/2010/The-Future-of-Nursing/Future%20of%20Nursing%202010%20Recommendations.pdf

Institute of Medicine. (2014). *Standing committee on credentialing research in nursing.* Retrieved from http://www.iom.edu/Activities/Workforce/NursingCredentialing

Josiah Macy Jr. Foundation. (2013). *Transforming patient care: Aligning interprofessional education with clinical practice redesign.* Conference recommendations. Retrieved from http://macyfoundation.org/publications/publication/aligning-interprofessional-education

Jost, T. S. (1997). *Regulation of the health professions.* Chicago: Health Administration Press.

Kohn, L. T., Corrigan, J. M., & Donaldson, M. S. (Eds.). (2000). *To err is human: Building a safer health care system.* Institute of Medicine of the National Academies. Washington, DC: National Academies Press.

Legal Information Institute. (n.d.). *Supremacy clause.* Retrieved from http://www.law.cornell.edu/wex/supremacy_clause

National Council of State Boards of Nursing. (1993). *Regulation of advanced nursing practice position paper.* Retrieved from https://www.ncsbn.org/1993_Position_Paper_on_the_Regulation_of_Advanced_Nursing_Practice.pdf

National Council of State Boards of Nursing. (1998, April). *Multi state regulation task force communiqué.* Chicago: Author.

National Council of State Boards of Nursing. (2002). *Uniform advanced practice registered nurse licensure/authority to practice requirements.* Retrieved from https://www.ncsbn.org/APRN_Uniform_requirements_revised_8_02.pdf

National Council of State Boards of Nursing. (2006). *Draft—Vision paper: The future regulation of advanced practice nursing.* Retrieved from https://www.ncsbn.org/Draft__Vision_Paper.pdf

National Council of State Boards of Nursing. (2008). *Contact a board of nursing.* Retrieved from https://www.ncsbn.org/515.htm

National Council of State Boards of Nursing. (2009). *Requirements for accrediting agencies and criteria for APRN certification programs.* Retrieved from https://www.ncsbn.org/428.htm

National Council of State Boards of Nursing. (2010). *APRN consensus model: Frequently-asked questions.* Retrieved from https://www.ncsbn.org/aprn.htm

National Council of State Boards of Nursing. (2011). *NCSBN model nursing practice act and model nursing administrative rules: Introduction to revised models.* Retrieved from https://www.ncsbn.org/nlc.htm

National Council of State Boards of Nursing. (2014a). *Map of NLC states.* Retrieved from http://www.ncsbn.org/nlc

National Council of State Boards of Nursing. (2014b). *Nurse practice act, rules & regulations.* Retrieved from https://www.ncsbn.org/1455.htm

Naylor, M. D., & Kurtzman, E. T. (2010). The role of nurse practitioners in reinventing primary care. *Health Affairs, 29*(5), 893–899. doi: 10.1377/hlthaff.2010.0440.

Nelson, R. (2006). NCSBN 'vision paper' ignites controversy. *American Journal of Nursing, 106*(7), 25–26.

O'Sullivan, J., Chaikind, H., Tilson, S., Boulanger, J., & Morgan, P. (2004). *Overview of the Medicare Prescription Drug, Improvement and Modernization Act of 2003.* Congressional Research Service. Order Code RL31966. Washington, DC: Library of Congress.

Pearson, L. J. (2002). Fourteenth annual legislative update. *Nurse Practitioner, 27*(1), 10–15.

Pew Health Professions Commission. (1994). *State strategies for health care workforce reform.* San Francisco: UCSF Center for the Health Professions.

Pew Health Professions Commission. (1995). *Report of task force on health care workforce regulation* (executive summary). San Francisco: UCSF Center for the Health Professions.

Phillips, S. J. (2014). 26th annual legislative update. *Nurse Practitioner, 39*(1), 29–52.

Roberts, M. J., & Clyde, A. T. (1993). *Your money or your life: The health care crisis explained.* New York: Doubleday.

Russell, K. A. (2012). Nurse practice acts guide and govern nursing practice. *Journal of Nursing Regulation, 3*(3), 36–42.

Safriet, B. J. (1992). Health care dollars and regulatory sense: The role of advanced practice nursing. *Yale Journal of Regulation, 9*(2), 419–488.

U.S. Department of Health and Human Services. (2013). *HHS awards $55.5 million to bolster America's health care workforce.* Retrieved from http://www.hhs.gov/news/press/2013pres/12/20131205a.html

U.S. Department of Health and Human Services. (2014). *The Affordable Care Act, section by section.* Retrieved from http://www.hhs.gov/healthcare/rights/law/

U.S. Department of Health and Human Services, Centers for Medicare & Medicaid Services. (2011). *Information for advanced practice registered nurses, anesthesiologist assistants, and physician assistants.* Medical Learning Network. ICN901623. Retrieved from http://www.cms.gov/Outreach-and-Education/Medicare-Learning-Network-MLN/MLNProducts/APNPA.html

Policy Design

Patricia Smart

Introduction

In today's world, it is imperative that healthcare providers be knowledge-able about the policy process and know how to play a key role in the changes that are occurring now and will continue to evolve. The purpose of this chapter is to examine the component of the policy process that involves the "tools" that government uses to get people to do what they might not ordinarily do.

The scope of government's involvement in social issues in the United States has expanded rapidly during the last 90 years. Federally funded health-care programs such as Medicare and Medicaid have made a major impact on how health care is implemented by providers and perceived by the public. The impact is even greater with the passage of the 2010 Affordable Care Act (ACA). As noted by Comer (2002), government involvement in health care has occurred at the state and local levels through program administration, educational preparation, licensing, and regulation of practice. As with most public issues, policies regarding health care are intentionally vague. Ambiguity provides states and municipalities flexibility in implementation; however, the vagueness complicates the implementation process and often results in a failed policy or an unintended consequence.

Health care is fraught with a multitude of factors that are difficult to identify and control, and the issue of healthcare reform has polarized the country. As noted by Eileen T. O'Grady (2010), there is massive misinformation and confusion about the many aspects of the Affordable Care Act: "It is like a giant root ball that cannot be understood without untangling and pulling apart each root" (p. 8). Public policy is by nature complicated. The root of public problems has no simple single answer; if it did, more than likely it would become a guideline, recommendation, or rule implemented by the private sector. Health care is perhaps the most convoluted of public issues because it is impacted by a multitude of factors such as national and international economies, social movements, education, resources, and religion. The intractability of most factors that lie within the healthcare field prevents uncomplicated, comprehensive, easily understandable solutions. One of the factors most inhibiting policy success is the inability to predict consumer behavior and participation in a program. The gap in matching desired behavior with appropriate government tools is discussed in this chapter. Advanced practice registered nurses (APRNs) are in a perfect position to help policymakers have a clear understanding of how target population participation can be maximized by choosing the appropriate tool. In this author's view, examining the tools that government chooses to use to achieve its desired goals in addressing a public issue is the most logical and simple way to determine policy success.

The United States has one of the most sophisticated healthcare systems (although challengers call it a "sick care system") in the world in terms of technology and preparation of healthcare professionals. Yet in many of the health indices designed to evaluate the overall health of a country, the United States rates comparatively low. For example, the average life expectancy for females in the United States is 80.9 years, whereas in many other developed countries such as Japan, Canada, and the Netherlands, a female's life expectancy is 86.1, 82.9, and 81.9 years, respectively (Central Intelligence Agency [CIA], 2009a). Infant mortality also is an important measure of a nation's health. The United States ranked 33rd among industrialized countries in 2009 and also had a high rate of low and very low birth weights, a major contributor to infant mortality (CIA, 2009b). The system is broken. It suffers from unwarranted variations in performance, effectiveness, and efficiency.

Efforts have been made by previous administrations to address the issues of cost, access, and quality, and those efforts were a reflection of the then-current political philosophies and ideologies. For example, the government programs in the 1960s reflected a democratic ideology where there was less concern with outcome-based planning and more concern with access. Then in the 1980s, under a Republican administration, regulatory efforts attempted to reduce costs through outcome-based choices, individual responsibility for cost, and less expansion.

Policies are usually designed to influence behavior and, as noted earlier, get people to do what they ordinarily might not do. Health policies address health concerns through laws, regulations, or programs that focus on health determinants including behavioral choices, the physical environment in which people live and work, and social factors. Although many studies regarding the policy process have been conducted, few have examined the process of policy design in issues of health care. The focus of most policy studies has been on the implementation of effective programs, and data have been gathered on statistical outcomes. This author argues that design considerations also should be a component to be considered during all phases of the policy process to promote policy success. For example, in the agenda-setting phase, the social issue must be stated in such a way that it will capture the attention of lawmakers and framed so that government response will be feasible and adaptable. During the implementation phase, the design of the policy provides guidance and also provides an overall picture of the plan by specifying the intended outcomes. During the evaluation phase (this phase should be specified in the design) the program objectives are clearly identified and measurable, or it would be difficult to determine that the focus is on an outcome that addresses the original issue.

The Policy Process

Policies reflect public opinion. The policy players are a collection of actors whose task is to find a solution to intractable problems. Policies that address social problems in the United States usually are formulated by a combination of legislators and aides, the executive branch, courts, and special-interest groups. Professional experts are often asked to serve as panel members or consultants or to serve on committees that provide input to policymakers, and so advanced practice registered nurses (APRNs) are asked to serve on committees that relate to health care. For example, nurse leaders were invited to sit at the table during the early 1990s when Hillary Clinton was proposing a national plan to change existing healthcare policies.

The proliferation of participants in policy formation makes systematic program design that is focused on outcomes difficult to achieve, which is also complicated by the fact that social problems are usually intractable and difficult to solve. Safriet (2002) reports that most social issues are not brought to the attention of policymakers until there is a crisis with multiple causative factors. It is well known that decision making with regard to relevant factors that relate to or have an impact on perceived social problems often is conducted hastily because of lack of information, constituency impatience, and lack of expertise.

Review of Policy Research

Notable work has been conducted regarding agenda setting, implementation, and evaluation, and many of the models stemming from this work are in use today in the study of the policy process. For example, in 1973 Pressman and Wildavsky noted the complexity of implementation and the difficulty in achieving policy success when many branches and divisions of government attempt to work together. Bardach (1977), in his classic work, identified certain relationships among policy actors that developed through game playing. He identified activities, such as bargaining and negotiating among players, that make a tremendous impact on policy success or failure. Bardach also noted that a good policy must begin with a design that incorporates scenarios that can anticipate games and "**fire alarms**." For example, in some states APNs have to be willing to allow a representative from the board of pharmacy or the board of medicine to be on the governing board that regulates nursing at the advanced level.

Several notable political scientists who have also contributed to the study of the policy process include Kingdon (1995); Cohen, March, and Olsen (1972); and Dryzek (1983). These researchers made significant contributions to the main body of knowledge of the policy process by examining the way decisions were made (e.g., loose coupling, garbage can model) and the complexity of the policy.

Recently, Bryan and O'Byrne (2012) wrote about using policy analysis framework when proposing a policy related to nondisclosure in Canada, using Leavitt, Mason, and Whelan's (2013) policy analysis framework. The framework included identifying several factors that should also be included when considering policy design, such as the setting and influencing components, forming taskforces composed of stakeholders, and including a values assessment component. Identifying these factors as being critical to the evaluation process is crucial when working in the design phase of policymaking.

Policy Links

During the 1980s, political scientists studied the content of policy with the intention of providing an understanding of the link between policy design and policy outcome (**policy links**). Their efforts hold importance for APRNs whose roles often require interpretation and implementation of policies. To improve the likelihood of policy success, APRNs must be able to critically analyze policy content; specifically, they must be able to understand what the original intent of the policy is and if the policy is designed in such a way as to assure the intended outcome.

Schneider and Ingram (1990) argued for a closer look at design and proposed a framework to examine behavioral assumptions and attributes of policy content that can be employed by APRNs to conduct the work of government. This framework was used by this author and also was used by Roch, Pitts, and Navarro (2010) to examine how racial and ethnic representation influences the tools public officials use in designing policies to address discipline in public schools. Schneider and Ingram (2005) note that "the laws that policy produces are the principle tools in securing the democratic process for all people" (p. 2). They also note that although public policy ensures all people certain entitlements, policy has also been responsible for creating "distinctive populations."

Government policies are subject to a wide scope of interpretation that depends on who brings problems to national attention and which legislative group attaches itself to problems and solutions. Policies are often vague, with unclear mandates. This is intentional, in order to provide more discretion in the implementation of policies. An opportunity exists for APRNs who recognize the value of vagueness; rather than waiting for clear directives, the nurse must learn and become comfortable with ambiguity because it allows discretion and flexibility in decision making and action, thereby enhancing the ability to individualize management.

The Design Issue

Unclear mandates often result in a mismatch between congressional intent and bureaucratic behavior. For example, federal money that is allocated to states for harm-reduction programs, such as smoking cessation during pregnancy, may reach a segment of the target group that may not need it. Many college-educated women will not smoke during pregnancy, yet private healthcare providers have access to as much federal money to develop an antismoking program as their public agency counterparts do.

Policy design became a focus of studies regarding the policy process over 30 years ago. For example, in 1987, Linder and Peters reported that poor policy design was a reason for policy failure. Describing some programs as crippled at birth, these scholars noted that the best bureaucracies in the world may not be able to achieve desired goals if an excessively ambitious policy is used (i.e., the problem is too complex for a single policy or agency). Also, if there is a misunderstanding of the nature of the problem, inappropriate policies may be formulated. Linder and Peters proposed that implementation should be examined, but only as one of the conditions that must be satisfied for successful policymaking. They maintain that by shifting the focus of study to policy design, a more reliable and explicit answer can be found regarding policy success.

Other scholars concurred with Linder and Peters. Ingraham (1987) argued that a systematic analysis of program design, rather than analysis using the garbage can model of agenda setting, could enhance policy success by allowing the option of considering alternative strategies and providing causal links, culminating in theory building. At that time, Ingraham focused her work on two areas of policy design: the level of design (sophistication of the design) and the location (exclusive to the legislative arena, exclusion of experts).

Upon reviewing the policy literature, it is apparent that the design phase of the policy process continues to be an area where few policy scholars choose to focus their efforts. However, there are a few policy studies that look at design when examining social policy. For example, in a study conducted to examine policy-instrument utilization to promote electricity-efficient household appliances and office equipment, Varone and Aebischer (2001) determined that the political climate in which a policy is implemented is a critical factor to be considered when choosing instruments. In addition, the work of Roch, Pitts, and Navarro (2010), as noted earlier, examined policy tools. In summary, policy design is an integral component of the policy process. An understanding of policy tools or instruments chosen for policy design and the underlying assumptions of policymakers during the design process is critical to an understanding of the overall policy process.

Policy Instruments (Government Tools)

The study of the instruments or tools by which the government achieves desired policy goals has allowed researchers to examine policies in relation to their intent and to begin to infer the predictive capabilities of tools. Two scholars proposed a framework for studying policy based on policy tools. Schneider and Ingram (1990) offer a framework to analyze implicit or explicit behavioral theories found in laws, regulations, and programs. Their analysis uses government tools or instruments and underlying behavioral assumptions as variables that guide policy decisions and choices. Their contention is that target group compliance and utilization are important forms of political behavior that should be examined closely. Combined with process variables such as competition, partisanship, and public opinion, Schneider and Ingram argue that the tools approach moves policy beyond considering the standard analysis and improved frameworks. They note that policy tools are substitutable and states often use a variety of tools to address a single problem. To understand which tools are most productive, emphasis should be placed on using them in conjunction with a particular policy design. APRNs can use their knowledge of policy tools to make suggestions and recommendations to government leaders who are designing policies and programs. Schneider and Ingram (1990) state that public policy almost always attempts to get or enable people to do things they would not have done otherwise, and policy tools are those methods chosen by policymakers to overcome barriers to policy-relevant actions. Large numbers of people in different situations are involved in policymaking. Actions required by these players include compliance with policy rules, utilization of policy opportunities, and self-initiated actions that promote policy goals. Schneider and Ingram suggest several issues that may affect failure to take actions needed to ameliorate social, economic, or political problems: (1) lack of incentives or capacity, (2) disagreement with the values implicit in the means or ends, or (3) the existence of high levels of uncertainty about the situation that make it unclear what people should do or how to motivate them. The researchers describe five specific policy tools used by governments in designing policy. In addition, they identify five broad categories of tools: authority, incentives, capacity building, symbolic or hortatory, and learning.

Authority Tools

Authority tools are used most frequently by governments to guide the behavior of agents and officials at lower levels. Authority tools are statements backed by the legitimate power of government that grant permission and prohibit or require action under designated circumstances. An example of an authority tool is a law, regulation, or mandate that requires that women qualify for prenatal services under regulated criteria.

Incentive Tools

Incentive tools assume individuals are utility maximizers and will not be motivated positively to take action without encouragement or coercion. Utility maximizers are those who want to get the greatest value for each expenditure. These tools rely on tangible payoffs (positive or negative) as motivating factors. Incentive policy tools manipulate tangible benefits, costs, and probabilities that policy designers assume are relevant to the situation. Incentives assume individuals have the "opportunity to make choices, recognize the opportunity, and have adequate information and decision-making skills to select from among alternatives that are in their best interests" (Schneider & Ingram, 1990, p. 516). An example of an incentive tool is coupons for free public transportation to prenatal clinics to encourage pregnant women to seek care. However, if the APRN assumes that lack of transportation is a barrier to accessing prenatal care (in that transportation options do not exist, regardless of cost), the outcome from an attempt to use this particular incentive may fail. The 2010 Affordable Care Act falls into this category, with a penalty to those individuals and businesses who do not adhere to the law.

Capacity-Building Tools

Capacity-building tools provide information, training, education, and resources to enable individuals, groups, or agencies to make decisions or carry out activities. These tools assume that incentives are not an issue and that target populations will be motivated adequately. For capacity-building tools to work, populations must be aware of the risk factors the tools possess and how these tools can help. Capacity-building tools focus on education. For example, information may point out the risks of smoking and drugs on a fetus, and information on such risk factors is distributed to the target population through brochures, email, YouTube videos, or other presentations. Another good example would be the extensive effort by the administration to inform the public about the Affordable Care Act. The underlying assumption is that information regarding the importance of smoking cessation is considered valuable to pregnant women and they will stop smoking to protect the health of their babies. Capacity-building tools also are used to encourage people to recognize the value of health care and to sign up for healthcare insurance.

Symbolic or Hortatory Tools

Symbolic or hortatory tools assume that people are motivated from within and decide whether to take policy-related actions on the basis of their beliefs and values. An example of this type of tool is a poster directed at adolescents that uses an adolescent model to issue advice or a warning. Such tools seek to gain the attention of the target population (adolescents) through use of peer imagery. Slogans also are symbolic and are used so that consumers link a positive or negative outcome to a particular behavior.

Learning Tools

These tools are used when the basis upon which target populations might be moved to take problem-solving action is unknown or uncertain. Policies that use learning tools often are open-ended in purpose and objectives and have broad goals. A needs assessment of the target population may be conducted by a taskforce, which provides knowledge and insight for policymakers and is an example of a learning tool. For example, if a community program related to addressing childhood obesity is to be proposed, a needs assessment must be conducted to determine what information is going to be needed before a proposal is presented to the county council.

Policy tools are important resources for the APRN because tools can be used to enlighten policymakers and persuade them to support or oppose a policy. Policy tools are similar to educational brochures and other materials that nurses provide to patients and families so that the patient can make informed decisions. For example, one of the primary goals of nursing is to provide the patient with comprehensive information regarding whether the patient has a chronic or acute illness or has undergone a stress-causing, life-changing event. Policy briefs, talking points, brochures about specific health conditions, and information about how the 2010 ACA will affect patient care often are given to policymakers to help them understand a health issue. More specific educational guidelines relating to health promotion behaviors and signs and symptoms of illness can reinforce information received from the care provider.

Behavioral Dimensions

In addition to understanding the types and the roles of tools in developing policy, the nurse in advanced practice must understand behavioral assumptions and the political context in which tools exist. The political climate in which social problems are addressed often prescribes the choice of tools to be implemented. Various tools are used when addressing similar social problems, and often these tools are interchanged, frequently resulting in differing outcomes when used by different agencies, states, or countries. In the United States, for example, liberal policymakers are inclined to use capacity-building tools when developing policies for poor and minority groups, whereas conservative policymakers might use the same types of tools in developing policies applicable to businesses.

Using Tools as a Looking Glass

Policy design is an integral component of the policy process. The choice of policy tools and the underlying assumptions of policymakers during the design process are critical to the success or failure of a policy. To help APRN students wrap their heads around how to analyze the policy process by looking at the tools used to address a policy, it might be useful to briefly discuss a study conducted by a nurse doctoral student studying health policy. The question was: If the United States is supposed to have the best healthcare system in the world, why do we have one of the highest infant mortality rates among developed countries? The research involved analyzing how two different countries address the issue of infant mortality; specifically, what tools did the government in the Netherlands use that had such a different outcome than that of a state in the United States (South Carolina)?

Political Culture

In the area of political culture, differences were evident. Even though South Carolina and the Netherlands are pluralist societies with democratically derived leadership and elected legislatures, many factors contribute to very different approaches to policymaking. The Constitution of the United States established a system of checks and balances that has led to a federal legislature that, even when dominated by the same party as the executive branch, has considerable autonomy and may be divided strongly on a given issue. This diffusion of power makes it difficult to enact and implement policies. The structure of federalism (a system of government that allows each state considerable room for decentralized development in terms of adapting to unique human and environmental circumstances) offers opportunities for bolder programs in states than at the national level. In addition, the cleavages and turf issues that exist in the United States present resistance to cooperation. Because of the growth of regulatory activities, policymaking has become more complex, with more interdependency and conflict. In contrast, the Dutch government is centralized with little discretion allowed to lower-level administrators in municipalities. This is the result of clear, specifically stated policies that limit administrative and management flexibility.

APRNs in the United States often work in settings where even small policy changes involve multiple disciplines or departments and actors. For example, in a primary care setting, such as a family planning center, a policy change relating to Medicaid payment would affect patient recordkeeping for the social worker, dietitian, physician, and business manager, as well as the nurse. The APRN must be prepared to assume a leadership role in the collaboration of the various disciplines in providing comprehensive care to the patient.

CASE STUDY 1: COMPARATIVE ANALYSIS OF PREGNANCY OUTCOMES IN TWO COUNTRIES

The study (Smart, 2008) looked at how different governments might approach the issue of infant mortality. South Carolina (in the United States) and the Netherlands were chosen as the foci of study, and the questions asked related to factors such as political culture, economies, government response, and policy participation. Although the state and national levels of government are different, they are appropriate for comparative analysis because of their bicameral political structures and relative similarity in size. The most revealing factors regarding the differences in pregnancy outcomes were related to the approaches taken by the two governments to address the issue.

Economies

The gap between equality and distribution of income is greater in the United States than in the Netherlands. Income in the Netherlands falls within a close range, and so the income gap between the rich and the poor is very narrow; this is as opposed to the United States, where the gap is large and getting larger with the current economic situation and the resulting increased number of unemployed. Sardell (1990) notes that access to health care among the poor and unemployed is a long-standing concern of proponents of maternal and infant care. Despite an unemployment rate that exceeds that of South Carolina, prenatal services are provided to all Dutch women, regardless of income, with minimal financial barriers to care.

Government Response

This research found that governments in both countries used tools similar to those described in Schneider and Ingram's framework (1990), although the policy environments differed a great deal. Policies and initiatives developed and implemented by policymakers were analyzed by applying policy tools used in the conceptualization and implementation of the policy. As noted by Schneider and Ingram, "Policy tools are used to overcome impediments to policy-relevant actions" (p. 510). Successful realization of policy goals requires active **participation** by the target population. If policymakers are not cognizant of motivating and deterring factors affecting the decision-making process of the target group, incorrect assumptions regarding participative behavior can result in an ineffective policy.

Although data relating to government responses to the problem of infant mortality revealed that policymakers in both countries were informed regarding beliefs and values of the target population, government-designed policies to address infant mortality in the United States have not been as successful in reducing the rate of infant mortality as in the Netherlands.

The area of family planning reflected the widest gap in the choice of tools. Several initiatives exist in most states, including South Carolina, that address family planning. All initiatives are activated through local and individualized programs, with no single program providing a clear and consistent framework to be followed by others. Although sex education is taught in the state-funded schools, each county may present the package in any form it chooses. Most key policymakers who are informed about the content of the sex-education curriculum practices around the state report that the content is often a very brief (15-minute) discussion each semester that covers broad concepts. In contrast, Dutch schools mandate a comprehensive sex education to all students beginning in the fifth grade. In addition, a government-funded family planning service is available through all general practitioners and midwives. The government is supported in these efforts by a majority of Dutch citizens and most of the clergy.

Policy Participation

The success of a policy or program is highly dependent upon whether the target population perceives the services provided by the program to be valuable enough to warrant participation. Policy participation in this study revealed that coproduction (assumption of the values and involvement of establishment of goals) of a policy is not coordinated in South Carolina, but that Dutch citizens are very involved with policy design and formulation. All Dutch citizens use the same healthcare system and, therefore, have greater vested interest.

(continues)

Utilization of services in South Carolina is poor, which informants suggest is the result of very little input regarding policy formulation from the target population. Dutch women fully participate in family planning and prenatal healthcare programs.

Policy-Process Variables

Policy-process variables may make a major impact on the success or failure of a policy or program. Process variables include partisanship, public opinion, interest group strength, homogeneity between policymakers and the target population, and influence of policy analysis. Partisanship is deeply embedded in the United States and affects decisions on policies addressing maternal and infant health. Democrats are disposed more favorably than Republicans toward capacity-building tools or positive inducements for populations such as the poor. The Netherlands, in contrast, is noted for its ability to provide an overarching relationship among political elites to provide harmony and stability. Lijphart (1977) notes that the Netherlands is "a dramatic example of the survival of a nation state as a stable democracy despite extreme social pluralism" (p. 103).

Public opinion regarding policies that address unwanted pregnancies in the United States is polarized. The divisions between those who favor open, factual, and consistent information regarding sexuality and sex education and those who feel that such an environment would foster more promiscuity and unwanted pregnancies are also reflected in the legislature. In the Netherlands, public opinion is strongly and cohesively in favor of open communication between adolescents and the community at large regarding unwanted pregnancies; not so in South Carolina. A gap exists in the United States between policymakers and the target population, and most informants state that this gap contributes to the relative lack of public support and the weakness of special-interest groups lobbying for prenatal care. Quite the opposite exists in the Netherlands. Political support is apathetic and inconsistent in South Carolina, yet is supportive, consistent, and proactive in the Netherlands.

Bringing Policy to the Classroom

It is exciting to watch students as they develop skills relating to the process of policy analysis. It is not uncommon to hear at the beginning of the semester that students do not necessarily like what they are seeing and hearing in the workplace, but they feel powerless to do anything about it except on a one-to-one basis with their patients and their families. However, as learners progress through the academic term and are required to go through various exercises relating to understanding and developing policy, educators can almost see a change in attitude about what they as APRNs can do to become significant actors in the policymaking area. Students in this faculty member's class are required to take on one health policy issue currently being discussed in the state legislature. They are asked to research the issue and identify what stage the policy is in (agenda setting, design, implementation, etc.), determine in which committee the issue is currently residing (to determine whether or not it is the right committee to address this issue), determine what and where the resistance is, research the resistance, and propose a solution or counterargument to the resistance. They are then required to visit with their legislator and present their position regarding the issue. These connected exercises help students identify an issue, learn about it to develop a position (by obtaining knowledge to support their position), and gain the confidence to articulate their position to a legislator. It is the challenge of meeting a legislator face-to-face that is often overwhelming. A majority of students cite this requirement as one of the most valuable skills they have developed in the program. Students have chosen fascinating topics, such as the effect of streetlights on a community, health care for the homeless, and the Medicare donut hole. In addition to studying local government, students are required to form groups and develop presentations related to a country of their choice and, using tools and policy factors, explore how healthcare policies are designed and implemented in other countries. Over the years, students have presented on countries around the globe, looking at wealthy, developed countries such as Canada, France, and Germany, as well as poor countries such as Nicaragua.

CASE STUDY 2: POLYPHARMACY PROBLEMS

Polypharmacy, a common problem in the United States' geriatric population, increases the risks of drug–drug interactions. APRNs and pharmacists are committed to providing compassionate, comprehensive, cost-effective health care that focuses on disease prevention, health promotion, and patient education, and the United States' elders need and deserve this quality of care. Some of the factors that exacerbate the problem include multiple health conditions requiring that multiple specialists attend a patient, the cost of medications leading to skipped doses, and use of multiple pharmacies. The use of computer-based recording might help reduce contraindicated drug use, but to date no national or state policies are in place to regulate and reduce the incidence of the practice of writing prescriptions that are inappropriate for use in older adults.

Discussion Points

1. Identify the goal of a policy written to reduce this practice.
2. What tools might be included in the design phase of the policy process to increase the probability of success?
3. What research from other countries could be helpful in addressing this issue?

CASE STUDY 3: TEEN PREGNANCY IN SOUTH CAROLINA

Concerned about the high rate of teen pregnancy in South Carolina (39.1 per 10,000 in 2011), five graduate nursing students (Philips, Bartee, Wittington, Voelker, & Coats, 2013) analyzed teen pregnancy using two types of criteria: evaluative criteria (to introduce values and philosophy into the policy analysis) and practical criteria (examining the process through adoption and implementation). In projecting outcomes, three alternatives were discussed: (1) do nothing (i.e., keep the current policy as it stands), (2) retain the current policy but add a mandate that addresses the issue, and (3) overhaul the current policy to address the issue from all sides. A detailed discussion ensued for each alternative that included economic and social attitudes and consumer behavior. Students began by looking at potential alternatives to address the social issue of teen pregnancy and subsequent economic and social implications, as well as the feasibility of government action and target group participation in each alternative. They delved into all factors that would potentially impact the outcome of each alternative. This comprehensive discussion is a very good example of how to set up a social issue and examine the issue and potential alternatives to policy success through the window of policy tools.

Discussion Points

1. Describe by example how tools and their underlying assumptions can affect the outcome of a policy to reduce teenage pregnancy.
2. Identify tools that might be included in the design phase of a policy to reduce teenage pregnancy to increase the opportunity of success.
3. Examine opportunities for healthcare professionals to work together in designing healthcare policies.
4. Analyze potential obstacles to policy success, and identify what strategies should be put in place to eliminate or bypass the obstacles.

Conclusion

As a component of advanced practice nursing, active participation in the policy process is essential in the formulation of policies designed to provide quality health care to all individuals. To be effective in the process, APRNs must understand how the process works and the points at which the greatest impact might be made. The design phase of the policy process is the point at which the original intent of a solution to a problem is understood and the appropriate tools are employed to achieve policy success. APRNs can be extremely effective in this phase as policy tools are considered and selected.

Discussion Points

1. Identify a health policy and the tools used by the institution/agency to implement the policy.
2. Using your understanding of the behavioral assumptions underlying the tools, predict the potential for success or failure of the policy. Identify policy variables that will affect success or failure.
3. Identify a policy (rule, regulation, etc.) that has been in use for several years, yet has had little success. Identify the variables that may be inhibiting success and offer possible solutions. Write or call your legislator to express your concerns (using data) and offer a proposal for revision. Explain why your proposal may increase success of the policy implementation and outcome.
4. How does the political climate affect the choice of policy tools and the behavioral assumptions made by policymakers?
5. Identify opportunities that are currently in place for APRNs to begin activity in policymaking.
6. Submit an article for publication to a refereed journal about a clinical problem based on the policy design process.

References

Bardach, E. (1977). *The implementation game: What happens after a bill becomes a law*. Cambridge: MA: MIT Press.

Bryan, A., & O'Byrne, P. (2012). A documentation policy development proposal for clinicians caring for people living with HIV/AIDS. *Policy, Politics and Nursing Practice, 13*(2), 98–104.

Central Intelligence Agency. (2009a). *Life expectancy: A comparison*. Retrieved from https://www.cia.gov/library/publications/the-world-factbook/rankorder/2012rank.html.

Central Intelligence Agency. (2009b). *Infant mortality: A comparison*. Retrieved from https://www.cia.gov/library/publications/the-world-factbook/rankorder/2091rank.html.

Cohen, M., March, J. G., & Olsen, J. P. (1972). A garbage can model of organizational choice. *Administrative Science Quarterly, 17*, 1–25.

Comer, M. E. (2002). Factors influencing organized political participation in nursing. *Power, Politics, and Policymaking*, 3(2), 97–107.

Dryzek, J. S. (1983). Don't toss coins in garbage cans: A prologue to policy design. *Journal of Public Policy*, 3(4), 345–368.

Ingraham, P. W. (1987). Toward more systematic consideration of policy design. *Policy Studies Journal*, 15(4), 611–628.

Kingdon, J. W. (1995). *Agendas, alternatives, and public policies*. Boston, MA: Little, Brown.

Leavitt, J., Mason, D., & Whelan, E. M. (2013). Political analysis and strategies. In: J. Leavitt, D. Mason, & E-M Whelan (Eds.), *Policy and politics in nursing and health care* (6th ed., pp. 65–76). St. Louis, MO: Elsevier.

Lijphart, A. (1977). *Democracy in plural societies*. New Haven, CT: Yale University Press.

Linder, S. H., & Peters, G. B. (1987). Design perspective on policy implementation: The fallacies of misplaced prescriptions. *Policy Studies Review*, 6(3), 459–475.

O'Grady, E. T. (2010). Rolling out reform despite political and legal challenges: The tug of war for public opinion. *Nurse Practitioner World News*, 15(11/12), 8–9.

Philips, J., Bartee, A., Wittington, R., Voelker., C., & Coats, R. (2013). *Health policy for nursing class*. College of Health and Human Development, School of Nursing, Clemson University.

Pressman, J., & Wildavsky, A. B. (1973). *Implementation: How great expectations in Washington are dashed in Oakland; Or, why it's amazing that federal programs work at all*. Berkeley, CA: University of California Press.

Roch, C. H., Pitts, D. W., & Navarro, I. (2010). Representative bureaucracy and policy tools: Ethnicity, student discipline, and representation in public schools. *Administration and Society*, 42(38), 38–65.

Safriet, B. J. (2002). Closing the gap between can and may in health-care providers' scopes of practice: A primer for policymakers. *Yale Journal on Regulation*, 19, 301–334.

Sardell, A. (1990). *The U.S. experiment in social medicine: The community health center program. 1965–1986*. Pittsburgh, PA: University of Pittsburgh Press.

Schneider, A., & Ingram, H. (1990). Behavioral assumptions of policy tools. *Journal of Politics*, 52(2), 510–529.

Schneider, A., & Ingram, H. (2005). *Public policy and the social construct of deservedness*. New York: Sage University Press.

Smart, P. A. (2008). Policy design. In J. Milstead (Ed.), *Health policy and politics: A nurse's guide* (3rd ed., pp. 129–155). Sudbury, MA: Jones and Bartlett.

Varone, F., & Aebischer, B. (2001). Energy efficiency: The challenges of policy design. *Energy Policy*, 29, 615–629.

CHAPTER 6

Policy Implementation

Marlene Wilken

KEY TERMS

Consensus: Collective judgment or belief; solidarity of opinion.

Deflection of goals: A type of maneuver used in policy implementation that creates changes in the original goals.

Dissipation of energies: Actions used by implementation players that can impede, delay, and/or cause the collapse of a program.

Diversion of resources: A type of maneuver used in policy implementation to win favor related to budget decisions.

Implementation of health policy: The process of putting a policy or program into effect.

Introduction

We have all been involved in situations where policy goals or outcomes were evaluated as successful, partially successful, or not successful. The relative success of a policy or program is heavily dependent upon what happened during the implementation process—that is, how the organization carried out the instructions indicated in the policy/program. The policymaking process is cyclical, dynamic, and imperfect. The process can be influenced by circumstances, events, and individuals. The preferences and influence of interest groups, political bargaining, and individual and organizational biases play a significant role in the policymaking process, especially during implementation.

After Congress passed and the president signed the Affordable Care Act (ACA) in 2010, it became the job of the U.S. Department of Health and Human Services and other federal agencies to implement the law, which is done mainly through the rulemaking or regulatory process. The laws passed by Congress are often broadly written, but the federal rules that interpret them are detailed outlines of how the laws will work. Agencies get their authority to issue regulations from laws (statutes) enacted by Congress. In some cases, the President may delegate existing presidential authority to an agency.

> Typically, when Congress passes a law to create an agency, it grants that agency general authority to regulate certain activities within our society. Congress may also pass a law that more specifically directs an agency to solve a particular problem or accomplish a certain goal. An agency must not take action that goes beyond its statutory authority or violates the Constitution. Agencies must follow an open public process when they issue regulations, according to the Administrative Procedures Act (APA). This includes publishing a statement of rulemaking authority in the *Federal Register* for all proposed and final rules. Congress may pass a law that directs an agency to take action on a certain subject and then set a schedule for the agency to follow in issuing rules. More often, an agency surveys its area of legal responsibility and then decides which issues or goals have priority for rule making. (*Federal Register*, 2013)

The politics that occurs among agencies related to implementation comes in many forms. For example, agency directors may reject taking on a program if the agency has little expertise to carry out the program objectives. An agency may choose to reject a program if it already has a full agenda of programs, especially successful ones, or does not have enough personnel or time available for another program. An agency not typically recognized as a "natural" site for a program may bargain with other agencies or policymakers to take on a program if it will bring an infusion of new money or if the new program will provide added prestige or visibility.

Successful implementation requires that the actors, organizations, procedures, and techniques work together to put the adopted policies into effect to attain the policy/program goals.

Implementation Research

The body of work in implementation research in health care is growing, including research that provides information about factors influencing nursing's implementation of evidence into practice. Implementation science research provides evidence of factors affecting implementation of evidence-based practice (EBP) and best practice guidelines that are cost effective and improve the quality of patient care and service delivery in the healthcare system. Organizations that want to make EBP and best practice guidelines the norm in practice need to be aware of complex and varied challenges for successful implementation. Factors affecting successful and unsuccessful implementation occur at three general levels: individual, organizational, and environmental. Further factors affecting implementation include the healthcare system; the practice, educational, social, and political environments; the practitioner; and the patient (Haines, Kuruvila, & Borchert, 2004).

Implementation is a social process involving change at the individual and organizational levels. Research to gain understanding of the interplay between the individual and the organization as it relates to behavior change is limited. Theories from the social and behavioral sciences provide frameworks to help address implementation challenges. A Consolidated Framework for Implementation Research (CFIR) was developed for advancing implementation science (Damschroder et al., 2009). The CFIR provides a pragmatic structure for identifying potential influences on implementation and organizing findings across studies. The CFIR also is used to complement process theories that guide how implementation should be planned, organized, and scheduled, and impact theories to develop hypotheses about how implementation activities will facilitate a desired change (Damschroder et al., 2009).

Research leading to the CFIR included a synthesis of 76 studies using social cognitive theories of behavior change related to implementation. The synthesis found that the Theory of Planned Behavior (TBP) model was most often used for intention and predicting the clinical behavior of health professionals (Damschroder et al., 2009). Essential activities of the implementation process common across organizational change models included planning, engaging, executing, reflecting, and evaluating.

The work of Ploeg, Davies, and colleagues (2007) offers the perceptions of administrators, staff, and project leaders about factors influencing implementation of nursing best practice guidelines at the individual, organizational, and environmental levels. The factors that helped facilitate implementation included learning about the guideline through group interactions, positive staff attitudes/beliefs, the presence of champions, support from leadership at all levels of the organization, and interprofessional teamwork and collaboration. In addition, financial support from professional associations and partnerships across agencies and sectors was important. The authors indicated that making changes incremental rather than radical helped facilitate implementation (Ploeg et al., 2007).

Barriers included negative staff attitudes and beliefs, limited integration of the guideline recommendations into organizational structure, and process, with the most common examples being inadequate staffing for implementation activities such as educational sessions and lack of integration into the policy, procedures, and documents. Time and resource constraints for implementers included a heavy workload, being short staffed, and feeling rushed due to the short timeline imposed by the funder. Consideration needs to be given regarding what other organizational changes might be occurring at the broader system level at the time of implementation. The findings suggest that factors influencing implementation are interlinked in complex ways not yet fully understood and are consistent with theoretical models that show the process of integrating research to be nonlinear, with complex interconnected relationships that are linked both vertically and horizontally among individuals, the environment, and the innovation (Ploeg et al., 2007).

Health care is big business, and the financial implications of implementing quality improvements are not well understood. Healthcare organizations are reluctant to support implementation of quality improvement unless it is accompanied by better payment or improved margins, or at least equal compensation. Until the reward for future benefits can be clearly identified, the current payment mechanisms will continue to reimburse for inferior health care (Leatherman, 2003).

The implementation process is a participatory endeavor that implies action and has start and end points. Health policies reflect the mix of public interest and self-influence, and often involve the choice of who will get health care and how, when, and where the health care will be delivered. Implementation is about who participates, the actors and organizations; why and how they participate, including procedures and techniques that reflect command, control, and incentives; and with what effect, meaning the extent to which the program goals were supported—the output and the measurable change (the outcome). The success or failure of implementation is judged against the specific policy goals. Hill and Hupe (2002) suggest that implementation should be considered in the context of organizational behavior or management. "Seldom is there a perfect fit between the problem defined by the policy makers, the design of the policy aimed at alleviating the problem, and the implementation delivered by the policy" (p. 5).

Knowing that policy implementation is imperfect, that it is almost impossible to separate policies from politics, and that many things can happen to impede successful implementation helps us appreciate why the U.S. public feels frustrated with government. The frustration is the perceived failure of government to turn promise into performance. Nurses are positioned to play a prominent role as healthcare reform is implemented in each state. The implementation of healthcare laws and policies can change the physical environment in which people live and work, affect behavior, affect human biology, and influence the availability and accessibility of health services (Longest, 2010). Nurses must be engaged in the implementation process because we all benefit from the nurse's voice; if our voice is missing, the American people lose.

Implementation: The Process

Variables

Implementation of health policy occurs when an individual, group, or community puts policy into use. Policies come in many forms: some are statutory and are the result of legislative enactment or permanent rule; others are nonstatutory in origin such as procedural manuals and institutional guidelines. Implementation of health policy is an essential part of effective, comprehensive client care for many documentable reasons. Successful implementation depends heavily on the manipulation of many variables. The extent of compliance with a policy is a frequently used measure of the success of the policy's implementation. During implementation, problem identification and problem solving occur in a cyclical pattern with a myriad of variables in play at any one time. The variables include private agencies and groups that are often contractors for carrying out policies; the target groups themselves; public attitudes; resources; the commitment and leadership of officials; and the socioeconomic, cultural, and political conditions in the environment in which policies are supposed to operate (Palumbo, Calista, & Policy Studies Organization, 1990). The presumption that once regulations and policies are enacted they are largely followed turns out to be unwarranted in many cases. The conscious or unconscious refusal to follow the policy directives can result in noncompliance, making the implementation process far from what the policymakers envisioned.

Control is at the core of actions taken by implementers. Control can be exercised in a variety of ways with the end result being decisions about withholding or delivering elements of the policy. Types of maneuvers that may occur during implementation include (1) **diversion of resources**, (2) **deflection of goals**, and (3) **dissipation of energies** (Bardach, 1977). The diversion of resources manifests itself in several ways. Organizations and individuals who receive government money tend to provide less in the way of exchange for services for that money. Playing the budget game is another diversion. Persons responsible for the budget do what they can to win favor in the eyes of those who have power over their funding. Incentives shaped for implementers by those who control their budgets influence what the implementers do with respect to executing policy mandates.

During the implementation phase, goals often undergo some change resulting in the second type of maneuver—deflection of goals. The change in the goals can be the result of (1) some feeling that the original goals were too ambiguous or too specific, (2) goals that were based on a weak **consensus**, (3) goals that were not thought out sufficiently, (4) an organization that realizes the program will impose a heavy workload, (5) a program that takes the organization into controversy, or (6) required tasks that are too difficult for the workers to perform. The agency will try to shift certain unattractive elements to different agencies. If nobody wants the responsibility, consumers get the runaround and each agency involved can claim it is not their problem (Bardach, 1977).

The third maneuver—dissipation of energy—wastes a great deal of the implementers' time. The dissipation of energy occurs when implementers avoid responsibility, defend themselves against others, and set themselves up for advantageous situations. Some may use their power to slow or stall the progress of the program until their own terms are met. This action can lead to delay, withdrawal of financial and political support, or the total collapse of a program. Public service workers, often referred to as "street-level bureaucrats," function as policy decision makers as they wield their considerable discretion in the day-to-day implementation of public programs.

There is little in the implementation literature to address how to improve compliance and minimize the types of maneuvers that implementers may use throughout the implementation process. Actions mentioned that may address these issues include building staff capacity to detect and correct noncompliant actions and having staff work with individuals to induce compliance (Deleon & Deleon, 2002).

The majority of problems that interfere with policy implementation are people problems, referring to those individuals who interact with the recipients of the policy or program. Personal attitudes and perceptions come into play during policy implementation. Nurses are often implementers faced with many of the dilemmas that can occur when interacting with clients. Implementers practice coping strategies such as negotiation and may find themselves in circumstances not foreseen or being confronted with rules that are often vague but within which they are compelled to act. They see themselves required to interpret the policy involved in a creative but justifiable way. Sometimes they are working with scarce resources. How often have you heard someone say, or even thought to yourself, "If they would just come down here and see how it is in the real world they wouldn't make policies that are impossible to carry out!" As a result, implementers may decide to alter the policy/procedure based on their perception of shortcomings in the policy. These perceptions of policy shortcomings may be based on a desire to enhance their professionalism, strengthen leadership, and perhaps restructure their organization (Hill & Hupe, 2002).

Implementing policies in ways that please everyone involved is incredibly difficult. When the results of a policy are determined to be disappointing or even worse, administrators are often quick to blame the implementers. When policymakers find out that the policy they wrote yields disappointing results, they may be inclined to take additional measures in hopes of ensuring tighter control. Both policymakers and administrators may add more (internal) rules and regulations. Successful policy can lead to more of the same policies with the idea that if this policy worked well, adding more policies may further improve implementation.

Gaps

Scholars of policy implementation offer reasons why gaps occur in policy implementation and result in less than optimal policy success; others offer recommendations to policymakers to help ensure policy success. The following list is a summary of the key elements to be considered when making policy and examining policy implementation. Think about a policy or program you have been involved in. Did it turn out the way you thought it would or should? Were there gaps in the implementation process that had an impact on outcomes? Take a look at the following list and see if you can identify with any of the reasons for implementation success or failure (Mazmanian & Sabatier, 1983, cited in Hill & Hupe, 2002):

1. Policy needs to be relevant, feasible, and based on sound theory with appropriate rationale that will correctly identify the design conditions and desired effect of the target groups.
2. Policy objectives need to be clear and consistent or, at a minimum, identify criteria for resolving goal conflict.
3. Policy should provide the persons in charge of implementation sufficient jurisdiction and leverage points over the target groups to help reach the desired goals.
4. Policy must maximize the likelihood that the implementing officials and target groups have sufficient resources to comply.
5. Policy needs to be examined periodically to ensure there is ongoing support from outside and within the agency/organization and that conditions have not changed over time that affect implementation.

Successful implementation depends on the fit between the organization and the objectives of the policies it must implement. "Fit is determined by whether (1) the organization is sympathetic to the policy's goals and objectives and (2) the organization has the necessary resources—authority, money, personnel, status or prestige, information and expertise, technology, and physical facilities and equipment to implement the policy effectively" (Longest, 2010, p. 135).

Finally, when policy implementation is examined or evaluated, one question that begs discussion is the notion of what is considered acceptable compliance? Is 100-percent compliance realistic? If not, what measures need to be taken to get closer to an acceptable compliance rate? Does the policy need to be reexamined? What are the implementers doing and reporting? Is this a policy, person, or systems problem? Do the measures of success need to be reconsidered or redefined? See **Exhibit 6-1**.

Exhibit 6-1   Policy Implementation Variables Related to the Affordable Care Act

The Patient Protection and Affordable Care Act (ACA), signed into law on March 23, 2010, allowed states to be largely responsible for implementation of both Medicaid expansion and private insurance coverage. The expectation was that governors and legislators would start working on how to implement the law that went into effect on October 1, 2013. Gawande (2013) indicated that some states worked toward the faithful implementation of the law, whereas other states worked to obstruct its implementation. Currently 25 states have expanded coverage for Medicaid and 4 other states are considering it (Kaiser Commission on Medicaid and the Uninsured, 2013). "Obstructionism has taken three forms. The first is a refusal by some states to accept federal funds to expand their Medicaid programs. Under the law, the funds cover a hundred per cent of state costs for three years and no less than ninety per cent thereafter" (Gawande, 2013, p. 25).

The ACA offered flexibility in terms of how the states implement the health exchanges that provide individuals with insurance options. States can implement a state-run exchange with maximum control, a joint partnership federal- or state-run exchange, or defer their exchange to the federal government completely. Currently, 16 states are opting for the federal government–run exchange with the remaining states opting for state-run exchanges (Gawande, 2013).

The ACA enables local health centers and other organizations to provide "navigators" to assist individuals in enrollment. Historically, Medicare has offered this service and there have been no documented complaints. More than a dozen states, however, passed measures subjecting health-exchange navigators to strict requirements: licensing exams, heavy licensing fees, insurance bonds, criminal background checks, fingerprinting, and hours of coursework (Gawande, 2013).

Conclusion

Policy implementation is the stage of the policy process immediately after passage of the law. The relationships between rule-making and operational activities involved with implementation are cyclical. The series of decisions and actions that occurs during implementation will impact the extent to which the program goals are supported and the measurable change that occurs. In this stage, the content of the policy, and its impact on those affected, may be modified substantially or even negated. In analyzing this stage in the policymaking process, one needs to examine how, when, and where particular policies have been implemented. Problems with policy implementation are widespread. During the implementation process the various forces of individuals, groups, organizations, and sometimes governmental bodies are at work. These various forces may be trying to change the policy to meet their own needs and control a part of the implementation process. When the implementers are not working in concert to meet the intended legislative goals, the recipients lose. Remember, the entire nursing community and other health professionals can affect implementation in both positive and negative ways.

Introduction to Case Studies

The United States is in the process of implementing healthcare policies that will transform its healthcare system, and nurses can and should play a fundamental role in this transformation. The Institute of Medicine (IOM) *Future of Nursing* report provides key messages that structured the discussion and recommendations presented in the report, including (1) nurses should practice to the full extent of their education and training; (2) nurses should be full partners, with physicians and other healthcare professionals, in redesigning health care in the United States; and that (3) effective workforce planning and policymaking require better data collection and an improved information infrastructure. Nurses should participate in, and sometimes lead, decision making and be engaged in healthcare reform-related implementation efforts. Nurses also should serve actively on advisory boards on which policy decisions are made to advance health systems and improve patient care. The implementation of health policy is complex with a variety of actors and organizations involved. The power to improve the current regulatory, business, and organizational conditions does not rest solely with any one entity, but rather requires that all must play a role. (Institute of Medicine [IOM], 2010).

Federal and state governments have a compelling interest in the regulatory environment for healthcare professions because of their responsibility to patients covered by federal programs including Medicare, Medicaid, the Veterans Administration, and the Bureau of Indian Affairs. Congress, the Federal Trade Commission, the Office of Personnel Management, and the Centers for Medicare and Medicaid Services each have specific authority over or responsibility for decisions that either could or must be made at the federal level to be consistent with state efforts to remove scope-of-practice barriers. Stakeholders involved in scope-of-practice barriers at the state level include state legislators, elected and appointed state officials, regulatory boards, insurance companies, and professional organizations. Equally important is our professional responsibility to all U.S. taxpayers who fund the care provided under these programs to ensure that their tax dollars are spent efficiently.

Despite the successes that have occurred in states related to scope-of-practice issues, a variety of barriers continue to hamper APRN practice. Legal, regulatory, institutional, and cultural barriers prevent many APRNs from practicing to the full extent of their education and training, despite the research that indicated that APRNs are equipped to deliver safe, effective care (IOM, 2010).

Programs and funding authorized by the Affordable Care Act support a number of emerging models, including nurse-led clinics and the primary care medical homes. Emerging models of primary care emphasize comprehensive, patient-centered, safe, and cost-effective care. The new paradigm models focus on interprofessional collaboration and patient-centered, team-based approaches that should provide for the highest level of APRN functioning in the interest of the public good (Health Affairs, 2013).

The case studies presented in this chapter will reflect the three IOM key messages:

1. Nurses should practice to the full extent of their education and training.
2. Nurses should be full partners, with physicians and other healthcare professionals, in the design and delivery of health care in the United States.
3. Effective workforce planning and policymaking require better data collection and an improved information infrastructure.

CASE STUDY 1: THE IMPACT OF EVIDENCE-BASED PRACTICE ON PATIENT SAFETY, QUALITY, AND COST

Organizations that want to make EBP and best practice guidelines the norms in practice need to be aware of complex and varied challenges for successful implementation. Implementation science research provides evidence of factors affecting implementation of evidence-based practice (EBP) and best practice guidelines that are cost effective and improve the quality of patient care and service delivery in the healthcare system. Factors affecting successful and unsuccessful implementation occur at three general levels: individual, organizational, and environmental. Further delineation of factors affecting implementation is identified in the healthcare system; the practice; the educational, social, and political environments; the practitioner; and the patient (Haines, Kuruvilla, & Borchert, 2004).

Implementation is a social process involving change at the individual and organizational levels. Research to gain understanding of the interplay between the individual and the organization as it relates to behavior change is limited. Theories from the social and behavioral sciences provide frameworks to help address implementation challenges. A Consolidated Framework for Implementation Science (CFIR) was developed for advancing implementation science (Damschroder et al., 2009). The CFIR provides a pragmatic structure for identifying potential influences on implementation and organizing findings across studies. CFIR also is used to complement process theories that guide how implementation should be planned, organized, and scheduled, and impact theories to develop hypotheses about how implementation activities will facilitate a desired change (Damschroder et al., 2009).

Research leading to the CFIR included was a synthesis of 76 studies using social cognitive theories of behavior change related to implementation. The synthesis found that the Theory of Planned Behavior (TPB) model was most often used for intention and predicting clinical behavior of health professional (Damschroder et al., 2009). Essential activities of the implementation process common across organizational change models include planning, engaging, executing, reflecting, and evaluating.

The work of Ploeg and colleagues (2007) offers perceptions of administrators, staff, and project leaders about factors influencing implementation of nursing best practice guidelines at the individual, organizational, and environmental levels. The factors that helped facilitate implementation included learning about the guideline through group interactions, positive staff attitudes/beliefs, the presence of champions, support from leadership at all levels of the organization, and interprofessional teamwork and collaboration. In addition, financial support from professional associations and partnerships across agencies and sectors was important. The authors indicated that making changes incremental rather than radical helped facilitate implementation (Ploeg et al., 2007).

Barriers included negative staff attitudes and beliefs, limited integration of the guideline recommendations into organizational structure and process with the most common examples of inadequate staffing for implementation activities such as educational sessions, and lack of integration into the policy, procedures, and documents. Time and resource constraints for implementers included heavy workload, being short staffed, and feeling rushed due to the short time line imposed by the funder. Consideration needs to be given to what other organizational changes might be occurring at the broader system level at time of implementation. The findings suggest that factors influencing implementation are interlinked in complex ways not yet fully understood. They are consistent with theoretical models that show the process of integrating research to be nonlinear, with complex interconnected relationships that are linked both vertically and horizontally among individuals, the environment, and the innovation (Ploeg et al., 2007).

Health care is big business and the financial implications of implementing quality improvements are not well understood. Healthcare organizations are reluctant to support implementation of quality improvement unless it is accompanied by better payment or improved margins, or at least equal compensation. Until the

(continues)

reward for future benefits can be clearly identified, the current payment mechanisms will continue to reimburse for inferior health care (Leatherman et.al., 2003)

Incentives to change behavior for individuals and organizations come in many forms. Based on the research addressing implementation of cost effective, quality health care respond to the following scenario.

Discussion Points

Evaluate the feasibility of implementing an evidence-based practice or best practice guideline in your work site.

1. Identify how the proposed innovation will result in improved care.
2. List the resources, including interprofessional teams, personnel, and economic resources, you will need for implementation.
3. What are the financial incentives?
4. What nonfinancial consequences matter?
5. Who at your site would need education about EBP? What resources would you use to conduct the education?

CASE STUDY 2: VHA INNOVATIVE MODEL

In 2010, the largest integrated delivery system, the U.S. Veterans Health Administration (VHA), launched a program to create patient-centered medical homes (PCMHs). The model organizes care around an interdisciplinary team of providers who work together to increase access and clinical effectiveness by identifying and removing barriers to high-quality care. The interdisciplinary teams are called patient-aligned care teams (PACTs) and include a primary care provider (either a physician, nurse practitioner, or physician's assistant), a registered nurse, a licensed practical nurse (LPN) or equivalent, and a medical clerk. Together they share responsibility for managing patients with support provided by pharmacists, social workers, nutritionists, psychologists, and disease management coaches. The PACTs are encouraged to test and implement new approaches, especially those that increase access and efficiency, while improving transitions between inpatient and outpatient care settings and patient hand-offs to providers. The VA has further increased capacity by having team physicians and nurse practitioners take a consultative and supervisory role—overseeing the care delivered by other team members—so the physicians and NPs can spend more time providing intensive services to the most clinically complex patients.

Two demonstration sites were selected for the implementation of the PCMH. Both demonstration sites focused on similar objectives: increasing continuity; enhancing patient engagement and satisfaction; improving the management, access, and coordination of the designated patient population; and advancing clinical improvement. In addition, both sites emphasized the importance of reassigning tasks normally handled by physicians to supporting team members.

In 2013, the U.S. Department of Veterans Affairs (DVA) was slated to implement a new policy for system-wide implementation that allows all APRNs who meet certain criteria to practice to the full extent of their education and training without direct physician supervision, even in states that do not recognize APRNs as independent practitioners.

The case study report by the Commonwealth Fund indicates that implementing the PCMH model has required extensive trust-building exercises to help physicians relinquish some control over patient care, as have new methods for monitoring quality and efficiency to ensure that the sharing of responsibility for care does not imperil patients. Problems were revealed with internal communication, which were not a surprise to staff. One doctor stated, "Physicians and nurses had not met as a group for more than five years; instead, they had conducted their own meetings, which exacerbated tensions between the two groups as each tended to blame problems in care on the other" (Klein, 2011, p. 13).

(continues)

Discussion Points

1. What is the role of APRNs who work in PCMHs?
2. Describe how the role of the APRNs and physicians complement each other.
3. What communication strategies would you use to support collaboration among the physicians and the APRNs, and the APRN and the other PACT members?
4. List four tactics you could use to bring together all members of the PACT.

CASE STUDY 3: NURSE MANAGED HEALTH CLINICS

Nurse managed health clinics (NMHCs) are authorized under Title III of the Public Health Service Act. NMHCs are healthcare delivery sites operated by APRNs and staffed by an interdisciplinary team of healthcare providers, which may include physicians, social workers, public health nurses, physician's assistants, pharmacists, and physical and occupational therapists. NMHCs provide primary care, health promotion, and disease prevention to individuals with limited access to care, regardless of their ability to pay. NMHCs serve as critical access points to keep patients out of the emergency room, saving the healthcare system millions of dollars annually (American Association of Colleges of Nursing, 2013).

The Affordable Care Act Nurse Managed Health Clinics (ACA NMHC) initiative provides federal funding to support the development and operation of NMHCs. The purposes of the NMHCs are to (1) improve access to comprehensive primary healthcare services and/or wellness services (disease prevention and health promotion) across the lifespan; (2) provide these services in medically underserved and/or vulnerable populations without regard to income or insurance status of the patient; (3) serve as valuable clinical training sites for students in primary care and, specifically, enhance nursing practice by increasing the number of structured clinical teaching sites for primary and community health graduate nursing students; and (4) establish or enhance electronic processes for establishing effective patient and workforce data collection systems. The focus of the funding supports the training and practice development site for nurse practitioners and other disciplines to build the capacity of the primary care provider workforce (Health Resources and Services Administration, 2013).

Discussion Points

You are writing a proposal seeking funding to establish an NMHC.

1. Describe the impact that APRNs could have or have had on vulnerable populations including the uninsured, elderly, children, and rural residents.
2. Provide evidence that APRN practice has addressed healthcare disparities across the life span.
3. Develop a one-page talking points document that helps professional groups including physicians, physician assistants, pharmacists, and physical and occupational therapists learn about NMHCs.

References

American Association of Colleges of Nursing. (2013). *Home Health Care Planning Improvement Act of 2013*. Retrieved July 10, 2014, from http://www.aacn.nche.edu/government-affairs/2013-Home-Health-Factsheet.pdf

Bardach, E. (1977). *The implementation game: What happens after a bill becomes a law.* Cambridge, MA: MIT Press.

Damschroder, L. J., Aron, D. C., Keith, R. E., Kirsh, S. R., Alexander, J. A., & Lowery, J. C. (2009). Fostering implementation of health services research findings into practice: A consolidated framework for advancing implementation science. *Implementation Science, 4*(1), 1–15. doi:10.1186/1748-5908-4-50

Deleon, L., & Deleon, P. (2002). What ever happened to policy implementation? An alternative approach. *Journal of Public Administration and Research, 12*(4), 467–492.

Federal Register. (2013). *A guide to the rulemaking process.* Retrieved from http://www .federalregister.gov/uploads/2011/01/the_rulemaking_process.pdf

Gawande, A. (2013). States of health. *The New Yorker, 89*(31), 25. Retrieved from http://www .newyorker.com/talk/comment/2013/10/07/131007taco_talk_gawande

Haines, A., Kuruvilla, S., & Borchert, M. (2004). Bridging the implementation gap between knowledge and action for health. *Bulletin of the World Health Organization, 82*(10), 724–731.

Health Affairs. (2013). *Nurse practitioners and primary care.* Retrieved from http://www .healthaffairs.org/healthpolicybriefs/brief.php?brief_id=79

Health Resources and Services Administration. (2013). *Affordable Care Act nurse managed health clinics, frequently asked questions.* Retrieved from http://bhpr.hrsa.gov/grants /nursemangfaq.pdf

Hill, M. J., & Hupe, P. L. (2002). *Implementing public policy: Governance in theory and in practice.* Thousand Oaks, CA: Sage.

Institute of Medicine. (2010). *The future of nursing: Leading change, advancing health.* Retrieved from http://iom.edu/~/media/Files/Report%20Files/2010/The-Future-of-Nursing /Future%20of%20Nursing%202010%20Report%20Brief.pdf

Kaiser Commission on Medicaid and the Uninsured. (2013, October). The coverage gap: Uninsured poor adults in states that do not expand Medicaid. Retrieved from http:// kaiserfamilyfoundation.files.wordpress.com/2013/10/8505-the-coverage-gap-uninsured-poor-adults8.pdf

Klein, S. (2011). *The Veterans Health Administration: Implementing patient-centered medical homes in the nation's largest integrated delivery system* (No. 1537). New York: Commonwealth Fund.

Leatherman, S., Berwick, D., Iles, D., Lewin, L. S., Davidoff, F., Nolan, T., & Bisognano, M. (2003). The business case for quality: Case studies and an analysis. *Health Affairs, 22*(2), 17–30.

Longest, B. (2010). *Health policy making in the United States* (5th ed.). Chicago, IL: Health Administration Press.

Mazmanian, D. A., & Sabatier, P. A. (1983). *Implementation and public policy.* Dallas, TX: Scott, Foresman.

Palumbo, D. J., Calista, D. J., & Policy Studies Organization. (1990). *Implementation and the policy process: Opening up the black box.* New York: Greenwood Press.

Ploeg, J., Davies, B., Edwards, N., Gifford, W., & Miller, P. E. (2007). Factors influencing best-practice guideline implementation: Lessons learned from administrators, nursing staff, and project leaders. *Worldviews on Evidence-Based Nursing, 4*(4), 210–219. doi:10.1111/j.1741-6787.2007.00106.x

CHAPTER 7

Program Evaluation

Ardith L. Sudduth

KEY TERMS

Evaluation report: A compilation of the findings of a program evaluation study. Reports are presented in a variety of formats depending upon the needs of those requesting the evaluation. Common formats include written reports, electronic transfer, oral presentations with multimedia enhancements, films, and videos.

Outcome evaluation: Assesses the extent to which a program achieves its outcome-oriented objectives. It focuses on outputs and outcomes to judge program effectiveness, but may assess a program's process to understand how outcomes are produced.

Policy: A purposeful, general plan of action that includes authoritative guidelines and is developed to respond to a problem. The plan directs human behavior toward specific goals.

Program evaluation: Analysis of social programs using a set of guidelines to gain an understanding of how well the intervention is meeting the objectives and goals set forth in the program's design.

Program evaluation design: The method selected to collect unbiased data for analysis to determine the extent to which a social program is meeting its designated goals, objectives, and outcomes and to assess the social program's merit and worth.

Public policy: A goal-directed plan, developed by a governmental body that provides a definitive course of action or nonaction.

Qualitative evaluation design: Evaluation methods that help the evaluator to determine the subjective meaning of a program and its interventions to the individual participants.

Quantitative evaluation design: Methods characterized as the "scientific model" of collecting measurable, objective data, with an emphasis on explanation based on well-defined expectations and observable events.

Social programs: Solutions developed to help solve an identified problem in society.

Theory: An idea used to design a program and its interventions and to explain and predict broad phenomena observed after data analysis.

Introduction

Advanced practice registered nurses (APRNs) such as nurse practitioners, clinical nurse specialists, and others have become key figures in the provision of health care or in healthcare management of persons enrolled in government-funded programs. APRN involvement will continue to grow as the demand for high quality care grows in conjunction with the changes occurring in the healthcare system, changing demographics created by the aging of the baby boomer generation, changes in the demographics of immigrants, and a growing concern for the rising costs of health care at all levels of government. Nearly all providers of health care, including APRNs, are impacted in some way by federal, state, or local health policy as it is interpreted into regulations and/or programs. APRNs and other healthcare providers who are delivering care in rural or inner-city clinics are often part of a program sponsored by the local, state, or federal government. All healthcare providers participate in governmental programs when they work with Medicare and Medicaid participants. Programs funded by governments, nonprofit organizations, and most private foundations require that these programs be evaluated regularly to meet a variety of criteria, including ensuring that the program is being conducted as developed, that there is fiscal responsibility, that goals and objectives are being met, and increasingly, that the outcomes are examined. To assist the APRN to meet the frequently mandated requirements for **program evaluation**, this chapter presents some of the components of policy and program evaluation, including conditions of evaluation, ethical considerations, potential design choices, and a few suggestions for reporting the results and recommendations of the evaluation. Healthcare providers who engage in programs sponsored by governments or organizations might also find this information useful as they evaluate the component of the programs in which they are involved. However, this chapter will be written using the APRN as the focus.

APRNs are not strangers to evaluation. They have long used evaluation in multiple clinical and healthcare settings, including the evaluation of a patient's response to a nursing intervention, use of outcome-based clinical evaluations, or a self-evaluation for promotion, and so the transition to using these skills to evaluate a program is a natural evolution of nursing practice. Understanding the process of policy and program evaluation can help the APRN contribute to the evaluation of social programs by bringing the unique perspective of nursing practice. The federal government has had a long-standing healthcare **policy** of funding hospitals and health care for the elderly. It has also developed policies that have supported the funding of programs to prepare APRNs. Healthcare policies are constantly being modified, and changes in healthcare policy continue to be very volatile issues as the public and government have grappled with the multiple issues facing the nation, including access to care, provision of quality care, and the cost to provide care. Further evaluation will be needed as healthcare providers work to meet the obligations of (or suggest changes to) the Affordable Care Act. To meet the healthcare needs of a population or to help solve a social problem in the community, the APRN may decide to seek funding from a government agency, foundation, or other resource to develop a new or unique service. Funding resources, including governments and nonprofit organizations, demand that the evaluation process be built into the proposal for funding (Environmental Protection Agency, 2010; Fredericks, Carman, & Birkland, 2002). Often an APRN is selected to study the needs of a social group and plan the program intervention, write the proposal in collaboration with other interested parties, and work to develop the evaluation process. This is particularly true in small, community-based programs.

Policy, Public Policy, and Social Programs

To start the discussion of the role of the APRN in the evaluation of a social program, it is helpful to define policy. A policy is a purposeful plan of action or inaction developed to deal with a problem or a matter of concern in either the public or private sector. A policy includes the authoritative guidelines that direct human behavior toward a set of specific goals and provides the structure to direct action, including guidelines to impose sanctions that affect the conduct of affairs (Mason, Leavitt, & Chaffee, 2012, p. 3). Policies can be determined by the private or public sector that together can have a significant and long-lasting impact on communities and individuals.

Public Policy

A **public policy** is a definitive course of action, or sometimes a nonaction, developed by a governmental body that addresses public concerns or public problems (Dye, 2008; Price, 2012). It is directed at a particular goal and does not occur by chance. Public policy is determined by legislative bodies as they make laws, by executive bodies as they administer the laws, and by judicial bodies as they interpret these laws (Dye, 2008). It is important to recognize that public policies are a result of the politics and values of those determining the policy (Mason, Leavitt, & Chaffee, 2012, pp. 4–6). Governments create public policy by making decisions regarding a health issue, such as requiring children to be immunized before entering school. Governments also may act negatively by adopting a laissez-faire, or hands-off, policy and do nothing about an issue, and the decision to do nothing may be as important as the decision to do something. In either case, some groups will be affected. Public policy provides direction to assist decision makers. Consider the thousands of decisions made by the Food and Drug Administration regarding the safety and efficacy of consumer goods sold in the United States, including the safety of drugs and vaccines, as well as the safety, purity, and nutritive value of foods (Law, 2010).

Public policies may be considered to be either positive or negative. Most programs that deal with the welfare of children; provision of safe water, food, and drugs; and public relief in times of disaster are considered quite favorably by the general public. However, public policies can also have negative effects and create problems.

Depending on one's point of view and individual circumstance, changes in healthcare policy resulting from the passage of the healthcare reform bill in 2010 may have a positive or negative impact on the lives of Americans. Some parents are pleased that their young adult children can be added to the family insurance plan or that their children cannot be denied insurance due to a preexisting condition. On the other hand, APRNs may be concerned about the changes in Medicare provider rates that reduce annual market basket updates and require payments for productivity (Henry J. Kaiser Family Foundation, 2011). It is important that the results of policy changes are carefully screened for the multiple outcomes that can be a result of what may appear to be a positive change.

Although public policy is developed by government bodies and officials, it is often influenced by multiple nongovernment persons and environmental factors and develops and changes over time. For example, in the 1960s there was increasing concern about the accessibility of affordable hospital care for the elderly. Families, labor unions, physicians, and many others were instrumental in creating the Medicare amendments to the Social Security Act. Over the years, numerous changes have been made to the initial amendments, many lobbied for by the American Nurses Association (ANA), but the overall goal of the federal policy of ensuring access to hospital and health care for the elderly, and now additional groups of citizens, has continued.

Another important dimension of public policy is that it is not limited to a specific law or legislative proposal. Public policy is a dynamic, evolving phenomenon with an ability to adapt as the needs and desires of its citizens change.

Healthcare policy has changed focus over time. In the 1940s and 1950s the focus was on access to care; in the 1970s the focus became cost containment. Healthcare policy of the new millennium focuses not only on access, but also on providing quality care at the lowest cost, which is determined by outcome and impact evaluations. **Outcome evaluations** focus on the benefits a program produces for the people who use the program (Thomas, Smith, & Wright-DeAguero, 2006). Impact evaluations, an important part of an outcome evaluation, are designed to examine the long-term effects of a program, such as a training program that has improved the participant's life as well as potentially improving the quality of life for future generations (Center for Nonprofit Management, 2014). An example of a program with an ongoing impact study that has been repeated many times since its launch in 1965 is the Head Start Program, which over the years has had both positive and negative evaluations, depending on the questions being evaluated

(Puma et al., 2012). Excellent impact evaluation case studies are presented at the Agency for Healthcare Research and Quality (AHRQ) website (AHRQ, n.d.).

Trends in health policy will continue to be driven by major movements in the healthcare delivery system, which "is becoming more managed and consolidated, more cost and quality accountable, more consumer focused, and more communication and information technology driven" (Jennings, 2001, p. 224). Another driving force in the dynamic nature of healthcare policy is public opinion validated by the increasing number of public opinion polls. Public opinion polling has become more important in policy development as the public has come to believe that governments should be responsive to public concerns and with the decline in public trust in government decision makers (Blendon et al., 2011, pp. 1–2).

Media can have a significant influence on healthcare policy. A national radio program picked up a story from a local outlet about a Medicare Part D plan denying a senior citizen life-saving hepatitis C medications. After the national broadcast it was only a matter of hours before the administrator of the Centers for Medicare and Medicaid Services reported the agency had updated its treatment guidelines for hepatitis C and this patient's Part D insurance had agreed to pay for the medications. Only time will tell what future guidelines will be established for allowing patients to receive this currently expensive medication treatment (Knox, 2014a, 2014b).

Nurses can play an important role in the development of policies, including healthcare policy. The ANA Code of Ethics for Nurses added a provision that states that nursing is "responsible for ... shaping and reshaping health care in our nation, specifically in areas of health care policy and legislation that affect accessibility, quality, and the cost of health care" (American Nurses Association, 2001, p. 94).

Social Programs

Social programs are public policy made visible. After a problem has come to the attention of the appropriate governmental body, suggestions are made on how to solve the problem. If the matter is of sufficient concern to the legislative body and if the program has support, legislation is passed to authorize the development of the program and to fund it. Often, at the legislative level the goals and objectives of a program are only general in nature, allowing the specifics to be designed by the developers of the program; this provides some flexibility for development postlegislation.

During the 1980s and 1990s, federal legislators began to return control of some policies to state and local governments. This allows states to determine how to use the resources with only minimal guidelines from the federal government. This shift of authority has increased the complexity of social programs and their evaluation because the policies are interpreted by multiple stakeholders such as state legislators, county boards of supervisors, municipal governments, and sometimes nonprofit, community-based organizations.

Program Evaluation

A social program is the set of resources and activities that have been directed toward one or more common goals. The resources and activities vary from program to program; some can be as small as a few activities with a small budget and a staff of one or two, whereas others can be very large with extensive resource allocation, complex activities, and implemented at several sites or two or more levels of government.

Public policy has generated multiple programs intended to improve the lives of a broad range of citizens, including health, education, environment, and social services. Over the last few decades, this growth of programs at all levels of government has resulted in the need for program evaluation; the importance of evaluation has been underscored by federal legislation that mandates the process, as well as supplying the funding needed to meet the evaluation requirements. The National Performance Review and the Government Performance and Results Act of 1993 (GPRA) were updated in 2010 to create a focus on the evaluation process: accountability, performance measurement, and results (Office of Management and Budget [OMB], 2011). States, because of funding matches with the federal government, also require that programs be evaluated. The need for evaluation and accountability is evident in many areas, such as the enormous outpouring of federal, state, local, and nonprofit dollars, expertise, and other scarce resources following the devastating natural disasters that have occurred in recent years.

Program evaluation follows a set of guidelines to provide information to assist others in making judgments about a program, service, policy, organization, or whatever is being evaluated (Centers for Disease Control and Prevention, 2011). Evaluation is used to examine programs to gain an understanding of it and how the human services policies and programs are solving the social problems that they were designed to alleviate (Sonpal-Valias, 2009; Westat, 2010). Some of the very practical reasons that program evaluation may be conducted include the following (Posavac & Carey, 1992; Westat, 2010):

- Determine the extent and severity of a problem
- Choose among possible programs
- Monitor program operations
- Determine if a program has resulted in desired change (outcomes)
- Document outcomes for program sustainability
- Account for funds
- Revise program interventions
- Answer requests for information
- Learn about unintended effects of a program
- Meet accreditation requirements

These topics will be discussed in the following sections.

Determining the Extent and Severity of a Problem

Evaluation designs are used to determine if a problem is severe enough or, according to opinion polls, important enough to a significant constituency to establish a program to help solve it. In today's world of scarce resources like time, money, trained personnel, and other valuable commodities, it is imperative that a well-documented program exists. Programs vie for resources, and the one that can show the best justification is the one most likely to be selected for implementation or continuation.

Choosing Among Possible Programs

Evaluation data may be used to help make difficult administrative decisions. Over the years, there has been an exponential growth in social programs; for example, in 2002 it was reported that there were more than 17,500 organizations providing youth programs (Lerner & Thompson, 2002). All of these programs must compete with multiple other social programs in a community.

Consider a situation in which several excellent social programs have been established and are functioning in a community. When a request comes to add another program, difficult decisions must be made in these days of limited resources. A city may be sponsoring a homeless healthcare clinic, an after-hours sports program for inner-city youth, and a lunch program for the elderly. When it becomes apparent that a program to deal with school violence may need to be added, it is possible that it can be added only if another program is eliminated. Program evaluation that provides systematic, reliable, and valid information will certainly assist the administrative staff in making difficult decisions. Unless there are good program evaluation data available, decisions are more likely to be made based upon perception, anecdotal evidence, or political pressure (Posavac & Carey, 1992; Royse, Thyer, & Padgett, 2010).

Monitoring Program Operations

The primary purpose of program monitoring is to systematically track and report on program outcomes using specified indicators, and then to provide feedback to the program stakeholders such as sponsors and the treatment team (United Nations World Food Programme, n.d., p. 9). In general, new social programs are supported by either authorizing legislation or private foundations. Rarely does the legislation or foundation specify in detail what the program should be or how it is to be implemented. The details of program design and implementation are left to the agency or organization that has the authority to administer the program. Demonstration projects are one example of programs that are frequently established to meet general goals and objectives. They focus on a new approach to solve a problem; if the demonstration project is successful, additional programs may be funded in other locations. Program monitoring is much easier when the program has been developed with clear and consistent operational objectives that allow for direct and reliable measurement and have been developed using sound evidence-based rationale. The results of monitoring the program can help program managers pay particular attention to a specific performance problem or recognize outstanding achievements of the program. Data resources frequently used for program monitoring include direct observation by the evaluator, program records, surveys of program participants (and nonparticipants), social media, community surveys, and public opinion polls (Blendon et al., 2011; Norman, n.d.; Rossi, Freeman, & Lipsy, 2004). Some program sponsors have timely reports that must be submitted for evaluation, whereas other program sponsors will allow the recipient of a grant to alter parts of the program as long as the overall intent is not changed; for example, if a school APRN developed a program to teach teenage fathers parenting skills and very few boys were enrolled in the program, the sponsoring agency might allow the program to be expanded to include teen mothers.

Determining If the Program Has Resulted in Desired Change

Legislative bodies, most nonprofit organizations, and philanthropic organizations request feedback about the program to determine if the program has achieved the stated goals. Organization officials want to know if the desired change has occurred—in other words, what are the outcomes of the program? This has become known as outcome-based evaluation. Outcomes are those benefits the participant receives from participating in the program. The United Way of Greater Richmond and Saint Petersburg (n.d.), for example, provides guidelines on the Web for determining best practices and conducting outcome-based evaluation

Documenting Outcomes for Program Sustainability

Periodic evaluation of the social program, including management, program outcomes, and financial solvency, becomes essential when a program has been designed to be maintained over a long period of time. Many programs sponsored by governments and other resources provide startup money, but with the expectation that the program will be designed so that the community, other interested parties, or the program itself will generate the financial, personnel, and other resources to keep it running long after the initial grant money has been used (LaPelle, Zapka, & Ockene, 2006). To ensure additional funding from the same source, or to enable a program to seek additional funding from different government or private agencies, the viability of the program must be established (Wallace, 2003). It is also wise for the staff to cultivate positive political and public support for the program. Keeping interested persons fully informed of the achievements of the program requires additional work by the program staff, but it may be very important in retaining the funding and other support needed to sustain the program. The program staff, including the APRN, cannot assume that political or public support will be there just because the program is doing a good job (Substance Abuse and Mental Health Services Administration [SAMHSA], 2012).

Accounting for Funds

Grant applications submitted to governmental resources and private foundations require that the program develop methods to ensure that the money being spent on the program is used as directed in the grant. Most government grants require that at least an annual audit report be submitted regarding the use of funds. Some sponsoring governmental groups will make site visits to review financial records and to ensure that everything documented can be verified. Other grant rules allow for the recipients of the grant to alter the use of funds with special permission from the granting agency, and some grants allow the principal program administrator to discuss the needs verbally, which should be followed by written documentation of the request according to the agency policies and procedures.

Revising Program Interventions

Program evaluation provides valuable feedback that can be used to make necessary revisions. Often, several months or years can elapse between the development of an idea for a program and the receipt of funding or other resources, and as time elapses situations change; personnel are recruited with differing backgrounds, personalities, strengths, and weaknesses, or the program is administered differently from the original design. It is important to evaluate periodically to ensure that the program is progressing as designed and, if change is needed, that revisions are made appropriately.

An excellent example of an intervention requiring revision occurred when a cost-effectiveness evaluation was conducted on a program for preventing perinatal human immunodeficiency virus (HIV) transmission (Stoto, 2001). Based on clinical trials published in 1994 that indicated that proper treatment of HIV in the mother could reduce perinatal transmission, specialists in preventive medicine and public health recommended counseling all women at risk of acquired immune deficiency syndrome (AIDS) on the benefits of universal and voluntary testing. This intervention was successful, but in 1996 Congress instructed the Institute of Medicine (IOM) to evaluate how successful states had been in reducing perinatal HIV transmission. Data revealed that only about 60 to 94 percent of women were offered HIV testing during pregnancy. After careful cost–benefit analysis, the IOM concluded that universal testing was cost effective and was the best intervention for preventing HIV transmission in the perinatal period. In 1999, the American College of Obstetricians and Gynecologists and the American Academy of Pediatrics issued a joint statement that adopted the universal testing approach of the IOM (Centers for Disease Control and Prevention, 2001). The Centers for Disease Control and Prevention (CDC) recommends universal HIV testing for all pregnant women using an opt-out approach rather than an opt-in approach, which leaves testing a voluntary decision by the pregnant woman (Delaware HIV Consortium Policy Committee and Planning Council, 2010). With the success of the opt-out approach with pregnant women, the state of Delaware in 2012 passed legislation that added HIV testing to the standard battery of tests using the opt-out approach for all individuals (State of Delaware, 2012). This example demonstrates how evaluation can alter interventions and make a difference in a health policy.

Answering Requests for Information

Program evaluation and careful maintenance of records enable the project director to more easily manage the large number of documents required by governmental agencies funding a social program. Periodic evaluation, along with meticulous recordkeeping, can provide a ready source for the data required; otherwise, the person completing the surveys may find that he or she will be required to spend many hours doing a search, either manually or digitally, through the program files.

Learning About Unintended Effects of the Program

Unintended effects are "unexpected effects that result from the politics surrounding a policy or the development and implementation of a policy" (Porche, 2012, p. 3). Program evaluations can help discover any unintended effects of an intervention. Program evaluations are particularly valuable when systems have been built to detect unanticipated and unwanted outcomes of the treatment intervention (Posavac & Carey, 1992).

Meeting Accreditation Requirements

Many healthcare facilities are required to evaluate their services to meet accreditation criteria, which usually have been authorized by legislation. Although meeting these standards may not predict the effectiveness of the programs offered, it does imply that the program meets the standards set by an official accrediting body, which serves to increase public trust. APRNs in their more advanced roles as nurse practitioners, clinical specialists, and the like often are asked to assume a key role in preparing the accreditation self-report and to ensure that the agency and its programs meet the standards.

Theory and Ethics: Valuable Tools in Evaluation

The use of **theory** in program evaluation provides a map to guide the evaluation process. Theory is defined in research and scientific inquiry as a set of interrelated concepts that explain and predict broad phenomena, whereas a concept is an abstract idea about a part of the phenomenon. The concepts may include definitions, empirical facts, or propositions that help explain and predict the phenomena observed. An ideal evaluation theory would describe and justify why certain evaluation practices lead to specific results across the many situations that program evaluators must confront (Shadish, Cook, & Leviton, 1995).

Program evaluation, by its very nature, evokes a sense of anxiety in most people who are in some way vulnerable. Questions are asked such as: How does the program measure up? Are we doing a good job? What happens if the evaluator finds a problem with the program? Will the clients lose the service? From these questions, it can be seen that the role of the evaluator can create stress and the potential for ethical dilemmas for all involved in the evaluation process. Good program evaluation will plan for the potential of ethical conflicts and either develop strategies to avoid them or deal with the conflicts as they arise.

Potential Areas of Ethical Conflict

Ethical issues must be considered whenever an evaluation design is planned or an evaluator conducts an evaluation. Posavac and Carey (1992) identify several major areas of ethical concern that include (1) the protection of the people treated, (2) the danger of role conflicts by providers, (3) threats to the quality of the evaluation, and (4) the discovery of any negative effects resulting from the evaluation. Put into a slightly different context by Sieber (1980), ethical dilemmas occur in three major areas: (1) conflict among the roles of researcher, administrator, and advocate; (2) conflict between the right to know and the right to privacy; and (3) conflict among the demands of the evaluator, political officials, and/or other significant stakeholders. In recent years it has become imperative to consider cultural differences between the evaluator and the individuals using the services of the program to reduce the potential for cultural conflict (American Evaluation Association, 2011).

Nurses have long recognized the need for ethical nursing care and developed a code of ethics that explicitly states the nurse's primary commitment "is to the patient, whether an individual, family, group, or community" (American Nurses Association, 2001). The newest code reflects on the importance of the nurse's responsibility to participate as an equal in ethical debates.

Protection from Harm: An Ethical Priority

A central ethical concern is that the evaluation should not harm the participant or anyone else involved in the program. One of the first areas of evaluation is to determine if the program does any harm to someone receiving the program's intervention or if the program harms the program staff in any way. For example, an evaluator must use the utmost care to follow the Health Insurance Portability and Accountability Act (HIPAA) guidelines so that program participants and staff do not have their privacy, anonymity, or confidentiality violated. Anonymity is often managed by the use of group data so individuals are not identifiable. If identification of the subject is possible, code numbers are used to protect the confidentiality and anonymity of the participant.

Informed consent is a recognized component of all care provided by the APRN and is a method frequently used to protect people from harm (Black, 2010). Participants in the evaluation process should be informed of the evaluation, told what it means, and offered a choice to participate or not (Royse et al., 2010). The APRN, whether participating as the evaluator or as a member of the program staff, should be certain that confidentiality and the privacy of participants and program staff have been secured in the design and implementation of the evaluation and its report.

The American Evaluation Association (2011) suggests that all evaluation protocols use approaches that are culturally appropriate to the situation; in some instances, such as when the participants have a concern about privacy or a have a low literacy rate, verbal consents may be appropriate.

Role Conflict: Potential for an Ethical Dilemma

There is potential for conflict at several levels in program development, implementation, and evaluation. The complexity of the institutional and political networks that have had to evolve in program development, funding, and evaluation is dynamic and has great potential for developing conflict and ethical dilemmas (Fredericks et al., 2002). People interested in the social program being evaluated may come from diverse groups, including the politicians who sponsored the funding legislation, the designers and recipients of the program, and supporting members of the community. These stakeholders may view the program very personally, as their "child," and may try to protect the program and the participants from outside scrutiny during the evaluation process and the sharing of evaluation results.

When the evaluator is also the administrator of the program, there is great potential for ethical conflict because it is very possible to have role conflict between the role of administrator and evaluator. The administrator's role is to ensure that the program runs smoothly with the least amount of interruption; the role of evaluator requires data to be collected to evaluate the program that may require record examination, interviewing recipients of the program, and discussing the evaluation with staff.

Objective Program Evaluation: An Ethical Responsibility

Program evaluators must try to provide the best, fair, and accurate description of the positive and negative outcomes of a program by selecting the methods and evaluation tools that are most appropriate. Making a mistake in accurately identifying the outcomes of a program, for example, might either allow the program to continue when it should be eliminated or, conversely, the program may be canceled when it should be continued. In both situations, the ethical dilemma is readily apparent.

Another area of ethical concern is to ensure that the evaluation design fits the needs of those who have requested the information (Posavac & Carey, 1992). If the evaluator cannot provide the answers needed, the evaluator must do the ethical thing and either decline to conduct the program evaluation or request that the evaluation tool be changed so that the evaluator can continue. For example, consider a program that has been designed to help people with diabetes alter their lifestyles to prolong their lives. At the end of 1 year, the APRN is asked to evaluate the program to determine if it has made a difference in life expectancy. This would be an impossible task; good program evaluation could not be designed to answer this question because 1 year is not long enough to determine life expectancy. To agree to conduct an evaluation to answer this question would create an ethical dilemma. A better question, albeit a very limited one, might be to request the evaluation tool be revised to determine improved disease control as measured by hemoglobin A1C, lipid profiles, incidence of delayed healing, and other such parameters over the 1-year period as a measure of improved self-care.

Reporting Negative Effects: An Ethical Requirement

An ethical dilemma occurs when the evaluator discovers that although many of the objectives of the program are being met, some aspects of the program may be having negative effects or may result in unintended consequences.

The question then becomes: How do you report these findings so that the data can be used by program administrators to alter the program? If the negative effect is judged to be serious enough that the harm outweighs the benefits, the program should be ended or revised.

Suggestions to Reduce Ethical Dilemmas in Program Evaluation

By the nature of social program evaluation, there is bound to be the potential for ethical dilemmas to arise. Some suggestions to reduce the incidence of an ethical dilemma include:

- The program evaluator can design an evaluation process that avoids ethical dilemmas. Good communication is essential throughout the evaluation process, but is invaluable when avoiding conflict, especially ethical conflicts. One suggestion is to establish written agreements among the evaluator, the program requesting evaluation, and any other significant stakeholders that have been identified in the evaluation design. A clause that provides a mechanism for either party to withdraw from the relationship should be included in case issues that cannot be resolved develop as the evaluation is conducted (Sieber, 1980).
- The evaluator must also be aware of his or her own strengths and weaknesses, as well as strong belief systems or cultural bias. An evaluator who firmly believes that all people who are homeless are lazy probably should not be the person participating in the evaluation of a homeless shelter.

Suggestions to Avoid Conflict

Program evaluation is complex and involves multiple stakeholders, who range from highly powerful political and social leaders to the program implementers and their support staff to the recipients of the program. All of the persons involved are interested in the program at various levels. Smith and associates (as cited in Clarke, 1999, p. 17) made five suggestions for program evaluators to help avoid conflict that are as applicable today as they were when first written.

First, recognize the potential for conflicts between multiple stakeholders and deal with them promptly and in a diplomatic, efficient manner. Attempt to identify the primary and secondary stakeholders.

Second, involve the multiple interest groups in the design of the evaluation study. If each group "owns" a portion of the design and is engaged as active participants in the process, there is less chance the varying groups of stakeholders will splinter off or create additional tensions in the evaluation process. Likewise, this approach recognizes the importance of each group and allows for compromises as needed.

Third, keep the multiple stakeholders and members of the evaluation team informed about the progress of the evaluation. It is easier to maintain cooperation among divergent groups if the groups are kept current with the project and are given the opportunity to provide feedback from their perspective. Communication may be enhanced by using technology to communicate the needs of the stakeholders and may be as diverse as a newsletter, email, Skype, wiki pages, or social media such as Facebook or Twitter.

Fourth, ensure that all stakeholders understand the goals and objectives of the program as they have been developed. This helps the stakeholders better understand exactly what the program was established to accomplish and identify the objectives that have been met, along with those that have not been met.

Fifth, identify the cultural, political, social, and organizational environmental conditions in which the evaluation is being conducted. These situational factors are important to understand throughout the evaluation process.

Program Evaluation Design Options

As discussed earlier, the environment in which program evaluation takes place often is complex and includes a large number of stakeholders who have been involved in some manner in the development and implementation of a social program. In designing a culturally sensitive evaluation, it is critical to the success of the evaluation that the stakeholders be involved in the process (Frierson, Hood, Hughes, & Thomas, 2010). In the past decade or so, designing, implementing, and evaluating programs that include a careful analysis of the cultural group that will be impacted by the social program has become essential. The focus of the social program will be much more successful if it considers all aspects of culture of the provider and the recipient (Frierson, Hood, Hughes, & Thomas, 2010). The American Evaluation Association (2011) cautions all evaluators that "evaluations cannot be culture free" (p. 3). The evaluator and the participants in a program bring their cultural belief system to the dialogue.

It is important to determine who holds the power to make decisions regarding evaluations, especially when there are multiple levels of stakeholders involved in the program. School-based programs are key examples of organizations with multiple stakeholders, all of whom interact with each other at varying levels. Federal, state, and local resources may be involved in significant ways, each level with their multiple layers of decision makers. When an APRN is asked to participate in the evaluation of a school-based health program, it is essential for the APRN to consider the personal and political priorities of the heads of the agencies sponsoring the program. Next, the school board and superintendent would be recognized as powerful decision makers. School principals, counselors, and teachers provide another layer of decision making, and parents have indirect authority because they can choose whether to allow their child to participate (Guzman & Feria, 2002). Students also influence the outcomes of the evaluation because they control the information that they share with the evaluator.

Early evaluation designs were based on a scientific approach that is founded on the principle of causation. The goal of **quantitative evaluation** is to collect sufficient data to rule out rival hypotheses by such means as control or comparison groups or by statistical adjustments (Fawcett & Garity, 2009). Quantitative evaluation methods seek to be precise and to identify all the relevant variables prior to the data collection. The method also seeks to minimize the role of the evaluator or data collector in the collection of the evaluation data.

As the complexity of social programs became apparent, additional evaluation designs were needed to determine how a program was affecting the individual recipients of the program interventions. Evaluation designs began to incorporate the **qualitative evaluation** approach, which has as its basis the belief that it is the quality or the subjective reality that has true meaning in the events, lives, and behaviors of individuals (Fine, Weiss, Weseen, & Wong, 2000; Polit & Beck, 2012). Evaluators using a qualitative approach attempt to seek an understanding of the meaning of public policy, its attendant programs, and interventions from the perspective of the recipients of the program, the staff, community, and other significant persons (Royse et al., 2010). Some evaluators find that combining the quantitative and qualitative designs allows for the best data collection and interpretation. To be successful in achieving an evaluation that is useful to the persons who have requested it and to be beneficial to the social program and its recipients, the design of the evaluation must receive careful planning. More detailed information regarding qualitative and quantitative designs may be found in many research texts. It must be repeated that **program evaluation designs** must be able to provide effective, culturally sensitive, useful, reliable, and valid information. Program evaluation also must be able to be conducted within the many constraints of real life, such as within the limitations of resources including time, money, personnel, and expertise.

Some down-to-earth suggestions by McNamera (2006) seem particularly useful to the novice APRN evaluator. His suggestions include the following:

- Don't fear evaluation—remember the 80/20 rule: The first 20% of the work will produce the first 80% of the plan, and this is a very good start.
- Remember that there is no perfect evaluation plan. Getting something done is better than waiting until every last detail has been identified.
- Include a few interviews in the evaluation methods. The stories provide powerful descriptions of the outcomes of the program.
- Don't review just successes—failures also give valuable insights into the function and outcomes of the program.
- Keep the evaluation data after the report has been written. These data may be useful as the program continues and changes over time.

Evaluation Reports: Sharing the Findings

After the social program has been evaluated, the results of the evaluation study need to be shared with those who have requested the evaluation, significant stakeholders, the staff of the program, the community, and/or sometimes the recipients of the program's interventions. Increasingly, **evaluation reports** are posted on the Internet, which allows for better access to the report by the public at large and the program stakeholders. A few guidelines suggested by Hendricks (1994) and SAMHSA (2012) for writing the final report help provide optimal information to those who have requested the evaluation and may enhance utilization of the report.

1. It is the responsibility of the evaluator to be the primary editor of the report and to ensure that it is presented in a timely, factual, unbiased, culturally sensitive, and appropriate format to meet the needs

of the program, its staff, and its sponsors (SAMHSA, 2012). Part of the evaluation plan should include plans for communication with members of the program and other interested persons. When possible, communication meetings should be planned and scheduled at mutually acceptable times and intervals. Evaluators must recognize that sometimes people associated with the program are fearful of the results of an evaluation; one technique to help alleviate some of the concerns of the key stakeholders is to provide an early idea of the results and recommendations of the evaluation. Face-to-face meetings or other means of communication such as conference calls, Skype, virtual meeting rooms, and the like can be used with the key players to provide valuable feedback among evaluator, program staff, and sponsors. After all inputs from the significant readers of the report are taken into account, a final report can be written.

2. Provide multiple opportunities for conveying the evaluation report's results. Some evaluation reports will be more useful if they are presented to multiple audiences. If the APRN has been selected to be the evaluator of a homeless shelter, the more audiences that can learn of the successes and areas of needed improvement, the more likely the APRN is to build support for the program. The APRN may seek to report to community groups, healthcare providers, city council members, and so forth to reach a larger audience regarding the results of the evaluation. Frequently, community projects need to keep many diverse interested groups informed so that they will remain supportive of a good social program that is meeting its goals and objectives. This becomes even more critical in times of limited budgets and available funding resources.

3. Reports should be succinct, with the major points presented clearly. Short, powerful sentences work best to grab the attention of decision makers (Jennings, 2003). The inclusion of an executive summary that gives a brief overview of the main findings and recommendations is appreciated (Royse et al., 2010).

   Reports should be written to meet the needs of the audience, including in the language that is best understood by the multiple stakeholders; therefore, there may be more than one report. For example, reports written for the sponsors and stakeholders may be best served by keeping technical terms to a minimum. Complex statistical interpretations may need to be simplified, depending on the audience. Detailed financial statements may be included for those sponsors that have provided money to the program; detailed statistical information may be needed if reporting to a group of researchers (SAMHSA, 2012).

It is wise to avoid using jargon, whether evaluation-related or technical, in the discussion because the readers of the report may not be familiar with the terms and tend to skip over the report without really reading it. A glossary of terms may be helpful to the readers. Many evaluators find that presenting findings in graph form is a useful method of communicating information in a condensed and visible way. Detailed additional information that is important to the total evaluation process may be put in appendices for those interested in a more complex and in-depth presentation.

4. Give direction and provide guidelines for action in the form of recommendations. The recipients of most evaluation reports want to learn about what is good about the program and what areas need improvement. Recommendations for action often are best received if the program staff reports them in identifiable, practical, and achievable terms. Unusual or unexpected outcomes must also be reported. If unusual outcomes are presented in a value-free, culturally sensitive approach, with several suggestions for change, the needs for improvement will be more readily acceptable.

The question can be asked: how specific should recommendations be? An absolute rule cannot be given to answer this question. In general, recommendations should always be presented as two or more options unless there is only one, very obvious, recommendation to be made. A specific topic with suggestions for the direction of change may be more effective because it gives those involved in the program direction and flexibility in choosing an approach or making a decision. It is also helpful if the suggestions include some indication of cost, acceptance, or the effects of the recommendations.

5. Use multiple communication techniques to disseminate results of the evaluation. Written reports may be delivered in printed or electronic formats. Videos, personal briefings, and community meetings are just a few examples of other methods of sharing the results of a program's evaluation. The technique(s) used should be appropriate to the audience or audiences.

Program evaluations may be used not only by those who have supported, developed, implemented, and/or utilized the program, but also by "policy entrepreneurs" who use the report as a resource to support new policy ideas (Cabatoff, 2000). A well-written report that defines the evaluation findings in clear, nonpartisan terms may be helpful to those engaged in seeking political support for changes in a broader public policy.

Conclusion

Advanced practice registered nurses, as well as all members of the healthcare team, have unlimited opportunities to participate in the development of public policy and program evaluation. Governments and the courts develop public policy via legislative bodies as they make laws, executive bodies as they administer the laws, and judicial bodies as they interpret these laws.

Although public policy is determined by governments, it is put into practice by the development of social programs. Most governmental and other agencies that sponsor social programs require that the programs be evaluated. Evaluation may take many forms, including studying the extent and severity of a problem, determining if the program is meeting its goals and objectives, conducting a financial audit, examining program outcomes and long-term impacts, verifying program outcomes, and seeking information about needed changes in the program.

The tools for evaluation include quantitative and qualitative methodologies that are carried out with rigor to meet the needs of the evaluation. Evaluation is expensive in terms of time, money, skilled personnel, and other scarce resources, so it is imperative that the evaluation study be done competently and efficiently to meet the diverse needs of multiple stakeholders.

After an evaluation has been conducted, the results of the study must be communicated. Some of the important principles of providing an evaluation report that is meaningful and useful include presenting the report to multiple audiences, providing multiple opportunities for others to learn about the evaluation report, writing the report succinctly with the interests of significant others included, giving guidelines for change, and using multiple presentation approaches when needed.

Evaluation of social programs is valuable and can provide very useful information to the APRN who is providing care through a funded or sponsored social program. Evaluation can present exciting challenges for any healthcare professional who participates in program evaluation and the presentation of the results.

Discussion Points

1. What are the advantages of having an APRN design and implement an evaluation of a healthcare program?
2. How might the APRN use the knowledge and expertise of members of the health team or members of the program staff in the evaluation process and dissemination of a final report?
3. Define how policy, public policy, and social programs may play a role in the APRN's practice.
4. List the reasons an APRN might be a participant in or conduct a program evaluation.
5. Under what conditions might the APRN use a quantitative evaluation design? Qualitative design? Combined quantitative and qualitative design?
6. As an APRN, what cultural considerations would you include in an evaluation as they apply to the stakeholders, including the participants?
7. Identify the conditions in program evaluation that might lead to ethical conflict.
8. How might the APRN avoid ethical conflict when participating in or conducting a program evaluation?
9. Draft a program evaluation report within the framework of the component parts.
10. Suggest several ways that APRNs might improve utilization of an evaluation report by the sponsors of the evaluation.

CASE STUDY 1: EVALUATING CLINIC SERVICES

The APRN has worked in a rural health clinic located in a small town of about 7,000 residents for several years. The clinic has been supported by a county tax and fee for service. The clinic provides care to a large number of individuals with Medicaid and Medicare and has a

(continues)

sliding fee schedule available for the uninsured. Due to budget constraints, county government officials are discussing closing the clinic to "get out of the business" of providing health care. The APRN has been asked to evaluate the services provided to determine if the clinic should continue to provide health care to the community.

Discussion Points

1. Where should the APRN begin?
2. What might be some of the role conflicts faced by the APRN?
3. How might the APRN gain support for the evaluation?
4. Who are the stakeholders? How should the APRN involve the stakeholders in the evaluation process?
5. What is the budget for the evaluation process?
6. Will the APRN get release time to conduct the evaluation process?
7. What type of research methodology will be needed?
8. Are there any ethical considerations that must be addressed prior to beginning the evaluation process?
9. How would you disseminate the report?

CASE STUDY 2: CLINIC: FOR EPISODIC OR CHRONIC CARE?

An inner-city clinic was established by a local, not-for-profit religious organization to provide health care for the poor and homeless at the request of the county government. It is located in the older part of town inhabited by the population that it serves. After a few years, it became apparent that the population served came only for episodic acute problems and did not keep follow-up appointments for chronic illness management. A study was conducted to evaluate this problem and identify possible solutions. The solution this agency chose was to offer only episodic, acute care to this population and refer them to university-sponsored clinics for management of chronic illnesses.

Discussion Points

1. As the APRN working in this clinic, would you agree with this decision?
2. What is the public policy that the clinic was established to meet?
3. Who should be hired to manage the evaluation?
4. Who will pay for the evaluation study? How should the data be collected?
5. What are some ethical questions that the board must consider when changing the mission of the healthcare clinic?
6. How might the funding of the clinic be impacted by a change in mission?
7. How will program success be measured in the future?
8. Who are the stakeholders?
9. How will the report be disseminated?

References

Agency for Healthcare Research and Quality (AHRQ). (n.d.). *All impact case studies.* Retrieved from http://www.ahrq.gov/policymakers/case-studies/All-AutoIndex.html

American Evaluation Association. (2011). *American Evaluation Association statement on cultural competence in evaluation.* Fairhaven, MA: Author. Retrieved from http://www.eval.org/p/cm/ld/fid=92

American Nurses Association. (2001). *Code of ethics for nurses with interpretive statements.* Washington, DC: Author. Retrieved from http://www.nursingworld.org/MainMenuCategories/EthicsStandards/CodeofEthicsforNurses

Black, B. (2010). Legal aspects of nursing. In K. Chitty & B. Black (Eds.), *Professional nursing: Concepts and challenges* (6th ed., pp. 60–76). Maryland Heights, MO: Saunders Elsevier.

Blendon, R., Brodie, M., Benson, J., Altman, D., Deane, C. & Buhr, T. (2011). Introduction: Public opinion on health policy. In R. Blendon, M. Brodie, J. Benson, & D. Altman (Eds.), *American public opinion and health care* (pp. 1–14). Washington, DC: CQ Press.

Cabatoff, K. (2000). Translating evaluation findings into "policy language." In R. K. Hoopson (Ed.), *New directions for evaluation: How and why language matters in evaluation* (pp. 43–54). San Francisco, CA: Jossey-Bass.

Center for Nonprofit Management. (2014). *What is the difference between process, outcome and impact evaluations?* Retrieved from http://nonprofitanswerguide.org/faq/evaluation/difference-between-process-outcome-and-impact-evaluations/

Centers for Disease Control and Prevention. (2001, November 9). *Revised recommendations for HIV screening of pregnant women.* Retrieved from http://www.cdc.gov/mmwr/preview /mmwrhtml/rr5019a2.htm

Centers for Disease Control and Prevention. (2011). *Introduction to program evaluation for public health programs: A self-study guide.* Retrieved from http://www.cdc.gov/eval/guide /CDCEvalManual.pdf

Clarke, A. (with Dawson, R.). (1999). *Evaluation research: An introduction to principles, methods, and practice.* London: Sage.

Delaware HIV Consortium Policy Committee and Planning Council. (2010). *Recommendations for adoption of routine opt-out HIV testing procedures for adolescents and adults 13–64 in health-care settings: White paper policy brief.* Retrieved July 29, 2014 from http://delawarehiv.org /content-positionpaper.html

Dye, T. (2008). *Understanding public policy.* Upper Saddle River, NJ: Pearson Prentice Hall.

Fawcett, J., & Garity, J. (2009). *Evaluating research for evidence-based nursing practice.* Philadelphia, PA: F.A. Davis.

Fine, M., Weiss, L., Weseen, S., & Wong, L. (2000). For Whom? Qualitative research, representations, and social responsibilities. In N. K. Denzin & Y. S. Lincoln (Eds.), *Handbook of qualitative research* (2nd ed., pp. 107–131). Thousand Oaks, CA: Sage.

Fredericks, K. A., Carman, J. G., & Birkland, T. A. (2002). Program evaluation in a challenging authorizing environment: Intergovernmental and interorganizational factors. In R. Mohan, D. Bernstein, & M. Whitsett (Eds.), *New directions for evaluation: Responding to sponsors and stakeholders in complex evaluation environments* (pp. 5–21). San Francisco, CA: Jossey-Bass.

Frierson, H. T., Hood, S., Hughes, G. B. & Thomas, V. G. (2010). A guide to conducting culturally responsive evaluations. In J. Westat (Ed.), *The 2010 user-friendly handbook for project evaluation* (pp. 75–96). Arlington, VA: National Science Foundation. Retrieved from http://coe .wayne.edu/engagement/theuserfriendlyprojectevaluationguide.pdf

Guzman, B. L., & Feria, A. (2002, Fall). Forces driving health care decisions. *Policy, Politics, and Nursing Practice, 3,* 35–42.

Hendricks, M. (1994). Making a splash: Reporting evaluation results effectively. In J. S. Wholey, H. P. Hatry, & K. E. Newomer (Eds.), *Handbook of practical program evaluation* (pp. 549–575). San Francisco, CA: Jossey-Bass.

Henry J. Kaiser Family Foundation. (2011). *Health reform implementation timeline.* Retrieved from http://healthreform.kff.org/timeline.aspx?gelid=CM3jhrOGtaYCFYtS2god01SzIg

Jennings, B. M. (2003). A half-dozen health policy hints. *Nursing Outlook, 51,* 92–93.

Jennings, C. P. (2001). The evolution of U.S. health policy and the impact of future trends. *Policy, Politics, and Nursing Practice, 2,* 218–227.

Knox, R. (2014a, May 12). *Medicare struggling with hepatitis-C cure costs.* Kaiser Health News. Retrieved from http://www.kaiserhealthnews.org/stories/2014/may/12/medicare-struggling-with-hepatitis-c-cure-costs.aspx

Knox, R. (2014b, May 15). *Medicare backs down on denying treatment for hepatitis patient.* NPR Shots. Retrieved from http://www.npr.org/blogs/health/2014/05/15/312828866 /medicare-backs-down-on-denying-treatment-for-hepatitis-patient

LaPelle, N., Zapka, J., & Ockene, J. (2006). Sustainability of public health programs: The example of tobacco treatment services in Massachusetts. *American Journal of Public Health*, *96*, 1363–1369.

Law, M. (2010). *History of food and drug regulation in the United States*. Retrieved from https://eh.net/?s=History+food+and+drug+regulation

Lerner, R. M., & Thompson, L. S. (2002). Promoting healthy adolescent behavior and development: Issues in the design and evaluation of effective youth programs. *Journal of Pediatric Nursing*, *17*, 338–344.

Mason, D. J., Leavitt, J. K., & Chaffee, M. W. (2012). A framework for action in policy and politics. In D. Mason, J. Leavitt, & M. Chaffee (Eds.), *Policy and politics in nursing and health care* (6th ed., pp. 1–18). St. Louis, MO: Saunders.

McNamera, C. (2006). *Basic guide to program evaluation (including outcomes evaluation)*. Retrieved from http://www.managementhelp.org/evaluatn/fnl_eval.htm

Norman, C. (n.d.). *Evaluation and social media*. Retrieved from https://www.ptcc-cfc.on.ca/common/pages/UserFile.aspx?fileId=120799

Office of Management and Budget. (2011). *Government Performance and Results Act (GPRA) related materials*. Retrieved from http://www.whitehouse.gov/omb/mgmt-gpra/index-gpra

Polit, D., & Beck, C. (2012). *Nursing research: Generating and assessing evidence for nursing practice*. Philadelphia, PA: Wolters Kluwer/Lippincott Williams & Wilkins.

Porche, D. (2012). *Health policy: Application for nurses and other healthcare professionals*. Burlington, MA: Jones & Bartlett Learning.

Posavac, E. J., & Carey, R. G. (1992). *Program evaluation: Methods and case studies* (4th ed.). Englewood Cliffs, NJ: Prentice Hall.

Price, L. (2012). Research as a political and policy tool. In D. Mason, J. Leavitt, & M. Chaffee (Eds.), *Policy and politics in nursing and health care* (6th ed., pp. 316–321.). St. Louis, MO: Elsevier Saunders.

Puma, M., Bell, S., Cook, R., Heid, C., Broene, P. Jenkins, F., et al. (2012). *Third grade follow-up to the Head Start impact study, Executive summary*. OPRE Report #2012-45b. Washington, DC: Office of Planning, Research and Evaluation, Administration for Children and Families, U.S. Department of Health and Human Services. Retrieved from http://www.acf.hhs.gov/sites/default/files/opre/head_start_executive_summary.pdf

Rossi, P. H., Freeman, H. E., & Lipsy, M. W. (2004). *Evaluation: A systematic approach* (7th ed.). New York: Random House.

Royse, D., Thyer, B., & Padgett, D. (2010). *Program evaluation: An introduction* (5th ed.). Belmont, CA: Wadsworth Cengage Learning.

Shadish, W. R., Jr., Cook, T. D., & Leviton, L. C. (1995). *Foundations of program evaluation: Theories of practice*. Newbury Park, CA: Sage.

Sieber, J. E. (1980). Being ethical: Professional and personal decisions in program evaluation. *New directions for program evaluation* (pp. 51–61). San Francisco, CA: Jossey-Bass.

Sonpal-Valias, N. (2009). *Outcome evaluation: Definition and overview*. Retrieved from http://www.acds.ca/PDF/Outcome%20Evaluations/MTD_Module_1_Outcome_Evaluation_Definition_and_Overview.pdf

State of Delaware. (2012). *Delaware SB 162: HIV testing now standard.* Retrieved from http://news.delaware.gov/2012/06/27/delaware-sb-162/

Stoto, M. A. (2001). Preventing perinatal transmission of HIV: Target programs, not people. In R. J. Light (Ed.), *New directions for evaluation: Evaluation findings that surprise* (pp. 41–53). San Francisco, CA: Jossey-Bass.

Substance Abuse and Mental Health Services Administration. (2012). *Non-researchers guide to evidence-based program evaluation.* Retrieved from http://nrepp.samhsa.gov/Courses/ProgramEvaluation/resources/NREPP_Evaluation_course.pdf

Thomas, C. W., Smith, B. D., & Wright-DeAguero, L. (2006). The program evaluation and monitoring evidence-based HIV prevention program processes and outcomes. *AIDS Education and Prevention, 18*(Suppl. A), 74–80.

United Nations World Food Programme. (n.d.). *Monitoring and evaluation guidelines.* Retrieved from http://documents.wfp.org/stellent/groups/public/documents/ko/mekb_module_10.pdf; http://documents.wfp.org/stellent/groups/public/documents/ko/mekb_module_7.pdf

United Way of Greater Richmond and Petersburg. (n.d.). *A guide to developing an outcome logic model and measurement plan.* Retrieved from http://www.yourunitedway.org/sites/uwaygrp.oneeach.org/files/Guide_for_Logic_Models_and_Measurements.pdf

U.S. Environmental Protection Agency. (2010). *General tips on writing a competitive grant proposal and preparing a budget.* Retrieved from http://www.epa.gov/ogd/recipient/tips.htm

Wallace, J. (2003). A policy analysis of the assistive technology alternative financing program in the United States. *Journal of Disability Policy Studies, 14*(2), 74–81.

Westat, J. F. (2010). *The 2010 user-friendly handbook for project evaluation.* National Science Foundation Directorate for Education & Human Resources, Division of Research, Evaluation, and Communication. Arlington, VA: National Science Foundation. Retrieved from http://coe.wayne.edu/engagement/theuserfriendlyprojectevaluationguide.pdf; http://www.westat.com/westat/pdf/news/ufhb.pdf

Online Resources

AcademyHealth: Provides links to health services researchers in health policy and practice. It fosters networking among a diverse membership. *http://www.academyhealth.org*

Agency for Healthcare Research and Quality (AHRQ): Provides links to multiple resources. The mission of the agency is to improve the quality, safety, efficiency, and effectiveness of health care for all Americans. *http://www.ahrq.gov*

American Evaluation Association: Free resources for program evaluation and social research methods. *http://gsociology.icaap.org/methods/*

Centers for Disease Control and Prevention (CDC), Program Performance and Evaluation Office (PPEO): Provides links to multiple resources for information or assistance in conducting an evaluation project. *http://www.cdc.gov/eval/resources/index.htm*

Free Management Library: Developed by Authenticity Consulting. Provides extensive online resources for program evaluation and personal, professional, and organization development, including many detailed guidelines, worksheets, and more. *http://www.managementhelp.org*

National Registry of Evidence-Based Programs and Practices: The focus of this site is on mental health. However, the module to develop and evaluate a program is well-organized, concise, and easy to read. *https://www.healthdata.gov/data/dataset/national-registry-evidence-based-programs-and-practices-nrepp*

National Science Foundation: The NSF is an independent government agency that is responsible for advancing science and engineering. In this role the NSF has developed multiple tools to use in the evaluation of programs that are applicable to a variety of programs. *http://www.nsf.gov/*

Social Media Information: A helpful resource that discusses how to use social media for evaluation and provides a website for training. The use of social media is increasing because it allows for interaction between the evaluator and the participants. *http://www.digitalgov.gov/category/socialmedia/*

United Nations World Food Programme: This resource focuses on the UN's food program. The site presents links to 14 modules providing step-by-step advice on monitoring and evaluation guidelines. A useful resource to review. *http://www.wfp.org/* and *http://documents.wfp.org/stellent/groups/public/documents/ko/mekb_module_15.pdf*

CHAPTER 8

The Impact of Social Media and the Internet on Healthcare Decisions

Elizabeth Barnhill and Troy Spicer

KEY TERMS

Asynchronously: Occurring at different times. For instance, a person can post to Facebook now, and a friend can respond at a later time. There is no requirement to be online at the same time for interaction to take place.

Big Data: The exponential growth of collected data. In health care, electronic records have tremendously increased the volume and speed of data collection. Current challenges include proper interpretation of the data and action taken for quality improvement.

Computerized provider order entry (CPOE): Electronic means of documenting patient orders that will disperse the information to the required areas such as pharmacy, radiology, or laboratory. Because the order is entered via the computer, illegibility issues and transmission delays should be minimized.

Data mining: Means of extracting information from an electronic document in order to gather individual information or aggregate the data for analysis and/or pattern identification.

Electronic health record (EHR): A computer-generated patient record with longitudinal information such as immunizations, allergies, and demographics of an individual that is designed to be accessed across healthcare systems. EHRs differ from the more detailed electronic medical record (EMR), which is an electronic legal record of an individual's specific encounter at a particular medical facility.

Electronic medical record (EMR): An electronic legal record of an individual's specific encounter at a particular medical facility. EMRs are more detailed than the longitudinal information contained in the EHR.

Healthcare literacy: The ability to search for and understand healthcare information.

Informatics: The study of information technology.

Really Simple Syndication (RSS): A means for a website to update information for distribution to interested parties who typically register to receive updates.

Superuser: An employee of a facility receiving new equipment, such as electronic documentation systems, who receives detailed, extensive training from the vendor in order to continue the training after the initial go-live phase is completed and the vendor trainers leave the facility.

Synchronously: Happening at the same time. For example, an online class that is synchronous meets at a specific time, with students and instructor logged on simultaneously.

Web 2.0: Also known as social networking and social media; an interactive way of communicating electronically as opposed to simply searching and reading posted webpages.

Introduction

Consider the widespread changes that have occurred relatively recently in how information is accessed and how people communicate. In just over 20 years, virtually all aspects of life, education, commerce, government, and the like have been changed by information technology. For instance, the original version of this chapter from 2013 contained information regarding Twitter as an example of new social media available at press time, but unfamiliar to many. At this writing, Twitter falls into the top 10 percent of websites in popularity (Statistic Brain, 2014). Moreover, new social networking sites such as Instagram and Tumblr continue to emerge. Keeping abreast of information technologies remains an ongoing challenge. The capacity to use technology has become a professional imperative for all healthcare providers, including advanced practice registered nurses (APRNs), as advances in technology are increasingly associated with how health-related information is accessed and used. In this environment of rapid change, APRNs must recognize the power of information technology in shaping the healthcare realm regarding both professional practice and healthcare policy. APRNs must adapt to these changes successfully.

Rapidly evolving technological advances in diagnosis and treatment have been wholly embraced by the healthcare sector, particularly in the past 50 years. Health care, however, has lagged behind other industries, such as entertainment, manufacturing, and transportation, in integrating advances in information technology into the fabric of the industry. Innovations such as *social networking*, a term often included in the overarching rubric **Web 2.0**, continue to accelerate the rate of change that influences APRN practice directly. The healthcare industry finds itself in the position of having to play catch-up. Even as the healthcare industry lags behind in taking advantage of healthcare information technology, healthcare information has nonetheless joined other types of Web-based content commonly created and used by the public. In the absence of authoritative sources creating sound content, a proliferation of questionable and inaccurate information has emerged. The challenge for APRNs is to take advantage of the information revolution in order to improve patient care and to continue to secure a voice in public policy.

To date, governmental policy regarding healthcare information technology has centered on security and access. Two important pieces of legislation that address and influence information technology are the Health Information Technology for Economic and Clinical Health (HITECH) Act of 2009 and the Health Insurance Portability and Accountability Act (HIPAA) of 1996. Both have had far-reaching effects on healthcare practice and healthcare information. With this legislation, along with other initiatives, the federal government in general, and the executive branch in particular, are taking strong positions regarding the promotion of patient safety, health-related information access, and health literacy among citizens with the objective of improving access to and the quality of health care (U.S. Department of Health and Human Services, 2011). From the APRN's perspective, successfully meeting these objectives hinges on the availability of and access to sound health-related information for both the provider and the patient.

Social Media: How They Have Changed Communication

Within the past 10 years, the Internet has evolved from a static yet immediate source of information into a more interactive entity. These innovations are described using the term *Web 2.0*. Web 2.0 is not a single application or platform, but rather suggests a new version of the Internet in which the consumer ceases to be like a patron at a library selecting discrete pieces of information. Instead, the user creates a personalized and interactive relationship with information and other users. This term is synonymous with the terms *social networking* and *social media*. Other expressions associated with social networking, such as texting, instant messaging, tweeting, instagramming, tagging, blogging, and skyping, have become synonymous with communicating. Because effective nursing is associated intimately with effective communication, becoming familiar with the "who, what, where, and how" of social media is essential for APRNs and their successful practices in the future.

What Are Social Media?

As social networking capabilities have expanded, the number and variety of sites have proliferated. Social websites such as Facebook focus on activities limited to friends and acquaintances (depending on individual privacy settings); Twitter and Instagram can include larger groups with more public access. Other sites concentrate on specific issues, such as WebMD for health-related information and LinkedIn, which connects professionals who have common interests. See **Table 8-1** for examples of social networking platforms.

Most social networking sites have multiple means of communicating information using media such as text, pictures, and video. Once the user accesses a particular site, different menu options can navigate the user to custom areas with specific interests. For instance, a search on WebMD for

■ Table 8-1 Examples of Social Media Sites and Characteristics

Website	Usage Statistics	Primary Purpose	Medium	Access	Capabilities
Facebook: http://www.facebook.com	1.23 billion active users (Facebook, 2014) 46.7%: > 34 years old 24.4%: 25–34 years old 23.3%: 18–24 years old 5.4%: 14–17 years old (Saul, 2014)	Social; support groups	Text and pictures; able to post videos	Both asynchronous and synchronous; various privacy settings available	Private chat; can leave private or public messages, blog; can post links to other websites
Twitter: http://www.twitter.com	Most users are 18–29 years old; minority use is greater than White use; increased use in urban areas (Bennett, 2013); almost 646,000 active users with 135,000 new registrants daily (Statistic Brain, 2014)	Social; posting updates, news, following interests	Short texts; can "drill down" to more detail with pictures and video	Primarily asynchronous	Public blog, can use screen name for privacy; messages limited to 140 characters; can receive updates via text messages
LinkedIn: http://www.linkedin.com	More than 277 million professionals from 200 countries and territories (LinkedIn Press Center, 2014)	Professional networking, career links	Text, profile pictures	Primarily asynchronous	Limits access unless permission from contact is granted; can create/join custom groups of professionals with similar interests/positions; can leave private messages for individuals

(continues)

■ Table 8-1 Examples of Social Media Sites and Characteristics *(continued)*

Website	Usage Statistics	Primary Purpose	Medium	Access	Capabilities
YouTube: http://www .youtube.com	> 1 billion views/month (YouTube Pressroom, n.d.)	Video sharing	Audiovisual	Asynchronous	Public forum
Instagram: http://www .instagram.com	150 million active users (Smith, 2013)	Picture sharing	Pictures	Asynchronous	Public, with ability to limit access with special privacy setting option
WebMD: http://www .wedmd.com	72% of Internet users pursue health information online (Pew Research, 2013)	Resource for health-related information	Text, pictures, some video	Asynchronous	Health information on specific disease sets; expert blogs; discussion groups; support

asthma information can reveal specific articles, expert advice, and interactive discussion groups geared toward this disease entity. An individual can then join a **Really Simple Syndication (RSS)** feed to receive instantaneous updates regarding asthma from WebMD or a host of other healthcare-related information sites. It is this ability to interact with and customize the Internet experience that is the hallmark of Web 2.0.

Who Uses Them?

With 1.23 billion active Facebook members and more than 1 billion daily hits on YouTube alone, social media has become the entertainment and information medium of choice for a multitude of people worldwide (Facebook, 2014; YouTube Pressroom, n.d.). A cottage industry has developed that studies user characteristics, allowing businesses to maximize their advertising dollars by sponsoring websites based on the demographics of their consumers (Bulik, 2009). Many politicians and public servants, realizing the significance of this widespread use, have started using social media as a means of communicating with constituents, campaigning, and fundraising (Dorsch & Greenberg, 2009).

Because of its universal accessibility, professionals who use social networking sites should proceed with caution. Dorsch and Greenberg (2009) recommend that personal and professional communication be kept completely separate. Bemis-Dougherty (2010) recognizes the advantages of using these sites, including the ease of communication with both colleagues and patients, but warns against violating patient confidentiality. Maintaining a professional demeanor by avoiding the temptation to vent is also paramount.

Speed of Communication

Posting information on social media occurs instantaneously, with most servers functioning both **synchronously** and **asynchronously**. With email alert options and increasingly sophisticated cellular phones with data plans, mobile updates can facilitate the speed of communication. This feature is a double-edged sword; however, important information can be posted immediately for the benefit of others, but once released, it becomes extremely difficult, if not impossible, to retract material because some sites, such as Facebook, maintain proprietary rights to all information (Bemis-Dougherty, 2010; Reid, 2009).

How Reliable Are the Postings?

Prior to the Internet and the advent of social networking, healthcare information was available through a variety of traditional sources such as newspapers, television, and journals (Nelson, 2008). The APRN had to be diligent in vetting the source of the material to ensure that it was reliable; analyzing information from social networking sites requires similar precautionary measures. The APRN needs to determine the origin of the content and understand that navigating different sites and following links can lead to unreliable information. Checking author credentials, dates, and the nature of the material (i.e., opinion vs. fact) is a basic guideline to heed.

Social Media and Healthcare Information: A Mixed Blessing

From a healthcare consumer standpoint, nothing may affect healthcare decision making in the future more than social media and the Internet. Everyone desires a more-informed healthcare consumer. The federal government has started a movement to emphasize the importance of improving **healthcare literacy** on a large scale (Benjamin, 2010; Institute of Medicine, 2011; Sarkar et al., 2010), and one means to this end is using information technologies. Government and industry leaders recognize that poor healthcare literacy and lack of access to appropriate information is a substantial impediment to creating a healthy populace.

Social media is an ideal venue for accomplishing the aim of improving healthcare literacy. Unfortunately, the sources and reliability of much of the healthcare information available on the Web in general, and on social networks in particular, are of dubious accuracy and questionable provenance. Information available to patients varies widely in basic readability (Pothier & Pothier, 2009). Due to the absence of a coordinated and concerted effort on the part of the government and the healthcare industry, the creation of timely, accurate, understandable, and efficacious information has been partially usurped by poorly informed, biased, or frankly mercenary sources. The Internet is full of websites that promote pseudoscience and quackery (Barrett, 2014).

In a 2012 survey, Pew Research (2013) found that patients are actively seeking and using information from the Internet and social networks regarding health care. Only 13 percent of patients start their healthcare information search on a site geared toward this topic, such as WebMD; the remainder begin their quest using general search engines such as Google and Bing. Obviously, using this approach affects the quality of the information ultimately retrieved. Healthcare providers, including APRNs, must be acutely attentive to the sources, quality, and accuracy of the healthcare information on which their patients rely. This will require an open dialogue with patients regarding the websites they are visiting. Better resources have developed and constitute an important source of information for patients, and legitimate blogs, illness-specific websites, and nonprofit websites all hold great promise in improving healthcare literacy and should be embraced by APRNs.

In the past few years, government and the private health industry have stepped up efforts to create sources of legitimate health information. MedlinePlus (2014), a government site, recommends checking the source of the website, determining if the research is subject to peer review, and ensuring that the information is current. Responsible purveyors of health information have taken initial steps to ensure better quality. One such effort is a nonprofit foundation called Health on the Net Foundation (HON). Organizations that meet HON's guidelines display the HON logo prominently on their websites (Health on the Net Foundation, 2014).

Consumer Uses

The first issue to emerge when discussing electronic information and social media is Internet penetration into U.S. households. According to the U.S. Department of Commerce (2011), Internet penetration into U.S. households is at best characterized as fair. According to Zickuhr (2013), 85 percent of people in the United States had broadband Internet access, a 17 percent increase over 2010. Disparities in access do exist, particularly with minorities and those who live in rural areas (U.S. Department of Commerce, 2011). Nonetheless, the Internet is an important source of health-related information for a large number of people (Fox, 2011).

One of the objectives of *Healthy People 2020* involves healthcare information technology and healthcare information strategies to improve health in both individuals and communities (U.S. Department of Health and Human Services, 2011). The premise is that technology and information have the power to influence the way society defines health and, as such, will be central to how the consumer and provider will negotiate healthcare decisions.

Explicit in these arguments is the declared objective to increase access to quality healthcare information via the Internet. A great deal of research demonstrates that poor health literacy is associated with poor health outcomes (Agency for Healthcare Research and Quality, 2007).

Consumers are already heavy users of Internet-related health information (Pew Research, 2013). Consumers are able to access a wide array of information from sources both legitimate and suspect. A variety of information is available to patients, including more traditional websites and articles, but there has been a rise in more interactive platforms that involve the exchange of information and opinion among people with like interests; these sites are in the form of blogs, discussion boards, and support groups. Some of the discussion boards are freestanding and some are associated with more established organizations, just as some are tightly moderated by experts in the field and some are more loosely monitored or not at all. Health issues, both common and esoteric, are addressed by these discussion boards. The quality of the information that is shared varies widely. **Table 8-2** offers a list of websites that are considered trustworthy and are geared toward consumers.

The introduction of social networking to healthcare venues and websites may be particularly helpful to those patients who are isolated due to physical or emotional infirmity or by geography. Support groups and interactive sites have the potential to overcome disparities such as those created by poverty, chronic conditions, conditions that limit mobility, or living in rural areas.

Healthcare Provider Uses

Healthcare providers, including APRNs, have a dual responsibility: to identify trustworthy information for both personal and patient use and to guide patients in accessing reliable consumer-targeted information, blogs, and support groups. APRNs have the related responsibility to recognize and counsel patients who are using, misusing, or misunderstanding existing information. APRNs can influence patient attitudes regarding information obtained over the Internet, because healthcare provider–patient conversations involving the Internet lead to higher confidence in the Internet as a resource by patients (Hong, 2008). By judiciously choosing appropriate patient-oriented Internet websites, discussion boards, blogs, and support groups, APRNs can contribute to increasing health literacy and improving patient outcomes.

■ Table 8-2 Selected Trustworthy Consumer Health Websites

Website Name and URL	Consumer Information	Blog/Discussion Board/Forum	Advocacy	Support Groups	RSS/ Twitter	HON Certified
Agency for Health Research and Quality http://www.ahrq.gov	✓	⊘	⊘	⊘	✓	⊘
American Cancer Society http://www.cancer.org	✓	✓	✓	✓	✓	✓
American Diabetes Association http://www.diabetes.org	✓	✓	✓	✓	✓	⊘
American Heart Association http://www.heart.org	✓	⊘	✓	⊘	✓	⊘
American Stroke Association http://www.strokeassociation.org	✓	⊘	✓	⊘	✓	⊘
American Lung Association http://www.lungusa.org	✓	⊘	✓	⊘	✓	⊘
Arthritis Foundation http://www.arthritis.org	✓	✓	✓	✓	✓	⊘

(continues)

■ Table 8-2   Selected Trustworthy Consumer Health Websites (*continued*)

Website Name and URL	Consumer Information	Blog/Discussion Board/Forum	Advocacy	Support Groups	RSS/Twitter	HON Certified
Centers for Disease Control and Prevention http://www.cdc.gov	✓	⊘	⊘	⊘	✓	⊘
Drugs.com http://www.drugs.com	✓	✓	⊘	⊘	✓	✓
Health on the Net (HON) http://www.hon.ch	✓	✓	✓	✓	✓	✓
National Institutes of Health http://www.nih.gov	✓	⊘	⊘	⊘	✓	⊘
National Kidney Foundation http://www.kidney.org	✓	✓	✓	✓	✓	✓
Mayo Clinic http://www.mayoclinic.com	✓	✓	⊘	⊘	✓	✓
Merck Manuals Home Edition http://www.merckmanuals.com/home/index.html	✓	⊘	⊘	⊘	⊘	⊘
WebMD http://www.webmd.com	✓	✓	⊘	⊘	✓	✓

In a time when a majority of adults in the United States look for health information online, a major consideration for the APRN is to determine what patients are doing with this information. The extent to which people feel that the Internet plays an important part in their lives influences their expectations that the health information they garner will make a difference (Leung, 2008). APRNs must realize that many patients will have consulted the Internet for answers; therefore, APRNs must be prepared to speak openly and frankly about the information. Patients might seek health care having a preset agenda or self-diagnosis, and they might also be seeking a specific diagnostic examination, laboratory workup, or medication.

Eventually, APRNs might find that patients are increasingly less challenging or, perhaps, more challenging to care for in light of ready access to health-related materials. Patients will solicit advice from APRNs regarding which Internet information sources and support groups the APRN recommends, and so APRNs should prepare in advance by thoroughly investigating healthcare websites, becoming familiar with all their functions, and revisiting the sites at regular intervals to know what has changed. A patient's trust will not be cultivated if a patient has the impression that the APRN is not fully familiar with the website he or she is recommending.

From a professional practice standpoint, health-related websites have great promise in making timely and important information available. Websites such as those for the Centers for Disease Control and Prevention (CDC) and Medscape, among many others, have the capacity to send emails with their latest recommendations. RSS technology allows APRNs to sign up for news releases and updates (CDC, 2008). RSS serves as a sort of electronic file cabinet that receives, categorizes, and stores electronic dispatches from healthcare agencies and professional organizations. APRNs need only to look for the orange RSS symbol on the website to sign up for the entity's dispatches. Other avenues for provider-related information include listservs (mass emails for groups of people with similar interests) and Facebook pages of colleagues or organizations. These resources have the potential to deliver highly specific and useful information to APRNs with great efficiency. These technologies also have the potential to decrease professional isolation. As always, however, the provider must be wary of the source of the information.

From a public policy standpoint, the Internet and social networking can be tools to influence public policy. Social media in particular can be a powerful tool in political organizing and issue advocacy, because communication with politicians and policymakers is easier with electronic resources. Political blogs and discussion boards often have healthcare-related areas. Platforms such as Twitter allow information to be received by an individual and then rebroadcast to friends, associates, and colleagues. As a result, the power to quickly disseminate information increases exponentially. Social media has the capacity to democratize access to policy-related information, to decrease professional isolation in rural areas, and to facilitate an individual's influence on policy.

APRNs must advocate for accurate and helpful information on the Internet. Healthcare information on the Internet can be targeted to specific audiences with specific health information at low cost. Web-based information is becoming increasingly more important as people spend more time online. New avenues for research using innovative methods that test new venues for patient education, peer and group support, assessment, and treatment will become more readily available.

The future of Internet healthcare information may lie in the integration of highly interactive platforms that combine elements from both the basic Web and social networking. Kaiser Permanente has begun using a tool, called KP Health Connect (Southeast Permanente Medical Group, 2012), that encourages patients to access their health records, appointments, scheduling, and email accounts that link them to their care provider. In addition, comprehensive medical records are immediately accessible to all members of a patient's healthcare team. A natural progression of a platform such as this would be the inclusion of health condition–related, moderated discussion boards and support groups. In another innovation to steer non-emergent patients to urgent care clinics, Blue Cross Blue Shield of Georgia has an audio tutorial, a 24/7 nurse helpline, and an urgent care locator powered by Google Maps (Williams, 2011).

Beyond Informatics: Electronic Health Records

The precursor of today's **electronic health records (EHRs)** emerged approximately 50 years ago (National Institutes of Health, 2006). Although fraught with technical difficulties, the original attempts to computerize medical information paved the way for current goals that include storing individual health data in usable formats and introducing interactive prompts to promote patient safety.

The HITECH Act was passed in 2009 as a subset of the American Recovery and Reinvestment Act (Tomes, 2010). This legislation created a deadline of 2015 for those medical facilities and eligible providers who receive Medicare reimbursement to employ EHRs in their systems. Criteria for successful implementation involve the degree of usefulness, or *meaningful use*, of the electronic documents.

Cost

The passage of the HITECH Act created a series of financial incentives paid over a 5-year period for those facilities and providers mandated to employ the EHR (Tomes, 2010). At first glance, this program might appear to offset the cost of compliance; however, this compensation does not necessarily remove all startup costs. For example, a physician can receive as much as $44,000 in total government reimbursements; however, one provider reported that a typical setup totaled $47,000 for the hardware package and service for the first year (BuyerZone, 2011). The desire to qualify for additional incentive payments for early implementation of the EHR might encourage impulsive decision making, ultimately creating the potential for "buyer's remorse" as facilities incur unexpected costs to supplement their systems.

Once the EHR is in place, a facility's clinical decision support team can help recoup costs by streamlining care and pinpointing areas of deficit through electronic retrieval of information via aggregate reports (Glaser, 2008). Literature reveals growing pains felt with EHR implementation in the form of increased costs of training staff, purchasing software, and a learning curve with new users, but the researchers also found decreased mortality rates among EHR facilities, attributed to interactive products employed to reduce medication errors. These facilities can expect increased savings as users become more proficient (knowIT, 2010).

Current Status of HITECH: Progression to Stage 2 of Meaningful Use

At press time, eligible providers and facilities that started early implementation of stage 1 meaningful use to earn the maximum incentives were in the process of meeting stage 2 criteria (Centers for Medicare and Medicaid Services, 2013). Stage 2 requires that eligible providers and facilities meet all core objectives and a selected number of menu objectives. In the interest of patient safety, the Centers for Medicare and Medicaid Services (CMS) added two core objectives to the original stage 2 list that involves secure electronic communication between patient and provider, as well as electronic medication tracking. Facilitating patient access to **electronic medical records (EMR)** is another mandate for successful completion of stage 2.

Efficiency

Despite the initial difficulty of incorporating the EHR, APRNs are already experiencing its advantages by accessing patient information remotely (Hosker, 2007). For example, not only can a fetal monitor tracing be accessed offsite, but medical records from previous admissions can be made available. **Computerized provider order entry (CPOE)** reduces duplication of orders, checks for drug allergies and interactions, and provides an interactive component that assists with clinical decision making (Lykowski & Mahoney, 2004). Efforts by the Office of the National Coordinator for Health Information Technology's Office of Science and Technology are underway to standardize and encrypt healthcare information to facilitate portability and accessibility of information (HealthIT.gov, n.d.). Once incompatibility issues are resolved, APRNs will have the ability to access a more complete longitudinal snapshot of their patients, creating safer, more streamlined care.

Besides facilitating individual efficiency, conversion to electronic record-keeping promises to increase performance on a larger scale. Patient data that are entered into an electronic format can be retrieved in the future using a process known as **data mining**. This activity allows analysis of patient safety measures, length of stay information, and other areas of opportunity, enabling both healthcare facilities and providers to improve areas of weakness (Mosby's Suite, 2014). Data mining also promises to identify potential fraud, waste, and abuse of the healthcare system.

On a broader scale, the advent of the EHR will create a huge depository for **Big Data**. Depending on personnel with appropriate analytical skills, healthcare facilities can use Big Data to monitor trends to create both clinical and financial improvement opportunities (Miliard, 2014). Some organizations are joining forces to take advantage of the various talents and capabilities available. For example, one surgical improvement program, the American College of Surgeons National Surgical Quality Improvement Program (ACS NSQIP), has been collecting surgical data from participating hospitals since the early 1990s. The data are collected and entered into a

Web-based data entry tool and ACS NSQIP is able to send participating facilities risk-adjusted reports to facilitate identification of trends (ACS NSQIP, 2014a). In recent years, participating hospitals have created collaboratives to share improvement projects and ideas (ACS NSQIP, 2014b). Originally geographically based, the collaboratives have expanded to a virtual venue, allowing all participating facilities to benefit from the experiences of others and to prevent re-creating the wheel during improvement efforts. Another product of Big Data collection is the creation of the ACS NSQIP online surgical risk calculator (Heitz, 2013). Surgeons can enter patient preoperative risk factors and the tool will interpret the information based on existing Big Data already in the system to predict the complication rate for that individual to allow better decision making. The future almost certainly holds the promise of decision making based on a body of evidence that is an order of magnitude more sophisticated than what is now available. An obvious challenge will be maintaining a commitment to individualized care that is deemed by the healthcare provider to be appropriate to a patient's particular circumstances. In other words, an APRN's recommendation and a patient's readiness to accept a recommendation for or against an intervention may run counter to advice that is solely data driven. This dilemma may be the latest manifestation of the dynamic nature of patient care that is both an art and a science.

Training

APRNs are a critical element when EHRs are introduced. As valuable end users, APRNs can provide input into both the selection and customization of the chosen product (Bernstein, McCreless, & Cote, 2007). As with any new program, successful implementation of EHRs involves a substantial investment for training. Both selection and customization activities demand full engagement of the participants in order to reap the maximum benefits from the new system. Most vendors, as part of the implementation costs, supply professional trainers or train existing staff as **superusers**, or onsite experts, to instruct other end users in the most efficient use possible.

With the proliferation of electronic information, nursing is beginning to recognize the importance of having a basic knowledge of **informatics** (Flanagan & Jones, 2007). Incorporating an informatics course into nursing curriculum can facilitate the transition to EHRs and provide insight into potential methods of abstracting data for use in research.

Information, Legislation, and Health Care

How the government approaches health care and the importance of health policy in influencing the government's decisions has never been more important. With political and policy information so readily available, there is no excuse for APRNs to be ill-informed. The speed with which information is disseminated has created a climate where information and interpretation are immediate; therefore, immediate responses are required because information is produced and consumed so rapidly that emerging policy is more unstable, dynamic, and susceptible to influence. Once again, the APRN needs to be diligent in vetting information sources because some websites that appear to be official can be deceptive. Relying on information that employs important-sounding monikers such as *The Society of ABC* or *The National Organization of XYZ* should not replace diligence in vetting the source.

The Institute of Medicine's (IOM) report on the future of nursing has acknowledged that nurses comprise the majority of healthcare providers and has called for facilitating maximum participation of this group (IOM, 2010). To achieve this goal, recommendations from the report include an emphasis on nurses becoming actively involved in healthcare issues and policies. APRNs must be involved in policy because, in reality, APRNs are the people who must cope with the changes that policy creates. Changes in governmental philosophies and priorities are important because the stakes are so high. The healthcare system in the United States has been routinely criticized as too expensive, with persistent pockets of disparities. In an effort to extend healthcare access to all Americans, the Affordable Care Act (ACA) of 2010 mandated that common barriers such as preexisting conditions and lifetime limits be eliminated (U.S. Department of Health and Human Services, 2014). Currently, implementing the healthcare law has benefited many without previous coverage, as well as children who can remain on a parent's policy until age 26. Conversely, the law has been fraught with challenges such as website failures and gaps in coverage of some individuals. The tone of the healthcare debate is emotionally charged and sometimes bitter. This should be no surprise because health care is such a large component of the U.S. gross domestic product and involves huge sums of money in an industry that essentially functions as an oligopoly composed of a few industries, such as insurance companies and hospitals. The immediate future of health care in the United States is frequently seen as obscured and in flux, so now more than ever, keeping track of health policy is an important aspect of professional practice.

Political activism can be as simple and personal as making a telephone call to a state legislator, or it can be as involved as volunteering to be a district policy coordinator for a state professional organization. Legislators appreciate nurses who are willing to volunteer as contacts regarding substantive issues such as school nursing or access to trauma care. This is especially true because legislators and their staffs are as likely as the general public to be exposed to poor quality health-related information.

Some politically active APRNs serve as liaisons between legislators and constituent nurses. State associations of nurses such as the American Association of Nurse Practitioners (2014) actively recruit nurses to participate and offer training for those who desire more involvement than telephone calling and letter writing. Although it would be expected that information technology would be a boon to both healthcare consumers and nurses seeking accurate information, electronic media have been exploited by some to distribute biased and misleading information, such as the myth of "death panels" during the healthcare debate of 2009 (Begley, Connolly, Kalb, & Yarett, 2009). Nurses will have to develop an equal measure of the technological savvy necessary to counter examples of demagoguery such as this.

Social media holds great promise in facilitating the political organization of nurses. Many of the state associations of nursing have Facebook pages. The American Nurses Association has taken an additional step of creating a social networking platform called *NurseSpace*, which allows nurses to share information and seek advice on nurse issues. The discussions are organized in terms of the various communities of nursing practice, geography, and the roles of the nurse, such as student, entrepreneur, and administrator. Of these discussion groups, one is devoted to politics and one to health policy.

The Internet and social media have fundamentally changed the practice of politics. Even though the Internet played a role in the 2000 and 2004 presidential elections, 2008 was quickly nicknamed the *Web 2.0 election*, such was the importance of information technology to both political parties (Germany, 2008). Campaign fundraising by politicians now commonly has an Internet component. The power of courting small donors was strikingly demonstrated by the historic fundraising success of the Obama presidential campaigns in 2008 (Hill, 2009) and 2012 (Tau, 2013).

Since the Supreme Court decision in *Citizens United v. FEC* in 2010, no time has been lost by SuperPACs in raising relatively unrestricted money to finance political campaigns. Until recently the ratio of spending by the national political parties compared to interest groups was roughly 50 to 1. In only two election cycles since the decision, this ratio has decreased to nearly 1 to 1 in federal elections (Franz, 2013). The ability of technologically savvy grassroots organizations and campaign teams to court massive numbers of small donors with success may be the best hope to counterbalance the financial power of the superrich.

The Future of Healthcare Policy in the Age of Social Media

The continuing explosion of social networking capabilities will certainly contribute to the dynamic nature of healthcare policy. Policymakers have been using websites such as Facebook and Twitter to monitor the pulse of their constituents. It is imperative for the APRN to remain current in these communication modalities in order to have a voice in decision making.

Agenda Setting and Implementation

Furlong (2008) describes several key components in agenda setting, including stakeholders, contextual dimensions, and windows of opportunity. With the growing use of interactive social networks among both the general public and public officials, the agenda-setting stage of the political process promises to become more fast-paced in future policymaking. A survey showed that although conventional means of communication remain the most influential, Facebook, Twitter, and YouTube are becoming increasingly popular and important among members of Congress and their senior staff (Eye on FDA, 2011). APRNs, as both individual constituents and members of professional organizations, have the opportunity to communicate ideas and concerns regarding future healthcare issues by using these networks. Because of the ease and speed of this new form of communication, APRNs must be especially vigilant at monitoring the accuracy of their information sources while they are attempting to affect change in policy.

Wilken (2008) describes common problems with policy implementation when policy criteria do not mirror real-life scenarios. The proliferation of social networking has the potential to reduce this issue as APRNs stay virtually connected with their colleagues by reporting problems, suggesting solutions, and creating an aura of supportiveness in a global manner. Because multiple entities, including policymakers, are connected to these networks, policy implementation efforts can be monitored with the ability to receive immediate feedback.

Implications for the Future

The increased flow of information through social media, along with the availability of remote access to medical records, will certainly raise concerns about privacy issues. Dorsch and Greenberg (2009) advise users to beware of potential hackers and to be aware of the terms of service for the different websites. For instance, Facebook policy states that all posted information belongs to the website (Reid, 2009); once information is posted, it is virtually impossible to retract. APRNs would be wise to stay apprised of the application and interpretation of current laws such as HIPAA, which is responsible for maintaining the security of health information, when using social networks and accessing medical records remotely. Information becomes more portable with smartphones and similar technology. Providers will need to become more cognizant of protecting patient information by implementing actions such as encryption and assessment of Wi-Fi security. Learning how to disable remote capabilities in the event of stolen or lost devices will be critical as well (Barrett, 2011).

Healthcare privacy policy is just one example of a healthcare issue in flux. Pay-for-performance, hospital-acquired conditions, core measure statistics, and health scorecards are other initiatives becoming publicly accessible and are designed to increase transparency in healthcare matters. Insurance companies, government agencies, healthcare consumers, and healthcare facilities are already becoming key players in this evolution. The climate for APRN participation in this new era of healthcare policy formation has never been more open than the present. Data are readily available, and the capability of immediate feedback with various stakeholders, including policymakers, promises to change the policy process in a more rapid fashion. APRNs need to become engaged in the process as well, in order to maintain a place at the decision-making table.

CASE STUDY 1: (IN)SECURE COMMUNICATION?

Annie Lewis, a registered nurse, takes a prescribed daily beta blocker to combat a rapid heart rate. Annie was running low with no refills on her prescription, so she called her primary care provider APRN, who provided her with a month's supply. At the same time, Annie scheduled her yearly wellness visit. When Annie arrived at the APRN's office, she was given instructions to access her records in the practice's new electronic record so she, the patient, could receive results and messages in a timely manner. Annie was examined, had routine labwork completed, and requested a refill of her beta blocker, although she did tell the APRN that she still had some medication remaining, so she wouldn't need the prescription called in yet. After about 2 days, Annie received her first email alerting her that there was new information in her electronic record. When she accessed the record, she found a narrative of her visit, with a diagnosis of dysuria. The next day another email arrived, and she found that her urine had been sent for a culture and came back positive, although she had no symptoms of a UTI. The day after that lab result, Annie received an automated call from the pharmacy that her prescription was ready. Thinking that the APRN had filled her beta blocker prescription early, she was tempted to ignore the pharmacy call. However, Annie did call the pharmacy and she learned that the prescription waiting for pickup was an antibiotic, apparently for her UTI. Knowing that it was a hassle to call regarding this, Annie decided to pick up the antibiotic and begin therapy, because she knew how to read the lab tests and assumed she should be treated for the UTI, despite having no physical symptoms. Annie never had any phone conversations with anyone from the APRN's office after her well-visit appointment. Another factor to note: the urine sample was collected in the APRN's office, not the lab, where Annie had labeled the specimen container in the lavatory using a black marker .

Discussion Points

1. Discuss what might have transpired if Annie did not have a nursing background.
2. List the breakdowns in communication that occurred and the potential ramifications.
3. Did the APRN's office fulfill the meaningful use stage 2 requirement of providing secure electronic communication between the patient and healthcare provider? Why or why not?

CASE STUDY 2: A DISCONNECT ABOUT VALUES/BELIEFS

In the course of interviewing the family of Jody Barrineau, a healthy 3-year-old presenting for routine checkup, the mother and father express unconventional beliefs regarding preventative health care. The APRN listens as both relate claims found on the Internet that vaccines are harmful to children. The mother says she is concerned by reports that, among other things, the measles/mumps/rubella (MMR) vaccine causes autism, the diphtheria/tetanus/acellular pertussis (DTAP) vaccine is associated with sudden infant death syndrome, and the influenza vaccine actually causes influenza. The father concurs and cites "authoritative" sources from the Internet including webpages and discussion groups that the APRN does not recognize. The APRN is faced with a family with deeply held beliefs than run counter to her own. These beliefs are made more intractable because the parents sincerely believe that they diligently researched the issue and that they are acting in the best interest of Jody.

(continues)

Discussion Points

1. Identify at least four Internet sites that offer legitimate health-related information and at least four Internet sites that offer questionable health-related information.
2. Discuss how the APRN can help a patient/family analyze information to ascertain its value and reliability.
3. Identify advantages and disadvantages of discussion boards and support groups on the Internet.
4. How can the APRN improve the quality of information found on the Internet?

CASE STUDY 3: ETHICS IN A CLINICAL SETTING

Sandra Martin, a woman in her mid-70s, was born with a deformity of her spine, which had never been a health issue until recently when arthritis began to impair her ability to compensate for her slightly shorter left leg. After consultation with an orthopedic surgeon, Ms. Martin agreed to have the deformity surgically corrected. Sandra's postoperative course was stormy, including complications with pneumonia that made a transfer to the intensive care unit necessary. Sandra's physician had prescribed a common antibiotic regimen used for the type of organism identified, but the patient seemed to be getting worse despite this intervention. William Girder, an APRN who worked with the pulmonary practice, was making rounds one afternoon. Sandra's daughter, Lucy, approached him with an Internet article she had found regarding an alternative therapy for this type of pneumonia. Lucy confided to William that she was glad he was the provider who was rounding that day, because she felt he would listen to her more than the attending physician would and advocate for her mother's well-being, especially because Sandra was showing no signs of improvement.

Discussion Points

1. Should William proceed with Lucy's request to try a different therapy?
2. How can William determine whether the article presented by Lucy has any merit? If William determines that the article is legitimate, what other steps are needed before deciding to switch the treatment approach?
3. Discuss the ethics of William's response to Lucy regarding the attending physician.

References

Agency for Healthcare Research and Quality. (2007). *Program brief: Health literacy.* AHRQ Publication No. 07-P010. Retrieved from http://www.ahrq.gov/research/healthlit.pdf

American Association of Nurse Practitioners. (2014). *Become an advocate.* Retrieved from http://www.aanp.org/legislation-regulation/policy

American College of Surgeons National Surgical Quality Improvement Program. (2014a). *About ACS NSQIP.* Retrieved from http://site.acsnsqip.org/about/

American College of Surgeons National Surgical Quality Improvement Program. (2014b). *Collaboratives.* Retrieved from http://site.acsnsqip.org/participants/collaboratives/

Barrett, C. (2011). *Healthcare providers may violate HIPAA by using mobile devices to communicate with patients.* Retrieved from http://www.americanbar.org/newsletter/publications /aba_health_esource_home/aba_health_law_esource_1110_barrett.ktml

Barrett, S. (2014). *Quackwatch mission statement.* Retrieved from http://www .quackwatch.com/00AboutQuackwatch/mission.html

Begley, S., Connolly, K., Kalb, C., & Yarett, I. (2009). The five biggest lies in the health care debate. *Newsweek, 154*(10), 42–43.

Bemis-Dougherty, A. (2010). Professionalism and social networking. *PT on Motion, 2*(5), 40–47.

Benjamin, R. M. (2010). Surgeon general's perspectives: Improving health by improving health literacy. *Public Health Reports, 125,* 784–785.

Bennett, S. (2013). *Who uses Twitter? 16% of Internet users, 18-29 year olds, minorities, men more than women.* Retrieved from https://www.mediabistro.com/alltwitter /twitter-demographics-2013_b36254

Bernstein, M. L., McCreless, T., & Cote, M. J. (2007). Five constants of information technology adoption in healthcare. *Hospital Topics: Research and Perspectives on Healthcare, 85*(1), 17–25.

Bulik, B. S. (2009). What your favorite social network says about you. *Advertising Age, 80*(25), 6.

BuyerZone. (2011). *Real-world EMR prices from BuyerZone buyers.* Retrieved from http://www.buyerzone.com/healthcare/electronic-medical-records/ar-prices-emr

Centers for Disease Control and Prevention. (2008). *RSS at CDC.* Retrieved from http://www2c.cdc.gov/podcasts/rsshelp.asp

Centers for Medicare and Medicaid Services. (2013). *Stage 2.* Retrieved from http://www.cms.gov/Regulations-and-Guidance/Legislation/EHRIncentivePrograms/Stage_2.html

Dorsch, M., & Greenberg, P. (2009). What you need to know about social networking. *State Legislatures, 35*(7), 62–64.

Eye on FDA. (2011, January 26). *Growing role of social media among policymakers.* Retrieved from http://www.eyeonfda.com/eye_on_fda/2011/01/growing-role-of-social-media-among-policymakers.html

Facebook. (2014). *Newsroom.* Retrieved from https://newsroom.fb.com/company-info

Flanagan, J., & Jones, D. A. (2007). Nursing language in a time of change: Capturing the focus of the discipline. *International Journal of Nursing Terminologies and Classifications, 18*(1), 1–2.

Fox, S. (2011). *Health topics.* Retrieved from http://www.pewinternet.org/2011/02/01/health-topics-2/

Franz, M. (2013). Bought and sold: The high price of the permanent campaign. *American Interest, 8*(6), 52–61.

Furlong, E. A. (2008). Agenda setting. In J. A. Milstead (Ed.), *Health policy and politics: A nurse's guide* (3rd ed., pp. 41–63). Sudbury, MA: Jones and Bartlett.

Germany, J. B. (2008). Changing political campaigns one voter at a time. *Insights on Law and Society, 9*(1), 15–16.

Glaser, J. (2008). Clinical decision support: The power behind the electronic health record. *Healthcare Financial Management, 62*(7), 46–48, 50–51.

HealthIT.gov. (n.d.). *Health information exchange: Standards and interoperability.* Retrieved from http://www.healthit.gov/providers-professionals/standards-interoperability

Health on the Net Foundation. (2014). *Medical professional.* Retrieved from http://www.hon.ch/med.html

Heitz, D. (2013). *Online calculator predicts risk of surgical complications.* Retrieved from http://site.acsnsqip.org/news/online-calculator-predicts-risk-of-surgical-complications/

Hill, S. (2009). World wide webbed: The Obama campaign's masterful use of the Internet. *Social Europe: The Journal of the European Left, 4*(2), 9–14.

Hong, T. (2008). Internet health information in the patient-provider dialog. *CyberPsychology and Behavior, 11*(5), 587–589.

Hosker, N. (2007). Exploiting the potential of informatics in health care. *Nurse Prescribing, 5*(9), 391–394.

Institute of Medicine. (2010). *The future of nursing: Leading change, advancing health.* Retrieved from http://www.iom.edu/Reports/2010/The-future-of-nursing-leading-change-advancing-health.aspx

Institute of Medicine. (2011). *Innovations in health literacy research: Workshop summary.* Washington, DC: National Academies Press.

knowIT. (2010). *Electronic medical records: A surprising short-term prognosis for cost savings.* Retrieved from http://knowledge.wpcarey.asu.edu/article.cfm?articleid=1912

Leung, L. (2008). Internet embeddedness: Links with online health information seeking, expectancy value/quality of health information websites, and Internet usage patterns. *CyberPsychology and Behavior, 11*(5), 565–569.

LinkedIn Press Center. (2014). *About LinkedIn.* Retrieved from http://press.linkedin.com/about

Lykowski, G., & Mahoney, D. (2004). Computerized provider order entry improves workflow and outcomes. *Nursing Management, 35*(2), 40G–40H.

MedlinePlus. (2014). *Evaluating health information.* Retrieved from http://www.nlm.nih.gov/medlineplus/evaluatinghealthinformation.html

Miliard, M. (2014). Big data is not just a numbers game. *Healthcare IT News.* Retrieved from http://www.healthcareitnews.com/news/big-data-not-just-numbers-game

Mosby's Suite. (2014). *Data mining in a healthcare setting.* Retrieved from http://www.confidenceconnected.com/connect/article/data_mining_in_a_healthcare_setting/

National Institutes of Health, National Center for Research Resources. (2006). *Electronic health records review.* Retrieved from http://www.himss.org/files/HIMSSorg/content/files/Code%20180%20MITRE%20Key%20Components%20of%20an%20EHR.pdf

Nelson, R. (2008). The Internet and healthcare policy information. In J. A. Milstead (Ed.), *Health policy and politics: A nurse's guide* (3rd ed., pp. 197–219). Sudbury, MA: Jones and Bartlett.

Pew Research. (2013). *Health fact sheet.* Retrieved from http://www.pewinternet.org/fact-sheets/health-fact-sheet/

Pothier, L., & Pothier, D. D. (2009). Patient-oriented websites on laryngectomy: Is their information readable? *European Journal of Cancer Care, 18,* 594–597.

Reid, C. K. (2009). Should business embrace social networking? *EContent, 32*(5), 34–39.

Sarkar, U., Karter, A. J., Liu, J. Y., Alder, N. E., Nguyen, R., López, A., et al. (2010). The literacy divide: Health literacy and the use of an Internet-based patient portal in an integrated health system—Results from the Diabetes Study of Northern California (DISTANCE). *Journal of Community Health, 15*(Suppl. 2), 183–196.

Saul, D. J. (2014). *3 million teens leave Facebook in 3 years; the 2014 Facebook demographic report.* Retrieved from http://istrategylabs.com/2014/01/3-million-teens-leave-facebook-in-3-years-the-2014-facebook-demographic-report/

Smith, C. (2014, January). By the numbers: 51 interesting Instagram statistics. Retrieved from http://expandedramblings.com/index.php/important-instagram-stats/

Southeast Permanente Medical Group. (2012). *Kaiser Permanente HealthConnect.* Retrieved from http://www.tspmg.com/index.php/innovation/kp-healthconnect

Statistic Brain. (2014). *Twitter statistics.* Retrieved from http://www.statisticbrain.com/twitter-statistics/

Tau, B. (2013). *Obama campaign final fundraising total: $1.1 billion.* Retrieved from http://www.politico.com/story/2013/01/obama-campaign-final-fundraising-total-1-billion-86445.html

Tomes, J. P. (2010). Avoiding the trap in the HITECH Act's incentive timeframe for implementing the EHR. *Journal of Health Care Finance, 37*(1), 91–100.

U.S. Department of Commerce. (2011). *Digital nation: Expanding Internet usage.* Retrieved from http://www.ntia.doc.gov/reports/2011/NTIA_Internet_Use_Report_February_2011.pdf

U.S. Department of Health and Human Services. (2011). *Healthy people 2020: Health communication and health information technology.* Retrieved from http://www.healthypeople.gov/2020/topicsobjectives2020/overview.aspx?topicid=18

U.S. Department of Health and Human Services. (2014). *About the law.* Retrieved from http://www.hhs.gov/healthcare/rights/

Wilken, M. (2008). Policy implementation. In J. A. Milstead (Ed.), *Health policy and politics: A nurse's guide* (3rd ed., pp. 157–169). Sudbury, MA: Jones and Bartlett.

Williams, M. (2011, March 22). Blue Cross taps technology to help steer consumers away from unnecessary ER visits. *Atlanta Journal and Constitution.* Retrieved from http://www.ajc.com/business/blue-cross-taps-technology-881465.html?cxtype=rss_news_81960

YouTube Pressroom. (n.d.). *Statistics.* Retrieved from http://www.youtube.com/yt/press/statistics.html

Zickuhr, K. (2013). *Who's not online and why.* Retrieved from http://www.pewinternet.org/2013/09/25/whos-not-online-and-why/

CHAPTER 9

Interprofessional Practice, Education, and Research

Kimberly Ann Galt, J.D. Polk, Patrick DeLeon,
and Jeri A. Milstead

INTRODUCTION

Health professionals in the United States have worked together when situations demanded it, but do not have a history of actually collaborating as a team in the organization of their practices. Traditionally, most practices are physician-led. Physicians may employ nurses, medical assistants, receptionists, and other support staff; some may have added advanced practice registered nurses (APRNs) and physician assistants (PAs) in recent years, but many still do not have pharmacists, behavioral health experts, dentists, dieticians, or occupational and physical therapists on board. Health care becomes fragmented as patients moved from one office to another or one provider to another in order to address the original (and emerging) issues.

Recent attempts to reform the U.S. sick care system (many do not refer to it as a healthcare system because the emphasis has been on curing and treating disease) has forced practitioners to reassess how care is provided. Health maintenance organizations (HMOs), independent provider organizations (IPOs), and other arrangements led to primary care as the starting place for patients to contact providers. Primary care offices became the sites for initial compilation of medical/health records, but care became disjointed when patients needed to be seen by specialists or providers other than the primary care generalists. Providers were not satisfied with this arrangement, and patients were not satisfied either. Reimbursement was made on the basis of the number of services delivered, which created an inefficient, expensive, duplicative system. The cost of care was skyrocketing out of control.

The concept of team-based provider practices got off to a slow start because the definition of team was narrow (i.e., physician-led). This definition ignored the importance of other professionals and did not offer the respect and recognition that "other" providers could bring to the scene. According to Heim and Golant (2007), the concept of team often is gender-biased; that is, roles learned in childhood have been different for boys and girls. Boys learn that there is a hierarchy, that team members follow orders, are competitive and goal oriented, take risks, and learn how to lose. Heim notes that girls learn that team play involves shared leadership, negotiation, fairness for all, dead-even power relationships, a focus on process not goals, and a win–win outcome. Because most physicians historically have been men, physician practices evolved within the perspective of a male concept of team. Physicians were responsible for diagnosing, recommending treatment, and evaluating patient "compliance" (a pejorative term that has underlying connotations of not following orders).

The concept of a team of professionals who respect the education of each other and the experience that each brings to the practice is relatively new. Patient-centered medical homes (PCMHs) are the most recent attempt to incorporate collaborative practice among various health professionals. An Ohio project emerged from legislation that resulted in 52 practices (4 of which were APRN-led) that adopted the PCMH model. Although originally unfunded, the project was placed under the direction of the director of the Ohio Department of Health (ODH) where the Department of Medicare provided funding. Goals were to control costs, improve patient outcomes, and enhance the patient experience. TransforMED, a proprietary company, was hired to provide direction, webinars, and other consultation to the practices. A governor-appointed PCMH Task Force and PCMH Education Advisory Group maintained guidance and oversight. An educational component was created through a proposed curriculum on the concepts of PCMHs. Choose Ohio First scholarships were provided to participating medical students and APRN students through the Ohio Board of Regents, with a stipulation that students work in PCMH practices for 3 to 5 years after graduation (Ohio Department of Health, n.d.). Practices currently are undergoing evaluation through the use of metrics determined by the practices. These types of practices hold hope for a more coherent, collaborative, cost-effective, accessible system of quality care.

The education component of the Ohio PCMH project is important. All 52 practices were required to have a formal relationship with a university that educated physicians and APRNs. Each college of nursing and college of medicine was required to implement a curriculum that focused on the basic concepts of a PCMH. Healthcare professionals need to learn what is meant by collaboration, negotiation, and coordination. Students must learn the concepts and then see them demonstrated in practices throughout their educational journey.

Interprofessional education does present challenges. Joanne Disch, PhD, RN, FAAN, president of the American Academy of Nursing, wrote that faculty who do not teach together in traditional healthcare programs must learn to partner with each other (2013). She notes a reticence that students in one program may not be at the same level (i.e., undergraduate vs. graduate or medical vs. nursing students), but insists that all students (and faculty) can learn about teamwork, power differentials, values, and goals in classrooms and clinical rounds. Disch suggests teams of students and professionals could follow a patient or group of patients, thereby learning and valuing the contributions that each brings to the patient situation.

Interprofessional organizations are a rarity—most organizations were created with members dedicated to specific missions and goals. For example, nurses developed nurse-focused associations, as did physicians, pharmacists, psychologists, and so on. These organizations had the effect of gathering comparable members, centering on a purpose, and protecting their participants. The thought of organizing a group of practitioners from many professions was not a common undertaking. As a result of the 2010 Institute of Medicine report, *The Future of Nursing: Leading Change, Advancing Health*, a group consisting of registered nurses, APRNs, physicians, physician assistants, pharmacists, and others incorporated in 2011 to form the Council for Ohio Health Care Advocacy (COHCA, n.d.). The focus was to join forces and approach legislators and other policymakers with one voice. COHCA required individual applicants to be members of at least one professional association. Issues are discussed via the Policy Committee by asking whether the issue: (1) focuses on patient-centered topics; (2) affects patient care and safety; (3) affects access, cost, or quality of health care; (4) promotes cross-professional practice/education; (5) has an effect/impact on providers; or (6) has a practical or timely interest. The committee makes recommendations to the board for action. To date, this group has had success in moving expanded prescriptive authority for APRNs and PAs, securing admitting privileges to hospitals for certain groups, and other issues.

Jan Lanier, RN, JD, served as a lobbyist for several years and is recognized throughout Ohio as a policy expert. She cautions that "taking credit" is a concept that causes some individuals and organizations to resist working interprofessionally. She notes that it is time to put aside individual effort if we really want to work together. She has said that when we reach a common goal the outcome probably involved many diverse opinions and solutions. She believes that the outcome is what matters—we should celebrate the goal and not try to one-up each other (i.e., we should leave our egos at home). This is a powerful lesson and one that clearly demonstrates that we honestly respect each other.

My personal thanks to Jones & Bartlett Learning for consenting to accept this new chapter that focuses on interprofessional practice, education, and research. Three of the most well-recognized leaders in their fields agreed to write about their experiences. They have been actively engaged in collaborating with others and have offered readers a glimpse of the rewards and challenges they have encountered. We welcome your comments.

Kimberly Galt, PharmD, PhD, FASHP, FNAP, is professor and assistant vice provost for Multidisciplinary Health Science Research and associate dean for research in the Schools of Dentistry, Nursing, Pharmacy, and the Health Professions at Creighton University, Omaha, Nebraska. Her early effort to provide courses that include students from all of the health professions was seminal and has become the model for interprofessional education (IPE).

J.D. Polk, DO, was flight surgeon and later medical director for the Space Medicine Division of the National Aeronautics and Space Administration (NASA). He was responsible for astronauts who lived in the space lab and was one of four professionals that NASA sent to Chile in 2013 when 33 miners were trapped underground. Dr. Polk later became assistant secretary for homeland security and currently is dean of the school of osteopathic medicine at Des Moines University, Des Moines, Iowa.

Pat DeLeon, PhD (Psychology), JD, MPH, was chief of staff to U.S. Senator Daniel K. Inouye (D-HI) and worked with the senator for more than 40 years. As a recent former president of the American Psychological Association, Dr. DeLeon continues to write a regular column for the APA newsletter—most columns focus on his long-time efforts to include psychologists and other therapists into the mainstream of U.S. health care. His special interest in prescriptive authority has borne fruit as today two states have included this aspect into legal practice acts. His vision for promoting nurses and APRNs is an example of his commitment to collaborative practice. Dr.

DeLeon currently is distinguished professor, Uniformed Services University of the Health Sciences.

This author hopes that the examples shared by these three professionals will inspire all who read this text and who work as healthcare professionals to seek collaboration with their colleagues to transform the healthcare system in this country.

References

Council for Ohio Health Care Advocacy. (n.d.). *Home page*. Retrieved from http://www.cohcaonline.org

Disch, J. (2013). Interprofessional education and collaborative practice. *Nursing Outlook*, *61*(1), 3–4.

Heim, P., & Golant, S. K. (2007). *Hardball for women: Winning the game of communications*. New York: Penguin.

Institute of Medicine. (2010). *The Future of Nursing: Leading Change, Advancing Health*. Retrieved from http://www.iom.edu/Reports/2010/the-future-of-nursing-leading-change-advancing-health.aspx

Ohio Department of Health. (n.d.). Retrieved from http://www.odh.ohio.gov/landing/medicalhomes/Choose%20Ohio%20First%20Scholarships.aspx

***

EXPERIENCES AND PERSPECTIVES ON INTERPROFESSIONAL EDUCATION

Kimberly Ann Galt

KEY TERMS

Collaborative practice: "When multiple health workers from different professional backgrounds provide comprehensive services by working together with patients, families, carers, and communities to deliver the highest quality of care across settings" (World Health Organization [WHO], 2010, p. 13).

Interprofessional education: "When two or more professions learn about, from and with each other to enable effective collaboration and improve health outcomes" (WHO, 2010, p. 13).
Interprofessional teamwork: "The levels of cooperation, coordination and collaboration characterizing the relationships between professions in delivering patient-centered care" (Interprofessional Education Collaborative Expert Panel, 2011, p. 2).

Why Interprofessional Education?

Providing safer and higher quality healthcare delivery in the United States requires that health professionals and administrators work together to achieve this common goal. In 1972, the Institute of Medicine envisioned that achieving this goal would require team-based education for the U.S. health professions and conducted an interprofessional conference to discuss key issues (Institute of Medicine, 1972). The 2000 Institute of Medicine (IOM) report, *To Err Is Human*, shed further light on the magnitude of the patient safety problem in the United States (Institute of Medicine [IOM], 2000). In a follow-up report, the IOM emphasized the need for patient safety education across the health professions and specifically identified the need for retraining the current healthcare workforce and establishing interprofessional learning approaches to prepare future healthcare practitioners post haste (IOM, 2001). Recommendations for organizations, administrators, educators, and national policymakers to achieve interprofessional team-based education and practice have emerged through the last 4 decades, calling for better teamwork and team-based care delivery at the individual, micro-system, organizational, educational, and policy levels (Baker, Gustafson, Beaubien, Salas, & Barach, 2005; King et al., 2008; O'Neil & the Pew Health Professions Commission, 1998).

Challenges Facing Interprofessional Education

Interprofessional education is critical to advancing the common goal of building patient-centered healthcare delivery systems that are safe and achieve high quality. Achieving this goal requires that we view healthcare delivery as a large system centered on patients and the communities in which they reside. To achieve successful **collaborative practice** we must train individuals across the professions by beginning in the classroom and in preclinical components of education (Galt et al., 2006). Our educational culture must promote interprofessional understanding and learning through early engagement of faculty and students in relevant areas of learning. During the college years we face culture and belief challenges among professors, temporal challenges in and across the curricula of the various learners among the professions, content selection challenges, and setting and educational workforce challenges.

Temporal challenges include timing the offering of education so that all professionals in training can participate to achieve the desired educational outcomes. This requires simultaneous attention to the structure and processes of the curriculum for students in different professions and at differing stages of training. Choosing content for interprofessional learning requires facing the challenges of both relevance and potential overlap within the respective roles and responsibilities of each health profession and responsiveness to accreditation and licensure standards for entry into the respective health professions. Setting challenges includes "space and place" problems, with too many students to simultaneously educate when we use traditional classroom arrangements and scheduling approaches. The natural problem that complements this is an inadequate volume of an expert professorial workforce to achieve simultaneous and interprofessional learning.

Overcoming the Challenges

Defining success is a critical step to building an interprofessional education effort on a university campus. Succeeding requires establishing a common vision and expected outcomes to be achieved with the interprofessional initiative. It makes sense to adopt paradigms for interprofessional education that work in real-life practice. Such a paradigm that resonates with all health professions is a patient-centered approach. Acting and thinking patient-centered plants a center stake in the ground that provides a common, fixed point for every profession from which roles and responsibilities can be viewed. Each professional can establish a view from the patient's perspective and have that view guide his or her own professional perspective. This outlook further creates an opportunity to examine and appreciate the contribution of each other's professional roles and responsibilities for achieving a safe and high quality outcome for the patient.

A complementary paradigm that guides health professionals of all backgrounds is a systems perspective on delivering care. Systems may be described as a set of things working together as parts of a mechanism or an interconnecting network. In traditional education for our professions we have studied most of our knowledge in the silo of our own programs, colleges, or schools. Interprofessional education should be designed to illustrate where our own work fits into the system of care delivery (i.e., how our independent and interdependent work complement each other by working together as parts to fulfill the holistic needs of the patient). We must share a common mental framework in healthcare practice to guide our own actions on behalf of the patient, toward the patient, and toward each other as care providers. Professors must understand this mental framework in healthcare practice and translate it within the classroom setting.

Using these two complementary paradigms—patient-centeredness and a healthcare systems approach to delivery—offers context to the profession-centric cultures and beliefs of each profession. Choosing these paradigms allows each profession to retain its own identity and professional norms, while expanding to include where overlaps and connections are needed to fulfill safe, quality, patient-centered care delivery. Although differing professional cultures and beliefs may exist, these must become minimized and take a secondary position as the professional responsibilities and roles required to meet patient-centered systems of care delivery emerge as primary.

CASE STUDY 1: MOVING TO A COMMON CORE INTERPROFESSIONAL PATIENT SAFETY CURRICULUM

All health professionals and administrators have a duty to prevent avoidable injury and harm to all patients who receive health care in the United States. "Declare the past, diagnose the present, foretell the future; practice these acts. As to diseases, make a habit of two things—to help, or at least to do no harm" (Hippocrates, *Epidemics*, Bk. 1, Sect. XI).

Students of the health professions need to understand the science of safety and the translation of new discoveries for safer care delivery into practice. Patient harm secondary to errors and mishaps results from system problems and failures. Systems have both technical and human components. Understanding this interface necessitates working together as health professionals to achieve systems improvement and reduce harm and injury. Current health professions education rarely delivers common core content about the science and application of safety principles.

Creighton University presently offers one of the most comprehensive interdisciplinary patient safety courses in the country, entitled Interprofessional Education 410: Foundations in Patient Safety. The course has been offered since 2005 and has reached more than 500 students in training (Abbott, Fuji, Galt, & Paschal, 2012; Fuji, Paschal, Galt, & Abbott, 2010; Galt et al., 2006); however, not all students and faculty are being reached through this elective approach. Patient Safety Day was organized to reach all pre-health professions and health professions–related students on campus with a core exposure to the science of safety. The daylong event is built on the elective interprofessional core curriculum course and is offered once in each of the spring and fall semesters. The objective is to provide students and faculty with training in the science of safety simultaneous with an introduction to basic patient safety science principles in an interprofessional educational delivery framework. Content was designed to illustrate how safety impacts both the overall healthcare system and the individual, and to apply lessons learned in a case-based interprofessional set of exercises. Three hundred fifty students participated in the first offering of our Patient Safety Day, including 70 from medicine, 95 from nursing, 35 from occupational therapy, 85 from pharmacy, 57 from physical therapy, and 8 from social work. Speakers, panelists, and faculty facilitators participated from Creighton University, the U.S. Department of Veterans Affairs, state government, and the local community.

"Today you made a difference" was the theme for this Patient Safety Day, and the focus was on the most personal and often tragic

(continues)

experiences of harm and injury of passionate leaders who conduct research, teach, implement research findings into practice, or use research findings to affect policy in patient safety. The keynote speaker, Evelyn McKnight, AuD, cofounder of HonorReform, presented the story of the hepatitis C outbreak in Fremont, Nebraska, and what needs to be done in practice and policy to prevent this "never event" from ever happening again. Content areas presented throughout the day included human factors, systems approaches to safety, and **interprofessional teamwork**.

Students were asked to reflect on the content presented during the Patient Safety Day and to complete a postevent questionnaire. This questionnaire solicited information about the value students placed on the day in the context of their professional learning and development. Descriptive analysis was conducted for quantitative responses, and thematic analysis was conducted for qualitative open-ended responses. Most students believed the material taught was essential core knowledge across the professions (78.6 percent). Similarly, students believed that the content should be required for all health professions students (77.4 percent). Students varied on the format they believed was best for learning: 40 percent would have preferred a full interprofessional course, 39 percent preferred the day-long program, and 21 percent indicated they would like to have it integrated with other content in their own disciplinary curriculums.

Students were asked to describe briefly what the most meaningful lessons were from the day. Three themes emerged, as follows, with a brief description and illustrative quote for each:

Theme 1: Errors can and do happen. Students were exposed to a variety of real-life stories shared by speakers. There was surprise and shock about the occurrence of harm-inducing errors. As one participant described, "It is heartbreaking that most of these are preventable and happened because of lapses at many different levels."

Theme 2: Mistakes are normal. Students came to the realization that mistakes and errors will happen regardless of a person's experience. They recognized that it is important to be vigilant and proactive on an individual level, and improve systems on an organizational level. As one student learned, "Being human we are all susceptible to error. It's inescapable."

Theme 3: Preventing errors is the responsibility of both individuals and teams. Students gained an understanding of the different expertise areas and roles of their health professions colleagues related to patient care. They recognized the need to speak up on an individual level and work together with other health professions to provide safe patient care. A few notable quotes from students were:

- "Communication is key! And we really need to check our attitude at the door."
- "We need to have the courage to speak up and advocate for our patient when we have concerns about care."
- "I don't want to get lost in the technical details and forget that I'm helping a real person."

Implications from the findings are that patient safety education is valued by most health professions students when they are exposed to this important content area. More important is the notion that the students had strong beliefs that learning about patient safety in an interprofessional manner, whether as a common day or as coursework, is essential. Students recognize the need for interprofessional dialogue and collaboration while learning about patient safety and prefer to learn the content in an interdisciplinary model. These observations present evidence of the need to develop an interdisciplinary mechanism for delivery of patient safety content to health professions students.

Since the first course implementation in 2005 and the subsequent addition of Patient Safety Days on campus, there have been national policy-level changes in organizations devoted to improving safe, quality health care. The various health professions accrediting bodies have standards for health programs accreditation. Many of these have adopted explicit training standards related to healthcare safety. The Institute for Healthcare Improvement launched the Open School in 2008 to provide students of nursing, medicine, public health, pharmacy, health administration, dentistry, and other allied health

(continues)

professions with core content learning online on the topics of patient safety and improvement at no charge to participants (Institute for Healthcare Improvement, n.d.). This powerful approach can facilitate academic institutions in the incorporation of safety content, although it does not offer educational strategy and techniques at the local level to enhance interprofessional learning. Local-level education still must be designed and facilitated through educators within the higher education professional programs.

Discussion Points

1. Why is it important that health professions share a common understanding of patient safety standards and practices?
2. What are the policy implications from accepting that "mistakes are normal and all humans err"?
3. How would you approach healthcare system leaders/employers about changing employment policies related to punitive action when errors occur?

Policy Implications

The university-wide implementation case offers important lessons to others nationally in healthcare education. Although the students in our case description have a strong sentiment toward receiving interprofessional education through shared work, we have not attained required core content across the professional training programs. We have seen growth in adoption of safety content; however, this content has remained relatively specific to each discipline and there is scattered overlap and discipline-specific foci as the prominent offering.

Although we see the advancement of incorporating educational content across health professions programs in the country, we still see disconnection between increasingly educated professionals (former students now in practice) and policy related to safety. Many healthcare organizations still maintain a blame culture that results in loss of employment for some individuals who make human errors despite employing best practices and genuinely doing their best while functioning in challenging and poorly designed care delivery systems. "Who is to blame?" all too often remains a key question in health care when someone is injured by preventable errors. Nurse professionals are often at the sharp edge of safety, and often are the last point of contact with a patient who ultimately has an upstream error committed in the care delivery system. When negative events occur, our professions often confront one another, rather than ask what we could have done differently to prevent this from occurring. We need to shift policy from blame to advocacy. That is, we must create policies and processes so that healthcare organizations and health professional employees respond to the question, "How can we make it so this never happens again?"

Education has been essential to enlightening health professionals, administrators, researchers, and policymakers. The Institute of Medicine has continued to advance our study of barriers to advancing safety in practice settings. The National Patient Safety Foundation continues to sponsor innovative projects to inform us about reducing harm and injury and to facilitate legislative and federal agendas. A key federal agency, the Agency for Healthcare Research and Quality (AHRQ), places improving the quality and safety of healthcare delivery systems as its primary focus for research and innovation and is a primary source of funding for research advances. These national and public initiatives are critical to the attainment of safe, quality health care. However, this goal will only be realized if health professionals advance patient centered systems approaches to delivering care and own the responsibility of reducing the risk of harm and injury through proactive interprofessional problem solving.

References

Abbott, A. A., Fuji, K. T., Galt, K. A., & Paschal, K. A. (2012). How baccalaureate nursing students value an interprofessional patient safety course for professional development. *ISRN Nursing* (Article ID 401358). doi:10.5402/2012/401358

Baker, D. P., Gustafson, S., Beaubien, J. M., Salas, E., & Barach, P. (2005). Medical team training programs in health care. *Advances in Patient Safety: From Research to Implementation*, 4, 253–267.

Fuji, K. T., Paschal, K. A., Galt, K. A., & Abbott, A. A. (2010). Pharmacy student attitudes toward an interprofessional patient safety course: An exploratory mixed methods study. *Currents in Pharmacy Teaching and Learning*, 2(4), 238–247.

Galt, K. A., Paschal, K. A., O'Brien, R. L., McQuillan, R. J., Graves, J. K., Harris, B., ... Sonnino, R. (2006). Description and evaluation of an interprofessional patient safety course for health professions and related sciences students. *Journal of Patient Safety*, 2(4), 207–216.

Hippocrates, *Epidemics*, Bk. 1, Sect. XI.

Institute for Healthcare Improvement. (n.d.). *Open school*. Retrieved from http://www.ihi.org /education/ihiopenschool/Pages/default.aspx

Institute of Medicine. (1972). *Educating for the health team*. Washington, DC: National Academy of Sciences.

Institute of Medicine. (2000). *To err is human: Building a safer health system*. Washington, DC: National Academy Press.

Institute of Medicine. (2001). *Crossing the quality chasm*. Washington, DC: National Academy Press.

Interprofessional Education Collaborative Expert Panel. (2011). *Core competencies for interprofessional collaborative practice: Report of an expert panel*. Washington, DC: Interprofessional Education Collaborative.

King, J. B., Battles, J., Baker, D. P., Alonso, A., Salas, E., & Webster, J. (2008). TEAMSTEPPS: Team strategies and tools to enhance performance and patient safety. *Advances in Patient Safety: New Directions and Alternative Approaches, 3*, 5–20.

O'Neil, E. H., & the Pew Health Professions Commission. (1998). *Recreating health professional practice for a new century—the fourth report of the Pew Health Professions Commission*. San Francisco, CA: Pew Health Professions Commission.

World Health Organization (WHO). (2010). *Framework for action on interprofessional education and collaborative practice*. Retrieved from http://www.who.int/hrh/resources /framework_action/en/

***

THE EVOLVING INTERPROFESSIONAL UNIVERSE

J.D. Polk

KEY TERM

Crowd source: Convening professionals from many disciplines to focus on a problem by means of innovative tactics.

What Is Interprofessional Collaboration?

By the time you read this chapter, the definition of interprofessional education (IPE) will have evolved. In the early outset of IPE the purpose was to show that healthcare providers other than the physician were just as important to the outcomes of the patient. Many would say that it was about teaching physicians they were no longer in charge. It has since evolved to a definition that looks more at all of the healthcare providers working as a team toward the end goal of better health outcomes for the patient (Aston et al., 2012).

But even this definition is too shallow. By the end of this chapter you will see that IPE is about a team approach to patient care and better health outcomes, but that the team is much larger than we currently think, and not restricted only to healthcare professionals. In fact, technology drives the access to and usability of information toward the patient outcome to such a degree that IPE and the collaboration of many partners has no bounds, and will continue to evolve and expand.

Core Attributes of Interprofessional Education

The need for and value of interprofessional education are not new concepts; IPE has been around for several decades. The World Health Organization put forward the idea of including IPE in medical education around the world in 1978, knowing that not all communities have physicians or access to quality medical care, and that the care and outcome of the patient depend on many caregivers, especially in third world countries (World Health Organization, 1978).

The Institute of Medicine soon followed with recommendations on incorporating IPE into medical education in its 2000 report, *To Err Is Human: Building a Safer Health System*, as well as in its 2003 report, *Health Professions Education: A Bridge to Quality* (Institute of Medicine, 2003). Much of the current IPE movement has centered on increasing quality through teaming, and it has been clear for some time that despite the United States being at the top of the scale in terms of healthcare spending, our patient care outcomes are still woefully behind many other countries that do a better job in regards to that team-based approach.

But the core attributes of what comprises interprofessional education vary depending on the institution and authorship. Many of the publications from the Health Resources and Services Administration (HRSA) and the Institute of Medicine (IOM) have focused on the need to have physician assistants, nurses, and advanced practice registered nurses fill the void that has come about due to a physician shortage in primary care, and the perceived inflection point that the Affordable Care Act requires more primary care providers. However, even that goal is too narrow and not quite holistic enough. Instead, all of the various incarnations and articles describing an attribute or core educational component can be boiled down to one succinct statement and goal: To teach all healthcare providers to partner and utilize any and all resources available, both medical and non-medical, to bring about a sustained positive outcome for the patient.

The following case study exemplifies this holistic concept and why we need to broaden our vision of IPE.

CASE STUDY 2: AN ADOLESCENT WITH DIABETES: TYPICAL TREATMENT OPTIONS?

A 13-year-old male presents to his primary care provider for his annual school physical and is noted to be grossly overweight. His vital signs show that he has a blood pressure of 138/70, pulse of 88, and respirations of 18, and he seems somewhat winded just walking from the waiting room to the exam room. His urine dip reveals trace protein and mild amounts of glucose and you suspect he is either already a type 2 diabetic or quickly on his way to becoming one. You arrange for a fasting glucose and HgA1C to be drawn. Knowing that his family can ill afford multiple physician visits, you determine that you will have him follow up with the nurse practitioner at the free clinic in his inner-city neighborhood, and you have also arranged for diet counseling with a nutritionist at the same clinic. You are quite proud of the fact that you have engaged your IPE partners and have worked toward a better outcome that is lower cost for the patient.

Discussion Points

1. Assess the probability that your plan will be successful. How can this scenario be altered so that it becomes an interprofessional plan?
2. Discuss implications about the fact that there is not a quality grocery near his home and that fresh produce is not readily available, but there is a fast food restaurant across the street from his home.
3. What about the fact that his school has soda and junk food vending machines on every floor and the lunch line considers pizza a vegetable?
4. What about the fact that his mother has never learned to prepare fresh fruits or vegetables, has never seen an avocado, and has never been taught how to prepare dinners that incorporate healthy foods?
5. What about the fact that his neighborhood is one in which jogging, running, or walking might not be the safest things to do, and as a result his exercise is highly curtailed?
6. What is the likelihood that this young man will have a positive health outcome in the years to come if the previous items are not addressed?

Reframing the Case Study: Treatment Options

In this case study, a partnership has to be forged not only with other healthcare providers, but also with the school, the child's mother, community leaders, private corporations, and public health departments.

Discussion Points

1. What kinds of public–private partnerships could you forge to change the access to fruits and vegetables and decrease the potential for disparities based on race, neighborhood, and countless other factors?

(continues)

2. What types of partnerships with local government and perhaps private entities might enable members to tear down several of the abandoned buildings and turn the lot into a park for recreation and exercise for the neighborhood?
3. What school and community leaders could be approached to eliminate the junk food and soda vending machines from the school?
4. What research could you bring to or interpret for a policymaker that would help the policymaker sell the idea to his or her colleagues?

Without changes such as those suggested in the discussion points, this child's destiny as a type 2 diabetic with metabolic syndrome will be very hard to change. The nurse practitioner, physician, and nutritional counselor could work together very well as a team and still never quite create a positive health outcome for this patient. There are just too many factors working against them. Such an endeavor will require true interprofessional collaboration, not only among healthcare providers but among all of the potential resources. IPE is about more than having the pharmacist, nutritional counselor, physician assistant, nurse practitioner, and physician work as a team. It is about utilizing every potential resource to bring about positive change in healthcare outcomes (U.S. Department of Health and Human Services, 2014).

The "Team 4" Concept

The National Aeronautics and Space Administration (NASA) is known for being innovative and collaborative, but also pretty smart. They are, after all, rocket scientists. But they also have a concept that aligns very well with IPE. I am sure that many of you have seen or recall the movie *Apollo 13* starring Tom Hanks (Howard, 1995).

There is a scene in the movie where the scientists at the NASA Space Center need to build a carbon dioxide scrubber, or at least alter the interface for it, in order to lower the CO_2 in the vehicle. The engineer puts all the equipment that is currently on board the spacecraft on the table and states "we need to make this fit into this, ... using only these" (Howard,

1995). You probably think that scene was a Hollywood invention meant to dramatize the movie; in reality, that is what actually occurred. But beyond that example, NASA has a concept even to this day that should serve as a potential example for IPE. Typically, for any space mission there are three shifts or teams in the flight control room. However, NASA also has a "Team 4." Team 4 is the problem solvers. It is a group of people from nearly every discipline that gets together to problem solve an issue that develops during a mission. The members are not just engineers. The team is collaborative, cross-cultural, and cross-disciplinary.

For example, one of the lights on the side of an astronaut's helmet had a fractured bracket. The light would not stay on the side of the helmet. The team got together to try to figure out what method they could use to affix the light to the helmet. Whatever solution they used had to withstand the vast 200-degree-Fahrenheit temperature variations between light and dark in space, as well as the vacuum of space. What did the team eventually come up with? They used dental cement that is typically used in the emergency department after a tooth fracture. The medical kit had this cement in it just in case an astronaut suffered a tooth fracture in orbit. The cement withstands hot and cold temperatures and is not bothered by the vacuum of space. The cement was used to adhere the light bracket to the helmet, and it worked perfectly (Simpson, 2007).

In another example, the thermal blanket that protects the space shuttle from extreme heat had become torn on entry. This could allow superhot gases to encroach on the vehicle during re-entry with catastrophic consequences. The Team 4 solution was less about engineering than it was about

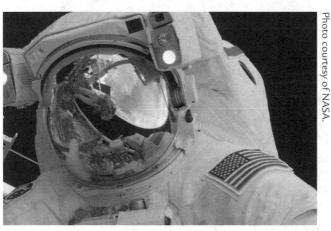

Photo courtesy of NASA.

An astronaut on a spacewalk. Note the light on his helmet.

simple patient care. Their solution was to perform a two-layer closure using skin staples and suture to repair the blanket, not unlike a surgeon would close a wound. The ideas and "solvers" for solutions sometimes come from unlikely sources, and NASA recognizes this. No idea is dismissed out of hand, and very often the solution comes from an unlikely source; in the previous two cases they came from the medical community and medical kits.

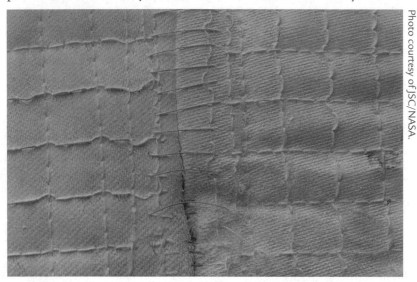

Photo courtesy of JSC/NASA.

A. Thermal blanket.

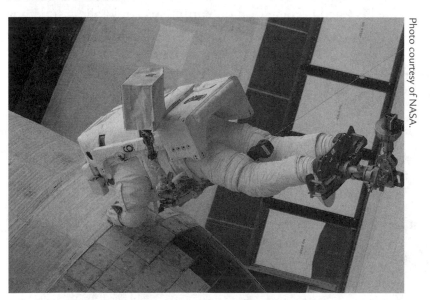

Photo courtesy of NASA.

B. Astronaut Danny Olivas performs a "surgical closure" on the thermal blanket.

What can we learn from NASA about teaming? In health care we tend to think of IPE as the physician, pharmacist, nurse, nurse practitioner, and physician assistant all getting along and working cohesively. NASA would say we were still thinking much too narrowly.

The business of innovation has taken a cue from NASA. InnoCentive (n.d.) is a private company that works to **crowd source** problems and challenges for customers using a worldwide network of solvers from many different walks of life, professions, and specialties in a host of countries (Allio, 2004).

Rather than sending out a chemistry problem to only chemists, the problem or challenge is crowd-sourced to a host of many different solvers. Sometimes, and in fact often, the answer comes from outside the specialty that would normally be looking at the problem. For example, an engineer who specializes in fluid mechanics might look at a problem much differently than the typical chemist would. He or she might offer a solution upon seeing similarities in their own world or work that the chemist would not have thought of. In 2007, InnoCentive helped the Oil Spill Recovery Institute post three challenges that all dealt with oil spill recovery issues. Who solved the first of the three challenges? It actually wasn't someone from the oil industry, but rather someone from the concrete industry, who looked at the problem in a whole new light.

CASE STUDY 3: INNOVATION AND IPE IN A CHILEAN MINE

The Chilean government took IPE to a whole new level after the collapse of one of its mines trapped 33 miners 2,400 feet below solid rock. The miners were trapped after 600,000 tons of rock collapsed in the 100-year-old mine in Copiapo, Chile. After 17 days of using a small drill to poke a hole into the caverns to see if the miners were alive or if they had perished, the miners were found alive.

The Chilean government did something that most governments would never think of doing. They crowd-sourced solutions and collaborated with multiple countries, industries, and teams in order to achieve their outcome. They threw off the cloak of bureaucracy, streamlined and flattened the leadership chain, and began an odyssey

(continues)

of interprofessional collaboration that was unmatched and never seen before in this type of problem and rescue. They invited NASA to participate and advise them because the space program is well versed at keeping people alive in enclosed spaces for prolonged periods of time, and also is known for their great engineering prowess. They invited the Chilean Navy, miners and drillers from every specialty, and a host of medical professions to help them problem solve the issues and complex problems related to feeding the miners, treating them for their ailments, drilling to rescue them, developing new drilling techniques, developing a rescue capsule, and inventing never-before-seen or -used procedures toward the successful rescue. Until their rescue, no miners had ever survived a collapse of this magnitude, so deep below the Earth, for so long a period. The multidisciplinary teams would bounce ideas off of each other, and the Chilean leadership would implement those ideas that they felt were the most promising. What was the result of their interprofessional collaboration? All 33 miners were rescued 69 days into their ordeal as the world watched.

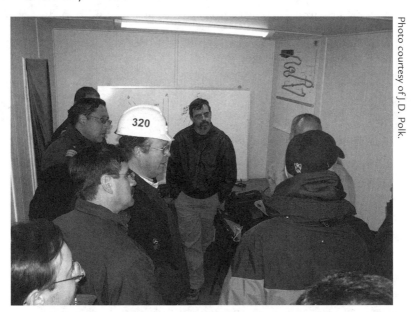

Photo courtesy of J.D. Polk.

Dr. J. D. Polk (center) at a team meeting among engineers, miners, doctors, and drilling experts from three different countries, the Chilean Navy, and NASA.

Discussion Points

1. What resources would you need when team members speak various languages?
2. What are the implications of a team composed of people from different cultures who are addressing a crisis such as the one described?
3. What health resources would you assemble in anticipation of bringing the miners to the surface?

The Future of IPE

Prior to 1967 there were no physician assistants, and prior to 1965 there were no nurse practitioners. The field of health care has grown in leaps and bounds since that time, and the need for multiple layers of care, and multiple team members to care for the many facets of a patient's needs to guarantee a positive outcome, has long been recognized. But this chapter should show you that creating the positive patient outcomes of the future may rely on more than the current subset of medical practitioners. It will require integration with public health, with industry, and with the private sector and touch virtually everything that the patient interacts with on some level. Technology will radically change how health care is delivered, and most especially change where patients get their information (Interprofessional Education Collaborative Expert Panel, 2011).

Today, most patients have surfed the web thoroughly before presenting to their caregiver's office. Imagine a vending machine in the future that recognizes that the customer is a diabetic by the bracelet worn or some other method, and suggests healthy choices tailored to the customer. Imagine point-of-care testing at home to test for a streptococcus infection. Technology will change how the patient interacts with the healthcare provider. It may also serve to connect and allow many disciplines to collaborate and crowd source what is best for the patient. A nurse practitioner in a rural area will be able to get a virtual consult from a specialist in a major city without much difficulty, and the idea of the patient always having to go to a tertiary care center to get specialized care will become a thing of the past.

References and Bibliography

Allio, R. J. (2004). CEO interview: The InnoCentive model of open innovation. *Strategy and Leadership, 32*(4), 4–9.

Aston, S. J., Rheault, W., Arenson, C., Tappert, S. K., Stoecker, J., Orzoff, J., ... Mackintosh, S. (2012). Interprofessional education: A review and analysis of programs from three academic health centers. *Academic Medicine, 87*(7), 949–955.

Howard, R., (1995). *Apollo 13* [Motion picture]. United States: Imagine Entertainment, distributed by Universal Pictures.

Institute of Medicine. (2003). *Health professions education: A bridge to quality.* Washington, DC: National Academy of Sciences. Retrieved from http://www.iom.edu/Reports/2003 /Health-Professions-Education-A-Bridge-to-Quality.aspx

InnoCentive. (n.d.). *What we do.* Retrieved from https://www.innocentive.com /about-innocentive

Interprofessional Education Collaborative Expert Panel. (2011). *Core competencies for interprofessional collaborative practice: Report of an expert panel.* Washington, DC: Interprofessional Education Collaborative.

Simpson, C. (2007). Atlantis completes spectacular mission. *Spaceflight, 49*(8), 293.

U.S. Department of Health and Human Services, Agency for Healthcare Research and Quality. (2014). *TeamSTEPPS®: National implementation.* Retrieved from http://teamstepps.ahrq. gov

World Health Organization. (1978). *Alma-Ata 1978: Primary health care, report of the International Conference on Primary Health Care. 6–12 September 1978; Alma-Ata, USSR.* Geneva, Switzerland: World Health Organization.

***

THE TRANSFORMATIVE JOURNEY

Patrick DeLeon

Vision, Persistence, Patience

Tip O'Neill, the former speaker of the House of Representatives, once opined: "All politics is local," which is perhaps the most critical message embedded in this chapter. The public policy process is an extraordinarily personal one, and those involved report, in retrospect, having experienced a life-changing journey rather than merely having a job or an interesting internship. To be successful, one needs vision, persistence, and presence;

that is, one must have an understanding of what it is that one wants to change or what new policy or program one wants to implement. We have learned over the years that change always takes time—often far longer than one might initially expect. Many are invested in the status quo, including those who were not expected to be that people had assumed would be proponents of the proposed changes. It is absolutely necessary to be personally committed to being involved in the public policy/political process for the long haul, and there are many avenues available for significant participation.

Meaningful public policy successes require more than short-term political advocacy efforts, as often proposed by one's professional association. We must appreciate that if change were easy, someone else would have undoubtedly instituted a particular idea long ago. In reality, what are sincerely proposed as "new ideas" often have been tried before. Accordingly one must be personally present and forever vigilant to be a successful change agent.

It is amazing how often serendipity plays a major role in shaping a national or local policy agenda. The media, in particular, can have a major impact in determining when substantive change will occur and the conditions necessary for it. Those involved in shaping public policy soon come to appreciate that steps taken by others in the past often laid the foundation for tomorrow's successes. Above all else, to be ultimately successful and to enjoy the unique journey, one must learn the language and nuances of the public policy process. There can be no question that thoughtful, involved, and prepared individuals can make a real difference in the lives of many (DeLeon, Rychnovsky, & Culp, 2011).

As highly educated members of society and as skilled healthcare practitioners, it is perhaps only natural to assume that the substance of one's issue is the critical factor for having it ultimately adopted by those who establish national or regional policy. With your extensive training and unique clinical expertise, you can see from the front line how society and patient care could be improved—if only... . Although the substance of an issue is definitely important, we would strongly suggest being very cautious about making generalized assumptions, including that others will see your issue in the same light as you do. At the federal level, for example, more than half of the elected officials are lawyers by training, with businesspeople representing the next largest group. Those professions have developed their own way of thinking and professional value system over the years that are quite different than those of healthcare practitioners. To assume that they appreciate the nuances of the healthcare environment of today would be naïve. The reality is that they will obtain most of their healthcare knowledge from the media and from personal experiences while accessing the system for themselves or members of their families.

Perspectives on Being Involved

Dr. Clifford Swensen, professor emeritus at Purdue University, said the following:

> Having been involved in politics, and for a long time in university politics, there are some things I have observed. (1) Any change hurts somebody. Who is being hurt and how can you ameliorate that? (2) The status quo has a lot of vested interests. Where are they and how can you alleviate their concerns? (3) Any change brings about unanticipated, undesirable side effects. How can you anticipate them as much as possible, but more important have in place means of coping with and ameliorating them? (4) Opponents are not evil enemies. They are people who have a vested interest somewhere and have a different point of view. (5) In any fight, the objective and overall purpose often gets lost, and the goal is simply to win the fight. The longer I observe, the more I am convinced that a lot of the conflict is based on the last item. (personal communication, April 2014)

Former American Psychological Association (APA) Congressional Science Fellow Neil Kirschner said the following when reflecting upon his year on Capitol Hill:

> More often than not, research findings in the legislative arena are only valued if consistent with conclusions based upon the more salient political decision factors. Thus, within the legislative setting, the research data are [sic] not used to drive decision-making decisions, but is more frequently used to support decisions made based upon other factors. As psychologists [and health care practitioners], we need to be aware of this basic difference between the role of research in science settings and the legislative world. It makes the role of the researcher who wants to put "into play" available research results into a public policy deliberation more complex. Data need to be introduced, explained or framed in a manner cognizant of the political exigencies. Furthermore, it emphasizes the importance of efforts to educate our legislators on the importance and long-term effectiveness of basing decisions on quality data.... If I've learned anything on the Hill, it is the importance of political advocacy if you desire a change in public policy." (Kirschner, 2003)

Nursing is particularly fortunate in that its national leadership has, for a prolonged period of time, appreciated the fundamental importance of training and mentorship in public policy program development. Today health policy is one of the required competencies within nursing education, and over 100 schools of nursing have stand-alone health policy courses in their basic curriculum. In stark contrast, it is quite rare to find a health policy course within psychology's educational programs. Le Ondra Clark Harvey is a psychologist working as a consultant to the California State Senate Committee on Business, Professions, and Economic Development.

> As I sit at my desk in the California Capitol, I am taking a moment to breathe and reflect on the past two weeks. I have been working on a number of controversial bills before the Senate. One of them is a bill that would require all mental health professionals to show evidence of suicide prevention training as a prerequisite for licensure. For those who are already practicing, they will have to take a onetime CE course on suicide prevention. As I examine the rationale provided for this bill, I am shocked. It appears that everyone has been so focused on the recent suicides that the media has highlighted that they have neglected to do a thorough review of the literature in this area. In moments like these, I realize that the unique research and clinical training I have been afforded aids me in bringing the empirical evidence to light via my analysis of the bill. Ultimately, it is up to the legislators to vote; but the analyses I write serve as a background and context for the decisions they make. How difficult it was for me to forge a path into the policy arena with no psychology mentors who were doing work in policy and no models for how to get into the policy arena. (personal communication, June 2014)

As these three perspectives indicate, there are many ways for concerned citizens to become effectively involved in the public policy process.

The Affordable Care Act

It is important to appreciate that the timing of the enactment of specific legislation frequently occurs seemingly as the result of "the stars finally lining up," rather than any specific activity initiated by those wishing change. At the same time, systematically developing foundational work clearly enhances the probability of one's success. The enactment of President Obama's landmark Patient Protection and Affordable Care Act (ACA) (P.L. 111-148) contains several exciting nurse-related provisions whose ideas, in retrospect, can be found discussed in various policy documents and previously introduced legislative bills. The essence of the President's vision was to provide incentives for the establishment of *systems* of patient-centered, interdisciplinary care that would capitalize on the unprecedented advances occurring within the communications and technology fields, as well as providing a priority for delivering gold-standard preventive and wellness-oriented care. Rather than focusing on specific clinical procedures, as had been done historically, the new reimbursement approach would emphasize developing measurable outcomes criteria, including the impact of providing long-neglected mental and behavioral health services that were now to be granted parity with physical healthcare interventions. Bringing the newest scientific knowledge to the practitioner at the bedside or in outpatient clinics in a timely fashion was to be a priority (i.e., translational research and competitive effectiveness research). This new approach would undoubtedly require a fundamental re-evaluation of the health professions requirements of the nation and, relatedly, the extent to which professional scope of practice issues and licensure mobility would best serve the needs of the nation. This new approach also required agreement negotiated among healthcare professionals, legislators and their staffs, and other interested parties.

Nurse-Managed Health Clinics

One example contained in the ACA that we are particularly familiar with is Section 330A-1, the Nurse-Managed Health Clinic provision of Title V— Health Care Workforce, Section 5208. Senator Daniel K. Inouye (D-HI) had long been supportive of enhanced nurse practice and over the years had been instrumental in sponsoring most, if not all, of the federal legislation resulting in direct payment to advanced practice registered nurses (APRNs) within a wide range of federal initiatives (including CHAMPUS, Medicaid, Medicare, and the Federal Employees Health Benefit [FEHB] programs), as well as introducing bills proposing nurse- and nursing school–managed health clinics. He had been quite impressed by the success of the School of Nursing at Vanderbilt University in running its clinics, under the leadership of Dean Colleen Conway Welch, in both providing needed health care and teaching their graduate students about the all-important financial aspects of health care. A provision ultimately included within the ACA would require the secretary of the Department of Health and Human Services (HHS) to establish a grant program to fund the operation of nurse-managed health clinics (NMHCs) that provide comprehensive primary health care and wellness services to vulnerable or underserved populations. To be eligible to receive a grant, an NMHC would have to submit an application to the secretary containing assurances that: (1) nurses are a major provider of services at the NMHC, (2) the NMHC will provide care to all patients regardless of income or insurance status, and (3) the NMHC will establish a community advisory committee in which the majority of the members are individuals served by the NMHC. All of the eligibility requirements were negotiated with input from nurses, agency staff (e.g., Department of Defense and others), and policymakers. When determining grant amounts, the secretary would be required to take into account the financial need of the NMHC, including other funding sources available to the NMHC, and other factors determined appropriate by the secretary. One might reasonably wonder how this far-reaching, visionary provision became public law.

Almost every U.S. President since Franklin D. Roosevelt, regardless of political affiliation, had proposed the enactment of comprehensive healthcare legislation during his tenure—whether to increase access, curtail escalating costs, or address national public health priorities. Many of the underlying principles contained within the ACA had been discussed for decades by various health policy think tanks, including the Institute of Medicine (IOM) of the National Academy of Sciences. The personal element of health policy was also notably present during the 111th Congress. Within President Obama's cabinet (as well as among his high-level appointees) there was considerable interest in comprehensively addressing the healthcare needs of the nation. For example, his first director of the Office of Management and Budget (OMB) was elected to the IOM in 2008; another member of the IOM, Dr. Mary Wakefield (a nurse), had been appointed administrator of the Health Resources and Services Administration (HRSA), which is the key federal agency for addressing the healthcare needs of the historically underserved.

The ACA would ultimately pass the U.S. Senate without any Republican votes, even though its original drafting drew heavily upon Republican ideas, including the successes in Massachusetts of the future Republican candidate for president, Governor Mitt Romney. As the political debates became increasingly partisan, the Senate Democratic majority leader made an unusually special effort to ensure that the personal priorities of his Democratic colleagues would be addressed in the final bill. There was never a question in anyone's mind that Senator Inouye would vote for the president's bill. The senator was one of the very few sitting elected officials who had voted for the original Medicare legislation and, over the years, had sponsored various national health insurance proposals introduced by Senator Kennedy and like-minded colleagues. Nevertheless, the leader's staff wanted to make absolutely sure that his personal interests would be taken into account.

At that time, Captain Jacqueline Rychnovsky (U.S. Navy) was serving as the Department of Defense Nursing Fellow in the Senator's office. Jacqueline staffed the meeting with the majority leader's office and reinforced their earlier appreciation for the senator's profound and long-time support for nursing as an autonomous profession. During that meeting she specifically proposed that the nurse-managed health clinic bill that Senator Inouye had earlier drafted be included in the leader's package of amendments. Not surprisingly, subsequent discussions elicited that organized medicine expressed considerable objections. Nevertheless, the leader ultimately prevailed and the provision became public law.

Again, the importance of the personal element of health policy was evident. During her year-long tenure, Rychnovsky had met with Senator Inouye on at least a daily basis, and he was very pleased to learn that she had the vision and presence to suggest that his nurse-managed health clinic provision be included in the ACA. As we noted earlier, success requires vision, persistence, and presence—all ably demonstrated that day by Rychnovsky. From a national public policy perspective, there can be no question that the inclusion of the nurse-managed health clinic provision in the ACA sent a powerful message to the entire healthcare community that, "Nurses should be full partners, with physicians and other health care professionals, in redesigning health care in the United States" (IOM, 2010, p. 4), as proclaimed in the IOM report, *The Future of Nursing: Leading Change, Advancing Health*. Rychnovsky was present at that critical meeting and possessed the scientific data to support her suggestion for national healthcare reform. She also was able to demonstrate that the NMHC provision had been modeled closely on the highly successful federally qualified health center (FQHC) program, which had been an integral component of President Lyndon Johnson's Great Society era, as well as the area health education center (AHEC) program within the HRSA. This new initiative had the potential to directly address the evolving questions surrounding the complex health professions personnel requirements of the nation as the ACA was steadily implemented. Rychnovsky personified two critical elements of the successful congressional staffer: she *listened* very carefully to Senator Inouye's passion for nursing and she did *not* require credit for her accomplishments.

Interdisciplinary Training

Throughout the ACA there are a number of provisions that actively encourage integrated and interdisciplinary care. Underlying this concept is the need for addressing at the health policy level what, if any, are the basic differences in the various disciplines and the closely related issue of whether their scope of practice statutes (i.e., licensure laws) are in line with the extent of their training. In 1985, Diane Kjervik of the American Association of Colleges of Nursing (AACN) noted:

> From a public policy frame of reference, the fundamental issues involved in defining the appropriate scope of practice for psychology are identical to those for nursing. The first and most basic issue is whether the profession is mature enough, has developed sufficient clinical skills, and has sufficient internal agreement regarding these matters to be able to define its own limits and to supervise its own practitioners. These considerations are reflected in the issue of whether the profession's practitioners should be deemed autonomous within the scope of their practice act, or whether it is necessary to legislate the active involvement or collaboration of members of another profession (i.e., medicine). The basic answer should be closely related to the stance of the educational institution involved . . . . Psychology and nursing would appear to be natural allies. Unfortunately, there has been only minimal organizational cooperation to date, especially at the state and practitioner level . . . . [F]rom a public policy perspective, the autonomous practice of psychology and nursing is a new evolution. As such, they have just begun to develop that "critical mass" of professionals (as well as clinical and scientific acceptance) that is necessary to truly affect our nation's health policy. (DeLeon, Kjervik, Kraut, & VandenBos, 1985, pp. 1153–1154, 1160–1161)

Her position is highly consistent with the visionary IOM recommendation that: "Nurses should practice to the full extent of their education and training [and that] nurses should achieve higher levels of education and training through an improved education system that promotes seamless academic progression" (IOM, 2010, p. 4).

In 2009, prior to the enactment of the ACA, six national education associations from schools of the health professions formed the Interprofessional Education Collaborative (IPEC) to promote and encourage constituent efforts that would advance substantive interprofessional learning experiences to help prepare future clinicians for the team-based care of patients. These organizations that represent higher education in nursing, medicine, dentistry, pharmacy, and public health would create core competencies for interprofessional collaborative practice that can guide curricula development at all health professions schools.

After being engaged in the public policy process at the federal level for nearly 4 decades, this author has come to appreciate that as long as one remains resolutely focused upon one's primary objective, there will always be many collegial supporters, often representing interests that one might not have originally thought about (DeLeon, Wakefield, Schultz, Williams, & VandenBos, 1989). The public policy world is actually quite small, and interactions are often described as reflecting the truism, "What goes around, comes around." At the Uniformed Services University of the Health Sciences (USUHS) within the Department of Defense, Professor Gloria Ramsey and I teach an interdisciplinary health policy course involving doctor of nursing practice (DNP) and psychology graduate students and faculty. As we expose our students to the experiences and views of a wide range of national policy experts, our presenters from time to time will inquire whether we might know of individuals who would be appropriate subject matter experts for their own areas of interest.

One of these discussions led to Professor Ramsey being invited to testify before the U.S. Senate Special Committee on Aging on the complex issues related to the question of respect for the person in the context of the patient's wishes and advanced care planning. This is an area in which Gloria is truly a national expert, having focused her education, clinical practice, policy, and research in this arena for more than 2 decades. She has worked closely with concerned policy stakeholders, such as government (Maryland State Advisory Council on Quality Care at the End of Life), colleagues within the American Bar Association (ABA) Commission on Law and Aging, and various national nursing organizations (American Nurses Association and the American Academy of Nursing), as well as other health policy organizations such as the Hastings Center, National Hospice and Palliative Care Organization; academic colleagues at the Duke University Institute on Care at the End of Life, NYU College of Nursing, Albert Einstein College of Medicine, and Montefiore Medical Center; and related advocacy groups. The senators on the committee were most impressed by her testimony and encouraged her to continue to work with them and their staff as they expanded their interest in this critical area over the next several congresses. Her nursing, bioethics, and legal background highlighted for the audience the unique contribution that advanced practice registered nurses (APRNs) and DNPs can make in the clinical and research arena in improving how we die in the United States. She is not only making an outstanding contribution to the health and well-being of our nation by being personally involved in the public policy process, but also serving as an inspirational role model for nursing's next generation. The one message that resonates for Gloria is that healthcare professionals, and nurses in particular, must remain vigilant in health policy efforts. "The ACA is a great example of how government reached out to health care providers to help with implementation. We must not let the ACA be the last effort that 'we' in the collective sense are able to influence. How we die is a public health concern and all of us share in making it better" (personal communication, July 2014).

The Importance of Personal Stories

Over the years, when discussing with members of Congress and/or their staff what impressed them the most about the need for a substantive change in policy (i.e., why they became personally engaged in a particular issue), it became quite clear that listening to an individual constituent, especially from their home state or district, talking about his or her aspirations and problems was the key. The "how" of change relies upon the elected official's expertise; the "why" for change is the personal experience of those whom they were elected to serve.

Senator Inouye would frequently talk about the personal obligation he felt to the Native Hawaiian people. His mother had been adopted by Native Hawaiians when she was a young child and had urged him to never forget them. Over the years he would listen to their concerns, spend hours listening to individuals and small groups, and preside at formal Congressional hearings that he initiated. He was the first elected member of the House of Representatives in the history of the State of Hawaii, and soon moved over to the U.S. Senate. Today, Hawaii is experiencing a Native Hawaiian renaissance, personified by the *Hokule'a*, an ancient voyaging canoe traveling around the world relying solely upon the winds, currents, and stars for its navigational inspiration. Senator Inouye was instrumental in modifying federal statutes over the years, authorizing special Native Hawaiian employment, education, and healthcare programs. Congressional staff estimate that these now account for $50–$60 million annually being appropriated to address the special needs and aspirations of these Native American peoples. Those personal stories and dreams make all the difference in the world to the elected official.

"The Times They Are A-Changin" (excerpts from DeLeon, P., June 2014, Let the Good Times Roll, APA Newsletter, Division 18)

The American Association of Colleges of Pharmacy (AACP) is engaged in a new venture, Professions Quest (PQ), in order to develop and produce serious educational games for the healthcare professions....PQ will release its first game, Mimyex, in January 2015. The competency framework...will be derived from the Core Competencies for Interprofessional Education released in May 2011 by the Interprofessional Education Collaborative (IPEC)....PQ will develop and publish virtual, interprofessional, and interactive multiplayer learning solutions targeted specifically towards health professions education institutions and health professions students.

The IOM Board on Children, Youth, and Families (BCYF)...[has] launched a nationwide video contest to help raise awareness among young athletes about the importance of taking concussions seriously. The "Play It Safe" video contest is open to anyone ages 13 to 22 interested in creating a 30- to 60-second public service announcement about sport-related concussions. Topics for the videos may include how youth can overcome a sports culture that often promotes "shaking it off" and getting back in the game, and how they can help teammates, coaches, and parents better recognize the signs, symptoms, and need for proper treatment of concussions. The IOM/NRC will pick three winners—one from each age group of middle school, high school, and post-high school—who will each receive a $300 gift card....As many as 1.6 million to 3.8 million sports- and recreation-related concussions and other traumatic injuries are reported each year in the United States.

A FANTASTIC ACCOMPLISHMENT

Illinois has now become the third state in the country in which licensed clinical psychologists with advanced, specialized training can prescribe medications for mental health disorders....[The] bill had been powerfully and effectively championed by [senators and representatives from both major political parties]....The rhetoric used against us had been fierce and unrelenting. The IPA team obtained support from the American Nurses'

Association-Illinois Chapter and the Illinois Society for Advanced Practice Nursing, and the American Nurses Association-Illinois, *and* were able to change the stance of the Illinois Psychiatric Society and the Illinois Medical Society from "oppose" to "neutral." What brought the state medical and psychiatric societies to the negotiating table were the psychologists' successive legislative victories in both the Senate and the House; the steady growth of psychology's support from state labor unions, statewide law enforcement associations, African American and Latino/a religious and advocacy networks, and other influential groups; and our steadfastness in staying the course.

While there are constraints in our law, currently, I have no doubt that these constraints will be lifted over time as our prescribing psychologists demonstrate not only safe prescribing, but effective prescribing. After all, prescribing psychologists have a full array of robust therapeutic (psychological as well as pharmacological) interventions that they can make.

Final Reflections

Being involved in the public policy process is a life-changing event. It requires, above all else, vision, persistence, and presence. There are many potential avenues through which dedicated nurses can make a real difference in the lives of our nation's citizens beyond providing direct clinical care. Passionately embracing a change in which one truly believes is an extremely rewarding experience. Supportive colleagues will often be found in the most unanticipated places, as long as one remains focused on the ultimate objective and does not require personal recognition or credit. Becoming a "social change agent" is a lifelong journey that begins with an appreciation that "all politics is local." Aloha.

Patrick H. DeLeon, PhD, JD, MPH
Uniformed Services University of the Health Sciences
Daniel K. Inouye Graduate School of Nursing
University of Hawaii
Former president, American Psychological Association

---

* The views expressed in this section are those of the author and do not reflect the official policy or position of the Uniformed Services University of the Health Sciences, the Department of Defense, or the United States Government.

References

DeLeon, P. H., Kjervik, D. K., Kraut, A. G., & VandenBos, G. R. (1985). Psychology and nursing: A natural alliance. *American Psychologist, 40*, 1153–1164.

DeLeon, P. H., Rychnovsky, J. D., & Culp, C. H. (2011). A maturing vision for the 21st century. *The Journal of Healthcare, Science and the Humanities: A Navy Medicine Publication, 1*(2), 149–153.

DeLeon, P. H., Wakefield, M., Schultz, A. J., Williams, J., & VandenBos, G. R. (1989). Rural America: Unique opportunities for health-care delivery and health-services research. *American Psychologist, 44*, 1298–1306.

Institute of Medicine (IOM). (2010). *The future of nursing: Leading change, advancing health*. Washington, DC: National Academy Press.

Kirschner, N. M. (2003, August). QMBs, SNFs and notch babies: A hippie banker tour. Presented at the 111th APA annual convention, Toronto, Ontario, Canada.

CONCLUSION

The authors who have contributed to the new chapter hope that if you are not involved in practice, education, or research with other healthcare professionals and patients/clients you will reconsider what you are doing and how you are doing it. Interprofessional work takes courage, respect, intention, and excellent communication skills. If the U.S. healthcare system is to be transformed, not just reorganized, all of us must set aside old biases and practices and focus on a common goal that will not just enable but inspire and embolden—and, yes, lead—organizations, government, and systems to move forward together in conceiving, writing, and implementing public policy.

CHAPTER 10

Overview: The Economics and Finance of Health Care

Nancy Munn Short

"Other people, including the politicians who make economic policy, know even less about economics than economists."

—HERBERT STEIN, *WASHINGTON BEDTIME STORIES*

KEY TERMS

Accountable care organization (ACO): A network of providers and hospitals that shares responsibility for providing coordinated care to Medicare patients. ACOs agree to manage all of the healthcare needs of a minimum of 5,000 Medicare beneficiaries for at least 3 years.

Adverse selection: A situation in which, as a result of private information, the insured are more likely to suffer a loss than the uninsured. A form of information asymmetry.

Affordable Care Act (ACA): The combination of the Patient Protection and Affordable Care Act of 2010 and the Health Care and Education Affordability Act of 2010. Also known as *Obamacare* or *O-Care*.

Coinsurance: The share of the costs of a covered healthcare service paid by the consumer, calculated as a percentage (for example, 20 percent) of the allowed amount for the service. The consumer pays coinsurance plus any deductibles owed. This should not be confused with a health plan that pays for a specific percentage of "essential health benefits."

Comparative effectiveness research (CER): A category of studies to determine the effectiveness of clinical interventions specifically when compared to differing treatments for the same condition, or for different subgroups of patients. The newly created Patient-Centered Outcomes Research Institute (PCORI) is charged with identifying priorities and carrying out CER.

Essential health benefits: A set of healthcare service categories that, starting in 2014, had to be covered by certain plans. Insurance policies must cover these benefits in order to be certified and offered in the health insurance marketplace. States expanding their Medicaid programs must provide these benefits to people newly eligible for Medicaid

Health insurance exchange (HIX): A market set up to facilitate the purchase of health insurance in accord with the Patient Protection and Affordable Care Act of 2010. Exchanges are either state, federal, or jointly run depending upon the state.

Information asymmetry: Occurs when some parties to business transactions have an information advantage over others. There is often information asymmetry between patients and providers regarding therapies and prices.

Means testing: A process undertaken to determine if a person's income qualifies him or her to participate in a social program. Often used to determine eligibility for Medicaid coverage of long-term care and to determine eligibility for subsidies for health insurance.

Moral hazard: The change in behavior as a result of a perceived reduction in the costs of misfortune (e.g., health insurance changes the costs of becoming ill or injured). A form of information asymmetry.

Opportunity costs: The value of the next best choice that one gives up when making a decision. Also called *economic costs*.

Quality adjusted life year (QALY): Calculated life expectancy adjusted for the quality of life, where quality of life is measured on a scale from 1 (full health) to 0 (dead). Originally developed as a broader measure of disease burden beyond mortality, QALYs are now used in cost-effectiveness analyses to aid coverage and reimbursement decisions worldwide.

Introduction

Three important concepts that form the framework for health policy discussions are quality/safety of care, access to care, and the cost of care. All health policy discussions boil down to one of these categories or the synergies between these categories. This chapter will focus on the "cost" category including some economic theories supporting current health policies and some of the structures created to implement these policies.

Health economics and the finance of health care are often erroneously used as interchangeable terms. How does health finance differ from health economics? In a nutshell, economics is the science that informs the processes of finance. The two disciplines share common ground such as cost–benefit analysis and analysis of risk, but they are not synonymous. Economics is amoral—that is, it is neither a moral science nor an immoral science. The science of health economics can suggest what makes a person, a population, a region, or a nation better off, but philosophy and ethics must be debated elsewhere and are represented by political trade-offs when policy is made. Similarly, the healthcare market as viewed by economists is amoral: When confronted with finite resources, there will be losers and winners. This is a tough concept for nurses to swallow.

Economic theory is based on the principle that all resources are scarce. Politics is the process for determining how scarce resources will be used and apportioned. Policy is the end result of the political process. Health policy is one type of policy determined in the political process and is made largely at the national level, but also at state and local levels of government. Health economics is a growing research field within the discipline of economics.

Economic science studies markets such as the labor market for nurses and physicians, the pharmaceutical market, and the insurance market. Together these markets form the universe that is termed the "healthcare market." Within the healthcare market are nonprofit organizations, government organizations, shareholder-owned corporations, and other financial entities. Economics informs policy and policy determines finance (see **Figure 10-1**).

Think about the supply and demand for oranges. When significant weather events affect the orange crop, prices go up for all products made from oranges. In response to price variation, consumers choose if they will continue to purchase orange juice or instead purchase a substitute such as apple juice. But what happens in health care when there are shortages

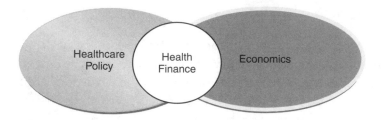

■ Figure 10-1 The intersection of health policy and health finance.

of resources? In 2010, intravenous oncology medications topped the list of drug shortages. (Pharmaceutical manufacturers tell the Food and Drug Administration [FDA] when there are shortages. See the FDA's Current Drug Shortage Index at http://www.fda.gov/drugs/drugsafety/drugshortages/ucm050792.htm.) Because pharmaceutical manufacturing is not owned and operated by the U.S. government, the government does not control choices of what and how much to produce. Can consumers choose to go without a medication or simply pay a higher price? They frequently do skip medications, sometimes at great risk. This added risk to health and life makes the healthcare market very different from all other economic markets. There are few ready-to-use substitutes for health care.

Economics: Opportunity Costs

There is no such thing as a free lunch: For every opportunity taken and for every option discarded there are trade-off costs. When you purchased the 2012 Oldsmobile Malibu, you did not purchase the 2014 Honda wagon. You also did not take a vacation, buy a new wardrobe, or pay off your college debt. Not acquiring the Honda, the vacation, or the new wardrobe or eliminating your debt are the opportunity costs of purchasing the Malibu.

Opportunity costs may also be described in terms of time spent on an activity (researching the safety of the Malibu) and other indirect measures or intangibles. An example of opportunity costs related to health policy is the current Medicare policy: 90 percent of Medicare funds are used for 10 percent of Medicare beneficiaries. Most Medicare dollars are expended in the final events of a person's life. Because there are finite funds available, policy directing payments for an elderly person's last weeks of life represent an opportunity cost. For example, the funds could also be used for preventive care of 30-year-olds, more school nurses, or health research. These are hard choices and are the core of perennial political debates at the federal, state, and local levels. The economic consequences of a policy may last for years and may be argued equally eloquently by economists who fall on both sides of an issue.

> The most important contribution economists can make to the operation of the health care system is to be relentless in pointing out that every choice involves a trade-off—that certain difficult questions regarding who gets what, and who must give up what, are inevitable and must be faced even when politicians, the public, and patients would rather avoid them. (Getzen, 2010, p. 429)

Finance: Does More Spending Buy Us Better Health?

Studies continue to show that there is no correlation between increased spending on health care in the United States and reductions in population mortality (Rothberg, Cohen, Lindenauer, Maselli, & Auerbach, 2010). In the 1900s, spending on infrastructure that provided clean water and hygiene, vaccination programs, and better access to health care resulted in large improvements in quality of life and life expectancy. As the United States approached $5,000 annual per capita spending on health care, gains in population health and life expectancy slowed. In 2010, spending reached $8,233 per capita (Central Intelligence Agency, 2013) and marginal gain to health became almost imperceptible. Nations tend to spend more money on health care simply because they have more money to spend (or the capacity to borrow money). Individuals spend more money on health care when they are ill. (See **Figure 10-2**, which illustrates a lack of correlation between life expectancy and per capita spending.) Routine indicators of health status, such as infant mortality and feeling that one has good health, also do not correlate to per capita spending on health care.

Economics: Health Insurance Market

Health insurance in the United States is a misnomer: what we are purchasing is *sickness* insurance. Like other forms of insurance, health insurance is a form of collectivism in which people pool their risk, in this case the risk

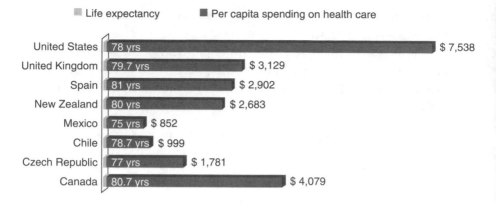

■ Figure 10-2 **Life expectancy in relation to per capita spending on health care.**

Source: Data from Life Expectancy data from the U.S. Central Intelligence Agency, *The World Factbook* (2013). Retrieved from https://www.cia.gov/library/publications/the-world-factbook/rankorder/2102rank.html; per capita expenditure data from the Kaiser Family Foundation (2010). Retrieved from http://kff.org/global-indicator/health-expenditure-per-capita/

of incurring medical expenses. Risk pooling is key to how insurance markets work: each participant with marginal or poor health and a high risk of accruing high expenses is financially "balanced" by several participants with good health and low risk of high expenses. Barring the participation of individuals who already have disease or injury (preexisting condition) allows insurers to manage adverse selection (which will be explained in a later section). The health insurance mandate in the ACA provides the enlargement and balance of the risk pool. Without the option to refuse to cover preexisting conditions or the increased risk pool created by the ACA's mandate the business model for the insurance market would collapse.

In general, the market for health insurance is divided into public and private insurance. Public insurance includes Medicare, Medicaid, State Children's Health Insurance Programs, and in some cases TriCare insurance for military families. Additionally, the industry is broken down into group and nongroup (or individual) insurance. More than 15 million Americans purchase individual insurance. The Kaiser Family Foundation (2013) reports that the average health insurance premium for an individual policy was

$5,884 per year and $16,351 for a family in 2013. The cost of monthly insurance premiums does not include out-of-pocket payments for deductibles, copays, noncovered treatments/medications, or other fees.

Finance: Health Insurance Exchanges

Introduced in October 2013, **health insurance exchanges (HIXs)** are intended to create a more organized and competitive market for health insurance by offering a choice of plans, establishing common rules regarding the offering and pricing of insurance, and providing information to help consumers better understand the options available to them. Depending upon the state, the HIX serving that state will be run by either the state government, the federal government, or jointly by both the state and the federal governments. The HIX marketplace is where people (individuals or small businesses) not covered through their employers or by public insurance may shop for health insurance at competitive rates. Private plans, outside of the HIXs, continue to be available; however, private plans are now more likely to be available for purchase only in designated "open enrollment" periods that coincide with those of the HIXs' open enrollment periods.

Insurance plans in the HIX marketplace are primarily separated into four health plan categories—Bronze, Silver, Gold, or Platinum—based on the percentage the plan pays of the average overall cost of providing essential health benefits to members. The plan category you choose affects the total amount you will spend for **essential health benefits** during the year. The percentages the plans will spend, on average, are 60 percent (Bronze), 70 percent (Silver), 80 percent (Gold), and 90 percent (Platinum). This isn't the same as **coinsurance**, in which you pay a specific percentage of the cost of a specific service.

The essential health benefits required by the ACA to be included in all qualified health insurance plans are:

- Well-baby and well-child care for children under age 21
- Oral health and vision services for children
- Preventative services and immunizations
- Ambulatory patient services including laboratory services
- Chronic disease management
- Mental health and substance abuse coverage at parity with physical ailment coverage

- Hospital/emergency services
- Rehabilitation and habilitative services and devices
- Prescription drug coverage
- Maternity care
- No cost sharing for these services

Additionally, insurers cannot impose annual or lifetime limits on health coverage and insurers must offer parents the choice of covering their children up to their 26th birthday through the parent's health insurance coverage. This also applies for those who age out of the foster care system and were covered by Medicaid.

Federal subsidies are available to help individuals pay for a qualified health plan. There are two kinds of subsidies: advance premium tax credits and cost sharing. Advance premium tax credits help to pay health insurance premiums each month for people with incomes 100–400 percent of the Federal Poverty Level (FPL). Cost sharing helps pay for all other health costs such as copayments, deductibles, and coinsurance for families with incomes 100–250 percent of the FPL who are enrolling in a silver-level plan in the marketplace. Both kinds of subsidies are determined based on a sliding scale (**means tested**). The subsidy is determined during the initial application based on the individual/family's annual projected income. There is no penalty for good faith estimates that are lower than the actual income at year's end.

As of 2014, the ACA requires citizens and legal immigrants to pay a penalty if they do not have a qualified health plan. A qualified health plan can be met if an individual has public health insurance coverage, employer-sponsored health insurance, or an individual health plan purchased from either the HIX marketplace or the private insurance market. The penalties for having no health insurance may be amended by the U.S. Department of Health and Human Services or Congress.

The small business health insurance options program (SHOP) opened to employers with 50 or fewer full-time equivalent (FTE) employees in 2014. (Note: 50 FTEs is not the same as 50 employees.) Beginning in 2016, all SHOPs will be open to employers with up to 100 FTEs. If a business wants to use SHOP, it must offer coverage to all of its full-time employees (generally those working 30 or more hours per week on average) *and* at least 70 percent of full-time employees must enroll in the business/SHOP plan (as opposed to being covered by a spouse's insurance or as an individual on the HIX).

Penalties for Not Having a Qualified Health Plan

2014 $95 per person or 1% of taxable income (whichever is greater)
2015 $325 per person or 2% of taxable income (whichever is greater)
2016 $695 per person or 2.5% of taxable income (whichever is greater)

- Children are assessed half of the penalty.
- Maximum penalty for a family is the amount they would have paid for the lowest cost Bronze plan.
- Penalties are paid when you file your taxes the following year.

If you have insurance outside of the marketplace, you will need to report your insurance coverage to the Internal Revenue Service every year when you file your taxes. Your insurer and your employer (if applicable) will provide you with the necessary proof of coverage to include in your tax return.

Exemptions from Penalties

1. Those who have to pay greater than 8% of their income for the lowest cost premium
2. People who do not pay taxes because their income is too low
3. People with certain religious exemptions
4. Prisoners, while incarcerated
5. Those experiencing a hardship (e.g., domestic violence victims, those being evicted, etc.)
6. Native Americans and/or Alaskan Natives
7. People who would have been covered had the state elected to expand Medicaid
8. Mixed status families (documented and undocumented immigrants within one nuclear family)

Finance: Healthcare Entitlement Programs

Medicare and Medicaid are publicly funded social entitlement programs. Anyone meeting the eligibility requirements for Medicare (Part A) or Medicaid is *entitled* to all of the promised benefits no matter the condition

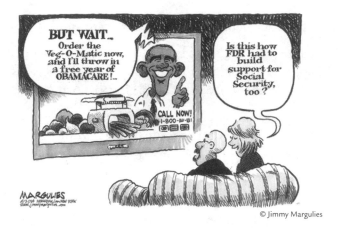

© Jimmy Margulies

■ Figure 10-3 Cartoon

of the government's (state or federal) finances. Think of this in terms of your personal budget: you plan for rent, transportation expenses, utilities, clothing, entertainment, gifts, and the like in your budget and you balance these amounts against your anticipated income to assure that your income covers your expenses. Expenses for Medicare and Medicaid are projected every year, but unlike your clothing allowance, if the government runs short of revenue (e.g., fewer taxes are collected during a down economy) there is no legal option to cut back on entitlement programs. Or if expenses for Medicare and Medicaid are higher than projected (e.g., perhaps more seniors are seriously ill), the government cannot choose not to provide payment for the overage in services. If the government fails to meet its obligation, beneficiaries are entitled to sue.

By law, state governments must balance their budgets; the federal government may run deficits up to a ceiling set by Congress. This is an important concept and explains much of the policies at the state and federal levels. In simple terms, Medicare is a federally funded program and Medicaid is funded by federal and state funds along with some local funds. The full reality is more complex but these generalities suffice for our discussion. Funding for Medicare comes primarily from general revenues (40 percent) and payroll taxes (38 percent), followed by premiums paid by beneficiaries (12 percent).

In 2012, the Kaiser Family Foundation reported that Medicare provided insurance coverage to 49.5 million people including those age 65 and over (if they or their spouse made payroll tax contributions for 10 or more years), and younger people with permanent disabilities (after 24 months of receiving Social Security Disability payments), end-stage renal disease, and amyotrophic lateral sclerosis (Lou Gehrig's disease). Medicare covers most healthcare services, but does not cover long-term care services such as nursing home care (Kaiser Family Foundation, 2012).

- Medicare Part A (Hospital Insurance Program) helps pay for inpatient hospitalizations, skilled nursing home care (up to 100 days), home health (limited posthospital), and hospice care. The beneficiary must pay a deductible.
- Medicare Part B (Supplementary Medical Insurance) is voluntary and covers 95 percent of all Part A beneficiaries. Part B helps pay for physician visits, outpatient hospital services, preventive services, mental health services, durable medical equipment, and home health. Beneficiaries pay a monthly premium plus some copays.
- Medicare Part C is also called Medicare Advantage. These are private health plans that receive payments from Medicare to provide Medicare-covered benefits to enrollees. Plans provide benefits covered under Parts A and B and often Part D.
- Medicare Part D is a voluntary program that helps pay for outpatient prescription drugs and is administered exclusively through private plans. Premiums and cost-sharing vary according to the plan purchased. The **Affordable Care Act** improves coverage by gradually closing the "donut hole"—an unusual gap in coverage in which 100 percent of costs become out-of-pocket. The cost of Part D is increasing at a faster rate than the rest of Medicare.

Prior to the implementation of the Affordable Care Act, Medicare served all eligible beneficiaries without regard to income or medical history. As health reform is rolled out, means testing will be applied to those with very high incomes. Note: Maryland has a waiver from the federal government to operationalize Medicare in a unique manner. The details are beyond the scope of this chapter; however, some economists believe that Maryland's reimbursement system may become the model for the rest of the nation.

Medicaid was enacted under the Social Security Act in 1965 as a companion to Medicare. It entitles participating states to federal matching funds on an open-ended basis, entitles eligible individuals to a set of specific benefits, is means tested, and allows states to provide broader coverage. In addition to providing health insurance coverage, Medicaid also provides assistance to low-income Medicare beneficiaries (dual-eligible), long-term care assistance (nursing home and in-home community-based services), support for the safety net system of health care, and is the largest source of federal funding to the states. Medicaid is the largest health insurance program in the United States.

Medicaid fills large gaps in our health insurance market, finances the lion's share of long-term care, and provides core support for the health centers and safety-net hospitals that serve the nation's uninsured and millions of others. Within broad federal guidelines, states design their own Medicaid programs. Medicaid reimburses private providers to provide services to beneficiaries. In 2009, the elderly and disabled accounted for 83.4 percent of all Medicaid expenditures. Medicaid reimburses private providers to provide services to beneficiaries. In 2009, the elderly and disabled accounted for 67 percent of all Medicaid expenditures, and the top 5 percent of enrollees accounted for over half of all Medicaid expenses. Of the 12 million Americans in long-term care, 87 percent are covered by Medicaid, making Medicaid the number-one program paying for long-term care (Kaiser Family Foundation, 2014).

Medicaid coverage prior to the implementation of the ACA, and currently in those states that opt out of the ACA Medicaid expansion plan, requires beneficiaries to have low incomes (defined by each state using the federal poverty guidelines) *and* to meet one of these categories of need:

- Pregnant or recent postpartum
- Younger than 18 years old
- Older than 65 years old and blind or disabled

Medically needy persons whose incomes are too high to be eligible for Medicaid may also be covered. (Each state determines eligibility.) Additionally, there are optional eligibility groups that may be defined by each state. In 2014 the Federal Poverty Level (FPL) for a family of four was $23,850 in the continental United States and a little higher in Alaska and Hawaii (U.S. Department of Health and Human Services, 2014). As of August 2014, 27 states had expanded Medicaid by eliminating medical need categories and providing coverage to those with incomes at or below 138 percent of the Federal Poverty Level. One of the arguments against

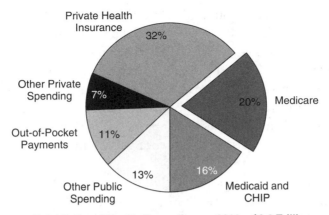

Total National Health Expenditures, 2010 = $2.6 Trillion

■ Figure 10-4 National health expenditures in the United States by source of payment, 2010.

Source: Data from Kaiser Family Foundation, *Medicare Chartbook*, Fourth edition, 2010. Slide date November 04, 2010. http://facts.kff.org/chartbook.aspx?cb=58

expanding Medicaid is a fear of increasing the overall health expenditures for the United States. See **Figure 10-4** for a look at the percentage paid by each type of payer in our healthcare system.

For more detail and analysis see the Centers for Medicare and Medicaid Services website at http://www.cms.gov.

Economics: Information Asymmetry

Information asymmetry is the term used by economists to point out that healthcare consumption differs from purchasing other goods and services because of the inability of patients, providers, or payers to possess all of the information needed for completely informed decision making. Optimal rational decision making requires "perfect information" where consumers are just as knowledgeable as sellers.

Think about when you buy a car. You gather all of the information that you can to eliminate any advantage the car seller may have in terms of the worth of this particular car. Being newly informed, you may choose to go to several dealerships before you find a seller that meets your expectations (or utility). Now think about your typical healthcare experience. You go to your primary care provider (PCP) for your annual physical and the PCP finds an abnormality and refers you to a specialist. Depending on your level of information, you will blindly trust the specialist or you may "shop around." You may be very hard pressed to learn about the quality or performance of either your primary care provider or the specialist. If you are referred to a hospital, you are probably unable to learn the nurse-to-patient ratio even though evidence shows that this is critical to your well-being. There is information asymmetry.

Healthcare professionals generally know what is "best" for patients, right? The problem of asymmetric information differs from a simple information problem in that one party possesses knowledge needed to enable rational decision making that the other party lacks.

However, the healthcare professional and the insurer have a potential conflict of interest because of the exchange of money. Benefiting monetarily from a decision may affect the decision-making process. In health care, the patient delegates much decision making to the healthcare professional (and sometimes even to the insurer).

Asymmetric information also affects healthcare professionals when patients conceal lifestyle information or state that they are compliant with a treatment when they are not. A patient's caregiver may also withhold or distort information that would be helpful to the provider. Insurers also face information asymmetry: Clients (buyers of insurance like you and me) know much more about the state of their health and their future plans than an insurer knows.

Two specific types of information asymmetry are adverse selection and moral hazard.

Economics: Adverse Selection and Moral Hazard

Economists use two terms, adverse selection and moral hazard, to describe the situations insurers face when consumers have greater information about their health than insurers or payers: (1) **adverse selection** occurs when a person participates in a health plan based *solely* on the likelihood that they will have higher than usual health expenses (e.g., planning to get pregnant), and (2) **moral hazard** occurs when a health plan member uses more health services than that person ordinarily would because he or she is insured (e.g., a person with orthodontic coverage gets braces on his teeth for cosmetic purposes only).

Insurers and payers may also lack sufficient information regarding the choices and decisions of providers and may be unable to ascertain if a procedure is medically necessary or not.

> The patient, who does not pay the bill, demands as much care as possible;… the insurance company maximizes profits by paying for as little as possible; and…it is very costly for either the patient or the insurance company to prove the "right" course of treatment. In short, information asymmetry makes health care different from the rest of the economy. (Wheelan, 2002, p. 86)

Imagine that you have consciously chosen not to purchase health insurance because you are young and enjoy good health—you decide it's cheaper to pay the annual penalty. Recall that insurers may no longer deny health insurance to those who have preexisting health conditions. Within a few months, you unexpectedly become pregnant and decide that you do not want to pay the full cost of prenatal care, delivery, and postpartum care, so you seek a private insurer such as Blue Cross & Blue Shield (BCBS) to purchase insurance. After the baby is born, and BCBS has paid for the costs of your pregnancy and delivery, you decide that you no longer need insurance and drop your coverage. This is an example of adverse selection. If millions of people made this choice, the insurance market would collapse. Insurance markets rely upon having a strong mix of those who will not require payouts for healthcare episodes and those who will. In other words, in the health insurance market the healthy subsidize the sick. If only the old, the sick, or the disabled purchased health insurance the market would collapse. This is similar to other insurances such as fire, life and automobile—those who don't use the benefits subsidize those who do. Mandating the purchase of health insurance is an economic strategy designed to create a sustainable risk pool of beneficiaries.

Many of the 48 million people who were uninsured in 2012 had preexisting conditions and were not eligible for regular public plans (Pear, 2013). In 2014, the ACA required that insurers eliminate coverage denials for preexisting conditions. When the ACA was passed, the hope was to provide insurance to approximately 33 million uninsured citizens and legal immigrants in the United States by expanding Medicaid eligibility and requiring the purchase of health insurance coverage. The goal of covering 33 million uninsured persons will not be reached because 23 states currently are not participating in Medicaid expansion.

Finance: Comparative Effectiveness Research and QALYs

Imagine a system of research in which new discoveries or approaches to reduce or eliminate disease are tested for effectiveness against doing nothing at all. The current gold standard for research in the United States is the randomized control trial (RCT), in which a group of subjects receives a treatment while another group receives no treatment. Effectiveness is decided by whether the disease or condition responded to the new approach, but the new approach is not compared to any other approach.

As a result of the 2009 American Recovery and Reinvestment Act (ARRA) and the 2010 ACA, the federal government made major investments in **comparative effectiveness research (CER)**. Comparative effectiveness research compares the overall benefits of one therapeutic approach with those of another for the majority of patients. These investments are likely to yield new information about which treatments work best for which population of patients. But how will this research be used beyond informing provider decisions?

Here is an example of a current dilemma: Solvadi is a new drug developed to treat hepatitis C, a life-threatening disease often unrecognized until the final stages. Solvadi costs $1,000 per dose, and a full treatment regimen costs $84,000. In March 2014, the high price led to street protests in San Francisco where health experts say that treating every person with advanced liver disease (from hepatitis C) in California would cost $6.3 billion. With a success rate of about 90 percent, Solvadi is an improvement over older drugs with regimens costing only $25,000. Should public insurance pay for Solvadi? Does a regimen of Solvadi have cost benefits when compared to a liver transplant and lifelong immunotherapy? Is avoiding chronic disease "worth" the cost? How many productive years of life are gained? If California's Medicaid program typically spends $3,500/beneficiary/year, how many new beneficiaries could be covered for the $6.3 billion? Economists and health services researchers tackle these types of questions by conducting CER and using a concept called **quality adjusted life years (QALYs)**.

QALY is an economic concept developed in the 1960s to facilitate cost-effectiveness analysis. Economists have attempted to include personal preferences regarding age and health conditions and have created a catalog known as the EQ-5D Index. For instance, if you have colon cancer and you are a 65-year-old, white female, your EQ-5D index for quality adjusted life years is 0.93. That is, if you live 1 year with colon cancer, it is only worth 93 percent of a year with full health and no diseases. If you have two conditions at the same time, perhaps colon cancer and neurotic disorder, your EQ-5D index is 0.79. Once they know how many QALYs a treatment is worth, economists can figure out its cost per QALY—the broadest measure of the cost-effectiveness of health care.

In general, a QALY carries an economic value of between $70,000 and $150,000 per quality life year gained by a treatment or approach (Anderson et al., 2014). Will CER be used to determine not only a treatment's effectiveness, but also the cost-effectiveness and ultimately payment decisions? CER findings can be translated into practice in a variety of ways, some of which may be more acceptable to the public than others. QALYs have been linked to CER in the United Kingdom by the National Institute for Clinical Excellence and have led to debates about rationing care. The "R" word represents a slippery slope for opponents of government funding for CER.

The Patient-Centered Outcomes Research Institute (PCORI) was created under the ACA to coordinate government activity around CER. The ACA does not include cost-effectiveness determination among the guidelines for PCORI. PCORI conducts research to provide information about the best available evidence to help patients and their healthcare providers make more informed decisions. PCORI's research is intended to give patients a better understanding of the prevention, treatment, and care options available, and the science that supports those options.

Finance: Bending the Healthcare Cost Curve Downward

Historically, physicians and hospitals have been paid for each procedure, test, visit, and consultation: more pay for doing "more" whether or not "more" results in good patient outcomes. This drives up costs for health care.

One of the ways the ACA seeks to reduce healthcare costs in the United States is by encouraging providers and hospitals to form networks to provide good quality care to Medicare beneficiaries while keeping down costs. Providers get paid more if they keep their patients well. An **accountable care organization (ACO)** brings together the different component parts of care for the patient—primary care, specialists, hospitals, home health care ... even private companies like Walgreen's—and ensures that all of the parts work well together. Although ACOs are touted as a way to help fix an inefficient payment system that rewards more, not better, care, some economists warn they could lead to greater consolidation in the healthcare industry, which could allow some providers to charge more if they are the only game in town. Consolidation of this type occurs when multiple hospitals and most provider practices in a geographic area financially merge into large integrated health systems.

How does a system become an ACO? Section 3022 of the PPACA outlines the following requirements for ACOs (Centers for Medicare and Medicaid Services, 2010; McClellan, McKethan, Lewis, Roski, & Fisher, 2010):

- The ACO becomes accountable for the quality, cost, and overall care of the Medicare fee-for-service beneficiaries assigned to it.
- The ACO must participate in the program for not less than a 3-year period.
- The ACO's formal legal structure must allow the organization to receive and distribute payments for shared savings to participating providers of services and suppliers.
- The ACO must include primary care professionals that are sufficient for the number of Medicare fee-for-service beneficiaries assigned to the ACO.
- At a minimum, the ACO must have 5,000 beneficiaries assigned to it in order to be eligible to participate.
- The ACO must have leadership and management structures that include clinical and administrative systems.
- The ACO must define processes to promote evidence-based medicine and patient engagement, report on quality and cost measures, and coordinate care.
- The ACO must demonstrate that it meets specific patient-centeredness criteria (such as the use of patient and caregiver assessments or the use of individualized care plans).

Table 10-1 provides a visual that explains the definition and purpose of key attributes required of ACOs.

One of the challenges for hospitals and providers is that the incentives are to reduce hospital stays, emergency room visits, and expensive specialist and testing services—all the ways that hospitals and physicians make

■ Table 10-1   Overview of Accountable Payment Models

Key Attributes	Bundled Payments	Value-Based Purchasing	Accountable Care Organizations (ACOs)
Definition	Purchaser disburses single payment to cover certain combination of hospital, physician, post-acute, or other services performed during an inpatient stay or across an episode of care; providers propose discounts, can gain share on any money saved	Pay-for-performance program differentially rewards or punishes hospitals (and likely ASCs and physicians in coming years) based on performance against predefined process and outcomes performance measures	Network of providers collectively accountable for the total cost and quality of care for a population of patients; ACOs are reimbursed through total cost payment structures, such as the shared savings model or capitation
Purpose	Incent multiple types of providers to coordinate care, reduce expenses associated with care episodes	Create material link between reimbursement and clinical quality, patient satisfaction scores	Reward providers for reducing total cost of care for patients through prevention, disease management, coordination

money in the current fee-for-service system. Unlike other industries, prices for health care vary dramatically depending on who is paying and on geography. The U.S. system is a bit like shopping in a department store where there are no prices marked on the goods. You check out and a few weeks later you receive a bill that reads, "Pay this." Growing movements toward price transparency in health care hope to empower patients to overcome information asymmetry, make wise choices, and increase competition that may lower prices. Physicians and hospitals that rarely competed on cost have been cushioned by third-party payers who pay the bulk of the bills. The advent of the Healthcare Bluebook aims to do what the Kelley Bluebook does for used cars. Some argue that true price transparency will destabilize the healthcare industry. Others think that transparency may confuse consumers (Beck, 2014).

Discussion Points

1. Discuss the role of economists in healthcare policy. Use Gail Wilensky, PhD, as a model of a health economist; watch clips of her presentations on her website (http://www.gailwilensky.com). Note that although she is not a clinician, she was a commissioner on the World Health Organization (WHO) Commission on the Social Determinants of Health and an elected member of the Institute of Medicine, where she served two terms on its governing council. She is a former chair of the board of directors of Academy Health and a former trustee of the American Heart Association. Identify factors that contribute to the influence of economists in health policy.

2. Read several issues of the journal *Health Affairs*. Access the journal's blog (http://www.healthaffairs.org/blog/) and use the keyword "economics" to search for the latest articles about healthcare economics.

3. Discuss the gross national product in terms of healthcare expenditures. What sorts of programs will not receive funding when health care consumes a large percentage of federal expenditures?

4. Read about social capital at the World Bank website (http://web .worldbank.org/WBSITE/EXTERNAL/TOPICS/EXTSOCIALDEVEL-OPMENT/EXTTSOCIALCAPITAL/0,,contentMDK:20642703~men uPK:401023~pagePK:148956~piPK:216618~theSitePK:401015,00 .html). How does social capital differ from economic capital? Discuss how you benefit from social capital in your own life. How does social capital determine or affect the health of populations?

5. Read about cost shifting in health care. Identify policies that use this method. Argue the benefits and losses of cost shifting. How might the ACA decrease cost shifting within hospitals?

6. Who finances most long-term care in the United States? Take a poll of your peers prior to researching this question to see what they think is the answer. Are nurses well informed about this economic issue, and does this meet your expectation?

7. How does QALY analysis benefit the young over the old?

8. What does the RAND Corporation do? Review its online series "Small Ideas for Saving Big Health Care Dollars" (http://www.rand.org/pubs/research_reports/RR390.html). Choose one idea for reducing healthcare spending and discuss three new things you learned, three things that surprised you, and how you can use this information in your own practice.

CASE STUDY 1: MEDICARE SUSTAINABLE GROWTH RATE FOR PHYSICIAN/NURSE PRACTITIONER PAYMENT

Management of chronic care needs, including care coordination between primary and specialty care clinicians, has received much attention lately, especially from legislators and federal regulators where Medicare beneficiaries are concerned. Can healthcare costs be lowered with better management of chronic conditions to keep patients stable and out of hospitals? Specifically, proposals on the sustainable growth rate (SGR) issue call for creation of a payment code for care management for individuals with chronic conditions, and in 2015 the Centers for Medicare and Medicaid Services (CMS) plans to establish additional payment codes for chronic care management services. Care for many older adults has long been fragmented, inefficient, and far from patient-centered.

Discussion Points

1. Define *Medicare SGR* in your own words. Why is SGR such a hot-potato topic?
2. How does physician payment policy affect patient access to care? How does physician payment policy affect medical student selection of specialties?
3. How will care coordination change if new payment codes are established for chronic care management? (Think about technologies, communication with patients, nontraditional management, etc.)

CASE STUDY 2: ECONOMIC VALUE OF BSN EDUCATION FOR RNS

Retrieve and read the study *Nurse Staffing and Education and Hospital Mortality in Nine European Countries: A Retrospective Observational Study* by Linda Aiken, PhD (and colleagues) of the Center for Health Outcomes and Policy Research at the University of Pennsylvania's School of Nursing. This study shows that an increase in a nurse's workload by one patient increased the likelihood of an inpatient dying within 30 days of admission by 7 percent (odds ratio 1.068, 95 percent, CI 1.031–1.106), and every 10 percent increase in bachelor's degree nurses was associated with a decrease in this likelihood by 7 percent (0.929, 0.886–0.973). These associations imply that patients in hospitals in which 60 percent of nurses had bachelor's degrees where nurses cared for an average of six patients would have almost 30 percent lower mortality than patients in hospitals in which only 30 percent of nurses had bachelor's degrees and nurses cared for an average of eight patients.

Discussion Points

1. State your interpretation of these data. Using these conclusions, discuss the implications for hospital leaders when making staffing decisions.
2. Discover the percentage of BSN-prepared nurses licensed in your state. If possible, discover the percentage of BSN-prepared nurses in a hospital or facility in your area.
3. How easily can an average person find out the RN:patient and BSN RN:patient ratio in hospitals? Why do you think this situation exists? What does it mean to you and your family? Who or what entities can change this situation?

CASE STUDY 3: ECONOMIC IMPACT OF STATES DECLINING MEDICAID EXPANSION

Recall that Medicaid is a joint federal and state entitlement health insurance program. The ACA of 2010 required all states to eliminate the use of categories to determine eligibility and expand the Medicaid program to all persons beneath the age of 65 with incomes at or below 138 percent of the Federal Poverty Level. However, in June 2012 the U.S. Supreme Court ruled that requiring states to expand their Medicaid programs was unconstitutional: each state could choose to expand the program or not. By 2014, 27 states and Washington, D.C., had opted to expand Medicaid; 23 states had declined expansion; and 4 states were undecided. Declining expansion means that Medicaid continues as it was pre-ACA with categorically based eligibility. The result of the Supreme Court ruling is a system that makes no sense: millions of people will remain uncovered by Medicaid in the states with no expansion because they are too poor to participate in the health insurance exchanges *and* don't fall into a need-based category to receive Medicaid. Under the ACA, 100 percent of the increased costs of covering more people on Medicaid will be borne by the federal government until 2016.

Discussion Points

1. Determine whether your state has expanded Medicaid.
2. Explain why a very poor person (income below FPL) living in one of the 23 states that declined Medicaid expansion is ineligible to participate in the health insurance exchanges.
3. What is the economic effect on the state (and on the hospital or site where you work or are being trained) of having a large population of uninsured people?
4. Why would a state choose not to participate in Medicaid expansion despite the federal promise of paying for the additional beneficiaries?

(continues)

5. Refer to Benjamin D. Sommers and Sara Rosenbaum (2011), "Issues in Health Reform: How Changes in Eligibility May Move Millions Back and Forth Between Medicaid and Insurance Exchanges." Answer the following questions: In terms of health insurance, what is churning? What effect does churning have on access to care and quality of care? What is the relationship among access to care, quality of care, and cost of care?

References

The Advisory Board Company. The Marketing and Planning Leadership Council's presentation. *Health Care Industry Trends 2013*. Retrieved from http://www.advisory.com/Research/Marketing-and-Planning-Leadership-Council/Resources/2013/Your-next-strategy-presentation-is-ready

Anderson, J. L., Heidenreich, P. A., Barnett, P. G., Creager, M. A., Fonarow, G. C., Gibbons, R. J., ... Shaw, L. J. (2014, March 27). ACC/AHA statement on cost/value methodology in clinical practice guidelines and performance measures: A report of the American College of Cardiology/American Heart Association Task Force on Performance Measures and Task Force on Practice Guidelines. *Circulation*. Retrieved from http://circ.ahajournals.org/lookup/doi/10.1161/CIR.0000000000000042

Beck, M. (2014, February 23). How to bring the price of health care into the open. *Wall Street Journal*. Retrieved from http://online.wsj.com/news/articles/SB10001424052702303650204579375242842086688

Centers for Medicare and Medicaid Services. (2010). *Medicare "accountable care organizations" shared savings program—New section 1899 of Title XVIII. Preliminary questions & answers.* Retrieved from https://www.aace.com/files/cmspremlimqa.pdf

Central Intelligence Agency. (2013). *The world factbook.* Retrieved from https://www.cia.gov/library/publications/the-world-factbook/rankorder/2012rank.html

Getzen, T. E. (2010). *Health economics and financing* (4th ed.) Hoboken, NJ: John Wiley & Sons.

Kaiser Family Foundation. (2012, Nov 14). Medicare at a glance. http://kff.org/medicare/fact-sheet/medicare-at-a-glance-fact-sheet/

Kaiser Family Foundation. (2013, August 20). *2013 employer health benefits survey*. Retrieved from http://kff.org/report-section/2013-summary-of-findings/

Kaiser Family Foundation. (2014, April 3). *Medicaid*. Retrieved from http://kff.org/medicaid/

McClellan, M., McKethan, A. N., Lewis, J. L., Roski, J., & Fisher, E. S. (2010). A national strategy to put accountable care into practice. *Health Affairs, 29*(5), 982–990. doi: 10.1377/hlthaff.2010.0194

Patient Protection and Affordable Care Act of 2010. Pub. L. No. 111-148, § 3022.

Pear, R. (2013, September 17). Percentage of Americans lacking health coverage falls again. *New York Times.*

Rothberg, M. B., Cohen, J., Lindenauer, P., Maselli, J., & Auerbach, A. (2010). Little evidence of correlation between growth in health care spending and reduced mortality. *Health Affairs, 29*(8), 1523–1531. doi: 10.1377/hlthaff.2009.0287

Sommers, B. D., & Rosenbaum, S. (2011). Issues in health reform: How changes in eligibility may move millions back and forth between Medicaid and insurance exchanges. *Health Affairs, 30*(2), 228–236.

Stein, H. (1986). *Washington Bedtime Stories: The Politics of Money and Jobs.* Free Press.

U.S. Department of Health and Human Services. (2014, January 22). *Annual update of the HHS poverty guidelines.* Retrieved from https://Federalregister.gov/a/2014-01303

Wheelan, C. (2002). *Naked economics: Undressing the dismal science.* New York: W. W. Norton.

Online Resources

Alliance for Health Reform: Nonpartisan, well-respected organization providing analytical materials and webcasts by health economists and other health experts. http://www.allhealth.org

America's Health Insurance Plans: http://www.ahip.org

California HealthCare Foundation: Annual chartbook provides a wealth of data and graphics. http://www.chcf.org

Centers for Medicare and Medicaid Services (CMS) Data Navigator: The purpose of the Data Navigator is to introduce healthcare data users to the Medicare and Medicaid program data maintained by CMS. Intended for use by researchers and analysts. http://www.cms.gov/home/rsds.asp

Commonwealth Fund: Supports independent research on healthcare issues and makes grants to improve healthcare practice and policy. http://www.commonwealthfund.org

Consumer Expenditure Survey (Bureau of Labor Statistics): Details of consumer healthcare expenditures. http://www.bls.gov/cex/

Consumer Price Indexes (Bureau of Labor Statistics): The CPI program produces monthly data on changes in the prices paid by urban consumers for a representative basket of goods and services. http://www.bls.gov/cpi/

Current Population Survey (U.S. Census Bureau): http://www.census.gov

Dartmouth Atlas of Health Care: The Atlas project brings together researchers in diverse disciplines—including epidemiology, economics, and statistics—and focuses on the accurate description of how medical resources are distributed and used in the United States. http://www.dartmouthatlas.org

Directory of Data Resources (U.S. Department of Health and Human Services): A compilation of information about virtually all major health data collection systems sponsored by the U.S. government. http://aspe.hhs.gov/datacncl/datadir/index.shtml

HealthCare.gov: Federal government website maintained by the U.S. Department of Health and Human Services. The web location for health insurance exchange information. http://www.healthcare.gov

Kaiser Family Foundation: Nonpartisan, nongovernmental organization in Washington, D.C., providing excellent data, facts, and analysis of healthcare issues and health policy. http://www.kff.org

National Health Expenditure Data (Centers for Medicare and Medicaid Services): http://www.cms.gov/NationalHealthExpendData/

Patient-Centered Outcomes Research Institution: http://www.pcori.org

CHAPTER 11

Global Connections

Jeri A. Milstead

KEY TERMS

Commission on Graduates of Foreign Nursing Schools (CGFNS): A group that offers services to evaluate and certify credentials of graduates from foreign nursing schools and education programs. It also offers a qualifying exam to test readiness for the National Council Licensing Exam for Registered Nurses (NCLEX-RN).

Emerging diseases: Those diseases that have "appeared in a population for the first time or that may have existed previously but [are] rapidly increasing in incidence or geographic range" (World Health Organization, 2011).

Milstead model: A way of organizing analysis of complex health issues in an international framework.

Introduction

McLuhan and Fiore (1968) described the world as a global village in which each person is affected by and affects all inhabitants. Franklin Shaffer (2014), chief executive officer of the **Commission on Graduates of Foreign Nursing Schools (CGFNS)**, reminds us that ". . . the world is gradually becoming a borderless society" (p. 3). Shaffer's thoughts call on us to consider health and illness as well as those who address health status, whether direct and indirect care providers or policymakers in a different way. This chapter considers the global reality of health care today. A brief presentation of health issues that have emerged around the world may stimulate the reader to consider how policy (or lack thereof) in one country is linked to policy in other countries. This chapter also explains the comparative approach to research and presents a model for the study of nursing and health policy at an international level.

Global Issues

Although few doubt that decisions made by policymakers in a country affect the health of its citizens and/or residents, have you considered how the health status of individuals or populations affects policymaking in a country? Certainly, the presence of conditions and illnesses such as communicable diseases (e.g., tuberculosis, malaria, influenza, HIV/AIDS, polio), environmental health concerns (e.g., natural and man-made disasters, access to potable water, food sources), and abuse (e.g., addictions and violence) direct how a nation allocates resources for attending to those health problems. In contrast, consider how a government's philosophy of social justice, ethics, personal responsibility, and political will can influence the management of epidemics, disasters, and healthcare delivery.

Communicable Diseases

Advanced practice registered nurses (APRNs) must think about the relationship between what they see in the clinic, school, or other practice sites and the incidence, prevalence, and treatment options available in other parts of the world. With the movement of people across continents and oceans quickly and often, APRNs must be alert to the possibility of vectors that transmit pathogens to humans and the possibility of contagion. Seasoned travelers know the potential health dangers of being in a foreign environment. Even traveling from one developed country to another can wreak havoc on one's digestive system, because food that is different or prepared differently with spices or condiments not usually found at home can affect the traveler's immediate health. When a traveler journeys to a country that is more or less developed than the home country, the likelihood of illness is even greater.

Healthcare professionals who work in countries other than their own, such as religious-based mission clinics, quickly become cognizant of disease transmission. For example, the incidence of Ebola in countries along the west coast of Africa quickly reached epidemic levels in 2014. Two healthcare workers from the United States contracted the disease, despite the lack of ease of transmission; they were flown to Emory University Hospital in Atlanta, Georgia for expert care. This represents the first documented incidence of Ebola in the western hemisphere or the United States. Great care will be exercised by those at the hospital and consultants from the U.S. Centers for Disease Control and Prevention to minimize the chances of spreading the disease.

Some diseases thought to have been eradicated can reappear, especially in poor or crowded areas. The World Health Organization (2011) defines an **emerging disease** as "one that has appeared in a population for the first time, or that may have existed previously but is rapidly increasing in incidence or geographic range." Examples of emerging diseases include polio and smallpox, which have reappeared in recent years. Measles and mumps are two diseases that were common to children in the 20th century but, for the most part, have been eradicated in the United States through childhood vaccines. However, both of these diseases became epidemics in 2014 in several states in that country. Public health officials suspect a large outbreak of mumps in Ohio may have been traced to several Amish families who had not vaccinated their children and who had traveled to the Philippines, were subjected to the disease, and brought it back to Ohio.

Public health policies that are no longer "on the books" may have to be restored or revised in order to address treatment and prevention. If enough time has elapsed since the last epidemic (and often only a few cases are defined by public health officers as an epidemic), officials may not remember the seriousness of or devastation caused by the disease. Without a historical perspective, officials may not understand the necessity of allocating funds or directing treatment personnel and resources. Some governments perceive a disease (e.g., HIV/AIDS) as so horrible or embarrassing that they will not acknowledge that the disease even exists in their countries, and they refuse to take steps to treat patients.

Environmental Disasters

Certainly many natural disasters, such as hurricanes, earthquakes, tsunamis, and droughts, create immediate and quickly compounded health problems. Lack of potable water, food, sanitation, and transportation are among the first major issues facing survivors. During the March 2011 earthquake and subsequent tsunami in Japan, entire regions were decimated, and the few people who survived were in desperate need of basic necessities. In some cases there were not enough survivors in some cities to bury the dead, and bodies that could not be buried led to an increase in rats and the transmission of disease to the living. People assigned to assist the survivors could not physically reach the area in a timely manner, and those living in the area had few resources (i.e., food, shelter, clothes) to help them eke out a meager existence.

The 2011 earthquake in Japan resulted in a crisis even greater than the tsunami—the potential for meltdown at several nuclear power plants in the area. Radiation leaks posed a huge problem. Government policy dictated that people who lived in the immediate area of the reactor should remain inside their homes, and those who lived within a 12-mile radius should evacuate their homes. For comparison, U.S. policy recommends that all people who live within a 50-mile radius of an actual or potential nuclear disaster center should evacuate. Residents of the area in Japan were confused; some stayed home, while others left. Those who left were told not to take any possessions because clothes and household goods were considered contaminated with radiation. Fear of immediate and long-term health concerns from radiation compounded the worries about lack of food, clothing, and water. Radiation had seeped into the ground and contaminated some vegetables and water.

People in other countries are concerned about the amount of radiation that will be airborne and be blown into their countries. The need for accurate information about the realities and fears is critical. Public health officials continue to offer advice and assistance in meeting these problems. Worldwide assistance on a long-term basis will be required to address these disasters.

Social Justice

Issues of social justice involve the fair treatment of humans and all living things. Social justice issues frequently involve health issues, such as in cases of clitoral circumcision or when preteenagers are force-fed by their mothers and other women of a tribe in order to make them appear more marriageable. These girls can reach weights over 400 pounds and have tremendous problems giving birth, and then are abandoned by the fathers of the babies because the girls are considered ugly and unworthy to be wives. Another issue of social injustice is human trafficking. For example, in Nepal, men, women, and children are abducted and taken to India, where they are forced to work as sex slaves. The abductors force the sex workers to use intravenous drugs, and when their work as slaves is no longer useful they are returned to Nepal, where they become the "untouchables." Untouchable status decreases or ignores access to health care for treatment of addictions, sexually transmitted diseases, and general health concerns.

Often there are no written policies that permit behavior that is considered atrocious in many other societies, but the customs continue with the silent acknowledgment of the tribal elders. Policies to outlaw these practices usually are met with strong resistance based on religious beliefs, tradition, lack of knowledge, or power; even when laws are enacted, they often are not enforced. Many examples of social injustice are revealed when members of a tribe escape or are brought to another country where the rituals may or may not be practiced.

The Importance of Understanding the Cultural Context

Nurses cannot work in any healthcare situation without grasping the importance of a basic understanding of the culture of the patient and the healthcare system. Philosophy about health, disease, customs, and traditions influence whether a person believes he or she has a health problem and, if so, how the problem should be acknowledged and treated. For example, the Hmong people, who live in mountainous regions of southeast Asia, believe that a person with epilepsy has a special gift and that, during seizures, the patient should be revered, not treated as if with a disease (Fadiman, 1997). When people from this region emigrate to another country and seek health care from a system that considers status epilepticus a medical emergency, there are major challenges for the patient/family and the provider.

Nurses are conducting research in international settings and developing models for cultural competence (Campinha-Bacote, 2009, 2011; Carver & Jessie, 2011; Purnell, 2000, n.d.; Villarruel, Gallegos, Cherry, & Refugio de Duran, 2003). One group of researchers has translated and validated a

French version of a tool to permit cross-cultural research in perinatal health (Goulet, Polomeno, Laizner, Marcil, & Lang, 2003). Ross (2000) described a "sister school" (hermanamiento) arrangement between Duquesne University in Pittsburgh, Pennsylvania, and the Universidad Politechnic (UPOLI) in Managua, Nicaragua. Students and faculty visit each others' nurse education programs, conduct research, and provide direct care that affects immersion in different cultures.

Researchers must be cognizant of cultural norms when planning to study a disease, population, or issue. For example, "'saving face' can imperil the research process" (Chen et al., 2013, p. 149) if researchers are not aware that on-site staff fear that participants might disclose something that might embarrass the study. Researchers also should realize that some cultures value individual effort less than collective effort; this can affect how the study results are written and disseminated.

Opportunities for publication of global research may be limited. In 2014 the *Journal of Nursing Scholarship* began a series of commentaries on the global state of nursing (Gennaro, 2014). The editorial board emphasized that all nurses must think globally while acting locally. This author challenges nurses to think globally and act globally to address health issues common to many countries.

A new journal, *Global Qualitative Nursing Research*, has been initiated by Sage Publications. As a peer-reviewed, "open-access, author-pays journal, GQNR will be published on-line only unrestricted by frequency or publication limits and governed solely by submission, editorial integrity, and content value." (Sage, n.d.). Open access refers to the "availability of authors' works in digital formats that are available online" (Broome, 2014, p. 70). Free of copyright or license restrictions by the publisher, anyone can use the work, although there may be charges from subscription-based journals.

The American Academy of Nursing (AAN), a prestigious group of nurse leaders, is organized through expert panels. The Expert Panel on Global Nursing and Health created a task force to examine cultural competence on a global level. The members of the task force had experience as nurses and researchers in many cultures and worked diligently to create a document without ethnocentric biases. The group worked with members of the Transcultural Nursing Society. (Some were members of both AAN and TNS.) The draft document was vetted by many individuals and groups with global knowledge and experience, and broad input was sought through a request for feedback in articles published in the *Journal of Transcultural*

Nursing (Douglas et al., 2009, 2011). The final version of the guidelines, published in the *Journal of Transcultural Nursing* (Douglas et al., 2014), was adopted by the International Council of Nurses and should be a valuable resource for nurses around the world.

The Nurse Shortage

One cannot write about global health issues without acknowledging the nurse and nurse faculty shortage. The AAN Expert Panel on Global Nursing and Health presented a white paper at the Sixth International Conference on Priorities in Health Care in Toronto, Ontario, Canada, in 2006: "The mission [of the Academy] is to serve the public and nursing profession by advancing health policy and practice through generation, synthesis, and dissemination of nursing knowledge" (American Academy of Nursing, 2007). Members of the global panel addressed the nurse shortage in the international arena through factors that included "stressful work environment, aging nurse population, decreasing school enrollments, increased career opportunities for women, inadequate salaries, and an increased demand for nursing services, especially in leadership and advanced practice" (American Nurses Association, 2006, p. 1).

The early practice of recruiting nurses from one country to another is unethical and does not "solve" the shortage (Zachary, 2001). Problems with immigration and comparability of nurse knowledge and skills have been addressed by the Commission on Graduates of Foreign Nursing Schools (CGFNS), which offers services that evaluate and verify credentials from the home country and nurse education program and administers a qualifying exam that predicts the probability of readiness to pass the National Council Licensing Exam for Registered Nurses (NCLEX-RN), the national exam required for licensure in the United States. The nurse faculty shortage is at epidemic proportions and does not seem to be abating. Nardi and Gyurko (2013) have written a thoughtful article on this subject and recommend some solutions for change.

Nurse education programs have worked for decades to raise the level of learning. In Europe, the Bologna Accords created a European Higher Education Area that was adopted by 47 countries. Participants agreed to standardize education by requiring the baccalaureate as the entry to professional nursing. This major decision eased the mobility of nurses from one country to another. Movement across borders and migration of nurses increases the diversity in programs but can raise issues in language and culture (Shaffer, 2014).

Nurse Involvement in Policy Decisions

To what extent have nurses been involved in influencing governmental policies that affect health, the delivery of care, and nursing practice? Nurses in Thailand who focus on elderly clients worked with policymakers to create mechanisms that are leading to recommendations for reform of the health insurance system for the elderly and the delivery of care (Sritanyarat, Aroonsang, Charoenchai, Limumnoilap, & Patanasri, 2004). Collaboration among nurses and other stakeholders in 14 countries in east, central, and southern Africa (ECSA) resulted in the creation of ECSACON (the East, Central, and Southern Africa College of Nursing), a professional advisory group that has adopted primary care as the official governmental approach to health care in those countries. ECSACON is an example of collaboration among the colleges of nursing that educate the largest group of professional healthcare providers on that continent, with nurses banding together to assess the status of health and health care, identify major problems, prioritize the high burden of disease in the region, and begin to change the system of healthcare delivery. The goal of the group is to assure quality care (Ndlovu, Phiri, Munjanja, Kibuka, & Fitzpatrick, 2003). Research conducted by Asp et al. (2014) has identified a lack of knowledge of neonatal danger signals among women in rural Uganda. Their research is providing opportunity for nurse interventions for neonates who otherwise might die. Asp and colleagues have determined a link between media exposure and birth preparedness among women in southwestern Uganda.

Similarly, nurses in Australia have worked with the Chief Nursing Officer to produce legislation that permits nurse practitioners to practice in that country (Adams & Della, 2005). Beginning with a Nurse Practitioner Committee in New South Wales in 1991, a working party developed pilot programs that reported in 1995 that nurse practitioners are "feasible safe, effective in their roles and provide quality health services" (p. 35). By 2004 legislation allowed legal authorization and protection for nurse practitioners by the New South Wales Nurse Registration Board (NP legislation, 2004). Persistence and courage characterize those in Australia who worked for better patient care through nurse practitioners.

Not all nurses have been successful in their efforts. Ferreira (2004) wrote that despite making great strides in getting technology incorporated into health care and attempts to improve access to care, Brazilian nurses were not able to bring together enough political and ideological power to accomplish a municipalization project in the district. A similar finding occurred in Botswana. Phaladze (2003) reported a study that described a lack of nurses in that country who participated in the process of developing healthcare public policy or resource allocation. The researcher noted that the "minimal participation ... resulted in implementation problems, thus compromising a service provision" (p. 22).

Teams of healthcare professionals can have a more powerful effect in addressing global health issues than a single type of professional. Consider which members of a team could have an impact on a health issue. Often physicians, nurses, dentists, and those who provide support services comprise teams that travel on mission trips. Although these teams treat serious health problems they usually do not become involved in underlying policy problems. Consider how a health problem in a country could be relieved if these mission teams could become involved in decisions that would address the problem or would work with the local population to advocate for themselves.

It is the responsibility of nurses to seek leadership positions in government and quasi-government institutions. Beverly Malone, PhD, RN, FAAN, is a former American Nurses Association (ANA) president; deputy assistant secretary for the U.S. Department of Health and Human Services; immediate past general secretary of the Royal College of Nursing of England, Scotland, and Northern Ireland; and currently chief executive officer for the National League for Nursing. She notes that most countries today still do not have nurse contacts in government (personal communication, June 10, 2014). This situation means that health-related grants, information, and policy ideas that are considered in various offices are never seen by a nurse. Dr. Malone agrees that nurses are always available to provide care, but are not at the policy table. She suggests that nurses in countries such as the United States who are in government positions must advocate at the World Health Assembly for access to care issues. Malone also urges nurses to exert leadership to assume positions that are recognized by governments and to pressure officials to appoint nurses to important government stations so that nurses can become policymakers.

To emphasize the importance of developing expertise in public policy, the American Association of Colleges of Nursing (AACN) designed a Doctor of Nursing Practice (DNP) degree that not only prepares practitioners at the highest level of direct care competence, but also offers students to focus on administration, healthcare policy, informatics, and population-based practice through the study of "aggregate/systems/organizational" (AACN, 2006, p. 18). Harrington, Crider, Benner, and Malone (2005) assert that nurses must have a very sophisticated comprehension of the policy process. These leaders urge that formal education is necessary to supplement any tangential experience nurses may have. DNP graduates are expected to serve as leaders and change agents at the macrosystems level that includes policy decisions.

Nurses throughout the world need to know how to maneuver through whatever political system is operating in their countries. Academic programs with the policy option of the DNP may attract nurses who come to the United States from other countries to obtain doctorates in nursing. Most countries outside the United States have set the standard for professional nursing at the baccalaureate level but have not yet developed doctoral programs; nurses with master's degrees frequently come to the United States to earn their doctorates. For example, the late King Hussein of Jordan, a landlocked, oil-poor country in the Middle East, determined that his country would be known for its exceptional educational system. The current King Abdullah II continues his father's legacy and directed the construction of universities throughout the country. The Ministry of Education supports master's-prepared academics in all fields to obtain doctorates in other countries until there are enough doctoral-prepared faculty and administrators in Jordan. As these well-prepared educators return to Jordan, they will accomplish the goals of their country related to conflict resolution, economic development, and education. The wife of King Abdullah II, Queen Rania, also supports education initiatives and has created scholarships for college students (Bio, 2014).

International health issues have economic, political, and sociocultural dimensions. The allocation of resources is at least a political decision. Today, advanced practice registered nurses must have a deep knowledge of health, illness, and wellness, plus an understanding of the broader social and political contexts in which these conditions exist. Issues of social justice, the relief of health disparities, and support for those with a stigmatized disease or disability are integral to APRN practices. Research is needed to help nurses and policymakers understand the extent of health problems, cultural and other variables that affect treatment, and political systems and players. There have been no comprehensive models for studying nursing and health policy from an international perspective.

This author has developed a model that may be useful for those who want to examine health issues in any country. The **Milstead model** was developed to guide researchers in analysis of complex health issues in an international framework. Essential components of the model include selecting the international setting, identifying the problem or policy, analyzing the sociocultural system, specifying the economic and political systems, and evaluating the specific health system.

Comparing issues and problems between and among countries can be an antidote to ethnocentrism, especially if the researcher is someone who is an outsider to the culture or who does not live in the situation. Commonly accepted values in a country are not necessarily universal, especially if the country is large or the values deeply ingrained. Comparative analysis searches for differences and diversity in addition to commonalities. Experimentation that is possible in a controlled laboratory is not possible in a human environment; "[t]he comparative method was perceived by John Stuart Mill, Auguste Comte, and Emile Durkheim as the best substitute for the experimental method in the social sciences" (Dogan & Pelassy, 1984, p. 13).

The Milstead model provides a comprehensive approach to the study of nursing and health policy issues within a country, or across countries and cultures, and integrates the policy components of political science with the roles of the nurse in advanced practice. The following case study will focus on a common global health issue, polio. Questions will guide the nurse through the model.

CASE STUDY: THE RESURGENCE OF POLIO

Imagine yourself in a rural clinic in Syria. You have completed an examination of a 10-year-old child who presented with a high fever (104°F) that has lasted for 2 days, pain and stiffness in all joints, and an inability to stand or walk. You suspect polio and recognize that the disease has had a resurgence in this country. Using the Milstead model, ask yourself the following questions.

(continues)

International Setting/Level of Analysis

1. Am I practicing in a country that offers the polio vaccine to everyone?
2. What governmental level offers the vaccine?
3. How do I find out about the government structure and function?
4. If I am not familiar with the type of government (parliamentary, monarchy, democracy, etc.), what resources are available to educate me?
5. What level of government is most likely to hear my concerns?
6. Are there governmental (i.e., public) policies that encourage or discourage vaccination for polio?

Policy Process

1. What component(s) of the policy process does this health problem most likely "fit"?
2. If this is a matter to put on the government agenda, what methods could I use when approaching officials?
3. How can I phrase the problem so that officials will pay attention?
4. Who would be important to enlist in expressing my concerns?
5. If this is a matter of getting government response, what are the formal and informal means of communicating with officials?
6. Is there a person with prestige or influence who will help carry my message to the government?
7. What policy tools can I use to design a government response to the problem? Is a law or regulation already in place that addresses this problem? If so, where was the breakdown in implementation?
8. Were the legal objectives clear when written? Were the program objectives changed during implementation?
9. Was the program or law ever evaluated? By whom? For what purpose?
10. Were any recommendations suggested? If so, were the recommendations followed?

Sociocultural System

Policies that are studied without regard to the human systems in which they function have little relevance. One must start by identifying the context, that is, the values of those who are affected and who affect the policy.

1. In the rural area in which you are practicing, is vaccination an accepted method of disease prevention? If not, what are the arguments against it?
2. If the procedure is accepted, was this child vaccinated? If not, why not?
3. Who was responsible for vaccinating the child?
4. Does polio hold a special meaning in this culture?
5. Is there a clear system of patriarchy or matriarchy? Does family hold a special meaning? Is the family a nuclear unit or an extended unit?
6. Is the patient/family part of a minority group that is treated differently from the majority? Is that person/family adherent in other areas of health care?
7. Are there religious or personal philosophical reasons why vaccination was not administered?
8. Are there myths about polio that keep some people from accepting vaccination? Do you believe these myths? If not, how can you help others dispel the myths?
9. Are there foods, clothing, sanitation practices, or language differences (vernacular phrases, intonations, regional or tribal accents) that could be barriers to vaccination? Is there geography or history that has contributed to the problem under study?

Economic and Political Systems

1. If there is a government mandate to vaccinate, was there funding available?
2. Was there enough vaccine available for the population?

(continues)

3. Were there other governmental priorities that superseded vaccination programs?
4. Is vaccine still available? Would pharmaceutical companies be asked to produce more vaccine for a small population? If so, what is the cost and who will pay for it?
5. What interest groups could be rallied to support a current government program? A new program?
6. What private resources could be tapped to assist with solving the problem?
7. Could resources such as the legal system, media, or interest groups be enlisted to address the problem?

The Health System

1. Is there a governmental health system available to help with the vaccination question?
2. At what level (national, regional/district, local/tribal) would this system exist? If not, how are children protected against common diseases?
3. Is there a national healthcare system? Is there a national health insurance system or other system of payment for healthcare services? What diseases or conditions does it cover? Do all citizens or residents have access to the health system? If the health system is religion-based, are services restricted to people of that faith?
4. Who are the healthcare providers? How does their education prepare them to address a potential epidemic? Are there enough of them to assist in a mass mobilization effort? Who would comprise your team and what resources would you need?
5. How is information about a health problem communicated to the population? Is there a sense of urgency about this problem?

Evaluating the Milstead Model

How useful was the model in dealing with the health problem you discovered? Which of the previously listed questions in the case study did you find especially helpful in addressing your particular issue? Were there other dimensions that were not addressed that are necessary in order to confront the problem?

Conclusion

This chapter introduces several global health issues. The importance of the role of the APRN in the formation of public policy, especially health policy, cannot be emphasized enough. Linking nurse expertise in health care with policy agenda-setting, design, implementation, and evaluation will affect the health of individuals and populations around the world. There is a powerful need for nurses to become involved with policymakers and stakeholders to eradicate pestilence and disease and to improve the quality of life of the Earth's inhabitants. There also is opportunity for teams of health professionals to exert not only their health expertise, but also their knowledge of policymaking to actually address the underlying reasons for health problems.

This chapter presents a model for analyzing nursing and health policy. The model is comprehensive and can serve as a framework for conceptualizing and implementing the process of inquiry into policy issues within and between countries. Advanced practice registered nurses are encouraged to cultivate an expansive intellect and consider all local health and nursing interests in the context of a global perspective. APRNs should use the model, evaluate the components, and validate the model's utility or improve it.

There is a dearth of policy research on nursing at the global level, and little comparative research has been done by nurses. The policy field is appropriate for APRNs who have integrated the multiple roles of the professional nurse into their practices. Nurses have an obligation to extend scientific inquiry beyond national borders and can serve as role models for those who are beginning to take an interest in a broader arena. Nurses are mentors and experts who are accountable to clients and consumers of health care, to nurse colleagues for authoring (Kennedy & Charles, 1997), and to other health professionals and policymakers for leadership in providing intelligent, insightful health care. The potential for contributing to knowledge of health, nursing, and public policy is unlimited.

Discussion Points

1. Discuss three reasons for conducting a comparative study of health problems.
2. Describe the type of government and general governmental structure in two countries in which you note a serious health problem. Identify resources you could use to obtain information about each country. At what level would your focus be most beneficial?
3. Compare the values of family, language, and food in two countries. What are the implications of your analysis in planning for health care in each country?
4. How might not including minorities of a country in a research study bias or skew the results of that study?
5. What resources does a researcher use in a country in which he or she does not know the language? What are the advantages and disadvantages of conducting a study under these circumstances?
6. In studying two countries with differing economic systems, what common indicators may be used to reduce variance?
7. In studying two countries with differing political systems, what common indicators may be used to reduce variance?
8. What other healthcare professionals would be useful to include in studying the health problem?
9. What indicators are useful in comparing two different healthcare systems?

References

Adams, E., & Della, P. (2005). Development of nurse practitioner roles in Western Australia. *Transplant Nurses' Journal, 14*(1), 21–24.

American Academy of Nursing. (2007). *Mission statement*. Washington, DC: Author.

American Association of Colleges of Nursing. (2006). *Essentials of Doctoral Education for Advanced Practice Nursing*. Washington, DC: Author.

American Nurses Association. (2006). *White paper on local nursing and health*. Washington, DC: Author.

Asp, G., Odberg Pettersson, K. O., Sandberg, J., Kalakyruga, J. K., & Agardh, L. A. (2014). Association between press media exposure and birth preparedness among women in SW Uganda: A community-based survey. *Global Health Action, 7*, 22904.

Bio. (2014). *Queen Rania*. Retrieved from http://www.biography.com/people/queen-rania-23468#awesm=oHO8jZcZLbqZQ

Broome, M. E. (2014). Open access publishing: A disruptive innovation. *Nursing Outlook, 62*, 69–71.

Campinha-Bacote, J. (2009). Culture and diversity issues: A culturally competent model of care for African Americans. *Journal of Urologic Nursing, 29*(1), 49–54.

Campinha-Bacote, J. (2011). Delivering patient-centered care in the midst of a cultural contest: The role of cultural competence. *Online Journal of Issues in Nursing, 16*(2), 5.

Carver, C., & Jessie, A. T. (2011, May 31). Patient-centered care in a medical home. *Online Journal of Issues in Nursing, 16*(2). Retrieved from www.nursingworld.org/MainMenuCategories/ANAMarketplace/ANAPeriodicals/OJIN/TableofContents/Vol-16-2011/No2-May-2011

Chen, W. T., Shiu, C. S., Simoni, J. M., Chuang, P., Zhao, H., Bao, M., & Lu, H. (2013). Challenges of cross-cultural research: Lessons from a U.S.-Asia HIV collaboration. *Nursing Outlook, 61*(3), 145–152.

Dogan, M., & Pelassy, D. (1984). *How to compare nations*. Chatham, NJ: Chatham House.

Douglas, M. K., Uhl Pierce, J., Rosenkoetter, M., Callister, L. C., Hattar-Pollara, M., Lauderdale, J., ... Pacquiao, D. (2009). Standards of practice for culturally competent nursing care: A discussion paper. *Journal of Transcultural Nursing, 20*(3), 257–269.

Douglas, M. K., Uhl Pierce, J., Rosenkoetter, M., Callister, L. C., Hattar-Pollara, M., Lauderdale, J., ... Pacquiao, D. (2011). Standards of practice for culturally competent nursing care. *Journal of Transcultural Nursing, 22*(4), 317–333.

Douglas, M. K., Rosenkoetter, M., Pacquiao, D., Callister, L. C., Hattar-Pollara, M., Lauderdale, J., Milstead, J. A., Nardi, D., & Purnell, L. (2014). Guidelines for implementing culturally competent care. *Journal of Transcultural Nursing, 25*(2), 109–121.

Fadiman, A. (1997). *The spirit catches you and you fall down*. New York: Farrar, Straus, & Giroux.

Ferreira, J. M. (2004). The health municipalization process from the perspective of the human being—nursing worker in the basic health network. *Revista Latino-Americana de Enfermagem, 12*(2), 212–220.

Gennaro, S. (2014). Commentaries on the global state of nursing. *Journal of Nursing Scholarship, 46*(3), 144.

Goulet, C., Polomeno, V., Laizner, A. M., Marcil, I., & Lang, A. (2003). Translation and validation of a French version of Brown's support behaviors inventory in perinatal health. *Western Journal of Nursing Research, 25*(5), 561–582.

Harrington, C., Crider, M. C., Benner, P. E., & Malone, R. E. (2005). Advanced nurse training in health policy: Designing and implementing a new program. *Policy, Politics, and Nursing Practice, 6*(2), 99–108.

Kennedy, E., & Charles, S. C. (1997). *Authority*. New York: Simon & Schuster.

McLuhan, M., & Fiore, Q. (1968). *War and peace in the global village*. New York: McGraw-Hill.

Nardi, D., & Gyurko, C. (2013). The global nursing faculty shortage: Status and solutions. *Journal of Nursing Scholarship, 45*(3), 317–326.

Ndlovu, R., Phiri, M. L., Munjanja, O. K., Kibuka, S., & Fitzpatrick, J. J. (2003). The East, Central, and Southern African College of Nursing: A collaborative endeavor for health policy and nursing practice. *Policy, Politics, and Nursing Practice, 4*(3), 221–226.

NP legislation amended act. (2004). Retrieved from www.acnp.org.au/history#34

Phaladze, N. S. (2003). The role of nurses in the human immunodeficiency virus/acquired immune deficiency syndrome policy process in Botswana. *International Nursing Review, 50*, 22–33.

Purnell, L. (2000). A description of the Purnell model for cultural competence. *Journal of Transcultural Nursing, 11*(1), 40–46.

Purnell, L. (n.d.). *Cultural competence in health care education and practice*. Retrieved from http://www.youtube.com/watch?v=03aZD3sEeW

Ross, C. A. (2000). Building bridges to promote globalization in nursing: The development of a Hermanamiento. *Journal of Transcultural Nursing, 11*(1), 64–67.

Sage. (n.d.). *Global qualitative nursing research*. Retrieved from www.uk.sagepub.com/journals/journal202291

Shaffer, F. (2014). Ensuring a global workforce: A challenge and opportunity. Guest editorial. *Nursing Outlook, 62*, 1–4.

Sritanyarat, W., Aroonsang, P., Charoenchai, A., Limumnoilap, S., & Patanasri, K. (2004). Health service system and health insurance for the elderly in Thailand: A knowledge synthesis. *Thai Journal of Nursing Research, 8*(2), 159–172.

Villarruel, A. M., Gallegos, E. C., Cherry, C. J., & Refugio de Duran, M. (2003). La uniendo de fronteras: Collaboration to develop HIV prevention strategies for Mexican and Latino youth. *Journal of Transcultural Nursing, 14*(3), 193–206.

World Health Organization. (2011). *Emerging diseases*. Retrieved from http://www.who.int/topics/emerging_diseases/en

Zachary, G. P. (2001, January 24). Shortage of nurses hits hardest where they are needed the most. *The Wall Street Journal*, A11–A12.

INDEX

Note: Page numbers followed by *f* or *t* indicate materials in figures or tables, respectively.

A

accelerated nurse education programs, 14
accountable care organization (ACO),
    123–124, 283, 299–301
accountable payment models, overview
    of, 301*t*
accreditation requirements, 200
ACO. *See* accountable care organization
ACS NSQIP. *See* American College of
    Surgeons National Surgical Quality
    Improvement Program
administrative practice acts (APAs), 109
Administrative Procedures Act (APA),
    99, 103, 172
    purpose of, 27
advanced practice registered nurses (APRNs),
    101, 152, 154, 155, 161, 190–191, 221, 228,
    232, 247, 279
    Consensus Model, 135–136
    definition, 1, 2
    delegation of medication administration
        by, 142–144
    history of, 23, 106–107
    multiple roles of, 32–33
    organizational involvement, 8
    regulation of, 111–112, 135–140
    reimbursement for, 121, 138
"advantaged" target population, 60
adverse selection, 283, 296–298
Affordable Care Act (ACA), 18, 20, 63,
    152, 159, 172, 179, 181, 186, 236, 262,
    273–274, 293
    definition, 283
    essential health benefits, 289–290
    fantastic accomplishment, 280–281
    interdisciplinary training, 277–279
    Nurse-Managed Health Clinics,
        274–277
    nursing provisions, 123
    personal stories, importance of, 279–280
    "Times They Are A-Changin, The," 280

African Americans, human research on, 32
Agency for Healthcare Research and Quality
    (AHRQ), 259
agency policies, 25
agenda setting
    case studies, 46–50
    definition, 45
    models, 50–61
    in policy process, 27–29
    social networking and, 238–239
AHEC program. *See* area health education
    center program
AHRQ. *See* Agency for Healthcare Research
    and Quality
AMA. *See* American Medical Association
American Academy of Nurse
    Practitioners, 112
American Academy of Nursing (AAN), 249
    annual meetings, 21
    Expert Panel on Global Nursing and
        Health, 314
    Raise the Voice campaign, 21
American Association of Colleges of Nursing
    (AACN), 276
    DNP program, 318
    educational models, 14
American Association of Colleges of Pharmacy
    (AACP), 280
American Association of Medical Colleges, 55
American Association of Nurse
    Anesthetists, 87
American Association of Nurse Anesthetists
    Council on Certification, 112
American Bar Association (ABA) Commission
    on Law and Aging, 278
American Cancer Society (website), 229*t*
American College of Nurse-Midwives
    Certification Council, 112
American College of Obstetricians and
    Gynecologists, 199

American College of Surgeons National Surgical Quality Improvement Program (ACS NSQIP), 234, 235
American Diabetes Association (website), 229t
American Heart Association (website), 229t
American Lung Association (website), 229t
American Medical Association (AMA), opposition to, 31
American Nurses Association (ANA), 20, 84–85, 106, 237
  PAC, 56
  social networking, 237
American Nurses Credentialing Center (ANCC), 112, 137
American Psychological Association (APA), 250
American Recovery and Reinvestment Act (ARRA), 233, 298
American Stroke Association (website), 229t
ANA. See American Nurses Association
"any willing provider" laws, 117
APA. See Administrative Procedures Act
APRNs. See advanced practice registered nurses
area health education center (AHEC) program, 276
ARRA. See American Recovery and Reinvestment Act
Arthritis Foundation (website), 229t
asynchronous interaction, 219, 225
authority tools for policy design, 158

B

bachelor of science in nursing (BSN), 13–14
bachelor's level educational programs
  policy process content in, 23
  as professional entry point, 14
"bandwagon approach" to implementation, 31
barriers, 174
BCBS. See Blue Cross & Blue Shield
behavioral dimensions in policy design, 160
Big Data, 234
bills becoming laws, process of, 102
  chief executive signature, 74–75
  committee consideration, 72–73
  conference committee, 74
  description, 71–72
  floor action, 73–74
bipartisan negotiation, 55
Black's Law Dictionary, 103
Blue Cross & Blue Shield (BCBS), 297

Blue Cross Blue Shield of Georgia, 232
board of pharmacy regulation, 118–119
boards of nursing (BONs), 102
  composition of, 113–114
  definition, 99
  licensure criteria establishment, 105–106
  overview, 113
  rule-making authority, 104
  serving on, 119–120
BONs. See boards of nursing
BSN. See bachelor of science in nursing
Bush, George W., 121

C

California Nurses Association (CNA), 20
capacity-building tools for policy design, 159
Capps, Lois, 36
case studies
  agenda setting, 46–50
  economics and finance of health care, 303–306
  implementation of public policy, 180–184
  Internet, consumer uses of, 240–241
  interprofessional education, 254–258, 262–264
  Milstead model, 319–323
  national policy, 61–62
  policy design, 162–164
  program evaluation, 211–212
CDC. See Centers for Disease Control and Prevention
Center for Beneficiary Choices, 121
Center for Medicaid and State Operations, 121
Center for Medicare Management, 121
Centers for Disease Control and Prevention (CDC), 199, 231
Centers for Medicare and Medicaid Services (CMS), 120, 181
CER. See comparative effectiveness research
certification, professional, 99, 109–110
CFIR. See Consolidated Framework for Implementation Research
CFR. See Code of Federal Regulations
CGFNS. See Commission on Graduates of Foreign Nursing Schools
Chilean mine, IPE in, 267–269
Christmas tree bills, 69, 71
chronic care services, episodic vs., 212
classroom, policy to, 165
clearance points, 31

client/patient, definition, 1, 2
clinic services, evaluating, 211–212
clinical nurse leaders (CNLs), 14–15
Clinton, Hillary, 154
CMS. *See* Centers for Medicare and Medicaid Services
CNLs. *See* clinical nurse leaders
Code of Federal Regulations (CFR), 126
coinsurance, 283, 289
collaborative practice, 253
 definition, 251
Commerce Clause of the U.S. Constitution, 122
Commission on Graduates of Foreign Nursing Schools (CGFNS), 309, 315
committee chairs, 75
committee hearings, 75
Commonwealth Fund, 185
communicable diseases, 310–311
communication, speed of, 225
comparative effectiveness research (CER), 284, 298–299
competency of nurses, monitoring, 115–116
complementary paradigms, 254
complexity science, 5
computerized provider order entry (CPOE), 219, 234
conference committee, 74
conflict, avoiding ethical, 204–205
Congress, 76
 definition, 69
congressional class, 57
Congressional Nursing Caucus, 36
congressional structure, 75
consensus, 171, 176
Consensus Model for APRN Regulation: Licensure, Accreditation, Certification, and Education, 136
Consensus Model for Regulation: Licensure, Accreditation, Certification, and Education (LACE), 111
Consolidated Framework for Implementation Research (CFIR), 173
constituents, 71
 definition of, 69
consumer health websites, trustworthy, 229t–230t
content, policy, 6
contextual dimensions
 definition, 45
 examples, 54–59
 importance of, 53–54
 list of, 53

Core Competencies for Interprofessional Education, 280
core interprofessional patient safety curriculum, case studies, 254–258
cost sharing, 290
Council for Ohio Health Care Advocacy (COHCA), 249
course syllabi, 6
court system, 26
CPOE. *See* computerized provider order entry
credentialing, professional
 future concerns, 135
 methods of, 108
crowd source, 267
 definition, 260
cultural context of global health care, 313–315

D
data mining, 219, 234
deflection of goals in policy implementation, 171, 176
delegated medical practice, 107
DeLeon, Pat, 250
Department of Health and Human Services (DHHS), 9, 274
"dependents" target population, 60
design issue, policy, 156–157
"deviants" target population, 60
DHHS. *See* Department of Health and Human Services
diabetes, adolescent with, 262–264
Disch, Joanne, 10
diseases
 communicable, 310–311
 emerging, 309, 311
disparities in health care
 economics and, 162
 nursing role in, 20
dissipation of energies in policy implementation, 171, 176
distance learning, 13
disunity, politics, 88
diversion of resources in policy implementation, 171, 176
divisiveness, politics, 88
Doctor of Nursing Practice (DNP), 6, 15, 278
doctoral level educational programs
 importance of, 318
 overview, 6
 policy process content in, 23

"donut hole" of Medicare coverage, 293
Drugs.com, 230*t*

E

e-CFR. *See* electronic Code of Federal
    Regulations
EBP. *See* evidence-based practice
economic costs, 284
economic theory, 285
economics and finance of health care
    ACO, 299–301
    adverse selection, 283, 296–298
    case studies, 303–306
    CER and, 284, 298–299
    health insurance exchanges, 289–291
    health insurance market, 287–289
    healthcare entitlement programs,
        291–295
    information asymmetry, 284, 295–298
    life expectancy *vs.* spending, 287
    moral hazard, 284, 296–298
    opportunity costs, 286–287
    overview, 285–286, 286*f*
    QALYs, 284, 298–299
    spending *vs.* life expectancy, 287
ECSACON, 316
ED nurses. *See* emergency department nurses
"Edge Runners," 21
education nurses, sustainable change, 13–15
educational culture, 253
educators, political selves, 33–34
EHRs. *See* electronic health records
elected officials, relationships with, 23
electronic Code of Federal Regulations
    (e-CFR), 126
electronic education, 13
electronic health records (EHRs), 219, 232
electronic medical record (EMR), 220, 234
emergency department (ED) nurses, 82
emergency regulations, 124
emerging diseases, 309, 311
EMR. *See* electronic medical record
entry point for nursing, 14
environmental disaster, 312
epilepsy, cultural context and, 313
episodic care services, chronic *vs.,* 212
EQ-5D index, 299
essential health benefits, 284, 289
ethics
    negative effects, reporting, 203–204
    program evaluation and, 191, 200–205
    protection from harm, 202
    role conflict, 202–203
ethnocentrism, 319
evaluation, policy and program
    definition, 31–32
    in policy process, 31–32
evaluation reports, 189, 191, 207–210
evidence-based practice (EBP), 173
    impact of, 182–184

F

Facebook, 223*t*
Faculty Loan Repayment Program, 123
federal and state health-related agencies, 9
federal deficit, 56
Federal Employees Health Benefit
    (FEHB), 274
federal lawmakers, 76
Federal Poverty Level (FPL), 290, 294
federal reform, 20
Federal Register
    definition, 99
    public comments and, 127
    purpose of, 124, 126
federal regulatory process
    emergency regulations, 124
    locating information, 124, 126–127
    need for, 120–131
    promulgation of, 124, 125*f*
    public comment period, 127, 129–130
    strengths and weaknesses of, 130–131
Federal Trade Commission (FTC), 9, 78
    Regulation Rules, 30
federally qualified health center (FQHC)
    program, 276
FEHB. *See* Federal Employees Health Benefit
Financial Reform bill, 78
fire alarms, 151, 154
"527 committees," 80
foreign nurse recruitment, 140
FPL. *See* Federal Poverty Level
FQHC program. *See* federally qualified health
    center program
"freedom of choice" laws, 117
FTC Trade Regulation Rules. *See* Federal
    Trade Commission
full-time equivalent (FTE), 290
funding agencies, accountability requirements
    of, 198–199
*Future of Nursing: Leading Change, Advancing
    Health, The,* 249, 276

impact of, 15–16
key messages and recommendations, 133, 180
Future Regulation of Advanced Practice Nursing, The, 135–136

G

Galt, Kimberly, 250
gaps in policy implementation, 178–179
geriatric population, polypharmacy and, 166
global connectivity of health care
communicable diseases, 310–311
cultural context, 313–315
environmental disasters, 312
nurse shortage, 315–316
public policy, nurse involvement in, 316–319
social justice, 312–313
goals, public policy *vs.,* 27
Government Printing Office (GPO), 126
government response to public problems, 29–30
government tools for policy design, 157–160, 163
GPO. *See* Government Printing Office
graduate education, 33
grassroots lobbyist, 85–86

H

harm, protection from, 202
HCFA. *See* Health Care Financing Administration
HCPs. *See* healthcare professionals; healthcare providers
health care. *See also* disparities in health care; economics and finance of health care
advances in, 17
life expectancy, 288*f*
regulation in transforming, 131–134
Health Care Financing Administration (HCFA), 120
health finance and health policy intersection, 286*f*
Health Information Technology for Economic and Clinical Health (HITECH) Act of 2009, 221, 233
health insurance exchanges (HIXs), 284, 289–291
health insurance market, 287–289
Health Insurance Portability and Accountability Act (HIPAA), 221

anonymity and, 202
social networking and, 239
health maintenance organizations (HMOs), 247
Health on the Internet (HON), 230*t*
Health on the Net Foundation (HON), 227
health policy, 273
and health finance intersection, 286*f*
organizations, 278
Health Professions Education: A Bridge to Quality, 261
health professions regulation, history of, 105–106
Health Research Extension Act of 1985, 48
Health Resources and Services Administration (HRSA), 262, 275
Health Systems Agencies, 55
health warnings, tobacco, 30
healthcare delivery systems, 259
healthcare entitlement programs, 291–295
healthcare information, social media and, 226–232
healthcare literacy, 220, 226
healthcare market, 285, 286
healthcare organizations, 258
healthcare policy, 194
in age of social media, 238–239
healthcare privacy policy, 239
healthcare professionals (HCPs), 46, 52–53
healthcare providers (HCPs)
definition, 1, 2
Internet use among, 220, 231–232
healthcare reform
nurse-driven campaigns, 21
politics and, 19
public policy process, 17–22
healthcare systems approach, 254
Healthy People 2020, 227
hearings, public, 100, 127
HHS. *See* Department of Health and Human Services
Hinshaw, Ada Sue, 54
HIPAA. *See* Health Insurance Portability and Accountability Act
HITECH Act of 2009. *See* Health Information Technology for Economic and Clinical Health Act of 2009
HIV transmission, perinatal care and, 199–200
HIXs. *See* health insurance exchanges
Hmong people, 313
HMOs. *See* Health maintenance organizations

HON. *See* Health on the Internet; Health on the Net Foundation
Hospital Insurance Program, 293
HRSA. *See* Health Resources and Services Administration

I

implementation of health policy
    definition, 171
    maneuvers, 176
    overview, 171–172
    process, 175–179
    research, 173–175
implementation of public policy
    case studies, 182–184
    gaps in, 178–179
    overview, 30–31
    social networking and, 237
incentive tools for policy design, 158
independent provider organizations (IPOs), 247
Indian Health Service, 122
infant mortality, 153
informatics, 220, 235
information asymmetry, 284, 295–298
informed consent, 202
InnoCentive, 267
Inouye, Daniel K., 274
Instagram, 224*t*
Institute for Healthcare Improvement, The, 257
Institute of Medicine (IOM), 180, 252, 259, 261, 262, 275
    program evaluation, 199
    publications, 15–16, 133
    report, 236
interdisciplinary health policy, 278
interest groups, 71
    definition, 69
    influence of, 58
    unity of, 55
Internet
    consumer uses, 227–228
    healthcare provider uses, 228, 231–232
    legislative and public policy issues, 127, 128–129
    penetration, 227
    trustworthy websites for consumers, 229*t*–230*t*
internships, political, 23
interprofessional education (IPE), 249, 252–254, 261

case studies, 254–258, 262–264
in Chilean mine, 267–269
definition, 252
future of, 269
overview, 252
Interprofessional Education Collaborative (IPEC), 277–278, 280
interprofessional learning, 253
interprofessional organizations, 249
interprofessional teamwork, 256
    definition, 252
interprofessional universe, evolving
    interprofessional collaboration, 261
    interprofessional education, core attributes of, 261–264
interstate compacts, 99, 134
IOM. *See* Institute of Medicine
IOM Board on Children, Youth, and Families (BCYF), 280
IPE. *See* interprofessional education
IPEC. *See* Interprofessional Education Collaborative
IPOs. *See* independent provider organizations
iron triangle, definition, 45, 51

J

Japanese earthquake and tsunami of 2011, 312
Johanns, Mike, 36
Johnson, Lyndon, 276
Josiah Macy Jr. Foundation, 134
judicial interpretation, 26

K

Kaiser Family Foundation, 288–289
Kaiser Permanente, 232
King Abdullah II of Jordan, 318
King Hussein of Jordan, 318
Kingdon model, 51–53, 61–63
Kirschner, Neil, 272
Kjervik, Diane, 277
KP Health Connect, 232

L

lame duck presidential terms, 56
lame duck sessions, 71
    definition, 69–70
Lanier, Jan, 250
laws. *See also* legislative process; specific laws
    implementation of, 101
    overtime, mandatory, 139

people in, making of, 75–78
in policy process, 25–26, 30
practice acts, 103
public policy *vs.*, 27
learning tools for policy design, 159–160
legislation
complexity of, 78
definition, 70
legislative process. *See also* laws
in policy process, 24, 28, 37
regulatory process *vs.*, 101–103
legislators, 70, 71
communicating with, 77
legislature, 70, 74
licensed practical nurse/licensed vocational
nurse (LPN/LVN) educational
programs, 104
licensure, 101
professional
definition and purpose, 99, 108–109
issues in, 131–135
multistate, 35
nurse shortage and, 138–140
life expectancy, healthcare spending and, 287
LinkedIn, 223*t*
lobbying and lobbyists, 71, 77–78
definition, 70
LPN/LVN educational programs. *See* licensed
practical nurse/licensed vocational nurse
educational programs

M

Madigan, Michael J., 52
Malone, Beverly, 10, 317
mandatory reporting, 115–116
master's level educational programs, 6, 14–15
Mayo Clinic (website), 230*t*
McLaughlin Group, The (television show), 36
means testing, 284, 290
Medicaid, 293–294
expansion, economic impact of, 305–306
Medicare, 193, 194
and Medicaid
health insurance market and, 288
reimbursement policies, 121
Medicare Advantage, 293
Medicare APRN reimbursement, discrepancies
in, 138
Medicare Part A, 293
Medicare Part B, 293
Medicare Part C, 293
Medicare Part D, 293

Medicare Prescription Drug, Improvement,
and Modernization Act (MMA), 121
Meet the Press (television show), 36
mental health disorders, medications for, 280
Merck Manual Home Edition (website), 230*t*
Merkley, Jeff, 36
Mikulski, Barbara, 36
military families, insurance for, 288
Milstead model, 309, 319–323
MMA. *See* Medicare Prescription Drug,
Improvement, and Modernization Act
monitoring, program, 197
moral hazard, 284, 296–298
multistate regulation, 123
definition, 100
overview, 134–135
mutual recognition, definition, 100
mutual recognition model of multistate
licensure, 134

N

NASA. *See* National Aeronautics and Space
Administration
National Aeronautics and Space
Administration (NASA), 264–267
National Center for Nursing Research
(NCNR) amendment
importance of, 50
Kingdon model and, 51–53
overview, 48–49
policy actors, stability of, 59–60
Schneider and Ingram model, 60–61
National Certification Board of Pediatric
Nurse Practitioners, 112
National Certification Corporation for the
Obstetric, Gynecologic, and Neonatal
Nursing Specialties, 112
National Council Licensing Exam for
Registered Nurses (NCLEX-RN), 14
National Council of State Boards of Nursing
(NCSBN), 100, 106
publications, 135
regulation of APRNs and, 111–112
National Institute of Nursing Research
(NINR), 49, 62
National Institutes of Health (NIH), 57, 58
National Kidney Foundation (website), 230*t*
National League for Nursing (NLN),
34–35, 106
National Nurses Organizing Committee
(NNOC), 20
National Patient Safety Foundation, The, 259

national policy, case studies, 61–62
national public policy perspective, 276
NCLEX-RN. *See* National Council Licensing Exam for Registered Nurses
NCNR amendment. *See* National Center for Nursing Research amendment
NCSBN. *See* National Council of State Boards of Nursing
Nebraska Nurses Association (NNA), 64
Nebraska, prenatal care policy in, 46–48
Netherlands, pregnancy outcomes in, 162
Nightingale, Florence, 3
NIH. *See* National Institutes of Health
NINR. *See* National Institute of Nursing Research
NLC model. *See* Nurse Licensure Compact model
NLN. *See* National League for Nursing
NMHCs. *See* nurse-managed health clinics
NNA. *See* Nebraska Nurses Association
NNOC. *See* National Nurses Organizing Committee
notice of proposed rulemaking (NPRM), 124
NPAs. *See* nurse practice acts
NPRM. *See* notice of proposed rulemaking
NPs. *See* nurse practitioners
nuclear power plants, environmental disasters and, 312
Nurse Aide Registry, 109
Nurse Corps Loan Repayment Program, 123
Nurse Licensure Compact (NLC) model, 134
nurse-managed health clinics (NMHCs), 186–187, 274–275
nurse practice acts (NPAs), 102, 113
Nurse Practitioner, The, 53, 107
nurse researchers, NIH grants and, 58
Nurse Scholarship Program, 123
nurse shortage
    accelerated nursing education programs and, 14
    global health and, 315–316
    regulation and licensure, impact on, 138–140
    statistics, 12
nurses. *See also* advanced practice registered nurses (APRNs)
    required skills, 22–23
    role of, 22–24
    sustainable change
        education, 13–15
        numbers, 12

    positive relationships, 15–17
    technology, 12–13
Nurse's Social Media Advantage, The, 22
NurseSpace, 237
nursing education
    accelerated, 14
    bachelor's level programs, 14
    changes in, 4–7
    distance learning, 13
    doctoral level programs, 6
    global health and, 315
    master's level programs, 6, 14–15
    political activism in, 33
    programs, proliferation of, 140
    technology, 12–13
nursing organizations. *See also* specific organizations
    certification examinations and, 112
    national, influence of, 49–50
    strengthening, 34–35
nursing practice, 7–8
nursing, requirement of, 103
nursing's agenda for health
    definition, 1–2
    required skills and, 23

O

objectives, public policy *vs.*, 27
obstructionism, 179
ODH. *See* Ohio Department of Health
Office of Management and Budget (OMB), 57, 275
official recognition, 100, 110
O'Grady, Eileen T., 152
Ohio Board of Regents, 248
Ohio Department of Health (ODH), 248
Ohio PCMH project, education component of, 249
Ohio project, 248
Oil Spill Recovery Institute, 267
Olivas, Danny, 266
OMB. *See* Office of Management and Budget
Omnibus Budget Reconciliation Act of 1987, 109
O'Neill, Tip, 270
online education, 13
opportunity costs, 284, 286–287
opposition, impact of, 31
O'Reilly Factor, The (television show), 36
organizational involvement, 8–10

organizations. *See also* nursing organizations; specific organizations
   new paradigm for, 17–18
outcome evaluations
   definition, 189, 193
   documentation, 198
overtime legislation, mandatory, 139

P

PACs. *See* political action committees
PACTs. *See* patient aligned care teams
participation policy, target population and, 151, 163
PAs. *See* physician assistants
patient-aligned care teams (PACTs), 184
patient-centered approach, 253
patient-centered medical homes (PCMHs), 248
Patient-Centered Outcomes Research Institute (PCORI), 299
patient-centered systems approaches, 259
patient-centeredness, 254
Patient Protection and Affordable Care Act (ACA). *See* Affordable Care Act (ACA)
Patient Safety Day, 255, 256
patient safety education, 257
patient simulators, 12
patient–provider interaction, 35
PCMHs. *See* patient-centered medical homes
PCORI. *See* Patient-Centered Outcomes Research Institute
PCP. *See* primary care provider
perinatal care, HIV transmission and, 199–200
persistence, public policy process, 270–272
Pew Health Professions Commission, 131–132
Pew Task Force on Health Care Workforce Regulation, 132
physician assistants (PAs), 247
physician/nurse practitioner payment, Medicare sustainable growth rate for, 303
policy
   definition, 189, 191
   overview, 192–194
policy actors, stability of, 59–60
Policy Committee, 249
policy content, 6
policy design
   case studies, 162–164
   issue, 156–157
   overview, 151–153
   tools for, 157–160
policy instruments, 157–160

policy links, 151, 155–156
policy participation, 163–164
policy process, 37. *See also* policy design
   definition, 2, 154
   overview, 28–32
   purpose of, 24–25
   role of nurse in, 23
   stages of, 27
policy research, review of, 154–156
policy streams, 51–52
policymaking process, money role in, 79
policy–process variables, 164
polio, resurgence of, 319–323
political action committees (PACs), 86
   ANA, 56
   definition, 70
political activism, 237
political astuteness, 85, 89
political contextual influence, 54–59
political culture, policy design and, 161
political participation, attitudes toward, 70
political role of nurses, developing, 22–24
political selves, educating, 33–34
political streams, 51–52
political system, working with, 35–36
politics
   as barrier to healthcare reform, 19
   coaching staff, 84–86
   defined, 285
   investment (time and money), 86–88
   players skills, 81, 84
   purse strings, 78–81
   strategizing for success, 81, 84–89
   team chemistry, 88–89
Polk, J.D., 250, 268
polypharmacy
   policy design in, 166
   problems, 166
Position Statement on the Practice Doctorate in nursing, 137
position statements, public policy *vs.*, 25, 27
practice acts, 103
pregnancy outcomes, policy design and, 162–164
prescriptive authority, 100, 104
   definition, 100
   examples, 104
primary care provider (PCP), 296
probability theory, 31
problem streams, 51–52
procedures, public policy *vs.*, 25
professional organizations, 9–10

Professional Standards Review Organization, 55
professional training programs, 258
program evaluation. *See also* outcome
    evaluations; social programs
        accountability in, 198–199
        case studies, 211–212
        definition, 189, 191
        ethics and, 200–205
        functions of, 195–196, 207
        objective, 203
        overview, 190–191
        qualitative, 206–207
        quantitative, 206–207
        reports, 207–209
        suggestions, 207
program evaluation design
        definition, 189, 207
        options, 205–207
program to create patient-centered medical
    homes (PCMHs), 184
public comment periods, 127, 129–130
public health insurance, 290
Public Health Service Act, 186
public hearings, 100, 127
public policy
        as an entity, 25–27
        definition, 2, 24, 190, 192
        global, nurse involvement in, 316–319
        overview, 192–194
        participation, 151, 163–164
        process, 7, 27–28
            healthcare reform, 17–22
        program development, 273
        research, 154–156

Q

QALYs. *See* quality adjusted life years
qualified health insurance plans, 289–290
qualified health plan, penalties for, 291
qualitative evaluation design, 190, 206–207
quality adjusted life years (QALYs), 284,
    298–299
Quality Chasm Series, 133
quantitative evaluation design, 190,
    206–207
quantum thinking, organizations and, 5–6

R

"R" word, 299
radiation exposure, environmental disasters
    and, 312

Raise the Voice campaign, 21
randomized control trial (RCT), 298
Reagan, Ronald, 56, 57
Really Simple Syndication (RSS) technology,
    220, 225, 231
recognition
        legislative, 105
        official, 100, 110
recruitment, foreign nurse, 140, 315
registered care technicians, opposition to, 31
registered nurses (RNs), 104
        economic value of BSN education
            for, 304
registration, professional, 100, 109
regulations (rules), 100
        changes in, 145–146
        definitions and purpose of, 100,
            103–105
        implementation of, 103
        issues in, 131–135
        monitoring, 117–119
        nurse shortage on, 138–140
        in policy process, 25–27, 30
        promulgation of, 116
regulatory process
        APRNs, history, 106–107
        definition, 100–101
        health professions, 103–112
        state level, 113–120
        strengths and weaknesses of, 130–131
        in transforming healthcare system,
            131–134
        workforce, 132
Rehabilitation Act of 1973, 26
reimbursement, 247–248
        of APRNs, 138
        policies, Medicare and Medicaid, 121
requests for information, 200
*Requirements for Accrediting Agencies and Criteria
    for APRN Certification Programs, The*
    (1995), 112
resolutions, public policy *vs.,* 27
RN. *See* registered nurse
Robert Wood Johnson Foundation (RWJF)
        funded projects, 16, 21
        publications, 133
Romney, Mitt, 275
Roosevelt, Franklin D., 275
RSS technology. *See* Really Simple Syndication
    technology
RWJF. *See* Robert Wood Johnson Foundation
Rychnovsky, Jacqueline, 276

S

SBTPE. *See* State Board Test Pool Examination

Schneider and Ingram model, 60–61

self-regulation, professional, 100, 110–111

Senate Nursing Caucus, 36

sick care system, 152

sickness insurance, 287

small business health insurance options program (SHOP), 290

Snowe, Olympia, 36

social constructions, 61

social justice, 312–313

social media. *See* social networking

social networking

    communication, impact on, 222, 225–226

    consumer uses, 227–228

    definitions, 221

    example sites, 223*t*–224*t*

    healthcare literacy, 226

    privacy issues, 239

social process, 173

social programs

    APRN in, 192

    choosing, 196–197

    definition, 190

    effects of unintended, 200

    interventions, revising, 199–200

    monitoring operations of, 197

    overview, 194–195

    periodic evaluation of, 198

    requests for information, 200

Social Security Act, 193, 293

sound bites, 29

South Carolina

    pregnancy outcomes in, 162

    teen pregnancy in, 166–167

"space and place" problems, 253

Space Medicine Division of the National Aeronautics and Space Administration (NASA), 250

speed of communication, 225

staffing issues, numbers *vs.* principles, 20

staffing patterns, 77

staffing ratios, 139

standing committees, 72

State Board Test Pool Examination (SBTPE), 106

State Children's Health Insurance Programs, 288

state regulatory process, 113

board meetings, 114–115

boards and commissions serving, 119–120

boards of nursing, 113–114

instituting state regulations, 116–117

nurses competency monitoring, 115–116

state regulations monitoring, 117–119

status epilepticus, cultural context and, 313

Stevenson, Joanne, 58

streams, definition, 45, 51–52

"street-level" bureaucrats, 177

structure of federalism, 161

"sunshine" laws, 114

superusers, 220, 235

Supplementary Medical Insurance, 293

Supremacy Clause of the U.S. Constitution, 122

Swensen, Clifford, 272

symbolic/hortatory tools for policy design, 159

synchronous interaction, 220, 225

T

target populations, 151, 163–164

    social construction of, 61

TBP model. *See* Theory of Planned Behavior model

"Team 4" concept, 264–267

    case studies, 267–268

team-based provider practices, concept of, 248

technology. *See also* Internet; social networking

    nurses, sustainable change, 12–13

    nursing education, 12–13

telehealth, 123

    multistate licensure and, 35

    overview, 13

television courses, 13

theory

    definition of, 190

    program evaluation, use in, 200–205

Theory of Planned Behavior (TBP) model, 173

"Third House of Congress," 30

This Week (television show), 36

To Err Is Human: Building a Safer Health System, 261

tobacco industry response to health warnings requirements, 30

TransforMED, 248

TriCare insurance, 288

Tuskegee experiment, 32

Twitter, 223*t*

U

UAP. *See* unlicensed assistive personnel
Uniformed Services University of the Health
    Sciences (USUHS), 278
United States
    health professionals in, 247
    national health expenditures, 295*f*
    RCT, 298
United States Congress, presidential
    interactions, 57
United States Constitution, 123
university-wide implementation case, 258
unlicensed assistive personnel (UAP), 132
    delegation and supervision of, 139
U.S. Department of Veterans Affairs, 185
U.S. healthcare reform, 139
U.S. Senate Special Committee on Aging, 278
U.S. sick care system, 247
U.S. Veterans Health Administration (VHA)
    innovative model, 184–185
USUHS. *See* Uniformed Services University of
    the Health Sciences

V

variables in policy implementation,
    175–177, 179
Veterans Health Administration, 122

veto-override votes, 58
VHA innovative model. *See* U.S. Veterans
    Health Administration innovative model
vision, public policy process, 270–272

W

Waxman, Henry, 57
Web 2.0. *See* social networking
WebMD (website), 224*t*, 230*t*
Whitfield, Ed, 36
window of opportunity, definition, 45, 51–52
word bites, 29
workforce regulation, 132
workplace safety, government response, 82–84
World Health Assembly, 317
World Health Organization, 261

Y

YouTube, 224*t*

select material from

SURVEY OF
ACCOUNTING

THIRD EDITION

Thomas P. Edmonds
University of Alabama–Birmingham

Frances M. McNair
Mississippi State University

Philip R. Olds
Virginia Commonwealth University

Bor-Yi Tsay
University of Alabama at Birmingham

A200: FOUNDATIONS OF ACCOUNTING

Mr. Rick Schrimper
Kelley School of Business
Indiana University

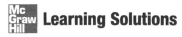 **Learning Solutions**

Boston Burr Ridge, IL Dubuque, IA New York San Francisco St. Louis
Bangkok Bogotá Caracas Lisbon London Madrid
Mexico City Milan New Delhi Seoul Singapore Sydney Taipei Toronto

The McGraw·Hill Companies

Select Material from
Survey of Accounting, Third Edition
A200: Foundations of Accounting
Mr. Rick Schrimper
Kelley School of Business
Indiana University

This book is a McGraw-Hill Learning Solutions textbook and contains select material from *Survey of Accounting*, Third Edition by Thomas P. Edmonds, Frances M. McNair, Philip R. Olds, and Bor-Yi Tsay. Copyright © 2012 by The McGraw-Hill Companies, Inc. Reprinted with permission of the publisher. Many custom published texts are modified versions or adaptations of our best-selling textbooks. Some adaptations are printed in black and white to keep prices at a minimum, while others are in color.

1 2 3 4 5 6 7 8 9 0   QDB QDB 13 12 11

ISBN-13: 978-0-07-754697-7
ISBN-10: 0-07-754697-0

Learning Solutions Representative: Ann Hayes
Production Editor: Nichole Birkenholz
Printer/Binder: Quad/Graphics

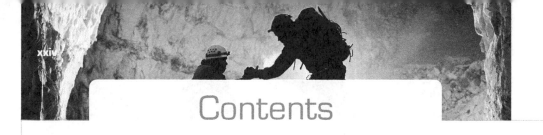

Contents

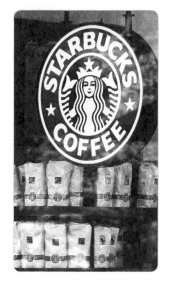

Chapter 1　An Introduction to Accounting　2

Chapter Opening　2

Role of Accounting in Society　4

*Using Free Markets to Set Resource
Priorities　4*

Accounting Provides Information　4

Types of Accounting Information　6

*Nonbusiness Resource
Usage　6*

Careers in Accounting　7

Measurement Rules　8

Reporting Entities　9

Elements of Financial Statements　10

*Using Accounts to Gather
Information　11*

Accounting Equation　12

**Recording Business Events under the
Accounting Equation　13**

Asset Source Transactions　13

Asset Exchange Transactions　14

*Another Asset Source
Transaction　15*

Asset Use Transactions　15

Summary of Transactions　17

Recap: Types of Transactions　17

Preparing Financial Statements　18

*Income Statement and the Matching
Concept　18*

*Statement of Changes in Stockholders'
Equity　20*

Balance Sheet　20

Statement of Cash Flows　21

The Closing Process　22

**The Horizontal Financial Statements
Model　23**

Real-World Financial Reports　24

*Annual Report for Target
Corporation　25*

*Special Terms in Real-World
Reports　25*

A Look Back　26

A Look Forward　26

Self-Study Review Problem　26

Key Terms　28

Questions　28

Multiple-choice Questions　29

Exercises　29

Problems　37

Analyze, Think, Communicate　41

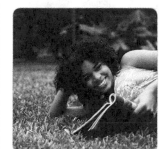

Chapter 2　Understanding the Accounting Cycle　44

Chapter Opening　44

Accrual Accounting　46

Accounting for Accounts Receivable　46

Other Events　47

*Accounting for Accrued Salary Expense
(Adjusting Entry)　47*

*Summary of Events and General
Ledger　49*

Vertical Statements Model　49

The Closing Process　52

Steps in an Accounting Cycle　52

The Matching Concept　53

The Conservatism Principle　53

Second Accounting Cycle　53

*Prepaid Items (Cost versus
Expense)　54*

*Accounting for Receipt of Unearned
Revenue　55*

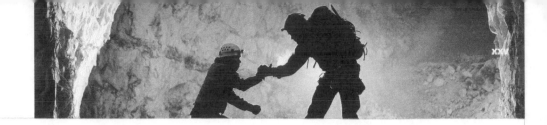

Accounting for Supplies Purchase   55

Other 2013 Events   55

Adjusting Entries   58

Accounting for Supplies (Adjusting Entry)   58

Accounting for Prepaid Rent (Adjusting Entry)   58

Accounting for Unearned Revenue (Adjusting Entry)   59

Accounting for Accrued Salary Expense (Adjusting Entry)   62

Summary of Events and General Ledger   62

Vertical Statements Model   62

Transaction Classification   66

A Look Back   66

A Look Forward   67

Self-Study Review Problem   67

Key Terms   68

Questions   69

Multiple-choice Questions   69

Exercises   70

Problems   78

Analyze, Think, Communicate   83

Chapter 3   Accounting for Merchandising Businesses   86

Chapter Opening   86

Product Costs Versus Selling and Administrative Costs   88

Allocating Inventory Cost between Asset and Expense Accounts   89

Perpetual Inventory System   89

Effects of 2012 Events on Financial Statements   90

Financial Statements for 2012   91

Transportation Cost, Purchase Returns and Allowances, and Cash Discounts Related to Inventory Purchases   92

Effects of 2013 Events on Financial Statements   92

Accounting for Purchase Returns and Allowances   93

Purchase Discounts   94

The Cost of Financing Inventory   94

Accounting for Transportation Costs   95

Recognizing Gains and Losses   98

Multistep Income Statement   98

Lost, Damaged, or Stolen Inventory   100

Adjustment for Lost, Damaged, or Stolen Inventory   101

Events Affecting Sales   101

Accounting for Sales Returns and Allowances   102

Accounting for Sales Discounts   102

Common Size Financial Statements   103

A Look Back   105

A Look Forward   106

Appendix   106

Self-Study Review Problem   107

Key Terms   109

Questions   109

Multiple-choice Questions   110

Exercises   110

Problems   117

Analyze, Think, Communicate   121

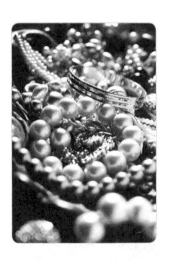

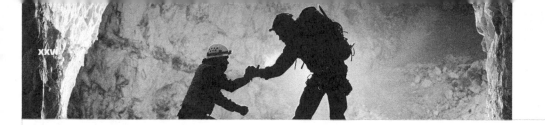

Chapter 4   Internal Controls, Accounting for Cash, and Ethics   124

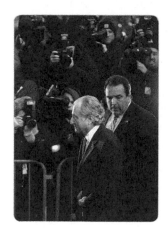

Chapter Opening   **124**

Key Features of Internal Control Systems   **126**

   Separation of Duties   *126*

   Quality of Employees   *127*

   Bonded Employees   *127*

   Required Absences   *127*

   Procedures Manual   *127*

   Authority and Responsibility   *127*

   Prenumbered Documents   *128*

   Physical Control   *128*

   Performance Evaluations   *128*

   Limitations   *128*

Accounting for Cash   **129**

   Controlling Cash   *129*

   Checking Account Documents   *130*

   Reconciling the Bank Account   *131*

   Determining True Cash Balance   *131*

   Illustrating a Bank Reconciliation   *134*

Importance of Ethics   **137**

   Common Features of Criminal and Ethical Misconduct   *137*

Role of the Independent Auditor   **139**

   The Financial Statement Audit   *140*

   Materiality and Financial Audits   *140*

   Types of Audit Opinions   *141*

   Confidentiality   *141*

A Look Back   **142**

A Look Forward   **143**

Self-Study Review Problem   **143**

Key Terms   **144**

Questions   **144**

Multiple-choice Questions   **145**

Exercises   **145**

Problems   **149**

Analyze, Think, Communicate   **153**

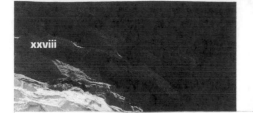

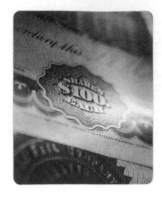

Chapter 8 Proprietorships, Partnerships, and Corporations 286

Chapter Opening 286

Forms of Business Organizations 288

Advantages and Disadvantages of Different Forms of Business Organization 288

    Regulation 288

    Double Taxation 289

    Limited Liability 289

    Continuity 290

    Transferability of Ownership 290

    Management Structure 290

    Ability to Raise Capital 291

Appearance of Capital Structure in Financial Statements 291

    Presentation of Equity in Proprietorships 291

    Presentation of Equity in Partnerships 292

    Presentation of Equity in Corporations 293

Characteristics of Capital Stock 293

    Par Value 293

    Stated Value 293

    Other Valuation Terminology 293

    Stock: Authorized, Issued, and Outstanding 293

    Classes of Stock 294

Accounting for Stock Transactions on the Day of Issue 296

    Issuing Par Value Stock 296

    Stock Classification 296

    Stock Issued at Stated Value 296

    Stock Issued with No Par Value 297

    Financial Statement Presentation 297

Stockholders' Equity Transactions after the Day of Issue 298

    Treasury Stock 298

    Cash Dividend 299

    Stock Dividend 300

    Stock Split 301

    Appropriation of Retained Earnings 301

Financial Statement Presentation

Investing in Common Stock 303

    Receiving Dividends 303

    Increasing the Price of Stock 303

    Exercising Control through Stock **302** *Ownership 304*

A Look Back 304

A Look Forward 305

Self-Study Review Problem 306

Key Terms 306

Questions 307

Multiple-choice Questions 308

Exercises 308

Problems 312

Analyze, Think, Communicate 315

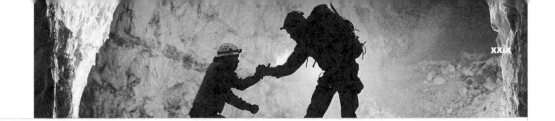

Chapter 10 An Introduction to Managerial Accounting 358

Chapter Opening   358

Differences between Managerial and Financial Accounting   360

Users and Types of Information   360

Level of Aggregation   360

Regulation   361

Information Characteristics   362

Time Horizon and Reporting Frequency   362

Product Costing in Manufacturing Companies   362

Tabor Manufacturing Company   362

Average Cost per Unit   362

Costs Can Be Assets or Expenses   363

Effect of Product Costs on Financial Statements   364

Materials Costs (Event 2)   365

Labor Costs (Event 4)   365

Overhead Costs (Event 8)   366

Total Product Cost   366

General, Selling, and Administrative Costs   367

Overhead Costs: A Closer Look   367

Manufacturing Product Cost Summary   369

Schedule of Cost of Goods Manufactured and Sold   370

Upstream and Downstream Costs   371

Just-in-Time Inventory   372

Just-in-Time Illustration   372

Statement of Ethical Professional Practice   374

A Look Back   375

A Look Forward   376

Appendix A   376

Self-Study Review Problem   378

Key Terms   380

Questions   381

Multiple-choice Questions   381

Exercises   381

Problems   388

Analyze, Think, Communicate   393

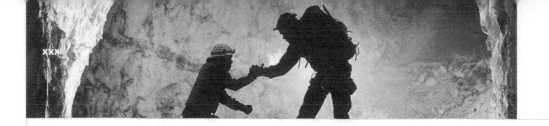

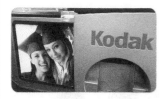

Chapter 11 Cost Behavior, Operating Leverage, and Profitability Analysis 396

Chapter Opening 396

Fixed Cost Behavior 398

Operating Leverage 398

Calculating Percentage Change 399

Risk and Reward Assessment 400

Variable Cost Behavior 401

Risk and Reward Assessment 401

An Income Statement under the Contribution Margin Approach 402

Measuring Operating Leverage Using Contribution Margin 403

Cost Behavior Summarized 404

Mixed Costs (Semivariable Costs) 405

The Relevant Range 405

Context-Sensitive Definitions of Fixed and Variable 405

Determining the Break-Even Point 406

Equation Method 407

Contribution Margin per Unit Method 408

Determining the Sales Volume Necessary to Reach a Desired Profit 409

Calculating the Margin of Safety 410

A Look Back 411

A Look Forward 412

Self-Study Review Problem 1 412

Self-Study Review Problem 2 414

Key Terms 415

Questions 415

Multiple-choice Questions 416

Exercises 416

Problems 422

Analyze, Think, Communicate 426

CHAPTER 1

An Introduction to Accounting

LEARNING OBJECTIVES

After you have mastered the material in this chapter, you will be able to:

1 Explain the role of accounting in society.

2 Construct an accounting equation using elements of financial statements terminology.

3 Record business events in general ledger accounts organized under an accounting equation.

4 Classify business events as asset source, use, or exchange transactions.

5 Use general ledger account information to prepare four financial statements.

6 Record business events using a horizontal financial statements model.

CHAPTER OPENING

Why should you study accounting? You should study accounting because it can help you succeed in business. Businesses use accounting to keep score. Imagine trying to play football without knowing how many points a touchdown is worth. Like sports, business is competitive. If you do not know how to keep score, you are not likely to succeed.

Accounting is an information system that reports on the economic activities and financial condition of a business or other organization. Do not underestimate the importance of accounting information. If you had information that enabled you to predict business success, you could become a very wealthy Wall Street investor. Communicating economic information is so important that accounting is frequently called the *language of business*.

The Curious Accountant

Who owns Starbucks? Who owns the American Cancer Society (ACS)? Many people and organizations other than owners are interested in the operations of Starbucks and the ACS. These parties are called *stakeholders*. Among others, they include lenders, employees, suppliers, customers, benefactors, research institutions, local governments, cancer patients, lawyers, bankers, financial analysts, and government agencies such as the Internal Revenue Service and the Securities and Exchange Commission. Organizations communicate information to stakeholders through *financial reports*.

How do you think the financial reports of Starbucks differ from those of the ACS? (Answer on page 11.)

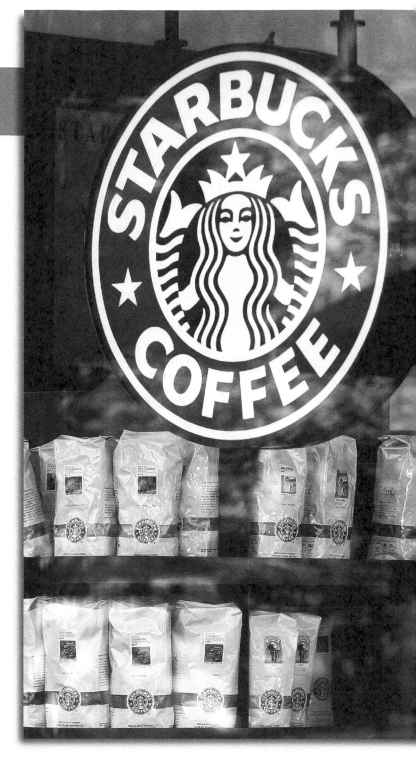

ROLE OF ACCOUNTING IN SOCIETY

Explain the role of accounting in society.

How should society allocate its resources? Should we spend more to harvest food or cure disease? Should we build computers or cars? Should we invest money in IBM or General Motors? Accounting provides information that helps answer such questions.

Using Free Markets to Set Resource Priorities

Suppose you want to start a business. You may have heard "you have to have money to make money." In fact, you will need more than just money to start and operate a business. You will likely need such resources as equipment, land, materials, and employees. If you do not have these resources, how can you get them? In the United States, you compete for resources in open markets.

A **market** is a group of people or entities organized to exchange items of value. The market for business resources involves three distinct participants: consumers, conversion agents, and resource owners. *Consumers* use resources. Resources are frequently not in a form consumers want. For example, nature provides trees but consumers want furniture. *Conversion agents* (businesses) transform resources such as trees into desirable products such as furniture. *Resource owners* control the distribution of resources to conversion agents. Thus resource owners provide resources (inputs) to conversion agents who provide goods and services (outputs) to consumers.

For example, a home builder (conversion agent) transforms labor and materials (inputs) into houses (output) that consumers use. The transformation adds value to the inputs, creating outputs worth more than the sum of the inputs. A house that required

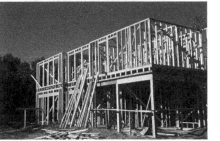

$220,000 of materials and labor to build could have a market value of $250,000.

Common terms for the added value created in the transformation process include **profit, income,** or **earnings.** Accountants measure the added value as the difference between the cost of a product or service and the selling price of that product or service. The profit on the house described above is $30,000, the difference between its $220,000 cost and $250,000 market value.

Conversion agents who successfully and efficiently (at low cost) satisfy consumer preferences are rewarded with high earnings. These earnings are shared with resource owners, so conversion agents who exhibit high earnings potential are more likely to compete successfully for resources.

Return to the original question. How can you get the resources you need to start a business? You must go to open markets and convince resource owners that you can produce profits. Exhibit 1.1 illustrates the market trilogy involved in resource allocation.

The specific resources businesses commonly use to satisfy consumer demand are financial resources, physical resources, and labor resources.

Financial Resources

Businesses (conversion agents) need **financial resources** (money) to get started and to operate. *Investors* and *creditors* provide financial resources.

- **Investors** provide financial resources in exchange for ownership interests in businesses. Owners expect businesses to return to them a share of the business income earned.

- **Creditors** lend financial resources to businesses. Instead of a share of business income, creditors expect businesses to repay borrowed resources at a future date.

The resources controlled by a business are called **assets.** If a business ceases to operate, its remaining assets are sold and the sale proceeds are returned to the investors and creditors through a process called business **liquidation.** Creditors have a priority claim on assets in business liquidations. After creditor claims are satisfied, any remaining assets are distributed to investors (owners).

EXHIBIT 1.1

Market Trilogy in Resource Allocation

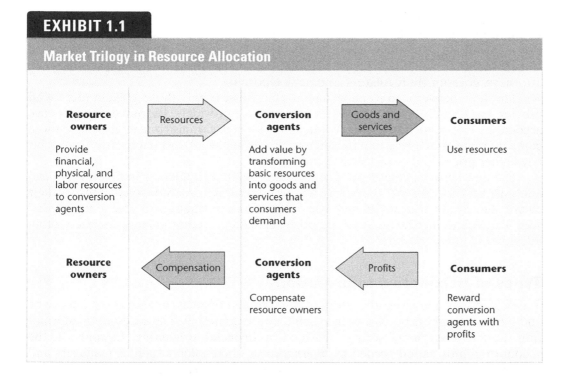

To illustrate, suppose a business acquired $100 cash from investors and $200 cash from creditors. Assume the business lost $75 and returned the remaining $225 ($300 − $75) to the resource providers. The creditors would receive $200; the owners would receive only $25. If the business lost $120, the creditors would receive only $180 ($300 − $120); the investors would receive nothing.

As this illustration suggests, both creditors and investors can lose resources when businesses fail. Creditors, however, are in a more secure position because of their priority claim on resources. In exchange for their more secure position, creditors normally do not share business profits. Instead, they receive a fixed amount of money called **interest.**

Investors and creditors prefer to provide financial resources to businesses with high earnings potential because such companies are better able to share profits and make interest payments. Profitable businesses are also less likely to experience bankruptcy and liquidation.

Physical Resources

In their most primitive form, **physical resources** are natural resources. Physical resources often move through numerous stages of transformation. For example, standing timber may be successively transformed into harvested logs, raw lumber, and finished furniture. Owners of physical resources seek to sell those resources to businesses with high earnings potential because profitable businesses are able to pay higher prices and make repeat purchases.

Labor Resources

Labor resources include both intellectual and physical labor. Like other resource providers, workers prefer businesses that have high income potential because these businesses are able to pay higher wages and offer continued employment.

Accounting Provides Information

How do providers of financial, physical, and labor resources identify conversion agents (businesses) with high profit potential? Investors, creditors, and workers rely heavily on accounting information to evaluate which businesses are worthy of receiving resources. In addition, other people and organizations have an interest in accounting information about businesses. The many **users** of accounting information are commonly called **stakeholders.** Stakeholders include resource providers, financial analysts, brokers, attorneys, government regulators, and news reporters.

The link between conversion agents (businesses) and those stakeholders who provide resources is direct: businesses pay resource providers. Resource providers use accounting information to identify companies with high earnings potential because those companies are more likely to return higher profits, make interest payments, repay debt, pay higher prices, and provide stable employment.

The link between conversion agents and other stakeholders is indirect. Financial analysts, brokers, and attorneys may use accounting information when advising their clients. Government agencies may use accounting information to assess companies' compliance with income tax laws and other regulations. Reporters may use accounting information in news reports.

Types of Accounting Information

Stakeholders such as investors, creditors, lawyers, and financial analysts exist outside of and separate from the businesses in which they are interested. The accounting information these *external users* need is provided by **financial accounting.** In contrast, the accounting information needed by *internal users,* stakeholders such as managers and employees who work within a business, is provided by **managerial accounting.**

The information needs of external and internal users frequently overlap. For example, external and internal users are both interested in the amount of income a business earns. Managerial accounting information, however, is usually more detailed than financial accounting reports. Investors are concerned about the overall profitability of Wendy's versus Burger King; a Wendy's regional manager is interested in the profits of individual Wendy's restaurants. In fact, a regional manager is also interested in non-financial measures, such as the number of employees needed to operate a restaurant, the times at which customer demand is high versus low, and measures of cleanliness and customer satisfaction.

Nonbusiness Resource Usage

The U.S. economy is not *purely* market based. Factors other than profitability often influence resource allocation priorities. For example, governments allocate resources to national defense, to redistribute wealth, or to protect the environment. Foundations, religious groups, the Peace Corps, and other benevolent organizations prioritize resource usage based on humanitarian concerns.

Like profit-oriented businesses, civic or humanitarian organizations add value through resource transformation. For example, a soup kitchen adds value to uncooked meats and vegetables by converting them into prepared meals. The individuals who consume the meals, however, are unable to pay for the kitchen's operating costs, much less for the added value. The soup kitchen's motivation is to meet humanitarian needs, not to earn profits. Organizations that are not motivated by profit are called **not-for-profit entities** (also called *nonprofit* or *nonbusiness organizations*).

Stakeholders interested in nonprofit organizations also need accounting information. Accounting systems measure the cost of the goods and services not-for-profit organizations provide, the efficiency and effectiveness of the organizations' operations, and the ability of the organizations to continue to provide goods and services. This information serves a host of stakeholders, including taxpayers, contributors, lenders, suppliers, employees, managers, financial analysts, attorneys, and beneficiaries.

The focus of accounting, therefore, is to provide information useful to making decisions for a variety of business and nonbusiness user groups. The different types of accounting information and the stakeholders that commonly use the information are summarized in Exhibit 1.2.

EXHIBIT 1.2

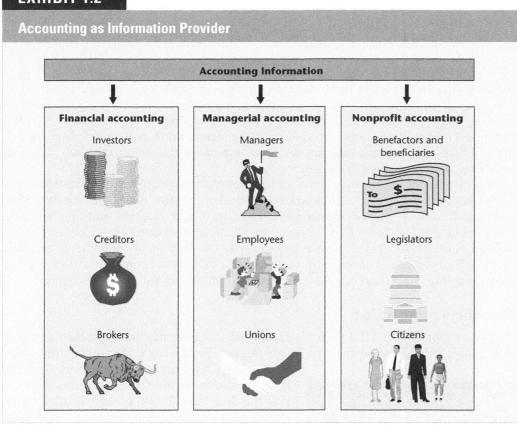

Accounting as Information Provider

Careers in Accounting

An accounting career can take you to the top of the business world. *BusinessWeek* studied the backgrounds of the chief executive officers (CEOs) of the 1,000 largest public corporations. More CEOs had backgrounds in finance and accounting than any other field. Exhibit 1.3 provides additional detail regarding the career paths followed by these executives.

What do accountants do? Accountants identify, record, analyze, and communicate information about the economic events that affect organizations. They may work in either public accounting or private accounting.

Public Accounting

You are probably familiar with the acronym CPA. CPA stands for certified *public* accountant. Public accountants provide services to various clients. They are usually paid a fee that varies depending on the service provided. Services typically offered by public accountants include (1) audit services, (2) tax services, and (3) consulting services.

- *Audit services* involve examining a company's accounting records in order to issue an opinion about whether the company's financial statements conform to generally accepted accounting principles. The auditor's opinion adds credibility to the statements, which are prepared by the company's management.

- *Tax services* include both determining the amount of tax due and tax planning to help companies minimize tax expense.

- *Consulting services* cover a wide range of activities that includes everything from installing sophisticated computerized accounting systems to providing personal financial advice.

EXHIBIT 1.3

Career Paths of Chief Executive Officers

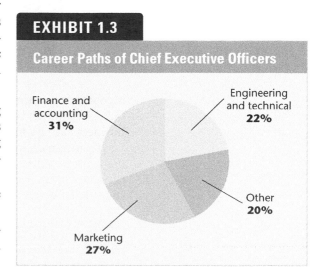

Finance and accounting 31%

Engineering and technical 22%

Other 20%

Marketing 27%

All public accountants are not certified. Each state government establishes certification requirements applicable in that state. Although the requirements vary from state to state, CPA candidates normally must have a college education, pass a demanding technical examination, and obtain work experience relevant to practicing public accounting.

Private Accounting

Accountants employed in the private sector usually work for a specific company or nonprofit organization. Private sector accountants perform a wide variety of functions for their employers. Their duties include classifying and recording transactions, billing customers and collecting amounts due, ordering merchandise, paying suppliers, preparing and analyzing financial statements, developing budgets, measuring costs, assessing performance, and making decisions.

Private accountants may earn any of several professional certifications. For example, the Institute of Certified Management Accountants issues the *Certified Management Accounting (CMA)* designation. The Institute of Internal Auditors issues the *Certified Internal Auditor (CIA)* designation. These designations are widely recognized indicators of technical competence and integrity on the part of individuals who hold them. All professional accounting certifications call for meeting education requirements, passing a technical examination, and obtaining relevant work experience.

Measurement Rules

Suppose a store sells a MP3 player in December to a customer who agrees to pay for it in January. Should the business *recognize* (report) the sale as a December transaction

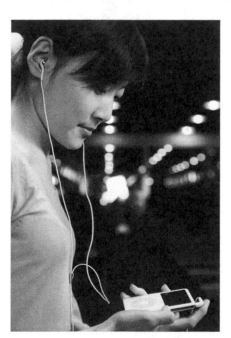

or as a January transaction? It really does not matter as long as the storeowner discloses the rule the decision is based on and applies it consistently to other transactions. Because businesses may use different reporting rules, however, clear communication also requires full and fair disclosure of the accounting rules chosen.

Communicating business results would be simpler if each type of business activity were reported using only one measurement method. World economies and financial reporting practices, however, have not evolved uniformly. Even in highly sophisticated countries such as the United States, companies exhibit significant diversity in reporting methods. Providers of accounting reports assume that users are educated about accounting practices.

The **Financial Accounting Standards Board (FASB)**[1] is a privately funded organization with the primary authority for establishing accounting standards in the United States. The measurement rules established by the FASB are called **generally accepted accounting principles (GAAP).** Financial reports issued to the public must follow GAAP. This textbook introduces these principles so you will be able to understand business activity reported by companies in the USA.

Companies are not required to follow GAAP when preparing *management accounting* reports. Although there is considerable overlap between financial and managerial accounting, managers are free to construct internal reports in whatever fashion best suits the effective operation of their companies.

---

[1]The FASB consists of seven full-time members appointed by the supporting organization, the Financial Accounting Foundation (FAF). The FAF membership is intended to represent the broad spectrum of individuals and institutions that have an interest in accounting and financial reporting. FAF members include representatives of the accounting profession, industry, financial institutions, the government, and the investing public.

FOCUS ON **INTERNATIONAL ISSUES**

IS THERE GLOBAL GAAP?

As explained in this chapter, accounting is a measurement and communication discipline based on rules referred to as *generally accepted accounting principles (GAAP)*. The rules described in this text are based on GAAP used in the United States, but what rules do the rest of the world use? Is there a global GAAP, or does each country establish its own unique GAAP?

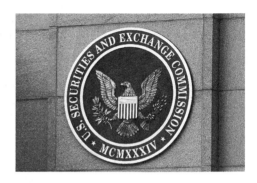

Not long ago each country developed its own unique GAAP. Global companies were required to prepare multiple sets of financial statements to satisfy each country's GAAP. The use of multiple accounting standards across the globe made comparing company performance difficult and expensive. To address the need for a common set of financial standards, the International Accounting Standards Committee was formed in 1973. The committee was reorganized as the **International Accounting Standards Board (IASB)** in 2001. The IASB issues **International Financial Reporting Standards (IFRS)**, which are rapidly gaining support worldwide. In 2005, companies in the countries who were members of the European Union were required to use the IFRS as established by the IASB, which is headquartered in London. Today, over 100 countries require or permit companies to prepare their financial statements using IFRS.

As of 2009 most of the major economic countries had either switched from their local GAAP to IFRS, or had rules in place to make the switch by 2012. One notable exception is the United States, but even here, the Securities and Exchange Commission announced in 2008 that it was seriously considering adopting rules that would allow U.S. companies to use either GAAP or IFRS. Although not finalized when this book was being prepared, many accountants in the United States believe this will occur. Additionally, there is an active process in place to reduce the differences between IFRS and U.S. GAAP.

There are many similarities between the IASB and the FASB. Both the FASB and the IASB are required to include members with a variety of backgrounds, including auditors, users of financial information, academics, and so forth. Also, both groups primarily require that their members work full-time for their respective boards; they cannot serve on the board while being compensated by another organization. (The IASB does allow up to three of its members to be part-time.) Members of each board serve five-year terms, and can be reappointed once. The funds to support both boards, and the large organizations that support them are obtained from a variety of sources, including selling publications and private contributions. To help maintain independence of the boards' members, fundraising is performed by separate sets of trustees.

There are significant differences between the IASB and the FASB, and one of these relates to size and geographic diversity. The FASB has only seven members, all from the United States. The IASB has fourteen members, and these must include at least four from Asia, four from Europe, four from North America, one from Africa, and one from South America.

Not only is the structure of the standards-setting boards different but the standards and principles they establish may also differ significantly. In this chapter, you will learn that GAAP employs the *historical cost concept.* This means that the assets of most U.S. companies are shown on the balance sheet at the amount for which they were purchased. For example, land owned by U.S. Steel, Inc., that has a market value of millions of dollars may be shown on US Steel's financial statements with a value of only a few hundred thousand dollars. This occurs because GAAP requires US Steel to show the land at its cost rather than its market value. In contrast, IFRS permits companies to show market values on their financial statements. This means that the exact same assets may show radically different values if the statements are prepared under IFRS rather than GAAP.

Throughout this text, where appropriate, we will note the differences between U.S. GAAP and IFRS. However, by the time you graduate, it is likely that among the major industrialized nations, there will be a global GAAP.

Reporting Entities

Think of accountants as you would of news reporters. A news reporter gathers and discloses information about some person, place, or thing. Likewise, an accountant gathers and discloses financial information about specific people or businesses. The people or businesses accountants report on are called **reporting entities.** When studying accounting you should think of yourself as an accountant. Your first step is to identify the person or business on which you are reporting. This is not always as easy as it may seem. To illustrate, consider the following scenario.

Jason Winston recently started a business. During the first few days of operation, Mr. Winston transferred cash from his personal account into a business account for a company he named Winston Enterprises. Mr. Winston's brother, George, invested cash in Winston Enterprises for which he received an ownership interest in the company. Winston Enterprises borrowed cash from First Federal Bank. Winston Enterprises paid cash to purchase a building from Commercial Properties, Inc. Winston Enterprises earned cash revenues from its customers and paid its employees cash for salaries expense.

How many reporting entities are described in this scenario? Assuming all of the customers are counted as a single entity and all of the employees are counted as a single entity, there are a total of seven entities named in the scenario. These entities include: (1) Jason Winston, (2) Winston Enterprises (3) George Winston, (4) First Federal Bank, (5) Commercial Properties, Inc., (6) the customers, and (7) the employees. A separate set of accounting records would be maintained for each entity.

Your ability to learn accounting will be greatly influenced by how you approach the entity concept. Based on your everyday experiences you likely think from the perspective of a customer. In contrast, this text is written from the perspective of a business entity. These opposing perspectives dramatically affect how you view business events. For example, as a customer you consider a sales discount a great bargain. The view is different from the perspective of the business granting the discount. A sales discount means an item did not sell at the expected price. To move the item, the business had to accept less money than it originally planned to receive. From this perspective, a sales discount is not a good thing. To understand accounting, train yourself to interpret transactions from the perspective of a business rather than a consumer. Each time you encounter an accounting event ask yourself, how does this affect the business?

✓ CHECK YOURSELF 1.1

In a recent business transaction, land was exchanged for cash. Did the amount of cash increase or decrease?

Answer   The answer depends on the reporting entity to which the question pertains. One entity sold land. The other entity bought land. For the entity that sold land, cash increased. For the entity that bought land, cash decreased.

ELEMENTS OF FINANCIAL STATEMENTS

LO 2

Construct an accounting equation using elements of financial statements terminology.

The individuals and organizations that need information about a business are called *stakeholders*. Stakeholders include owners, lenders, government agencies, employees, news reporters, and others. Businesses communicate information to stakeholders through four financial statements:[2] (1) an income statement, (2) a statement of changes in equity, (3) a balance sheet, and (4) a statement of cash flows.

The information reported in **financial statements** is organized into ten categories known as **elements.** Eight financial statement elements are discussed in this chapter: assets, liabilities, equity, contributed capital, revenue, expenses, distributions, and net income. The other two elements, gains and losses, are discussed in a later chapter. In practice, the business world uses various titles to identify several of the financial statement elements. For example, business people use net income, net *earnings,* and net *profit* interchangeably to describe the same element. Contributed capital may be called *common stock* and equity

---

[2]In practice these statements have alternate names. For example, the income statement may be called *results of operations* or *statement of earnings.* The balance sheet is sometimes called the *statement of financial position.* The statement of changes in equity might be called *statement of capital* or *statement of stockholders' equity.* Since the Financial Accounting Standards Board (FASB) called for the title *statement of cash flows,* companies do not use alternate names for that statement.

Answers to The Curious Accountant

Anyone who owns stock in Starbucks owns a part of the company. Starbucks has many owners. In contrast, nobody actually owns the American Cancer Society (ACS). The ACS has a board of directors that is responsible for overseeing its operations, but the board is not its owner.

Ultimately, the purpose of a business entity is to increase the wealth of its owners. To this end, it "spends money to make money." The expense that Starbucks incurs for advertising is a cost incurred in the hope that it will generate revenues when it sells coffee. The financial statements of a business show, among other things, whether and how the company made a profit during the current year. For example, Starbucks' income statements show how much revenue was generated from "company-owned retail"operations versus from "licensing operations."

The ACS is a not-for-profit entity. It operates to provide services to society at large, not to make a profit. It cannot increase the wealth of its owners, because it has no owners. When the ACS spends money to assist cancer patients, it does not spend this money in the expectation that it will generate revenues. The revenues of the ACS come from contributors who wish to support efforts related to fighting cancer. Because the ACS does not spend money to make money, it has no reason to prepare an *income statement* like that of Starbucks. The ACS's statement of activities shows how much revenue was received from "contributions" versus from "special events."

Not-for-profit entities do prepare financial statements that are similar in appearance to those of commercial enterprises. The financial statements of not-for-profit entities are called the *statement of financial position,* the *statement of activities,* and the *cash flow statement.*

may be called *stockholders' equity, owner's capital,* and *partners' equity.* Furthermore, the transfer of assets from a business to its owners may be called *distributions, withdrawals,* or *dividends.* Think of accounting as a language. Different terms can describe the same business event. Detailed definitions of the elements and their placement on financial statements will be discussed in the following sections of the chapter.

Using Accounts to Gather Information

Detailed information about the elements is maintained in records commonly called **accounts.** For example, information regarding the element *assets* may be organized in separate accounts for cash, equipment, buildings, land, and so forth. The types and number of accounts used by a business depends on the information needs of its stakeholders. Some businesses provide very detailed information; others report highly summarized information. The more detail desired, the greater number of accounts needed. Think of accounts like the notebooks students keep for their classes. Some students keep detailed notes about every class they take in a separate notebook. Other students keep only the key points for all of their classes in a single notebook. Similarly, some businesses use more accounts than other businesses.

Diversity also exists regarding the names used for various accounts. For example, employee pay may be called salaries, wages, commissions, and so forth. Do not become frustrated with the diversity of terms used in accounting. Remember, accounting is a language. The same word can have different meanings. Similarly, different words can be used to describe the same phenomenon. The more you study and use accounting, the more familiar it will become to you.

Accounting Equation

The resources that a business uses to produce earnings are called *assets*. Examples of assets include land, buildings, equipment, materials, and supplies. Assets result from historical events. For example, if a business owns a truck that it purchased in a past transaction, the truck is an asset of the business. A truck that a business *plans* to purchase in the future, however, is not an asset of that business, no matter how certain the future purchase might be.

The resource providers (creditors and investors) have potential **claims**[3] on the assets owned by a business. The relationship between the assets and the providers' claims is described by the **accounting equation:**

$$\text{Assets} = \text{Claims}$$

Creditor claims are called **liabilities** and investor claims are called **equity.** Substituting these terms into the accounting equation produces the following expanded form:

$$\overbrace{\text{Assets} = \text{Liabilities} + \text{Equity}}^{\text{Claims}}$$

Liabilities can also be viewed as future *obligations of the enterprise.* To settle the obligations, the business will probably either relinquish some of its assets (e.g., pay off its debts with cash), provide services to its creditors (e.g., work off its debts), or accept other obligations (e.g., trade short-term debt for long-term debt).

As indicated by the accounting equation, the amount of total assets is equal to the total of the liabilities plus the equity. To illustrate, assume that Hagan Company has assets of $500, liabilities of $200, and equity of $300. These amounts appear in the accounting equation as follows:

$$\overbrace{\begin{matrix} \text{Assets} = & \text{Liabilities} + & \text{Equity} \\ \$500 = & \$200 + & \$300 \end{matrix}}^{\text{Claims}}$$

The claims side of the accounting equation (liabilities plus equity) may also be viewed as listing the sources of the assets. For example, when a bank loans assets (money) to a business, it establishes a claim to have those assets returned at some future date. Liabilities can therefore be viewed as sources of assets.

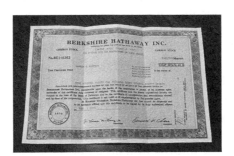

Equity can also be viewed as a source of assets. In fact, equity represents two distinct sources of assets. First, businesses typically acquire assets from their owners (investors). Many businesses issue **common stock**[4] certificates as receipts to acknowledge assets received from owners. The owners of such businesses are often called **stockholders,** and the ownership interest in the business is called **stockholders' equity.**

Second, businesses usually obtain assets through their earnings activities (the business acquires assets by working for them). Assets a business has earned can either be distributed to the owners or kept in the business. The portion of assets that has been provided by earnings activities and not returned as dividends is called **retained earnings.** Since stockholders own the business, they are entitled to assets acquired through its earnings activities. Retained earnings is therefore a component of stockholders' equity. Further

---

[3]A claim is a legal action to obtain money, property, or the enforcement of a right against another party.

[4]This presentation assumes the business is organized as a corporation. Other forms of business organization include proprietorships and partnerships. The treatment of equity for these types of businesses is slightly different from that of corporations. A detailed discussion of the differences is included in a later chapter of the text.

expansion of the accounting equation can show the three sources of assets (liabilities, common stock, and retained earnings):

$$\text{Assets} = \text{Liabilities} + \overbrace{\text{Common stock} + \text{Retained earnings}}^{\text{Stockholders' equity}}$$

✓ CHECK YOURSELF 1.2

Gupta Company has $250,000 of assets, $60,000 of liabilities, and $90,000 of common stock. What percentage of the assets was provided by retained earnings?

Answer   First, using algebra, determine the dollar amount of retained earnings:

Assets = Liabilities + Common stock + Retained earnings
Retained earnings = Assets − Liabilities − Common stock
Retained earnings = $250,000 − $60,000 − $90,000
Retained earnings = $100,000

Second, determine the percentage:

Percentage of assets provided by retained earnings = Retained earnings/Total assets
Percentage of assets provided by retained earnings = $100,000/$250,000 = 40%

RECORDING BUSINESS EVENTS UNDER THE ACCOUNTING EQUATION

An **accounting event** is an economic occurrence that changes an enterprise's assets, liabilities, or stockholders' equity. A **transaction** is a particular kind of event that involves transferring something of value between two entities. Examples of transactions include acquiring assets from owners, borrowing money from creditors, and purchasing or selling goods and services. The following section of the text explains how several different types of accounting events affect a company's accounting equation.

Record business events in general ledger accounts organized under an accounting equation.

Asset Source Transactions

As previously mentioned, businesses obtain assets (resources) from three sources. They acquire assets from owners (stockholders); they borrow assets from creditors; and they earn assets through profitable operations. Asset source transactions increase total assets and total claims. A more detailed discussion of the effects of asset source transactions is provided below:

EVENT 1   Rustic Camp Sites (RCS) was formed on January 1, 2012, when it acquired $120,000 cash from issuing common stock.

When RCS issued stock, it received cash and gave each investor (owner) a stock certificate as a receipt. Since this transaction provided $120,000 of assets (cash) to the business, it is an **asset source transaction.** It increases the business's assets (cash) and its stockholders' equity (common stock).

	Assets		=	Liab.	+	Stockholders' Equity	
	Cash	+ Land	=	N. Pay.	+	Com. Stk.	+ Ret. Earn.
Acquired cash through stock issue	120,000	+ NA	=	NA	+	120,000	+ NA

Notice the elements have been divided into accounts. For example, the element *assets* is divided into a Cash account and a Land account. Do not be concerned if some of these account titles are unfamiliar. They will be explained as new transactions are presented. Recall that the number of accounts a company uses depends on the nature of its business and the level of detail management needs to operate the business. For example, Sears would have an account called Cost of Goods Sold although GEICO Insurance would not. Why? Because Sears sells goods (merchandise) but GEICO does not.

Also, notice that a stock issue transaction affects the accounting equation in two places, both under an asset (cash) and also under the source of that asset (common stock). All transactions affect the accounting equation in at least two places. It is from this practice that the **double-entry bookkeeping** system derives its name.

EVENT 2   RCS acquired an additional $400,000 of cash by borrowing from a creditor.

This transaction is also an asset source transaction. It increases assets (cash) and liability claims (notes payable). The account title Notes Payable is used because the borrower (RCS) is required to issue a promissory note to the creditor (a bank). A promissory note describes, among other things, the amount of interest RCS will pay and for how long it will borrow the money.[5] The effect of the borrowing transaction on the accounting equation is indicated below.

	Assets			=	Liab.	+	Stockholders' Equity		
	Cash	+	Land	=	N. Pay.	+	Com. Stk.	+	Ret. Earn.
Beginning balances	120,000	+	NA	=	NA	+	120,000	+	NA
Acquired cash by issuing note	400,000	+	NA	=	400,000	+	NA	+	NA
Ending balances	520,000	+	NA	=	400,000	+	120,000	+	NA

The beginning balances above came from the ending balances produced by the prior transaction. This practice is followed throughout the illustration.

Asset Exchange Transactions

Businesses frequently trade one asset for another asset. In such cases, the amount of one asset decreases and the amount of the other asset increases. Total assets are unaffected by asset exchange transactions. Event 3 is an asset exchange transaction.

EVENT 3   RCS paid $500,000 cash to purchase land.

This asset exchange transaction reduces the asset account Cash and increases the asset account Land. The amount of total assets is not affected. An **asset exchange transaction** simply reflects changes in the composition of assets. In this case, the company traded cash for land. The amount of cash decreased by $500,000 and the amount of land increased by the same amount.

	Assets			=	Liab.	+	Stockholders' Equity		
	Cash	+	Land	=	N. Pay.	+	Com. Stk.	+	Ret. Earn.
Beginning balances	520,000	+	NA	=	400,000	+	120,000	+	NA
Paid cash to buy land	(500,000)	+	500,000	=	NA	+	NA	+	NA
Ending balances	20,000	+	500,000	=	400,000	+	120,000	+	NA

---

[5]For simplicity, the effects of interest are ignored in this chapter. We discuss accounting for interest in future chapters.

Another Asset Source Transaction

EVENT 4   RCS obtained $85,000 cash by leasing camp sites to customers.

Revenue represents an economic benefit a company obtains by providing customers with goods and services. In this example the economic benefit is an increase in the asset cash. Revenue transactions can therefore be viewed as *asset source transactions*. The asset increase is balanced by an increase in the retained earnings section of stockholders' equity because producing revenue increases the amount of earnings that can be retained in the business.

	Assets			=	Liab.	+	Stockholders' Equity				
	Cash	+	Land	=	N. Pay.	+	Com. Stk.	+	Ret. Earn.	Acct. Title
Beginning balances	20,000	+	500,000	=	400,000	+	120,000	+	NA	
Acquired cash by earning revenue	85,000	+	NA	=	NA	+	NA	+	85,000	Revenue
Ending balances	105,000	+	500,000	=	400,000	+	120,000	+	85,000	

Note carefully that the $85,000 ending balance in the retained earnings column is *not* in the Retained Earnings account. It is in the Revenue account. It will be transferred to the Retained Earnings account at the end of the accounting period. Transferring the Revenue account balance to the Retained Earnings account is part of a process called *closing the accounts*.

Asset Use Transactions

Businesses use assets for a variety of purposes. For example, assets may be used to pay off liabilities or they may be transferred to owners. Assets may also be used in the process of generating earnings. All **asset use transactions** decrease the total amount of assets and the total amount of claims on assets (liabilities or stockholders' equity).

EVENT 5   RCS paid $50,000 cash for operating expenses such as salaries, rent, and interest. (RCS could establish a separate account for each type of expense. However, the management team does not currently desire this level of detail. Remember, the number of accounts a business uses depends on the level of information managers need to make decisions.)

In the normal course of generating revenue, a business consumes various assets and services. The assets and services consumed to generate revenue are called **expenses.** Revenue results from providing goods and services to customers. In exchange, the business acquires assets from its customers. Since the owners bear the ultimate risk and reap the rewards of operating the business, revenues increase stockholders' equity (retained earnings), and expenses decrease retained earnings. In this case, the asset account, Cash, decreased. This decrease is balanced by a decrease in the retained earnings section of stockholders' equity because expenses decrease the amount of earnings retained in the business.

	Assets			=	Liab.	+	Stockholders' Equity				
	Cash	+	Land	=	N. Pay.	+	Com. Stk.	+	Ret. Earn.	Acct. Title
Beginning balances	105,000	+	500,000	=	400,000	+	120,000	+	85,000	
Used cash to pay expenses	(50,000)	+	NA	=	NA	+	NA	+	(50,000)	Expense
Ending balances	55,000	+	500,000	=	400,000	+	120,000	+	35,000	

Like revenues, expenses are not recorded directly into the Retained Earnings account. The $50,000 of expense is recorded in the Expense account. It will be transferred to the Retained Earnings account at the end of the accounting period as part of the closing process. The $35,000 ending balance in the retained earnings column shows what would be in the Retained Earnings account after the balances in the Revenue and Expense accounts have been closed. The current balance in the Retained Earnings account is zero.

EVENT 6   RCS paid $4,000 in cash dividends to its owners.

To this point the enterprise's total assets and equity have increased by $35,000 ($85,000 of revenue − $50,000 of expense) as a result of its earnings activities. RCS can keep the additional assets in the business or transfer them to the owners. If a business transfers some or all of its earned assets to owners, the transfer is frequently called a **dividend.** Since assets distributed to stockholders are not used for the purpose of generating revenue, *dividends are not expenses.* Furthermore, dividends are a transfer of *earnings,* not a return of the assets acquired from the issue of common stock.

	Assets			=	Liab.	+	Stockholders' Equity			
	Cash	+	Land	=	N. Pay.	+	Com. Stk.	+	Ret. Earn.	Acct. Title
Beginning balances	55,000	+	500,000	=	400,000	+	120,000	+	35,000	
Used cash to pay dividends	(4,000)	+	NA	=	NA	+	NA	+	(4,000)	Dividends
Ending balances	51,000	+	500,000	=	400,000	+	120,000	+	31,000	

Like revenues and expenses, dividends are not recorded directly into the Retained Earnings account. The $4,000 dividend is recorded in the Dividends account. It will be transferred to retained earnings at the end of the accounting period as part of the closing process. The $31,000 ending balance in the retained earnings column shows what would be in the Retained Earnings account after the balances in the Revenue, Expense, and Dividend accounts have been closed. The current balance in the Retained Earnings account is zero.

EVENT 7   The land that RCS paid $500,000 to purchase had an appraised market value of $525,000 on December 31, 2012.

Although the appraised value of the land is higher than the original cost, RCS will not increase the amount recorded in its accounting records above the land's $500,000 historical cost. In general, accountants do not recognize changes in market value. The **historical cost concept** requires that most assets be reported at the amount paid for them (their historical cost) regardless of increases in market value.

Surely investors would rather know what an asset is worth instead of how much it originally cost. So why do accountants maintain records and report financial information based on historical cost? Accountants rely heavily on the **reliability concept.** Information is reliable if it can be independently verified. For example, two people looking at the legal documents associated with RCS's land purchase will both conclude that RCS paid $500,000 for the land. That historical cost is a verifiable fact. The appraised value, in contrast, is an opinion. Even two persons who are experienced appraisers are not likely to come up with the same amount for the land's market value. Accountants do not report market values in financial statements because such values are not reliable.

Accountants recognize the conflict between *relevance* and *reliability.* As a result, there are exceptions to the application of the historical cost rule. When market value can be clearly established, GAAP not only permits but requires its use. For example, securities that are traded on the New York Stock Exchange must be shown at market value rather than historical cost. We will discuss other notable exceptions to the historical cost principle later in the text. However, as a general rule you should assume that assets shown in a company's financial statements are valued at historical cost.

EXHIBIT 1.4

Accounting Events

1.	RCS issued common stock, acquiring $120,000 cash from its owners.
2.	RCS borrowed $400,000 cash.
3.	RCS paid $500,000 cash to purchase land.
4.	RCS received $85,000 cash from earning revenue.
5.	RCS paid $50,000 cash for expenses.
6.	RCS paid dividends of $4,000 cash to the owners.
7.	The land that RCS paid $500,000 to purchase had an appraised market value of $525,000 on December 31, 2012.

General Ledger Accounts Organized Under the Accounting Equation

Event No.	Assets			=	Liabilities	+	Stockholders' Equity				Other Account Titles
	Cash	+	Land	=	Not es Payable	+	Common Stock	+	Retained Earnings		
Beg. bal.	0		0		0		0		0		
1.	120,000						120,000				
2.	400,000				400,000						
3.	(500,000)		500,000								
4.	85,000								85,000		Revenue
5.	(50,000)								(50,000)		Expense
6.	(4,000)								(4,000)		Dividend
7.	NA		NA		NA		NA		NA		
	51,000	+	500,000	=	400,000	+	120,000	+	31,000		

Summary of Transactions

The complete collection of a company's accounts is called the **general ledger.** A summary of the accounting events and the general ledger account information for RCS's 2012 accounting period is shown in Exhibit 1.4. The revenue, expense, and dividend account data appear in the retained earnings column. These account titles are shown immediately to the right of the dollar amounts listed in the retained earnings column.

RECAP: TYPES OF TRANSACTIONS

The transactions described above have each been classified into one of three categories: (1) asset source transactions; (2) asset exchange transactions; and (3) asset use transactions. A fourth category, claims exchange transactions, is introduced in a later chapter. In summary

Classify business events as asset source, use, or exchange transactions.

- *Asset source transactions* increase the total amount of assets and increase the total amount of claims. In its first year of operation, RCS acquired assets from three sources: first, from owners (Event 1); next, by borrowing (Event 2); and finally, through earnings activities (Event 4).

- *Asset exchange transactions* decrease one asset and increase another asset. The total amount of assets is unchanged by asset exchange transactions. RCS experienced one asset exchange transaction; it used cash to purchase land (Event 3).

- *Asset use transactions* decrease the total amount of assets and the total amount of claims. RCS used assets to pay expenses (Event 5) and to pay dividends (Event 6).

As you proceed through this text, practice classifying transactions into one of the four categories. Businesses engage in thousands of transactions every day. It is far more effective to learn how to classify the transactions into meaningful categories than to attempt to memorize the effects of thousands of transactions.

PREPARING FINANCIAL STATEMENTS

LO 5

Use general ledger account information to prepare four financial statements.

As indicated earlier, accounting information is normally presented to external users in four general-purpose financial statements. The information in the ledger accounts is used to prepare these financial statements. The data in the ledger accounts in Exhibit 1.4 are color coded to help you understand the source of information in the financial statements. The numbers in *green* are used in the *statement of cash flows.* The numbers in *red* are used to prepare the *balance sheet.* Finally, the numbers in *blue* are used to prepare the *income statement.* The numbers reported in the statement of changes in stockholders' equity have not been color coded because they appear in more than one statement. The next section explains how the information in the accounts is presented in financial statements.

The financial statements for RCS are shown in Exhibit 1.5. The information used to prepare these statements was drawn from the ledger accounts. Information in one statement may relate to information in another statement. For example, the amount of net income reported on the income statement also appears on the statement of changes in stockholders' equity. Accountants use the term **articulation** to describe the interrelationships among the various elements of the financial statements. The key articulated relationships in RCS's financial statements are highlighted with arrows (Exhibit 1.5). A description of each statement follows.

Income Statement and the Matching Concept

A business must make sacrifices in order to obtain benefits. For example, RCS must sacrifice cash to pay for employee salaries, rent, and interest. In turn, RCS receives a benefit when it collects cash from its customers. As this example implies, sacrifices are defined as decreases in assets; and benefits are increases in assets. In accounting terms sacrifices are called expenses; and benefits are called revenues. *Therefore, expenses are decreases in assets; and revenues are increases in assets.*[6]

The **income statement** matches the expenses with the revenues that occur when operating a business. If revenues exceed expenses, the difference is called **net income.** If expenses are greater than revenues, the difference is called **net loss.** The practice of pairing revenues with expenses on the income statement is called the **matching concept.**

The income statement in Exhibit 1.5 indicates that RCS has earned more assets than it has used. The statement shows that RCS has increased its assets by $35,000 (net income) as a result of operating its business. Observe the phrase *For the Year Ended December 31, 2012,* in the heading of the income statement. Income is measured for a span of time called the **accounting period.** While accounting periods of one year are normal for external financial reporting, income can be measured weekly, monthly, quarterly, semiannually, or over any other desired time period. Notice that the cash RCS paid to its stockholders (dividends) is not reported as expense. The decrease in assets for dividend payments is not incurred for the purpose of generating revenue. Instead, dividends are transfers of wealth to the owners of the business. Dividend payments are not reported on the income statement.

---

[6]The definitions for revenue and expense is expanded in subsequent chapters as additional relationships among the elements of financial statements are introduced.

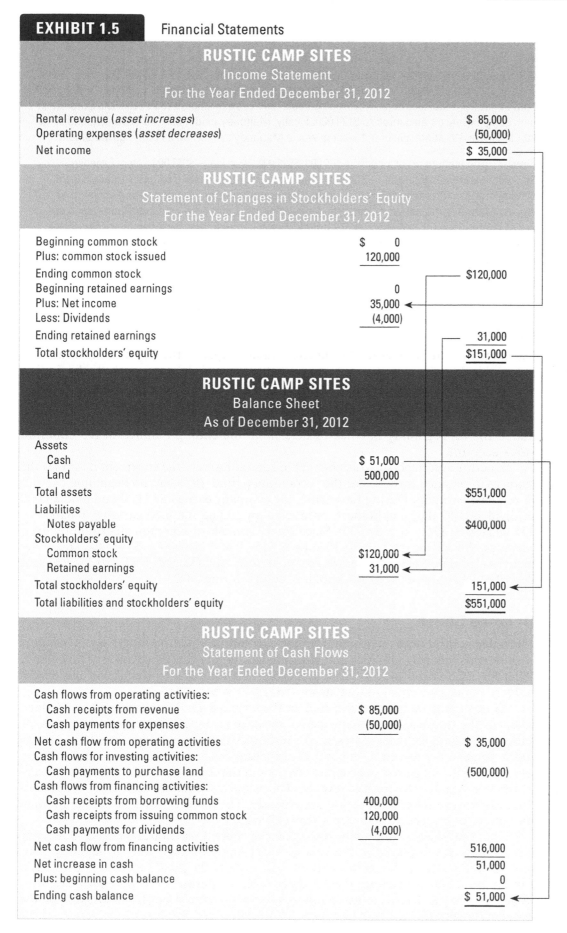

EXHIBIT 1.5   Financial Statements

RUSTIC CAMP SITES
Income Statement
For the Year Ended December 31, 2012

Rental revenue (*asset increases*)	$ 85,000
Operating expenses (*asset decreases*)	(50,000)
Net income	$ 35,000

RUSTIC CAMP SITES
Statement of Changes in Stockholders' Equity
For the Year Ended December 31, 2012

Beginning common stock	$ 0	
Plus: common stock issued	120,000	
Ending common stock		$120,000
Beginning retained earnings	0	
Plus: Net income	35,000	
Less: Dividends	(4,000)	
Ending retained earnings		31,000
Total stockholders' equity		$151,000

RUSTIC CAMP SITES
Balance Sheet
As of December 31, 2012

Assets		
Cash	$ 51,000	
Land	500,000	
Total assets		$551,000
Liabilities		
Notes payable		$400,000
Stockholders' equity		
Common stock	$120,000	
Retained earnings	31,000	
Total stockholders' equity		151,000
Total liabilities and stockholders' equity		$551,000

RUSTIC CAMP SITES
Statement of Cash Flows
For the Year Ended December 31, 2012

Cash flows from operating activities:		
Cash receipts from revenue	$ 85,000	
Cash payments for expenses	(50,000)	
Net cash flow from operating activities		$ 35,000
Cash flows for investing activities:		
Cash payments to purchase land		(500,000)
Cash flows from financing activities:		
Cash receipts from borrowing funds	400,000	
Cash receipts from issuing common stock	120,000	
Cash payments for dividends	(4,000)	
Net cash flow from financing activities		516,000
Net increase in cash		51,000
Plus: beginning cash balance		0
Ending cash balance		$ 51,000

✓ CHECK YOURSELF 1.3

Mahoney, Inc., was started when it issued common stock to its owners for $300,000. During its first year of operation Mahoney received $523,000 cash for services provided to customers. Mahoney paid employees $233,000 cash. Advertising costs paid in cash amounted to $102,000. Other cash operating expenses amounted to $124,000. Finally, Mahoney paid a $25,000 cash dividend to its stockholders. What amount of net income would Mahoney's report on its earnings statement?

Answer   The amount of net income is $64,000 ($523,000 Revenue − $233,000 Salary Expense − $102,000 Advertising Expense − $124,000 Other Operating Expenses). The cash received from issuing stock is not revenue because it was not acquired from earnings activities. In other words, Mahoney did not work (perform services) for this money; it was contributed by owners of the business. The dividends are not expenses because the decrease in cash was not incurred for the purpose of generating revenue. Instead, the dividends represent a transfer of wealth to the owners.

Statement of Changes in Stockholders' Equity

The **statement of changes in stockholders' equity** explains the effects of transactions on stockholders' equity during the accounting period. It starts with the beginning balance in the common stock account. In the case of RCS, the beginning balance in the common stock account is zero because the company did not exist before the 2012 accounting period. The $120,000 of stock issued during the accounting period is added to the beginning balance to determine the ending balance in the common stock account.

In addition to reporting the changes in common stock, the statement describes the changes in retained earnings for the accounting period. RCS had no beginning balance in retained earnings. During the period, the company earned $35,000 and paid $4,000 in dividends to the stockholders, producing an ending retained earnings balance of $31,000 ($0 + $35,000 − $4,000). Since equity consists of common stock and retained earnings, the ending total equity balance is $151,000 ($120,000 + $31,000). This statement is also dated with the phrase *For the Year Ended December 31, 2012,* because it describes what happened to stockholders' equity during 2012.

Balance Sheet

The **balance sheet** draws its name from the accounting equation. Total assets balances with (equals) claims (liabilities and stockholders' equity) on those assets. The balance sheet for RCS is shown in Exhibit 1.5. Note that total claims (liabilities plus stockholders' equity) are equal to total assets ($551,000 = $551,000).

At this point we take a closer look at the term *assets*. Previously, we have defined assets as the resources a company uses to produce revenues. More precisely, the assets shown on a balance sheet represent the resources that a company plans to use *in the future* to generate revenues. In contrast, expenses represent the assets that have been used in the current period to generate revenues in the current period. In summary, businesses use resources to produce revenue. The resources that *have been sacrificed* to produce revenues in the current period are expenses. The resources that *will be sacrificed* in the future to produce future revenues are called assets.

Note the order of the assets in the balance sheet. Cash appears first, followed by land. Assets are displayed in the balance sheet based on their level of **liquidity.** This means that assets are listed in order of how rapidly they will be converted to cash. Finally, note that the balance sheet is dated with the phrase *As of December 31, 2012,* indicating that it describes the company's financial condition on the last day of the accounting period.

✓ CHECK YOURSELF 1.4

To gain a clear understanding of the balance sheet, try to create one that describes your personal financial condition. First list your assets, then your liabilities. Determine the amount of your equity by subtracting your liabilities from your assets.

Answer   Answers for this exercise will vary depending on the particular assets and liabilities each student identifies. Common student assets include automobiles, computers, stereos, TVs, phones, MP3 players, clothes, and textbooks. Common student liabilities include car loans, mortgages, student loans, and credit card debt. The difference between the assets and the liabilities is the equity.

Statement of Cash Flows

The **statement of cash flows** explains how a company obtained and used *cash* during the accounting period. Receipts of cash are called *cash inflows,* and payments are *cash outflows.* The statement classifies cash receipts (inflows) and payments (outflows) into three categories: financing activities, investing activities, and operating activities.

Businesses normally start with an idea. Implementing the idea usually requires cash. For example, suppose you decide to start an apartment rental business. First, you would need cash to buy the apartments. Acquiring cash to start a business is a financing activity. **Financing activities** include obtaining cash (inflow) from owners or paying cash (outflow) to owners (dividends). Financing activities also include borrowing cash (inflow) from creditors and repaying the principal (outflow) to creditors. Because interest on borrowed money is an expense, however, cash paid to creditors for interest is reported in the operating activities section of the statement of cash flows.

After obtaining cash from financing activities, you would invest the money by building or buying apartments. **Investing activities** involve paying cash (outflow) to purchase long-term assets or receiving cash (inflow) from selling long-term assets. Long-term assets are normally used for more than one year. Cash outflows to purchase land or cash inflows from selling a building are examples of investing activities.

After investing in the productive assets (apartments), you would engage in operating activities. **Operating activities** involve receiving cash (inflow) from revenue and paying cash (outflow) for expenses. Note that cash spent to purchase short-term assets such as office supplies is reported in the operating activities section because the office supplies would likely be used (expensed) within a single accounting period.

The primary cash inflows and outflows related to the types of business activity introduced in this chapter are summarized in Exhibit 1.6. The exhibit will be expanded as additional types of events are introduced in subsequent chapters.

The statement of cash flows for Rustic Camp Sites in Exhibit 1.5 shows that the amount of cash increased by $51,000 during the year. The beginning balance in the Cash account was zero; adding the $51,000 increase to the beginning balance results in a $51,000 ending balance. Notice that the $51,000 ending cash balance on the statement of cash flows is the same as the amount of cash reported in the asset section on the December 31 year-end balance sheet. Also, note that the statement of cash flows is dated with the phrase *For the Year Ended December 31, 2012,* because it describes what happened to cash over the span of the year.

EXHIBIT 1.6

Classification Scheme for Statement of Cash Flows

Cash flows from operating activities:
   Cash receipts (inflows) from customers
   Cash payments (outflows) to suppliers

Cash flows from investing activities:
   Cash receipts (inflows) from the sale of long-term assets
   Cash payments (outflows) for the purchase of long-term assets

Cash flows from financing activities:
   Cash receipts (inflows) from borrowing funds
   Cash receipts (inflows) from issuing common stock
   Cash payments (outflows) to repay borrowed funds
   Cash payments (outflows) for dividends

✓ CHECK YOURSELF 1.5

Classify each of the following cash flows as an operating activity, investing activity, or financing activity.

1. Acquired cash from owners.
2. Borrowed cash from creditors.
3. Paid cash to purchase land.
4. Earned cash revenue.
5. Paid cash for salary expenses.
6. Paid cash dividend.
7. Paid cash for interest.

Answer (1) financing activity; (2) financing activity; (3) investing activity; (4) operating activity; (5) operating activity; (6) financing activity; (7) operating activity.

The Closing Process

As previously indicated transaction data are recorded in the Revenue, Expense, and Dividend accounts during the accounting period. At the end of the accounting period the data in theses accounts is transferred to the Retained Earnings account. The process of transferring the balances is called **closing.** Since the Revenue, Expense, and Dividend accounts are closed each period, they are called **temporary accounts.** At the beginning of each new accounting period, the temporary accounts have zero balances. The Retained Earnings account carries forward from one accounting period to the next. Since this account is not closed, it is called a **permanent account.**

Since RCS started operations on January 1, 2012, the beginning Retained Earnings account balance was zero. In other words, there were no previous earnings available to be retained by the business. During 2012, amounts were recorded in the Revenue, Expense, and Dividend accounts. Since the Retained Earnings account is separate from the Revenue, Expense, and Dividend accounts, the entries in these temporary accounts did not affect the Retained Earnings balance. Specifically, the *before closing* balance in the Retained Earnings account on December 31, 2012, is still zero. In contrast, the Revenue account has a balance of $85,000; the Expense account has a balance of $50,000; and the Dividends account has a balance of $4,000. The closing process transfers the balances in the Revenue, Expense, and Dividend accounts to the Retained Earnings account. Therefore, *after closing* the balance in the Retained Earnings account is $31,000 ($85,000 − $50,000 − $4,000) and the Revenue, Expense, and Dividend accounts have zero balances.

Since the asset, liability, common stock, and retained earnings accounts are permanent accounts, they are not closed at the end of the accounting period. After the closing account process, RCS's general ledger will contain the following account balances as of December 31, 2012.

Cash	+	Land	=	Notes Payable	+	Common Stock	+	Retained Earnings
51,000	+	500,000	=	400,000	+	120,000	+	31,000

Take note that the December 31, 2012, ending account balances become the January 1, 2013, beginning account balances. So, RCS will start the 2013 accounting period with these same accounts balances. In other words, the current period's after closing ending balances become the next period's beginning balances.

✓ CHECK YOURSELF 1.6

After closing on December 31, 2012, Walston Company had $4,600 of assets, $2,000 of liabilities, and $700 of common stock. During January of 2013, Walston earned $750 of revenue and incurred $300 of expense. Walston closes it books each year on December 31.

1. Determine the balance in the Retained Earnings account as of December 31, 2012.
2. Determine the balance in the Retained Earnings account as of January 1, 2013.
3. Determine the balance in the Retained Earnings account as of January 31, 2013.

Answer

1. Assets = Liabilities + Common Stock + Retained Earnings

   $4,600 = $2,000 + $700 + Retained Earnings

   Retained Earnings = $1,900

2. The balance in the Retained Earnings account on January 1, 2013, is the same as it was on December 31, 2012. This year's ending balance becomes next year's beginning balance. Therefore, the balance in the Retained Earnings account on January 1, 2013, is $1,900.

3. The balance in the Retained Earnings account on January 31, 2013, is still $1,900. The revenue earned and expenses incurred during January are not recorded in the Retained Earnings account. Revenue is recorded in a Revenue account and expenses are recorded in an Expense account during the accounting period. The balances in the Revenue and Expense accounts are transferred to the Retained Earnings account during the closing process at the end of the accounting period (December 31, 2013).

THE HORIZONTAL FINANCIAL STATEMENTS MODEL

Financial statements are the scorecard for business activity. If you want to succeed in business, you must know how your business decisions affect your company's financial statements. This text uses a **horizontal statements model** to help you understand how business events affect financial statements. This model shows a set of financial statements horizontally across a single page of paper. The balance sheet is displayed first, adjacent to the income statement, and then the statement of cash flows. Because the effects of equity transactions can be analyzed by referring to certain balance sheet columns, and because of limited space, the statement of changes in stockholders' equity is not shown in the horizontal statements model.

Record business events using a horizontal financial statements model.

The model frequently uses abbreviations. For example, activity classifications in the statement of cash flows are identified using OA for operating activities, IA for investing activities, and FA for financing activities. NC designates the net change in cash. The statements model uses "NA" when an account is not affected by an event. The background of the *balance sheet* is red, the *income statement* is blue, and the *statement of cash flows* is green. To demonstrate the usefulness of the horizontal statements model, we use it to display the seven accounting events that RCS experienced during its first year of operation (2012).

1. RCS acquired $120,000 cash from the issuance of common stock.
2. RCS borrowed $400,000 cash.
3. RCS paid $500,000 cash to purchase land.
4. RCS received $85,000 cash from earning revenue.
5. RCS paid $50,000 cash for expenses.
6. RCS paid $4,000 of cash dividends to the owners.
7. The market value of the land owned by RCS was appraised at $525,000 on December 31, 2012.

Event No.	Balance Sheet											Income Statement							Statement of Cash Flows	
	Assets			=	Liab.	+	Stockholders' Equity													
	Cash	+	Land	=	N. Pay.	+	Com. Stk.	+	Ret. Earn.			Rev.	−	Exp.	=	Net Inc.				
Beg. bal.	0	+	0	=	0	+	0	+	0			0	−	0	=	0			NA	
1.	120,000	+	NA	=	NA	+	120,000	+	NA			NA	−	NA	=	NA			120,000	FA
2.	400,000	+	NA	=	400,000	+	NA	+	NA			NA	−	NA	=	NA			400,000	FA
3.	(500,000)	+	500,000	=	NA	+	NA	+	NA			NA	−	NA	=	NA			(500,000)	IA
4.	85,000	+	NA	=	NA	+	NA	+	85,000			85,000	−	NA	=	85,000			85,000	OA
5.	(50,000)	+	NA	=	NA	+	NA	+	(50,000)			NA	−	50,000	=	(50,000)			(50,000)	OA
6.	(4,000)	+	NA	=	NA	+	NA	+	(4,000)			NA	−	NA	=	NA			(4,000)	FA
7.	NA	+	NA	=	NA	+	NA	+	NA			NA	−	NA	=	NA			NA	
Totals	51,000	+	500,000	=	400,000	+	120,000	+	31,000			85,000	−	50,000	=	35,000			51,000	NC

Recognize that statements models are learning tools. Because they are helpful in understanding how accounting events affect financial statements, they are used extensively in this book. However, the models omit many of the details used in published financial statements. For example, the horizontal model shows only a partial set of statements. Also, since the statements are presented in aggregate, the description of dates (i.e., "as of" versus "for the period ended") does not distinguish periodic from cumulative data.

REAL-WORLD FINANCIAL REPORTS

As previously indicated, organizations exist in many different forms, including *business* entities and *not-for-profit* entities. Business entities are typically service, merchandising, or manufacturing companies. **Service businesses,** which include doctors, attorneys, accountants, dry cleaners, and maids, provide services to their customers. **Merchandising businesses,** sometimes called *retail* or *wholesale companies,* sell goods to customers that other entities make. **Manufacturing businesses** make the goods that they sell to their customers.

Some business operations include combinations of these three categories. For example, an automotive repair shop might change oil (service function), sell parts such as oil filters (retail function), and rebuild engines (manufacturing function). The nature of the reporting entity affects the form and content of the information reported in an entity's financial statements. For example, governmental entities provide statements of revenues, expenditures, and changes in fund equity while business entities provide income statements. Similarly, income statements of retail companies show an expense

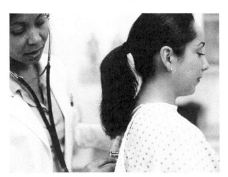

Service

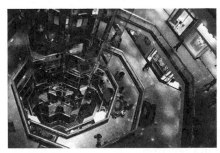

Merchandising

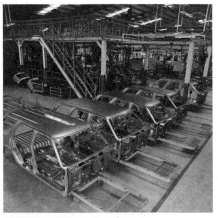

Manufacturing

REALITY BYTES

On April 19, 2010, the stock of BP, Plc. (formally known as British Petroleum) was trading at $59.48 per share. On that same day, the stock of Chevron Corp. was trading at $81.32 and the stock of Exxon Mobil Corp. was trading at $68.23. About six weeks later, on June 4, 2010, these companies' stocks had fallen to $37.16, $71.28, and $59.53 per share, respectively. Why did this happen? Did the companies report a large drop in their net earnings during these six weeks? No. What happened was that on April 20, 2010, the Deepwater Horizon oil well, owned by BP, failed and began discharging 60,000 barrels of oil daily into the Gulf of Mexico.

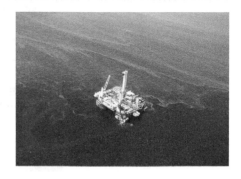

While it is easy to see why this event could cause BP's stock to lose 38 percent of its value, why would this cause Chevron's stock to fall 12 percent and Exxon's stock to fall 13 percent? These two companies did not have any oil spills during this time. One reason that the stock price of most oil companies declined significantly after BP's problems was that investors were concerned the failure would result in tighter regulation of all oil companies. Additionally, there was the concern that the government would ban, or seriously reduce, all future deepwater drilling. More regulations, and certainly a ban on future drilling, could drastically reduce the future earnings potential of all oil companies, not just BP.

As this situation illustrates, investors frequently use information not yet reported in a company's annual report. The annual report focuses on historical data, but investors are more concerned about the future. The historical information contained in the annual report is important because the past is frequently a strong predictor of the future. However, current negative news, such as an oil spill, may give investors more information about a company's furture than last year's annual report. For example, while the oil spill was bad news for the oil companies, it was, in financial terms, good news for companies that manufacture the oil-booms used to prevent oil from reaching the beaches. Similarly, a new company, that has never earned a profit, may have an idea that is so innovative investors rush to buy it stock, even though they expect it to be a few years to have positive earnings. Also, investors and creditors may be motivated by nonfinancial considerations such as social consciousness, humanitarian concerns, or personal preferences. While accounting information is critically important, it is only one dimension of the information pool that investors and creditors use to make decisions.

---

item called *cost of goods sold,* but service companies that do not sell goods have no such item in their income statements. You should expect some diversity when reviewing real-world financial statements.

Annual Report for Target Corporation

Organizations normally provide information, including financial statements, to *stakeholders* yearly in a document known as an **annual report.** The annual report for Target Corporation is reproduced in Appendix B of this text. This report includes the company's financial statements. Immediately following the statements are footnotes that provide additional details about the items described in the statements. The annual report contains commentary describing management's assessment of significant events that affected the company during the reporting period. This commentary is called *management's discussion and analysis* (MD&A).

The U.S. Securities and Exchange Commission (SEC) requires public companies to file an annual report in a document known as a 10-K. Even though the annual report is usually flashier (contains more color and pictures) than the 10-K, the 10-K is normally more comprehensive with respect to content. As a result, the 10-K report frequently substitutes for the annual report, but the annual report cannot substitute for the 10-K. In an effort to reduce costs, many companies now use the 10-K report as their annual report.

Special Terms in Real-World Reports

The financial statements of real-world companies include numerous items relating to advanced topics that are not covered in survey accounting textbooks, especially the first chapter of a survey accounting textbook. Do not, however, be discouraged from browsing through real-world annual reports. You will significantly enhance your learning if you look at many annual reports and attempt to identify as many items as you can. As your accounting knowledge grows, you will likely experience increased interest in real-world financial reports and the businesses they describe.

We encourage you to look for annual reports in the library or ask your employer for a copy of your company's report. The Internet is another excellent source for obtaining annual reports. Most companies provide links to their annual reports on their home pages. Look for links labeled "about the company" or "investor relations" or other phrases that logically lead to the company's financial reports. The best way to learn accounting is to use it. Accounting is the language of business. Learning the language will serve you well in almost any area of business that you pursue.

A Look Back

This chapter introduced the role of accounting in society and business: to provide information helpful in operating and evaluating the performance of organizations. Accounting is a measurement discipline. To communicate effectively, users of accounting must agree on the rules of measurement. *Generally accepted accounting principles (GAAP)* constitute the rules used by the accounting profession in the United States to govern financial reporting. GAAP is a work in progress that continues to evolve.

This chapter has discussed eight elements of financial statements: *assets, liabilities, equity, common stock (contributed capital), revenue, expenses, dividends (distributions),* and *net income.* The elements represent broad classifications reported on financial statements. Four basic financial statements appear in the reports of public companies: the *balance sheet,* the *income statement,* the *statement of changes in stockholders' equity,* and the *statement of cash flows.* The chapter discussed the form and content of each statement as well as the interrelationships among the statements.

This chapter introduced a *horizontal financial statements model* as a tool to help you understand how business events affect a set of financial statements. This model is used throughout the text. You should carefully study this model before proceeding to Chapter 2.

>> A Look Forward

To keep matters as simple as possible and to focus on the interrelationships among financial statements, this chapter considered only cash events. Obviously, many real-world events do not involve an immediate exchange of cash. For example, customers use telephone service throughout the month without paying for it until the next month. Such phone usage represents an expense in one month with a cash exchange in the following month. Events such as this are called *accruals.* Understanding the effects that accrual events have on the financial statements is included in Chapter 2.

A step-by-step audio-narrated series of slides is provided on the text website at www.mhhe.com/edmondssurvey3e.

 SELF-STUDY REVIEW PROBLEM

During 2013 Rustic Camp Sites experienced the following transactions.

1. RCS acquired $32,000 cash by issuing common stock.
2. RCS received $116,000 cash for providing services to customers (leasing camp sites).
3. RCS paid $13,000 cash for salaries expense.
4. RCS paid a $9,000 cash dividend to the owners.

5. RCS sold land that had cost $100,000 for $100,000 cash.
6. RCS paid $47,000 cash for other operating expenses.

Required

a. Record the transaction data in a horizontal financial statements model like the following one. In the Cash Flow column, classify the cash flows as operating activities (OA), investing activities (IA), or financing activities (FA). The beginning balances have been recorded as an example. They are the ending balances shown on RCS's December 31, 2012, financial statements illustrated in the chapter. Note that the revenue and expense accounts have a zero beginning balance. Amounts in these accounts apply only to a single accounting period. Revenue and expense account balances are not carried forward from one accounting period to the next.

	Balance Sheet								Income Statement					
	Assets		=	Liab.	+	Stockholders' Equity								
Event No.	Cash	+ Land	=	N. Pay.	+	Com. Stk.	+	Ret. Earn.	Rev.	−	Exp.	=	Net Inc.	Statement of Cash Flows
Beg. bal.	51,000	+ 500,000	=	400,000	+	120,000	+	31,000	NA	−	NA	=	NA	NA

b. Explain why there are no beginning balances in the Income Statement columns.
c. What amount of net income will RCS report on the 2013 income statement?
d. What amount of total assets will RCS report on the December 31, 2013, balance sheet?
e. What amount of retained earnings will RCS report on the December 31, 2013, balance sheet?
f. What amount of net cash flow from operating activities will RCS report on the 2013 statement of cash flows?

Solution

a.

	Balance Sheet								Income Statement					
	Assets		=	Liab.	+	Stockholders' Equity								
Event No.	Cash	+ Land	=	N. Pay.	+	Com. Stk.	+	Ret. Earn.	Rev.	−	Exp.	=	Net Inc.	Statement of Cash Flows
Beg. bal.	51,000	+ 500,000	=	400,000	+	120,000	+	31,000	NA	−	NA	=	NA	NA
1.	32,000	+ NA	=	NA	+	32,000	+	NA	NA	−	NA	=	NA	32,000 FA
2.	116,000	+ NA	=	NA	+	NA	+	116,000	116,000	−	NA	=	116,000	116,000 OA
3.	(13,000)	+ NA	=	NA	+	NA	+	(13,000)	NA	−	13,000	=	(13,000)	(13,000) OA
4.	(9,000)	+ NA	=	NA	+	NA	+	(9,000)	NA	−	NA	=	NA	(9,000) FA
5.	100,000	+ (100,000)	=	NA	+	NA	+	NA	NA	−	NA	=	NA	100,000 IA
6.	(47,000)	+ NA	=	NA	+	NA	+	(47,000)	NA	−	47,000	=	(47,000)	(47,000) OA
Totals	230,000	+ 400,000	=	400,000	+	152,000	+	78,000	116,000	−	60,000	=	56,000	179,000 NC*

*The letters NC on the last line of the column designate the net change in cash.

b. The revenue and expense accounts are temporary accounts used to capture data for a single accounting period. They are closed (amounts removed from the accounts) to retained earnings at the end of the accounting period and therefore always have zero balances at the beginning of the accounting cycle.

c. RCS will report net income of $56,000 on the 2013 income statement. Compute this amount by subtracting the expenses from the revenue ($116,000 Revenue − $13,000 Salaries expense − $47,000 Other operating expense).

d. RCS will report total assets of $630,000 on the December 31, 2013, balance sheet. Compute total assets by adding the cash amount to the land amount ($230,000 Cash + $400,000 Land).

e. RCS will report retained earnings of $78,000 on the December 31, 2013, balance sheet. Compute this amount using the following formula: Beginning retained earnings + Net income − Dividends = Ending retained earnings. In this case, $31,000 + $56,000 − $9,000 = $78,000.

f. Net cash flow from operating activities is the difference between the amount of cash collected from revenue and the amount of cash spent for expenses. In this case, $116,000 cash inflow from revenue − $13,000 cash outflow for salaries expense − $47,000 cash outflow for other operating expenses = $56,000 net cash inflow from operating activities.

KEY TERMS

accounting 2
accounting equation 12
accounting event 13
accounting period 15
accounts 11
annual report 25
articulation 18
asset exchange transaction 14
asset source transaction 13
asset use transaction 15
assets 4
balance sheet 9
claims 4
closing 22
common stock 12
creditors 4
dividend 16
double-entry bookkeeping 14
earnings 4
elements 10
equity 12
expenses 15
financial accounting 6
Financial Accounting Standards
    Board (FASB) 8

financial resources 4
financial statements 10
financing activities 21
general ledger 17
generally accepted accounting
    principles (GAAP) 8
historical cost concept 16
horizontal statements
    model 23
income 4
income statement 18
International Accounting
    Standards Board (IASB) 9
International Financial
    Reporting Standards
    (IFRS) 9
interest 5
investing activities 21
investors 4
labor resources 4
liabilities 10
liquidation 4
liquidity 20
managerial accounting 6
manufacturing businesses 24

market 4
matching concept 18
merchandising
    businesses 24
net income 18
net loss 18
not-for-profit entities 6
operating activities 21
permanent accounts 22
physical resources 5
profit 4
reliability concept 16
reporting entities 9
retained earnings 12
revenue 10
service businesses 24
stakeholders 6
statement of cash flows 10
statement of changes in
    stockholders' equity 10
stockholders 12
stockholders' equity 12
temporary accounts 22
transaction 12
users 6

QUESTIONS

1. Explain the term *stakeholder.* Distinguish between stakeholders with a direct versus an indirect interest in the companies that issue accounting reports.

2. Why is accounting called the *language of business?*

3. What is the primary mechanism used to allocate resources in the United States?

4. In a business context, what does the term *market* mean?

5. What market trilogy components are involved in the process of transforming resources into finished products?

6. Give an example of a financial resource, a physical resource, and a labor resource.

7. What type of return does an investor expect to receive in exchange for providing financial resources to a business? What type of return does a creditor expect from

providing financial resources to an organization or business?

8. How do financial and managerial accounting differ?

9. Describe a not-for-profit or nonprofit enterprise. What is the motivation for this type of entity?

10. What are the U.S. rules of accounting information measurement called?

11. Explain how a career in public accounting differs from a career in private accounting.

12. Distinguish between elements of financial statements and accounts.

13. What role do assets play in business profitability?

14. To whom do the assets of a business belong?

15. What is the nature of creditors' claims on assets?

16. What term describes creditors' claims on the assets of a business?

17. What is the accounting equation? Describe each of its three components.

18. Who ultimately bears the risk and collects the rewards associated with operating a business?

19. What does a *double-entry bookkeeping system* mean?

20. How does acquiring capital from owners affect the accounting equation?

21. What is the difference between assets that are acquired by issuing common stock and those that are acquired using retained earnings?

22. How does earning revenue affect the accounting equation?

23. What are the three primary sources of assets?

24. What is the source of retained earnings?

25. How does distributing assets (paying dividends) to owners affect the accounting equation?

26. What are the similarities and differences between dividends and expenses?

27. What four general-purpose financial statements do business enterprises use?

28. Which of the general-purpose financial statements provides information about the enterprise at a specific designated date?

29. What causes a net loss?

30. What three categories of cash receipts and cash payments do businesses report on the statement of cash flows? Explain the types of cash flows reported in each category.

31. How are asset accounts usually arranged in the balance sheet?

32. Discuss the term *articulation* as it relates to financial statements.

33. How do temporary accounts differ from permanent accounts? Name three temporary accounts. Is retained earnings a temporary or a permanent account?

34. What is the historical cost concept and how does it relate to the reliability concept?

35. Identify the three types of accounting transactions discussed in this chapter. Provide an example of each type of transaction, and explain how it affects the accounting equation.

36. What type of information does a business typically include in its annual report?

37. What is U.S. GAAP? What is IFRS?

 ## MULTIPLE-CHOICE QUESTIONS

Multiple-choice questions are provided on the text website at www.mhhe.com/edmondssurvey3e.

EXERCISES

All applicable Exercises are available with McGraw-Hill's *Connect Accounting.*

Exercise 1-1   *The role of accounting in society*

Free economies use open markets to allocate resources.

LO 1

Required

Identify the three participants in a free business market. Write a brief memo explaining how these participants interact to ensure that goods and services are distributed in a manner that satisfies consumers. Your memo should include answers to the following questions: If you work as a public accountant, what role would you play in the allocation of resources? Which professional certification would be most appropriate to your career?

Exercise 1-2   *Distributions in a business liquidation*

Assume that Kennedy Company acquires $1,600 cash from creditors and $1,800 cash from investors.

LO 1

Required

a. Explain the primary differences between investors and creditors.

b. If Kennedy has a net loss of $1,600 cash and then liquidates, what amount of cash will the creditors receive? What amount of cash will the investors receive?

c. If Kennedy has net income of $1,600 and then liquidates, what amount of cash will the creditors receive? What amount of cash will the investors receive?

LO 1

Exercise 1-3   *Careers in accounting*

Accounting is commonly divided into two sectors. One sector is called public accounting. The other sector is called private accounting.

Required

a. Identify three areas of service provided by public accountants.
b. Describe the common duties performed by private accountants.

LO 1

Exercise 1-4   *Identifying the reporting entities*

Kenneth Chang recently started a business. During the first few days of operation, Mr. Chang transferred $30,000 from his personal account into a business account for a company he named Chang Enterprises. Chang Enterprises borrowed $40,000 from First Bank. Mr. Chang's father-in-law, Jim Harwood, invested $64,000 into the business for which he received a 25 percent ownership interest. Chang Enterprises purchased a building from Morton Realty Company. The building cost $120,000 cash. Chang Enterprises earned $28,000 in revenue from the company's customers and paid its employees $25,000 for salaries expense.

Required

Identify the entities that were mentioned in the scenario and explain what happened to the cash accounts of each entity that you identify.

LO 2

Exercise 1-5   *Titles and accounts appearing on financial statements*

Annual reports normally include an income statement, a statement of changes in stockholders' equity, a balance sheet, and a statement of cash flows.

Required

Identify the financial statements on which each of the following titles or accounts would appear. If a title or an account appears on more than one statement, list all statements that would include it.

a. Common Stock
b. Land
c. Ending Cash Balance
d. Beginning Cash Balance
e. Notes Payable
f. Retained Earnings
g. Revenue
h. Cash Dividends
i. Financing Activities
j. Salaries Expense

LO 2

Exercise 1-6   *Components of the accounting equation*

Required

The following three requirements are independent of each other.

a. Craig's Cars has assets of $4,550 and stockholders' equity of $3,200. What is the amount of liabilities? What is the amount of claims?
b. Heavenly Bakery has liabilities of $4,800 and stockholders' equity of $5,400. What is the amount of assets?
c. Bell's Candy Co. has assets of $49,200 and liabilities of $28,200. What is the amount of stockholders' equity?

LO 2

Exercise 1-7   *Missing information in the accounting equation*

Required

Calculate the missing amounts in the following table.

Company	Assets	=	Liabilities	+	Stockholders' Equity Common Stock	+	Retained Earnings
A	$?		$25,000		$48,000		$50,000
B	40,000		?		7,000		30,000
C	75,000		15,000		?		42,000
D	125,000		45,000		60,000		?

Exercise 1-8 *Missing information in the accounting equation*

As of December 31, 2012, Eber Company had total assets of $156,000, total liabilities of $85,600, and common stock of $52,400. During 2013 Eber earned $36,000 of cash revenue, paid $20,000 for cash expenses, and paid a $2,000 cash dividend to the stockholders.

Required

a. Determine the amount of retained earnings as of December 31, 2012, after closing.
b. Determine the amount of net income earned in 2013.
c. Determine the amount of retained earnings as of December 31, 2013, after closing.
d. Determine the amount of cash that is in the retained earnings account as of December 31, 2013.

Exercise 1-9 *Missing information for determining net income*

The December 31, 2012, balance sheet for Classic Company showed total stockholders' equity of $82,500. Total stockholders' equity increased by $53,400 between December 31, 2012, and December 31, 2013. During 2013 Classic Company acquired $13,000 cash from the issue of common stock. Classic Company paid an $8,000 cash dividend to the stockholders during 2013.

Required

Determine the amount of net income or loss Classic reported on its 2013 income statement. (*Hint:* Remember that stock issues, net income, and dividends all change total stockholders' equity.)

Exercise 1-10 *Effect of events on the accounting equation*

Olive Enterprises experienced the following events during 2012.

1. Acquired cash from the issue of common stock.
2. Paid cash to reduce the principal on a bank note.
3. Sold land for cash at an amount equal to its cost.
4. Provided services to clients for cash.
5. Paid utilities expenses with cash.
6. Paid a cash dividend to the stockholders.

Required

Explain how each of the events would affect the accounting equation by writing the letter I for increase, the letter D for decrease, and NA for does not affect under each of the components of the accounting equation. The first event is shown as an example.

Event Number	Assets	=	Liabilities	+	Stockholders' Equity Common Stock	+	Retained Earnings
1	I		NA		I		NA

LO 2, 3

Exercise 1-11   *Effects of issuing stock*

Shiloh Company was started in 2012 when it acquired $15,000 cash by issuing common stock. The cash acquisition was the only event that affected the business in 2012.

Required

Write an accounting equation, and record the effects of the stock issue under the appropriate general ledger account headings.

LO 2, 3

Exercise 1-12   *Effects of borrowing*

Marcum Company was started in 2012 when it issued a note to borrow $6,200 cash.

Required

Write an accounting equation, and record the effects of the borrowing transaction under the appropriate general ledger account headings.

LO 2, 3

Exercise 1-13   *Effects of revenue, expense, dividend, and the closing process*

Rhodes Company was started on January 1, 2011. During 2012, the company experienced the following three accounting events: (1) earned cash revenues of $13,500, (2) paid cash expenses of $9,200, and (3) paid a $500 cash dividend to its stockholders. These were the only events that affected the company during 2012.

Required

a. Write an accounting equation, and record the effects of each accounting event under the appropriate general ledger account headings.
b. Prepare an income statement for the 2012 accounting period and a balance sheet at the end of 2012 for Rhodes Company.
c. What is the balance in the Retained Earnings account immediately after the cash revenue is recognized?
d. What is the balance in the Retained Earnings account after the closing process is complete?

LO 2, 3

Exercise 1-14   *Effect of transactions on general ledger accounts*

At the beginning of 2012, J & J Corp.'s accounting records had the following general ledger accounts and balances.

J & J CORP. **Accounting Equation**								
Event	Assets		=	Liabilities	+	Stockholders' Equity		Acct. Titles for RE
	Cash	Land		Notes Payable		Common Stock	Retained Earnings	
Balance 1/1/2012	10,000	20,000		12,000		7,000	11,000	

J & J Corp. completed the following transactions during 2012.

1. Purchased land for $5,000 cash.
2. Acquired $25,000 cash from the issue of common stock.
3. Received $75,000 cash for providing services to customers.
4. Paid cash operating expenses of $42,000.
5. Borrowed $10,000 cash from the bank.
6. Paid a $5,000 cash dividend to the stockholders.
7. Determined that the market value of the land is $35,000.

Required

a. Record the transactions in the appropriate general ledger accounts. Record the amounts of revenue, expense, and dividends in the Retained Earnings column. Provide the appropriate titles for these accounts in the last column of the table.

b. Determine the net cash flow from financing activities.

c. What is the balance in the Retained Earnings account as of January 1, 2013?

Exercise 1-15   *Classifying events as asset source, use, or exchange*   **LO 4**

BJ's Business Services experienced the following events during its first year of operations.

1. Acquired $10,000 cash from the issue of common stock.
2. Borrowed $8,000 cash from First Bank.
3. Paid $4,000 cash to purchase land.
4. Received $5,000 cash for providing boarding services.
5. Acquired an additional $2,000 cash from the issue of common stock.
6. Purchased additional land for $3,500 cash.
7. Paid $2,500 cash for salary expense.
8. Signed a contract to provide additional services in the future.
9. Paid $1,000 cash for rent expense.
10. Paid a $1,000 cash dividend to the stockholders.
11. Determined the market value of the land to be $8,000 at the end of the accounting period.

Required

Classify each event as an asset source, use, or exchange transaction or as not applicable (NA).

Exercise 1-16   *Classifying items for the statement of cash flows*   **LO 5**

Required

Indicate how each of the following would be classified on the statement of cash flows as operating activities (OA), investing activities (IA), financing activities (FA), or not applicable (NA).

a. Paid $4,000 cash for salary expense.
b. Borrowed $8,000 cash from State Bank.
c. Received $30,000 cash from the issue of common stock.
d. Purchased land for $8,000 cash.
e. Performed services for $14,000 cash.
f. Paid $4,200 cash for utilities expense.
g. Sold land for $7,000 cash.
h. Paid a cash dividend of $1,000 to the stockholders.
i. Hired an accountant to keep the books.
j. Paid $3,000 cash on the loan from State Bank.

Exercise 1-17   *Preparing financial statements*   **LO 2, 3, 5**

Montana Company experienced the following events during 2012.

1. Acquired $30,000 cash from the issue of common stock.
2. Paid $12,000 cash to purchase land.
3. Borrowed $10,000 cash.
4. Provided services for $20,000 cash.
5. Paid $1,000 cash for rent expense.
6. Paid $15,000 cash for other operating expenses.
7. Paid a $2,000 cash dividend to the stockholders.
8. Determined that the market value of the land purchased in Event 2 is now $12,700.

Required

a. The January 1, 2012, general ledger account balances are shown in the following accounting equation. Record the eight events in the appropriate general ledger accounts. Record the amounts of revenue, expense, and dividends in the Retained Earnings column. Provide the appropriate titles for these accounts in the last column of the table. The first event is shown as an example.

MONTANA COMPANY
Accounting Equation

Event	Assets		=	Liabilities	+	Stockholders' Equity		Acct. Titles for RE
	Cash	Land		Notes Payable		Common Stock	Retained Earnings	
Balance 1/1/2012 1.	2,000 30,000	12,000		0		6,000 30,000	8,000	

b. Prepare an income statement, statement of changes in equity, year-end balance sheet, and statement of cash flows for the 2012 accounting period.

c. Determine the percentage of assets that were provided by retained earnings. How much cash is in the retained earnings account?

LO 5

Exercise 1-18   *Retained earnings and the closing process*

Davis Company was started on January 1, 2012. During the month of January, Davis earned $4,600 of revenue and incurred $3,000 of expense. Davis closes its books on December 31 of each year.

Required

a. Determine the balance in the Retained Earnings account as of January 31, 2012.

b. Comment on whether retained earnings is an element of financial statements or an account.

c. What happens to the Retained Earnings account at the time expenses are recognized?

LO 5

Exercise 1-19   *Relationship between assets and retained earnings*

Washington Company was organized when it acquired $2,000 cash from the issue of common stock. During its first accounting period the company earned $800 of cash revenue and incurred $500 of cash expenses. Also, during the accounting period the company paid its owners a $200 cash dividend.

Required

a. Determine the balance in the Retained Earnings account before and after the temporary accounts are closed.

b. As of the end of the accounting period, determine what percentage of total assets were provided by retained earnings.

LO 5

Exercise 1-20   *Historical cost versus market value*

Hilltop, Inc., purchased land in January 2009 at a cost of $270,000. The estimated market value of the land is $350,000 as of December 31, 2012.

Required

a. Name the December 31, 2012, financial statement(s) on which the land will be shown.

b. At what dollar amount will the land be shown in the financial statement(s)?

c. Name the key concept that will be used in determining the dollar amount that will be reported for land that is shown in the financial statement(s).

Exercise 1-21   *Relating accounting events to entities*

Wright Company was started in 2012 when it acquired $25,000 cash by issuing common stock to Cal Wright.

Required

a. Was this event an asset source, use, or exchange transaction for Wright Company?

b. Was this event an asset source, use, or exchange transaction for Cal Wright?

c. Was the cash flow an operating, investing, or a financing activity on Wright Company's 2012 statement of cash flows?

d. Was the cash flow an operating, investing, or a financing activity on Cal Wright's 2012 statement of cash flows?

Exercise 1-22   *Effect of events on a horizontal financial statements model*

City Consulting Services experienced the following events during 2012.

1. Acquired cash by issuing common stock.
2. Collected cash for providing tutoring services to clients.
3. Borrowed cash from a local government small business foundation.
4. Purchased land for cash.
5. Paid cash for operating expenses.
6. Paid a cash dividend to the stockholders.
7. Determined that the market value of the land is higher than its historical cost.

Required

Use a horizontal statements model to show how each event affects the balance sheet, income statement, and statement of cash flows. Indicate whether the event increases (I), decreases (D), or does not affect (NA) each element of the financial statements. Also, in the Cash Flows column, classify the cash flows as operating activities (OA), investing activities (IA), or financing activities (FA). The first transaction is shown as an example.

Event No.	Cash	+	Land	=	N. Pay	+	C. Stock.	+	Ret. Ear.	Rev.	−	Exp.	=	Net Inc.	Statement of Cash Flows
					Balance Sheet						Income Statement				
1.	I	+	NA	=	NA	+	I	+	NA	NA	−	NA	=	NA	I FA

Exercise 1-23   *Record events in the horizontal statements model*

Expo Co. was started in 2012. During 2012, the company (1) acquired $11,000 cash from the issue of common stock, (2) earned cash revenue of $18,000, (3) paid cash expenses of $10,500, and (4) paid a $1,000 cash dividend to the stockholders.

Required

a. Record these four events in a horizontal statements model. Also, in the Cash Flows column, classify the cash flows as operating activities (OA), investing activities (IA), or financing activities (FA). The first event is shown as an example.

Event No.	Cash	=	N. Pay	+	C. Stock.	+	Ret. Ear.	Rev.	−	Exp.	=	Net Inc.	Statement of Cash Flows
			Balance Sheet						Income Statement				
1.	11,000	=	NA	+	11,000	+	NA	NA	−	NA	=	NA	11,000 FA

b. What does the income statement tell you about the assets of this business?

LO 6

Exercise 1-24 *Effect of events on a horizontal statements model*

Solito, Inc., was started on January 1, 2012. The company experienced the following events during its first year of operation.

1. Acquired $50,000 cash from the issue of common stock.
2. Paid $12,000 cash to purchase land.
3. Received $50,000 cash for providing tax services to customers.
4. Paid $9,500 cash for salary expense.
5. Acquired $5,000 cash from the issue of additional common stock.
6. Borrowed $10,000 cash from the bank.
7. Purchased additional land for $10,000 cash.
8. Paid $8,000 cash for other operating expenses.
9. Paid a $2,800 cash dividend to the stockholders.
10. Determined that the market value of the land is $25,000.

Required

a. Record these events in a horizontal statements model. Also, in the Cash Flows column, classify the cash flows as operating activities (OA), investing activities (IA), or financing activities (FA). The first event is shown as an example.

Event No.	Balance Sheet									Income Statement					Statement of Cash Flows
	Cash	+	Land	=	N. Pay	+	C. Stock.	+	Ret. Ear.	Rev.	−	Exp.	=	Net Inc.	
1.	50,000	+	NA	=	NA	+	50,000	+	NA	NA	−	NA	=	NA	50,000 FA

b. What is the net income earned in 2012?
c. What is the amount of total assets at the end of 2012?
d. What is the net cash flow from operating activities for 2012?
e. What is the net cash flow from investing activities for 2012?
f. What is the net cash flow from financing activities for 2012?
g. What is the cash balance at the end of 2012?
h. As of the end of the year 2012, what percentage of total assets were provided by creditors, investors, and retained earnings?
i. What is the balance in the Retained Earnings account immediately after Event 4 is recorded?

LO 4, 6

Exercise 1-25 *Types of transactions and the horizontal statements model*

Partner's Pet Store experienced the following events during its first year of operations, 2012.

1. Acquired cash by issuing common stock.
2. Purchased land with cash.
3. Borrowed cash from a bank.
4. Signed a contract to provide services in the future.
5. Paid a cash dividend to the stockholders.
6. Paid cash for operating expenses.
7. Determined that the market value of the land is higher than the historical cost.

Required

a. Indicate whether each event is an asset source, use, or exchange transaction.
b. Use a horizontal statements model to show how each event affects the balance sheet, income statement, and statement of cash flows. Indicate whether the event increases (I), decreases (D), or does not affect (NA) each element of the financial statements. Also, in the Cash

Flows column, classify the cash flows as operating activities (OA), investing activities (IA), or financing activities (FA). The first transaction is shown as an example.

Event No.	Balance Sheet																	Income Statement							Statement of Cash Flows
	Cash	+	Land	=	N. Pay	+	C. Stock.	+	Ret. Ear.									Rev.	−	Exp.	=	Net Inc.			
1.	I	+	NA	=	NA	+	I	+	NA									NA	−	NA	=	NA			I FA

Exercise 1-26 *International Financial Reporting Standards*

IFRS

Seacrest Company is a U.S.–based company that develops its financial statements under GAAP. The total amount of the company's assets shown on its December 31, 2012, balance sheet was approximately $225 million. The president of Seacrest is considering the possibility of relocating the company to a country that practices accounting under IFRS. The president has hired an international accounting firm to determine what the company's statements would look like if they were prepared under IFRS. One striking difference is that under IFRS the assets shown on the balance sheet would be valued at approximately $275 million.

Required

a. Would Seacrest's assets really be worth $50 million more if it moves its headquarters?
b. Discuss the underlying conceptual differences between U.S. GAAP and IFRS that cause the difference in the reported asset values.

PROBLEMS

All applicable Problems are available with McGraw-Hill's *Connect Accounting*.

connect
|ACCOUNTING

Problem 1-27 *Accounting's role in not-for-profits*

LO 1

Teresa Hill is struggling to pass her introductory accounting course. Teresa is intelligent but she likes to party. Studying is a low priority for Teresa. When one of her friends tells her that she is going to have trouble in business if she doesn't learn accounting, Teresa responds that she doesn't plan to go into business. She says that she is arts oriented and plans someday to be a director of a museum. She is in the school of business to develop her social skills, not her quantitative skills. Teresa says she won't have to worry about accounting, since museums are not intended to make a profit.

Required

a. Write a brief memo explaining whether you agree or disagree with Teresa's position regarding accounting and not-for-profit organizations.
b. Distinguish between financial accounting and managerial accounting.
c. Identify some of the stakeholders of not-for-profit institutions that would expect to receive financial accounting reports.
d. Identify some of the stakeholders of not-for-profit institutions that would expect to receive managerial accounting reports.

Problem 1-28 *Accounting entities*

LO 1

The following business scenarios are independent from one another.

1. Beth Mays purchased an automobile from Mills Bros. Auto Sales for $9,000.
2. Bill Becham loaned $15,000 to the business in which he is a stockholder.
3. First State Bank paid interest to Levi Co. on a certificate of deposit that Levi Co. has invested at First State Bank.
4. Southside Restaurant paid the current utility bill of $128 to Midwest Utilities.
5. Filmore, Inc., borrowed $50,000 from City National Bank and used the funds to purchase land from Tuchols Realty.

CHECK FIGURE
1. Entities mentioned: Beth Mays and Mills Bros. Auto Sales

6. Jing Chu purchased $10,000 of common stock of International Sales Corporation from the corporation.

7. Bill Mann loaned $4,000 cash to his daughter.

8. Research Service Co. earned $5,000 in cash revenue.

9. Yang Imports paid $1,500 for salaries to each of its four employees.

10. Meyers Inc. paid a cash dividend of $3,000 to its sole shareholder, Mark Meyers.

Required

a. For each scenario, create a list of all of the entities that are mentioned in the description.

b. Describe what happens to the cash account of each entity that you identified in Requirement *a*.

LO 2, 5

Problem 1-29 *Relating titles and accounts to financial statements*

Required

Identify the financial statements on which each of the following items (titles, date descriptions, and accounts) appears by placing a check mark in the appropriate column. If an item appears on more than one statement, place a check mark in every applicable column.

Item	Income Statement	Statement of Changes in Stockholders' Equity	Balance Sheet	Statement of Cash Flows
Notes payable				
Beginning common stock				
Service revenue				
Utility expense				
Cash from stock issue				
Operating activities				
For the period ended (date)				
Net income				
Investing activities				
Net loss				
Ending cash balance				
Salary expense				
Consulting revenue				
Dividends				
Financing activities				
Ending common stock				
Interest expense				
As of (date)				
Land				
Beginning cash balance				

LO 2, 3, 5, 6

Problem 1-30 *Preparing financial statements for two complete accounting cycles*

Webster Consulting experienced the following transactions for 2012, its first year of operations, and 2013. *Assume that all transactions involve the receipt or payment of cash.*

Transactions for 2012

1. Acquired $20,000 by issuing common stock.
2. Received $35,000 cash for providing services to customers.
3. Borrowed $25,000 cash from creditors.
4. Paid expenses amounting to $22,000.
5. Purchased land for $30,000 cash.

Transactions for 2013

Beginning account balances for 2013 are:

Cash	$28,000
Land	30,000
Notes payable	25,000
Common stock	20,000
Retained earnings	13,000

1. Acquired an additional $24,000 from the issue of common stock.
2. Received $95,000 for providing services.
3. Paid $15,000 to creditors to reduce loan.
4. Paid expenses amounting to $71,500.
5. Paid a $3,000 dividend to the stockholders.
6. Determined that the market value of the land is $47,000.

Required

a. Write an accounting equation, and record the effects of each accounting event under the appropriate headings for each year. Record the amounts of revenue, expense, and dividends in the Retained Earnings column. Provide appropriate titles for these accounts in the last column of the table.

b. Prepare an income statement, statement of changes in stockholders' equity, year-end balance sheet, and statement of cash flows for each year.

c. Determine the amount of cash that is in the retained earnings account at the end of 2012 and 2013.

d. Examine the balance sheets for the two years. How did assets change from 2012 to 2013?

e. Determine the balance in the Retained Earnings account immediately after Event 2 in 2012 and in 2013 are recorded.

Problem 1-31   *Interrelationships among financial statements*

Gofish Enterprises started the 2012 accounting period with $50,000 of assets (all cash), $18,000 of liabilities, and $4,000 of common stock. During the year, Gofish earned cash revenues of $38,000, paid cash expenses of $32,000, and paid a cash dividend to stockholders of $2,000. Gofish also acquired $15,000 of additional cash from the sale of common stock and paid $10,000 cash to reduce the liability owed to a bank.

Required

a. Prepare an income statement, statement of changes in stockholders' equity, period-end balance sheet, and statement of cash flows for the 2012 accounting period. (*Hint:* Determine the amount of beginning retained earnings before considering the effects of the current period events. It also might help to record all events under an accounting equation before preparing the statements.)

b. Determine the percentage of total assets that were provided by creditors, investors, and retained earnings.

CHECK FIGURES
b. Net Income 2012: $13,000
b. Retained Earnings 2013: $33,500

LO 2, 3, 5, 6

CHECK FIGURE
a. Net Income: $6,000
   Total Assets: $59,000

LO 4

Problem 1-32 *Classifying events as asset source, use, or exchange*

The following unrelated events are typical of those experienced by business entities.

1. Acquire cash by issuing common stock.
2. Purchase land with cash.
3. Purchase equipment with cash.
4. Pay monthly rent on an office building.
5. Hire a new office manager.
6. Borrow cash from a bank.
7. Pay a cash dividend to stockholders.
8. Pay cash for operating expenses.
9. Pay an office manager's salary with cash.
10. Receive cash for services that have been performed.
11. Pay cash for utilities expense.
12. Acquire land by accepting a liability (financing the purchase).
13. Pay cash to purchase a new office building.
14. Discuss plans for a new office building with an architect.
15. Repay part of a bank loan.

Required

Identify each of the events as an asset source, use, or exchange transaction. If an event would not be recorded under generally accepted accounting principles, identify it as not applicable (NA). Also indicate for each event whether total assets would increase, decrease, or remain unchanged. Organize your answer according to the following table. The first event is shown in the table as an example.

Event No.	Type of Event	Effect on Total Assets
1	Asset source	Increase

LO 6

Problem 1-33 *Recording the effect of events in a horizontal statements model*

Texas Corporation experienced the following transactions during 2012.

1. Paid a cash dividend to the stockholders.
2. Acquired cash by issuing additional common stock.
3. Signed a contract to perform services in the future.
4. Performed services for cash.
5. Paid cash expenses.
6. Sold land for cash at an amount equal to its cost.
7. Borrowed cash from a bank.
8. Determined that the market value of the land is higher than its historical cost.

Required

Use a horizontal statements model to show how each event affects the balance sheet, income statement, and statement of cash flows. Indicate whether the event increases (I), decreases (D), or does not affect (NA) each element of the financial statements. Also, in the Cash Flows column, classify the cash flows as operating activities (OA), investing activities (IA), or financing activities (FA). The first transaction is shown as an example.

Event No.		Balance Sheet								Income Statement				Statement of Cash Flows
	Cash	+	Land	=	N. Pay	+	C. Stock.	+	Ret. Ear.	Rev.	−	Exp.	=	Net Inc.	
1.	D	+	NA	=	NA	+	NA	+	D	NA	−	NA	=	NA	D FA

Problem 1-34   *Recording events in a horizontal statements model*

Cooley Company was started on January 1, 2012, and experienced the following events during its first year of operation.

1. Acquired $30,000 cash from the issue of common stock.
2. Borrowed $40,000 cash from National Bank.
3. Earned cash revenues of $48,000 for performing services.
4. Paid cash expenses of $45,000.
5. Paid a $1,000 cash dividend to the stockholders.
6. Acquired an additional $20,000 cash from the issue of common stock.
7. Paid $10,000 cash to reduce the principal balance of the bank note.
8. Paid $53,000 cash to purchase land.
9. Determined that the market value of the land is $75,000.

Required

a. Record the preceding transactions in the horizontal statements model. Also, in the Cash Flows column, classify the cash flows as operating activities (OA), investing activities (IA), or financing activities (FA). The first event is shown as an example.

Event No.	Balance Sheet																Income Statement						Statement of Cash Flows
	Cash	+	Land	=	N. Pay	+	C. Stock.	+	Ret. Ear.	Rev.	−	Exp.	=	Net Inc.	
1.	30,000	+	NA	=	NA	+	30,000	+	NA	NA	−	NA	=	NA	30,000 FA

b. Determine the amount of total assets that Cooley would report on the December 31, 2012, balance sheet.

c. Identify the asset source transactions and related amounts for 2012.

d. Determine the net income that Cooley would report on the 2012 income statement. Explain why dividends do not appear on the income statement.

e. Determine the net cash flows from operating activities, financing activities, and investing activities that Cooley would report on the 2012 statement of cash flows.

f. Determine the percentage of assets that were provided by investors, creditors, and retained earnings.

g. What is the balance in the Retained Earnings account immediately after Event 3 is recorded?

ANALYZE, THINK, COMMUNICATE

ATC 1-1   Business Applications Case   *Understanding real-world annual reports*

Required

Use the Target Corporation's annual report in Appendix B to answer the following questions. Note that net income and net earnings are synonymous terms.

Target Corporation

a. What was Target's net income for 2009?
b. Did Target's net income increase or decrease from 2008 to 2009, and by how much?
c. What was Target's accounting equation for 2009?
d. Which of the following had the largest percentage change from 2008 to 2009: net sales, cost of sales, or selling, general, and administrative expenses? Show all computations.

ATC 1-2   Group Assignment   *Missing information*

The following selected financial information is available for HAS, Inc. Amounts are in millions of dollars.

Income Statements	2014	2013	2012	2011
Revenue	$ 860	$1,520	$ (a)	$1,200
Cost and expenses	(a)	(a)	(2,400)	(860)
Income from continuing operations	(b)	450	320	(a)
Unusual items	-0-	175	(b)	(b)
Net income	$ 20	$ (b)	$ 175	$ 300
Balance Sheets				
Assets				
Cash and marketable securities	$ 350	$1,720	$ (c)	$ 940
Other assets	1,900	(c)	2,500	(c)
Total assets	2,250	$2,900	$ (d)	$3,500
Liabilities	$ (c)	$ (d)	$1,001	$ (d)
Stockholders' equity				
Common stock	880	720	(e)	800
Retained earnings	(d)	(e)	800	(e)
Total stockholders' equity	1,520	1,345	(f)	2,200
Total liabilities and stockholders' equity	$2,250	$ (f)	$3,250	$3,500

Required

a. Divide the class into groups of four or five students each. Organize the groups into four sections. Assign Task 1 to the first section of groups, Task 2 to the second section, Task 3 to the third section, and Task 4 to the fourth section.

Group Tasks

(1) Fill in the missing information for 2011.
(2) Fill in the missing information for 2012.
(3) Fill in the missing information for 2013.
(4) Fill in the missing information for 2014.

b. Each section should select two representatives. One representative is to put the financial statements assigned to that section on the board, underlining the missing amounts. The second representative is to explain to the class how the missing amounts were determined.

c. Each section should list events that could have caused the unusual items category on the income statement.

ATC 1-3   Research Assignment   *Finding real-world accounting information*

This chapter introduced the basic four financial statements companies use annually to keep their stakeholders informed of their accomplishments and financial situation. Complete the requirements below using the most recent (20xx) financial statements available on the McDonald Corporation's website. Obtain the statements on the Internet by following the steps below. (The formatting of the company's website may have changed since these instructions were written.)

1. Go to www.mcdonalds.com.
2. Click on the "Corporate" link at the bottom of the page. (Most companies have a link titled "investors relations" that leads to their financial statements; McDonald's uses "corporate" instead.)
3. Click on the "INVESTORS" link at the top of the page.

4. Click on "*McDonald's 20xx Annual Report*" and then on "*20xx Financial Report.*"
5. Go to the company's financial statements that begin on page 45 of the annual report.

Required

a. What was the company's net income in each of the last 3 years?

b. What amount of total assets did the company have at the end of the most recent year?

c. How much retained earnings did the company have at the end of the most recent year?

d. For the most recent year, what was the company's cash flow from operating activities, cash flow from investing activities, and cash flow from financing activities?

ATC 1-4   Writing Assignment   *Elements of financial statements defined*

Sam and his sister Blair both attend the state university. As a reward for their successful completion of the past year (Sam had a 3.2 GPA in business, and Blair had a 3.7 GPA in art), their father gave each of them 100 shares of The Walt Disney Company stock. They have just received their first annual report. Blair does not understand what the information means and has asked Sam to explain it to her. Sam is currently taking an accounting course, and she knows he will understand the financial statements.

Required

Assume that you are Sam. Write Blair a memo explaining the following financial statement items to her. In your explanation, describe each of the two financial statements and explain the financial information each contains. Also define each of the elements listed for each financial statement and explain what it means.

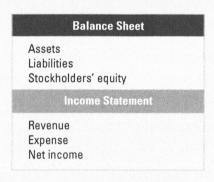

Balance Sheet
Assets
Liabilities
Stockholders' equity
Income Statement
Revenue
Expense
Net income

CHAPTER 2

Understanding the Accounting Cycle

LEARNING OBJECTIVES

After you have mastered the material in this chapter, you will be able to:

1 Record basic accrual and deferral events in a horizontal financial statements model.

2 Organize general ledger accounts under an accounting equation.

3 Prepare financial statements based on accrual accounting.

4 Describe the closing process, the accounting cycle, and the matching concept.

5 Explain how business events affect financial statements over multiple accounting cycles.

6 Classify accounting events into one of four categories:

a. asset source transactions.

b. asset use transactions.

c. asset exchange transactions.

d. claims exchange transactions.

CHAPTER OPENING

Users of financial statements must distinguish between the terms *recognition* and *realization*. **Recognition** means formally *reporting* an economic item or event in the financial statements. **Realization** refers to collecting money, generally from the sale of products or services. Companies may recognize (report) revenue in the income statement in a different accounting period from the period in which they collect the cash related to the revenue. Furthermore, companies frequently make cash payments for expenses in accounting periods other than the periods in which the expenses are recognized in the income statement.

To illustrate assume Johnson Company provides services to customers in 2012 but collects cash for those services in 2013. In this case, realization occurs in 2013. When should Johnson recognize the services revenue?

Users of *cash basis* accounting recognize (report) revenues and expenses in the period in which cash is collected or paid. Under cash basis accounting Johnson would recognize the revenue in 2013. When it collects the cash. In contrast, users of **accrual accounting** recognize revenues and expenses in the period in which they occur, regardless of when cash is collected or paid. Under accrual accounting Johnson would recognize the revenue in 2012 (the period in which it performed the services) even though it does not collect (realize) the cash until 2013.

Accrual accounting is required by generally accepted accounting principles. Virtually all major companies operating in the United States use it. Its two distinguishing features are called *accruals* and *deferrals*

- The term **accrual** describes a revenue or an expense event that is recognized *before* cash is exchanged. Johnson's recognition of revenue in 2012 related to cash realized in 2013 is an example of an accrual.
- The term **deferral** describes a revenue or an expense event that is recognized *after* cash has been exchanged. Suppose Johnson pays cash in 2012 to purchase office supplies it uses in 2013. In this case the cash payment occurs in 2012 although supplies expense is recognized in 2013. This example is a deferral.

The Curious Accountant

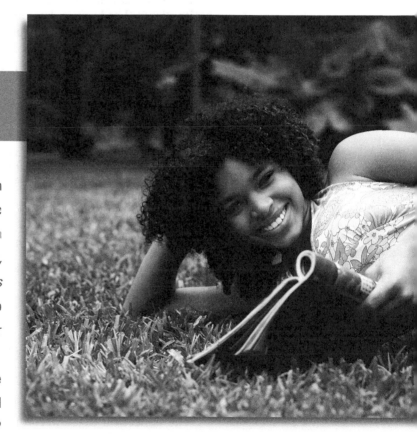

Suppose Arno Forst wishes to purchase a subscription to *Fitness magazine* for his sister for her birthday. He pays $12 for a one-year subscription to the Meredith Corporation, the company that publishes *Fitness, American Baby, Better Homes and Gardens, The Ladies Home Journal,* and several other magazines. It also owns 12 television stations. His sister will receive her first issue of the magazine in October.

How should Meredith Corporation account for the receipt of this cash? How would this event be reported on its December 31, 2012, financial statements? (Answer on page 60.)

ACCRUAL ACCOUNTING

Record basic accrual and deferral events in a horizontal financial statements model.

The next section of the text describes seven events experienced by Cato Consultants, a training services company that uses accrual accounting.

EVENT 1   Cato Consultants was started on January 1, 2012, when it acquired $5,000 cash by issuing common stock.

The issue of stock for cash is an **asset source transaction.** It increases the company's assets (cash) and its equity (common stock). The transaction does not affect the income statement. The cash inflow is classified as a financing activity (acquisition from owners). These effects are shown in the following financial statements model:

Assets	=	Liab.	+		Stockholders' Equity							
Cash	=			Com. Stk.	+	Ret. Earn.	Rev.	−	Exp.	=	Net Inc.	Cash Flow
5,000	=	NA	+	5,000	+	NA	NA	−	NA	=	NA	5,000 FA

Accounting for Accounts Receivable

EVENT 2   During 2012 Cato Consultants provided $84,000 of consulting services to its clients. The business has completed the work and sent bills to the clients, but not yet collected any cash. This type of transaction is frequently described as providing services *on account*.

Accrual accounting requires companies to recognize revenue in the period in which the work is done regardless of when cash is collected. In this case, revenue is recognized in 2012 even though cash has not been realized (collected). Recall that revenue represents the economic benefit that results in an increase in assets from providing goods and services to customers. The specific asset that increases is called **Accounts Receivable.** The balance in Accounts Receivable represents the amount of cash the company expects to collect in the future. Since the revenue recognition causes assets (accounts receivable) to increase, it is classified as an asset source transaction. Its effect on the financial statements follows.

		Assets		=	Liab.	+		Stockholders' Equity							
Cash	+	Accts. Rec.	=				Com. Stk.	+	Ret. Earn.	Rev.	−	Exp.	=	Net Inc.	Cash Flow
NA	+	84,000	=	NA	+	NA	+	84,000	84,000	−	NA	=	84,000	NA

Notice that the event affects the income statement but not the statement of cash flows. The statement of cash flows will be affected in the future when cash is collected.

EVENT 3   Cato collected $60,000 cash from customers in partial settlement of its accounts receivable.

The collection of an account receivable is an **asset exchange transaction.** One asset account (Cash) increases and another asset account (Accounts Receivable) decreases. The amount of total assets is unchanged. The effect of the $60,000 collection of receivables on the financial statements is as follows.

		Assets		=	Liab.	+		Stockholders' Equity							
Cash	+	Accts. Rec.	=				Com. Stk.	+	Ret. Earn.	Rev.	−	Exp.	=	Net Inc.	Cash Flow
60,000	+	(60,000)	=	NA	+	NA	+	NA	NA	−	NA	=	NA	60,000 OA

Notice that collecting the cash did not affect the income statement. The revenue was recognized when the work was done (see Event 2). Revenue would be double counted if it were recognized again when the cash is collected. The statement of cash flows reflects a cash inflow from operating activities.

Other Events

EVENT 4   Cato paid the instructor $10,000 for teaching training courses (salary expense).

Cash payment for salary expense is an **asset use transaction.** Both the asset account Cash and the equity account Retained Earnings decrease by $10,000. Recognizing the expense decreases net income on the income statement. Since Cato paid cash for the expense, the statement of cash flows reflects a cash outflow from operating activities. These effects on the financial statements follow.

Assets			=	Liab.	+	Stockholders' Equity							
Cash	+	Accts. Rec.	=			Com. Stk.	+	Ret. Earn.	Rev.	−	Exp.	=	Net Inc.	Cash Flow
(10,000)	+	NA	=	NA	+	NA	+	(10,000)	NA	−	10,000	=	(10,000)	(10,000) OA

EVENT 5   Cato paid $2,000 cash for advertising costs. The advertisements appeared in 2012.

Cash payments for advertising expenses are asset use transactions. Both the asset account Cash and the equity account Retained Earnings decrease by $2,000. Recognizing the expense decreases net income on the income statement. Since the expense was paid with cash, the statement of cash flows reflects a cash outflow from operating activities. These effects on the financial statements follow.

Assets			=	Liab.	+	Stockholders' Equity							
Cash	+	Accts. Rec.	=			Com. Stk.	+	Ret. Earn.	Rev.	−	Exp.	=	Net Inc.	Cash Flow
(2,000)	+	NA	=	NA	+	NA	+	(2,000)	NA	−	2,000	=	(2,000)	(2,000) OA

EVENT 6   Cato signed contracts for $42,000 of consulting services to be performed in 2013.

The $42,000 for consulting services to be performed in 2013 is not recognized in the 2012 financial statements. Revenue is recognized for work actually completed, *not* work expected to be completed. This event does not affect any of the financial statements.

Assets			=	Liab.	+	Stockholders' Equity							
Cash	+	Accts. Rec.	=			Com. Stk.	+	Ret. Earn.	Rev.	−	Exp.	=	Net Inc.	Cash Flow
NA	+	NA	=	NA	+	NA	+	NA	NA	−	NA	=	NA	NA

Accounting for Accrued Salary Expense (Adjusting Entry)

It is impractical to record many business events as they occur. For example, Cato incurs salary expense continually as the instructor teaches courses. Imagine the impossibility of trying to record salary expense second by second! Companies normally record transactions when it is most convenient. The most convenient time to record many expenses is when they are paid. Often, however, a single business transaction pertains to more than one accounting period. To provide accurate financial reports in such cases, companies may need to recognize some expenses before paying cash for them. Expenses that are recognized before cash is paid are called **accrued expenses.** The accounting for Event 7 illustrates the effect of recognizing accrued salary expense.

EVENT 7   At the end of 2012. Cato recorded accrued salary expense of $6,000 (the salary expense is for courses the instructor taught in 2012 that Cato will pay cash for in 2013).

Accrual accounting requires that companies recognize expenses in the period in which they are incurred regardless of when cash is paid. Cato must recognize all salary expense in the period in which the instructor worked (2012) even though Cato will not pay the instructor again until 2013. Cato must also recognize the obligation (liability) it has to pay the instructor. To accurately report all 2012 salary expense and year-end obligations, Cato must record the unpaid salary expense and salary liability before preparing its financial statements. The entry to recognize the accrued salary expense is called an **adjusting entry.** Like all adjusting entries, it is only to update the accounting records; it does not affect cash.

This adjusting entry decreases stockholders' equity (retained earnings) and increases a liability account called **Salaries Payable.** The balance in the Salaries Payable account represents the amount of cash the company is obligated to pay the instructor in the future. The effect of the expense recognition on the financial statements follows.

Assets			=	Liab.	+	Stockholders' Equity							
Cash	+	Accts. Rec.	=	Sal. Pay.	+	Com. Stk.	+	Ret. Earn.	Rev.	−	Exp.	=	Net Inc.	Cash Flow
NA	+	NA	=	6,000	+	NA	+	(6,000)	NA	−	6,000	=	(6,000)	NA

This event is a **claims exchange transaction.** The claims of creditors (liabilities) increase and the claims of stockholders (retained earnings) decrease. Total claims remain unchanged. The salary expense is reported on the income statement. The statement of cash flows is not affected.

Be careful not to confuse liabilities with expenses. Although liabilities may increase when a company recognizes expenses, liabilities are not expenses. Liabilities are obligations. They can arise from acquiring assets as well as recognizing expenses. For example, when a business borrows money from a bank, it recognizes an increase in assets (cash) and liabilities (notes payable). The borrowing transaction does not affect expenses.

✓ CHECK YOURSELF 2.1

During 2012, Anwar Company earned $345,000 of revenue on account and collected $320,000 cash from accounts receivable. Anwar paid cash expenses of $300,000 and cash dividends of $12,000. Determine the amount of net income Anwar should report on the 2012 income statement and the amount of cash flow from operating activities Anwar should report on the 2012 statement of cash flows.

Answer   Net income is $45,000 ($345,000 revenue − $300,000 expenses). The cash flow from operating activities is $20,000, the amount of revenue collected in cash from customers (accounts receivable) minus the cash paid for expenses ($320,000 − $300,000). Dividend payments are classified as financing activities and do not affect the determination of either net income or cash flow from operating activities.

EXHIBIT 2.1

Transaction Data for 2012 Recorded in General Ledger Accounts

1	Cato Consultants acquired $5,000 cash by issuing common stock.
2	Cato provided $84,000 of consulting services on account.
3	Cato collected $60,000 cash from customers in partial settlement of its accounts receivable.
4	Cato paid $10,000 cash for salary expense.
5	Cato paid $2,000 cash for 2012 advertising costs.
6	Cato signed contracts for $42,000 of consulting services to be performed in 2013.
7	Cato recognized $6,000 of accrued salary expense.

	Assets			=	Liabilities	+	Stockholders' Equity				
Event No.	Cash	+	Accounts Receivable	=	Salaries Payable	+	Common Stock	+	Retained Earnings		Other Account Titles
Beg. bal.	0		0		0		0		0		
1	5,000						5,000				
2			84,000						84,000		Consulting revenue
3	60,000		(60,000)								
4	(10,000)								(10,000)		Salary expense
5	(2,000)								(2,000)		Advertising expense
6											
7					6,000				(6,000)		Salary Expense
End bal.	53,000	+	24,000	=	6,000	+	5,000	+	66,000		

Summary of Events and General Ledger

The previous section of this chapter described seven events Cato Consultants experienced during the 2012 accounting period. These events are summarized in Exhibit 2.1. The associated general ledger accounts are also shown in the exhibit. The information in these accounts is used to prepare the financial statements. The revenue and expense items appear in the Retained Earnings column with their account titles immediately to the right of the dollar amounts. The amounts are color coded to help you trace the data to the financial statements. Data in red appear on the balance sheet, data in blue on the income statement, and data in green on the statement of cash flows.

Organize general ledger accounts under an accounting equation.

Vertical Statements Model

The financial statements for Cato Consultants' 2012 accounting period are represented in a vertical statements model in Exhibit 2.2. A vertical statements model arranges a set of financial statement information vertically on a single page. Like horizontal statements models, vertical statements models are learning tools. They illustrate interrelationships among financial statements. The models do not, however, portray the full, formal presentation formats companies use in published financial statements. For example, statements models may use summarized formats with abbreviated titles and dates. As you read the following explanations of each financial statement, trace the color coded financial data from Exhibit 2.1 to Exhibit 2.2.

Prepare financial statements based on accrual accounting.

Prepare a vertical financial statements model.

EXHIBIT 2.2	Vertical Statements Model

CATO CONSULTANTS
Financial Statements*
Income Statement
For the Year Ended December 31, 2012

Consulting revenue	$84,000
Salary expense	(16,000)
Advertising expense	(2,000)
Net income	$66,000

Statement of Changes in Stockholders' Equity
For the Year Ended December 31, 2012

Beginning common stock	$ 0	
Plus: Common stock issued	5,000	
Ending common stock		$ 5,000
Beginning retained earnings	0	
Plus: Net income	66,000	
Less: Dividends	0	
Ending retained earnings		66,000
Total stockholders' equity		$71,000

Balance Sheet
As of December 31, 2012

Assets		
Cash	$53,000	
Accounts receivable	24,000	
Total assets		$77,000
Liabilities		
Salaries payable		$ 6,000
Stockholders' equity		
Common stock	$ 5,000	
Retained earnings	66,000	
Total stockholders' equity		71,000
Total liabilities and stockholders' equity		$77,000

Statement of Cash Flows
For the Year Ended December 31, 2012

Cash flows from operating activities		
Cash receipts from customers	$60,000	
Cash payments for salary expense	(10,000)	
Cash payments for advertising expenses	(2,000)	
Net cash flow from operating activities		$48,000
Cash flow from investing activities		0
Cash flows from financing activities		
Cash receipt from issuing common stock	5,000	
Net cash flow from financing activities		5,000
Net change in cash		53,000
Plus: Beginning cash balance		0
Ending cash balance		$53,000

*In real-world annual reports, financial statements are normally presented separately with appropriate descriptions of the date to indicate whether the statement applies to the entire accounting period or a specific point in time.

Income Statement

The income statement reflects accrual accounting. Consulting revenue represents the price Cato charged for all the services it performed in 2012, even though Cato had not by the end of the year received cash for some of the services performed. Expenses include all costs incurred to produce revenue, whether paid for by year-end or not. We can now expand the definition of expenses introduced in Chapter 1. Expenses were previously defined as assets consumed in the process of generating revenue. Cato's adjusting entry to recognize accrued salaries expense did not reflect consuming assets. Instead of a decrease in assets, Cato recorded an increase in liabilities (salaries payable). An **expense** can therefore be more precisely defined as *a decrease in assets or an increase in liabilities resulting from operating activities undertaken to generate revenue.*

Statement of Changes in Stockholders' Equity

The statement of changes in stockholders' equity reports the effects on equity of issuing common stock, earning net income, and paying dividends to stockholders. It identifies how an entity's equity increased and decreased during the period as a result of transactions with stockholders and operating the business. In the Cato case, the statement shows that equity increased when the business acquired $5,000 cash by issuing common stock. The statement also reports that equity increased by $66,000 from earning income and that none of the $66,000 of net earnings was distributed to owners (no dividends were paid). Equity at the end of the year is $71,000 ($5,000 + $66,000).

Balance Sheet

The balance sheet discloses an entity's assets, liabilities, and stockholders' equity at a particular point in time. Cato Consultants had two assets at the end of the 2012 accounting period: cash of $53,000 and accounts receivable of $24,000. These assets are listed on the balance sheet in order of liquidity. Of the $77,000 in total assets, creditors have a $6,000 claim, leaving stockholders with a $71,000 claim.

Statement of Cash Flows

The statement of cash flows explains the change in cash from the beginning to the end of the accounting period. It can be prepared by analyzing the Cash account. Since Cato Consultants was established in 2012, its beginning cash balance was zero. By the end of the year, the cash balance was $53,000. The statement of cash flows explains this increase. The Cash account increased because Cato collected $60,000 from customers and decreased because Cato paid $12,000 for expenses. As a result, Cato's net cash inflow from operating activities was $48,000. Also, the business acquired $5,000 cash through the financing activity of issuing common stock, for a cumulative cash increase of $53,000 ($48,000 + $5,000) during 2012.

Comparing Cash Flow from Operating Activities with Net Income

The amount of net income measured using accrual accounting differs from the amount of cash flow from operating activities. For Cato Consulting in 2012, the differences are summarized below.

	Accrual Accounting	Cash Flow
Consulting revenue	$84,000	$60,000
Salary expense	(16,000)	(10,000)
Advertising expense	(2,000)	(2,000)
Net income	$66,000	$48,000

Many students begin their first accounting class with the misconception that revenue and expense items are cash equivalents. The Cato illustration demonstrates that a company may recognize a revenue or expense without a corresponding cash collection or payment in the same accounting period.

The Closing Process

LO 4

Describe the closing process, the accounting cycle, and the matching concept.

Recall that the temporary accounts (revenue, expense, and dividend) are closed prior to the start of the next accounting cycle. The closing process transfers the amount in each of these accounts to the Retained Earnings account, leaving each temporary account with a zero balance.

Exhibit 2.3 shows the general ledger accounts for Cato Consultants after the revenue and expense accounts have been closed to retained earnings. The closing entry labeled Cl.1 transfers the balance in the Consulting Revenue account to the Retained Earnings account. Closing entries Cl.2 and Cl.3 transfer the balances in the expense accounts to retained earnings.

EXHIBIT 2.3

General Ledger Accounts for Cato Consultants

Assets		=	Liabilities		+	Stockholders' Equity	
Cash			**Salaries Payable**			**Common Stock**	
(1)	5,000		(7)	6,000		(1)	5,000
(3)	60,000		Bal.	6,000			
(4)	(10,000)					**Retained Earnings**	
(5)	(2,000)					Cl.1	84,000
Bal.	53,000					Cl.2	(16,000)
						Cl.3	(2,000)
Accounts Receivable						Bal.	66,000
(2)	84,000						
(3)	(60,000)					**Consulting Revenue**	
Bal.	24,000					(2)	84,000
						Cl.1	(84,000)
						Bal.	0
						Salary Expense	
						(4)	(10,000)
						(7)	(6,000)
						Cl.2	16,000
						Bal.	0
						Advertising Expense	
						(5)	(2,000)
						Cl.3	2,000
						Bal.	0

Steps in an Accounting Cycle

An accounting cycle, which is represented graphically in Exhibit 2.4, involves several steps. The four steps identified to this point are (1) recording transactions; (2) adjusting the accounts; (3) preparing financial statements; and (4) closing the temporary accounts. The first step occurs continually throughout the accounting period. Steps 2, 3, and 4 normally occur at the end of the accounting period.

The Matching Concept

Cash basis accounting can distort reported net income because it sometimes fails to match expenses with the revenues they produce. To illustrate, consider the $6,000 of accrued salary expense that Cato Consultants recognized at the end of 2012. The instructor's teaching produced revenue in 2012. If Cato waited until 2013 (when it paid the instructor) to recognize $6,000 of the total $16,000 salary expense, then $6,000 of the expense would not be matched with the revenue it generated. By using accrual accounting, Cato recognized all the salary expense in the same accounting period in which the consulting revenue was recognized. A primary goal of accrual accounting is to appropriately match expenses with revenues, the **matching concept.**

Appropriately matching expenses with revenues can be difficult even when using accrual accounting. For example, consider Cato's advertising expense. Money spent on advertising may generate revenue in future accounting periods as well as in the current period. A prospective customer could save an advertising brochure for several years before calling Cato for training services. It is difficult to know when and to what extent advertising produces revenue. When the connection between an expense and the corresponding revenue is vague, accountants commonly match the expense with the period in which it is incurred. Cato matched (recognized) the entire $2,000 of advertising cost with the 2012 accounting period even though some of that cost might generate revenue in future accounting periods. Expenses that are matched with the period in which they are incurred are frequently called **period costs.**

Matching is not perfect. Although it would be more accurate to match expenses with revenues than with periods, there is sometimes no obvious direct connection between expenses and revenue. Accountants must exercise judgment to select the accounting period in which to recognize revenues and expenses. The concept of conservatism influences such judgment calls.

The Conservatism Principle

When faced with a recognition dilemma, **conservatism** guides accountants to select the alternative that produces the lowest amount of net income. In uncertain circumstances, accountants tend to delay revenue recognition and accelerate expense recognition. The conservatism principle holds that it is better to understate net income than to overstate it. If subsequent developments suggest that net income should have been higher, investors will respond more favorably than if they learn it was really lower. This practice explains why Cato recognized all of the advertising cost as expense in 2012 even though some of that cost may generate revenue in future accounting periods.

SECOND ACCOUNTING CYCLE

The effects of Cato Consultants' 2013 events are as follows:

EVENT 1   Cato paid $6,000 to the intructor to settle the salaries payable obligation.

Cash payments to creditors are *asset use transactions.* When Cato pays the instructor, both the asset account Cash and the liability account Salaries Payable decrease. The

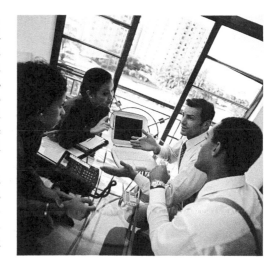

LO 5

Explain how business events affect financial statements over multiple accounting cycles.

cash payment does not affect the income statement. The salary expense was recognized in 2012 when the instructor taught the classes. The statement of cash flows reflects a cash outflow from operating activities. The effects of this transaction on the financial statements are shown here.

Assets	=	Liab.	+	Stk. Equity		Rev.	−	Exp.	=	Net Inc.	Cash Flow	
Cash	=	Sal. Pay.										
(6,000)	=	(6,000)	+	NA		NA	−	NA	=	NA	(6,000)	OA

Prepaid Items (Cost versus Expense)

EVENT 2 On March 1, 2013, Cato signed a one-year lease agreement and paid $12,000 cash in advance to rent office space. The one-year lease term began on March 1.

Accrual accounting draws a distinction between the terms *cost* and *expense*. A cost *might be either an asset or an expense*. If a company has already consumed a purchased resource in the process of earning revenue, the cost of the resource is an *expense*. For example, companies normally pay for electricity the month after using it. The cost of electric utilities is therefore usually recorded as an expense. In contrast, if a company purchases a resource it will use in the future to generate revenue, the cost of the resource represents an *asset*. Accountants record such a cost in an asset account and **defer** recognizing an expense until the resource is used to produce revenue. Deferring the expense recognition provides more accurate **matching** of revenues and expenses.

The cost of the office space Cato leased in Event 2 is an asset. It is recorded in the asset account *Prepaid Rent*. Cato expects to benefit from incurring this cost for the next twelve months. Expense recognition is deferred until Cato uses the office space to help generate revenue. Other common deferred expenses include *prepaid insurance* and *prepaid taxes*. As these titles imply, deferred expenses are frequently called **prepaid items.** Exhibit 2.5 illustrates the relationship between costs, assets, and expenses.

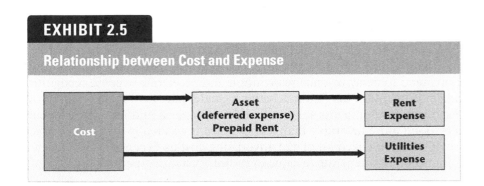

EXHIBIT 2.5

Relationship between Cost and Expense

Cost → Asset (deferred expense) Prepaid Rent → Rent Expense

Cost → Utilities Expense

Purchasing prepaid rent is an asset exchange transaction. The asset account Cash decreases and the asset account Prepaid Rent increases. The amount of total assets is unaffected. The income statement is unaffected. Expense recognition is deferred until the office space is used. The statement of cash flows reflects a cash outflow from operating activities. The effects of this transaction on the financial statements are shown here.

Assets			= Liab. + Stk. Equity						
Cash	+	Prep. Rent			Rev.	−	Exp.	=	Net Inc.	Cash Flow
(12,000)	+	12,000	= NA + NA		NA	−	NA	=	NA	(12,000) OA

Accounting for Receipt of Unearned Revenue

EVENT 3   Cato received $18,000 cash in advance from Westberry Company for consulting services Cato agreed to perform over a one-year period beginning June 1, 2013.

Cato must defer (delay) recognizing any revenue until it performs (does the work) the consulting services for Westberry. From Cato's point of view, the deferred revenue is a liability because Cato is obligated to perform services in the future. The liability is called **unearned revenue.** The cash receipt is an *asset source transaction.* The asset account Cash and the liability account Unearned Revenue both increase. Collecting the cash has no effect on the income statement. The revenue will be reported on the income statement after Cato performs the services. The statement of cash flows reflects a cash inflow from operating activities. The effects of this transaction on the financial statements are shown here.

Assets	=	Liab.	+	Stk. Equity		Rev.	−	Exp.	=	Net Inc.	Cash Flow
Cash	=	Unearn. Rev.				Rev.	−	Exp.	=	Net Inc.	Cash Flow
18,000	=	18,000	+	NA		NA	−	NA	=	NA	18,000 OA

Accounting for Supplies Purchase

EVENT 4   Cato purchased $800 of supplies on account.

The purchase of supplies on account is an *asset source transaction.* The asset account Supplies and the liability account Accounts Payable increase. The income statement is unaffected. Expense recognition is deferred until the supplies are used. The statement of cash flows is not affected. The effects of this transaction on the financial statements are shown here.

Assets	=	Liab.	+	Stk. Equity		Rev.	−	Exp.	=	Net Inc.	Cash Flow
Supplies	=	Accts. Pay.				Rev.	−	Exp.	=	Net Inc.	Cash Flow
800	=	800	+	NA		NA	−	NA	=	NA	NA

Other 2013 Events

EVENT 5   Cato provided $96,400 of consulting services on account.

Providing services on account is an *asset source transaction.* The asset account Accounts Receivable and the stockholders' equity account Retained Earnings increase.

Revenue and net income increase. The statement of cash flows is not affected. The effects of this transaction on the financial statements are shown here.

Assets	=	Liab.	+	Stk. Equity						
Accts. Rec.	=			Ret. Earn.	Rev.	−	Exp.	=	Net Inc.	Cash Flow
96,400	=	NA	+	96,400	96,400	−	NA	=	96,400	NA

EVENT 6 Cato collected $105,000 cash from customers as partial settlement of accounts receivable.

Collecting money from customers who are paying accounts receivable is an *asset exchange transaction.* One asset account (Cash) increases and another asset account (Accounts Receivable) decreases. The amount of total assets is unchanged. The income statement is not affected. The statement of cash flows reports a cash inflow from operating activities. The effects of this transaction on the financial statements are shown here.

Assets			=	Liab.	+	Stk. Equity					
Cash	+	Accts. Rec.					Rev.	−	Exp.	=	Net Inc.	Cash Flow
105,000	+	(105,000)	=	NA	+	NA	NA	−	NA	=	NA	105,000 OA

EVENT 7 Cato paid $32,000 cash for salary expense.

Cash payments for salary expense are *asset use transactions.* Both the asset account Cash and the equity account Retained Earnings decrease by $32,000. Recognizing the expense decreases net income on the income statement. The statement of cash flows reflects a cash outflow from operating activities. The effects of this transaction on the financial statements are shown here.

Assets	=	Liab.	+	Stk. Equity						
Cash	=			Ret. Earn.	Rev.	−	Exp.	=	Net Inc.	Cash Flow
(32,000)	=	NA	+	(32,000)	NA	−	32,000	=	(32,000)	(32,000) OA

EVENT 8 Cato incurred $21,000 of other operating expenses on account.

Recognizing expenses incurred on account are *claims exchange transactions.* One claims account (Accounts Payable) increases and another claims account (Retained Earnings) decreases. The amount of total claims is not affected. Recognizing the expenses decreases net income. The statement of cash flows is not affected. The effects of this transaction on the financial statements are shown here.

Assets	=	Liab.	+	Stk. Equity						
		Accts. Pay.	+	Ret. Earn.	Rev.	−	Exp.	=	Net Inc.	Cash Flow
NA	=	21,000	+	(21,000)	NA	−	21,000	=	(21,000)	NA

EVENT 9   Cato paid $18,200 in partial settlement of accounts payable.

Paying accounts payable is an *asset use transaction.* The asset account Cash and the liability account Accounts Payable decrease. The statement of cash flows reports a cash outflow for operating activities. The income statement is not affected. The effects of this transaction on the financial statements are shown here.

Assets	=	Liab.	+	Stk. Equity		Rev.	–	Exp.	=	Net Inc.	Cash Flow
Cash	=	Accts. Pay.				Rev.	–	Exp.	=	Net Inc.	Cash Flow
(18,200)	=	(18,200)	+	NA		NA	–	NA	=	NA	(18,200) OA

EVENT 10   Cato paid $79,500 to purchase land it planned to use in the future as a building site for its home office.

Purchasing land with cash is an *asset exchange transaction.* One asset account, Cash, decreases and another asset account, Land, increases. The amount of total assets is unchanged. The income statement is not affected. The statement of cash flows reports a cash outflow for investing activities. The effects of this transaction on the financial statements are shown here.

Assets			=	Liab.	+	Stk. Equity		Rev.	–	Exp.	=	Net Inc.	Cash Flow
Cash	+	Land						Rev.	–	Exp.	=	Net Inc.	Cash Flow
(79,500)	+	79,500	=	NA	+	NA		NA	–	NA	=	NA	(79,500) IA

EVENT 11   Cato paid $21,000 in cash dividends to its stockholders.

Cash payments for dividends are *asset use transactions.* Both the asset account Cash and the equity account Retained Earnings decrease. Recall that dividends are wealth transfers from the business to the stockholders, not expenses. They are not incurred in the process of generating revenue. They do not affect the income statement. The statement of cash flows reflects a cash outflow from financing activities. The effects of this transaction on the financial statements are shown here.

Assets	=	Liab.	+	Stk. Equity		Rev.	–	Exp.	=	Net Inc.	Cash Flow
Cash	=			Ret. Earn.		Rev.	–	Exp.	=	Net Inc.	Cash Flow
(21,000)	=	NA	+	(21,000)		NA	–	NA	=	NA	(21,000) FA

EVENT 12   Cato acquired $2,000 cash from issuing additional shares of common stock.

Issuing common stock is an *asset source transaction.* The asset account Cash and the stockholders' equity account Common Stock increase. The income statement is unaffected. The statement of cash flows reports a cash inflow from financing activities. The effects of this transaction on the financial statements are shown here.

Assets	=	Liab.	+	Stk. Equity		Rev.	–	Exp.	=	Net Inc.	Cash Flow
Cash	=			Com. Stk.		Rev.	–	Exp.	=	Net Inc.	Cash Flow
2,000	=	NA	+	2,000		NA	–	NA	=	NA	2,000 FA

Adjusting Entries

Recall that companies make adjusting entries at the end of an accounting period to update the account balances before preparing the financial statements. Adjusting entries ensure that companies report revenues and expenses in the appropriate accounting period; adjusting entries never affect the Cash account.

Accounting for Supplies (Adjusting Entry)

EVENT 13   After determining through a physical count that it had $150 of unused supplies on hand as of December 31, Cato recognized supplies expense.

Companies would find the cost of recording supplies expense each time a pencil, piece of paper, envelope, or other supply item is used to far outweigh the benefit derived from such tedious recordkeeping. Instead, accountants transfer to expense the total cost of all supplies used during the entire accounting period in a single year-end adjusting entry. The cost of supplies used is determined as follows.

Beginning supplies balance + Supplies purchased = Supplies available for use

Supplies available for use − Ending supplies balance = Supplies used

Companies determine the ending supplies balance by physically counting the supplies on hand at the end of the period. Cato used $650 of supplies during the year (zero beginning balance + $800 supplies purchase = $800 available for use; $800 available for use − $150 ending balance = $650). Recognizing Cato's supplies expense is an *asset use transaction.* The asset account Supplies and the stockholders' equity account Retained Earnings decrease. Recognizing supplies expense reduces net income. The statement of cash flows is not affected. The effects of this transaction on the financial statements are shown here.

Assets	=	Liab.	+	Stk. Equity						
Supplies	=			Ret. Earn.	Rev.	−	Exp.	=	Net Inc.	Cash Flow
(650)	=	NA	+	(650)	NA	−	650	=	(650)	NA

Accounting for Prepaid Rent (Adjusting Entry)

EVENT 14   Cato recognized rent expense for the office space used during the accounting period.

Recall that Cato paid $12,000 on March 1, 2013, to rent office space for one year (see Event 2). The portion of the lease cost that represents using office space from March 1 through December 31 is computed as follows.

$12,000 Cost of annual lease ÷ 12 Months = $1,000 Cost per month

$1,000 Cost per month × 10 Months used = $10,000 Rent expense

Recognizing the rent expense decreases the asset account Prepaid Rent and the stockholders' equity account Retained Earnings. Recognizing rent expense reduces net income. The statement of cash flows is not affected. The cash flow effect was recorded in the March 1 event. These effects on the financial statements follow.

Assets	=	Liab.	+	Stk. Equity						
Prep. Rent	=			Ret. Earn.	Rev.	−	Exp.	=	Net Inc.	Cash Flow
(10,000)	=	NA	+	(10,000)	NA	−	10,000	=	(10,000)	NA

✓ CHECK YOURSELF 2.2

Rujoub Inc. paid $18,000 cash for one year of insurance coverage that began on November 1, 2012. Based on this information alone, determine the cash flow from operating activities that Rujoub would report on the 2012 and 2013 statements of cash flows. Also, determine the amount of insurance expense Rujoub would report on the 2012 income statement and the amount of prepaid insurance (an asset) that Rujoub would report on the December 31, 2012, balance sheet.

Answer   Since Rujoub paid all of the cash in 2012, the 2012 statement of cash flows would report an $18,000 cash outflow from operating activities. The 2013 statement of cash flows would report zero cash flow from operating activities. The expense would be recognized in the periods in which the insurance is used. In this case, insurance expense is recognized at the rate of $1,500 per month ($18,000 ÷ 12 months). Rujoub used two months of insurance coverage in 2012 and therefore would report $3,000 (2 months × $1,500) of insurance expense on the 2012 income statement. Rujoub would report a $15,000 (10 months × $1,500) asset, prepaid insurance, on the December 31, 2012, balance sheet. The $15,000 of prepaid insurance would be recognized as insurance expese in 2013 when the insurance coverage is used.

Accounting for Unearned Revenue (Adjusting Entry)

EVENT 15   Cato recognized the portion of the unearned revenue it earned during the accounting period.

Recall that Cato received an $18,000 cash advance from Westberry Company to provide consulting services from June 1, 2013, to May 31, 2014 (see Event 3). By December 31, Cato had earned 7 months (June 1 through December 31) of the revenue related to this contract. Rather than recording the revenue continuously as it performed the consulting services, Cato can simply recognize the amount earned in a single adjustment to the accounting records at the end of the accounting period. The amount of the adjustment is computed as follows.

$$\$18,000 \div 12 \text{ months} = \$1,500 \text{ revenue earned per month}$$

$$\$1,500 \times 7 \text{ months} = \$10,500 \text{ revenue to be recognized in 2013}$$

The adjusting entry moves $10,500 from the Unearned Revenue account to the Consulting Revenue account. This entry is a *claims exchange transaction.* The liability account Unearned Revenue decreases and the equity account Retained Earnings increases. The effects of this transaction on the financial statements are shown here.

Assets	=	Liab.	+	Stk. Equity						
		Unearn. Rev.	+	Ret. Earn.	Rev.	−	Exp.	=	Net Inc.	Cash Flow
NA	=	(10,500)	+	10,500	10,500	−	NA	=	10,500	NA

Recall that revenue was previously defined as an economic benefit a company obtains by providing customers with goods and services. In this case the economic benefit is a decrease in the liability account Unearned Revenue. **Revenue** can therefore be more precisely defined as *an increase in assets or a decrease in liabilities that a company obtains by providing customers with goods or services.*

✓ CHECK YOURSELF 2.3

Sanderson & Associates received a $24,000 cash advance as a retainer to provide legal services to a client. The contract called for Sanderson to render services during a one-year period beginning October 1, 2012. Based on this information alone, determine the cash flow from operating activities Sanderson would report on the 2012 and 2013 statements of cash flows. Also determine the amount of revenue Sanderson would report on the 2012 and 2013 income statements.

Answer   Since Sanderson collected all of the cash in 2012, the 2012 statement of cash flows would report a $24,000 cash inflow from operating activities. The 2013 statement of cash flows would report zero cash flow from operating activities. Revenue is recognized in the period in which it is earned. In this case revenue is earned at the rate of $2,000 per month ($24,000 ÷ 12 months = $2,000 per month). Sanderson rendered services for three months in 2012 and nine months in 2013. Sanderson would report $6,000 (3 months × $2,000) of revenue on the 2012 income statement and $18,000 (9 months × $2,000) of revenue on the 2013 income statement.

Answers to The Curious Accountant

Because the Meredith Corporation receives cash from customers before actually providing any magazines to them, the company has not earned any revenue when it receives the cash. Thus, Meredith has a liability called *unearned revenue.* If it closed its books on December 31, then $3 of Arno's subscription would be recognized as revenue in 2012. The remaining $9 would appear on the balance sheet as a liability.

Meredith Corporation actually ends its accounting year on June 30 each year. A copy of the 2009 balance sheet for the company is presented in Exhibit 2.6. The liability for unearned subscription revenue was $319.1 ($170.7 + $148.4) million—which represented about 30.1 percent of Meredith's total liabilities!

Will Meredith need cash to pay these subscription liabilities? Not exactly. The liabilities will not be paid directly with cash. Instead, they will be satisfied by providing magazines to the subscribers. However, Meredith will need cash to pay for producing and distributing the magazines supplied to the customers. Even so, the amount of cash required to provide magazines will probably differ significantly from the amount of unearned revenues. In most cases, subscription fees do not cover the cost of producing and distributing magazines. By collecting significant amounts of advertising revenue, publishers can provide magazines to customers at prices well below the cost of publication. The amount of unearned revenue is not likely to coincide with the amount of cash needed to cover the cost of satisfying the company's obligation to produce and distribute magazines. Even though the association between unearned revenues and the cost of providing magazines to customers is not direct, a knowledgeable financial analyst can use the information to make estimates of future cash flows and revenue recognition.

| **EXHIBIT 2.6** | Balance Sheet for Meredith Corporation |

CONSOLIDATED BALANCE SHEETS
Meredith Corporation and Subsidiaries
As of June 30 (amounts in thousands)

	2009	2008
Assets		
Current assets		
Cash and cash equivalents	$ 27,910	$ 37,644
Accounts receivable		
(net of allowances of $13,810 in 2009 and $23,944 in 2008)	192,367	230,978
Inventories	28,151	44,085
Current portion of subscription acquisition costs	60,017	59,939
Current portion of broadcast rights	8,297	10,779
Deferred income taxes	—	2,118
Other current assets	23,398	17,547
Total current assets	340,140	403,090
Property, plant, and equipment		
Land	19,500	20,027
Buildings and improvements	125,779	122,977
Machinery and equipment	276,376	273,633
Leasehold improvements	14,208	12,840
Construction in progress	9,041	17,458
Total property, plant, and equipment	444,904	446,935
Less accumulated depreciation	(253,597)	(247,147)
Net property, plant, and equipment	191,307	199,788
Subscription acquisition costs	63,444	60,958
Broadcast rights	4,545	7,826
Other assets	45,907	74,472
Intangible assets, net	561,581	781,154
Goodwill	462,379	532,332
Total assets	$1,669,303	$2,059,620
Liabilities and Shareholders' Equity		
Current liabilities		
Current portion of long-term debt	$ —	$ 75,000
Current portion of long-term broadcast rights payable	10,560	11,141
Accounts payable	86,381	79,028
Accrued expenses		
Compensation and benefits	42,667	40,894
Distribution expenses	12,224	13,890
Other taxes and expenses	26,653	47,923
Total accrued expenses	81,544	102,707
Current portion of unearned subscription revenues	170,731	175,261
Total current liabilities	349,216	443,137
Long-term debt	380,000	410,000
Long-term broadcast rights payable	11,851	17,186
Unearned subscription revenues	148,393	157,872
Deferred income taxes	64,322	139,598
Other noncurrent liabilities	106,138	103,972
Total liabilities	1,059,920	1,271,765
Shareholders' equity		
Series preferred stock, par value $1 per share	—	—
Common stock, par value $1 per share	35,934	36,295
Class B stock, par value $1 per share, convertible to common stock	9,133	9,181
Additional paid-in capital	53,938	52,693
Retained earnings	542,006	701,205
Accumulated other comprehensive income (loss)	(31,628)	(11,519)
Total shareholders' equity	609,383	787,855
Total liabilities and shareholder' equity	$1,669,303	$2,059,620

Accounting for Accrued Salary Expense (Adjusting Entry)

EVENT 16   Cato recognized $4,000 of accrued salary expense.

The adjusting entry to recognize the accrued salary expense is a *claims exchange transaction.* One claims account, Retained Earnings, decreases and another claims account, Salaries Payable, increases. The expense recognition reduces net income. The statement of cash flows is not affected. The effects of this transaction on the financial statements are shown here.

Assets	=	Liab.	+	Stk. Equity						
		Sal. Pay.	+	Ret. Earn.	Rev.	−	Exp.	=	Net Inc.	Cash Flow
NA	=	4,000	+	(4,000)	NA	−	4,000	=	(4,000)	NA

Summary of Events and General Ledger

The previous section of this chapter described sixteen events Cato Consultants experienced the during the 2013 accounting period. These events are summarized in Exhibit 2.7 on page 63. The associated general ledger accounts are also shown in the exhibit. The account balances at the end of 2012; shown in Exhibit 2.3, become the beginning balances for the 2013 accounting period. The 2013 transaction data are referenced to the accounting events with numbers in parentheses. The information in the ledger accounts is the basis for the financial statements in Exhibit 2.8 on pages 64 and 65. Before reading further, trace each event in the summary of events into Exhibit 2.7.

Vertical Statements Model

Financial statement users obtain helpful insights by analyzing company trends over multiple accounting cycles. Exhibit 2.8 presents for Cato Consultants a multicycle **vertical statements model** of 2012 and 2013 accounting data. To conserve space, we have combined all the expenses for each year into single amounts labeled "Operating Expenses," determined as follows.

	2012	2013
Other operating expenses	$ 0	$21,000
Salary expense	16,000	36,000
Rent expense	0	10,000
Advertising expense	2,000	0
Supplies expense	0	650
Total operating expenses	$18,000	$67,650

Similarly, we combined the cash payments for operating expenses on the statement of cash flows as follows.

	2012	2013
Supplies and other operating expenses	$ 0	$18,200*
Salary expense	10,000	38,000
Rent expense	0	12,000
Advertising expense	2,000	0
Total cash payments for operating expenses	$12,000	$68,200

*Amount paid in partial settlement of accounts payable

EXHIBIT 2.7

Ledger Accounts with 2013 Trnsaction Data

1. Cato paid $6,000 to the instructor to settle the salaries payable obligation.
2. On March 1, Cato paid $12,000 cash to lease office space for one year.
3. Cato received $18,000 cash in advance from Westberry Company for consulting services to be performed for one year beginning June 1.
4. Cato purchased $800 of supplies on account.
5. Cato provided $96,400 of consulting services on account.
6. Cato collected $105,000 cash from customers as partial settlement of accounts receivable.
7. Cato paid $32,000 cash for salary expense.
8. Cato incurred $21,000 of other operating expenses on account.
9. Cato paid $18,200 in partial settlement of accounts payable.
10. Cato paid $79,500 to purchase land it planned to use in the future as a building site for its home office.
11. Cato paid $21,000 in cash dividends to its stockholders.
12. Cato acquired $2,000 cash from issuing additional shares of common stock.

The year-end adjustments are:

13. After determining through a physical count that it had $150 of unused supplies on hand as of December 31, Cato recognized supplies expense.
14. Cato recognized rent expense for the office space used during the accounting period.
15. Cato recognized the portion of the unearned revenue it earned during the accounting period.
16. Cato recognized $4,000 of accrued salary expense.

| | Assets | | = | Liabilities | + | | Stockholders' Equity |

Assets

Cash		Prepaid Rent	
Bal.	53,000	Bal.	0
(1)	(6,000)	(2)	12,000
(2)	(12,000)	(14)	(10,000)
(3)	18,000	Bal.	2,000
(6)	105,000		
(7)	(32,000)	**Land**	
(9)	(18,200)	Bal.	0
(10)	(79,500)	(10)	79,500
(11)	(21,000)	Bal.	79,500
(12)	2,000		
Bal.	9,300		

Accounts Receivable	
Bal.	24,000
(5)	96,400
(6)	(105,000)
Bal.	15,400

Supplies	
Bal.	0
(4)	800
(13)	(650)
Bal.	150

Liabilities

Accounts Payable	
Bal.	0
(4)	800
(8)	21,000
(9)	(18,200)
Bal.	3,600

Unearned Revenue	
Bal.	0
(3)	18,000
(15)	(10,500)
Bal.	7,500

Salaries Payable	
Bal.	6,000
(1)	(6,000)
(16)	4,000
Bal.	4,000

Stockholders' Equity

Common Stock	
Bal.	5,000
(12)	2,000
Bal.	7,000

Retained Earnings	
Bal.	66,000

Dividends	
Bal.	0
(11)	(21,000)
Bal.	(21,000)

Consulting Revenue	
Bal.	0
(5)	96,400
(15)	10,500
Bal.	106,900

Other Operating Expenses	
Bal.	0
(8)	(21,000)
Bal.	(21,000)

Salary Expense	
Bal.	0
(7)	(32,000)
(16)	(4,000)
Bal.	(36,000)

Rent Expense	
Bal.	0
(14)	(10,000)
Bal.	(10,000)

Supplies Expense	
Bal.	0
(13)	(650)
Bal.	(650)

EXHIBIT 2.8   Vertical Statements Model

CATO CONSULTANTS
Financial Statements
Income Statements
For the Years Ended December 31

	2012	2013
Consulting revenue	$84,000	$106,900
Operating expenses	(18,000)	(67,650)
Net income	$66,000	$ 39,250

Statements of Changes in Stockholders' Equity
For the Years Ended December 31

	2012	2013
Beginning common stock	$ 0	$ 5,000
Plus: Common stock issued	5,000	2,000
Ending common stock	5,000	7,000
Beginning retained earnings	0	66,000
Plus: Net income	66,000	39,250
Less: Dividends	0	(21,000)
Ending retained earnings	66,000	84,250
Total stockholders' equity	$71,000	$ 91,250

Balance Sheets
As of December 31

	2012	2013
Assets		
Cash	$53,000	$ 9,300
Accounts receivable	24,000	15,400
Supplies	0	150
Prepaid rent	0	2,000
Land	0	79,500
Total assets	$77,000	$106,350
Liabilities		
Accounts payable	$ 0	$ 3,600
Unearned revenue	0	7,500
Salaries payable	6,000	4,000
Total liabilities	6,000	15,100
Stockholders' equity		
Common stock	5,000	7,000
Retained earnings	66,000	84,250
Total stockholders' equity	71,000	91,250
Total liabilities and stockholders' equity	$77,000	$106,350

continued

EXHIBIT 2.8   *Concluded*

Statements of Cash Flows
For the Years Ended December 31

	2012	2013
Cash Flows from Operating Activities		
Cash receipts from customers	$60,000	$123,000
Cash payments for operating expenses	(12,000)	(68,200)
Net cash flow from operating activities	48,000	54,800
Cash Flows from Investing Activities		
Cash payment to purchase land	0	(79,500)
Cash Flows from Financing Activities		
Cash receipts from issuing common stock	5,000	2,000
Cash payments for dividends	0	(21,000)
Net cash flow from financing activities	5,000	(19,000)
Net change in cash	53,000	(43,700)
Plus: Beginning cash balance	0	53,000
Ending cash balance	$53,000	$ 9,300

Recall that the level of detail reported in financial statements depends on user information needs. Most real-world companies combine many account balances together to report highly summarized totals under each financial statement caption. Before reading further, trace the remaining financial statement items from the ledger accounts in Exhibit 2.7 to where they are reported in Exhibit 2.8.

The vertical statements model in Exhibit 2.8 shows significant interrelationships among the financial statements. For each year, trace the amount of net income from the income statement to the statement of changes in stockholders' equity. Next, trace the ending balances of common stock and retained earnings reported on the statement of changes in stockholders' equity to the stockholders' equity section of the balance sheet. Also, confirm that the amount of cash reported on the balance sheet equals the ending cash balance on the statement of cash flows.

Other relationships connect the two accounting periods. For example, trace the ending retained earnings balance from the 2012 statement of stockholders' equity to the beginning retained earnings balance on the 2013 statement of stockholders' equity. Also, trace the ending cash balance on the 2012 statement of cash flows to the beginning cash balance on the 2013 statement of cash flows. Finally, confirm that the change in cash between the 2012 and 2013 balance sheets ($53,000 − $9,300 = $43,700 decrease) agrees with the net change in cash reported on the 2013 statement of cash flows.

✓ CHECK YOURSELF 2.4

Treadmore Company started the 2012 accounting period with $580 of supplies on hand. During 2012 the company paid cash to purchase $2,200 of supplies. A physical count of supplies indicated that there was $420 of supplies on hand at the end of 2012. Treadmore pays cash for supplies at the time they are purchased. Based on this information alone, determine the amount of supplies expense to be recognized on the income statement and the amount of cash flow to be shown in the operating activities section of the statement of cash flows.

Answer The amount of supplies expense recognized on the income statement is the amount of supplies that were used during the accounting period. This amount is computed below.

$580 Beginning balance + $2,200 Supplies purchases = $2,780 Supplies available for use

$2,780 Supplies available for use − $420 Ending supplies balance = $2,360 supplies used

The cash flow from operating activities is the amount of cash paid for supplies during the accounting period. In this case, Treadmore paid $2,200 cash to purchase supplies. This amount would be shown as a cash outflow.

TRANSACTION CLASSIFICATION

LO 6

Classify accounting events into one of four categories:

a. asset source transactions.
b. asset use transactions.
c. asset exchange transactions.
d. claims exchange transactions.

Chapters 1 and 2 introduced four types of transactions. Although businesses engage in an infinite number of different transactions, all transactions fall into one of four types. By learning to identify transactions by type, you can understand how unfamiliar events affect financial statements. The four types of transactions are

1. *Asset source transactions:* An asset account increases, and a corresponding claims account increases.
2. *Asset use transactions:* An asset account decreases, and a corresponding claims account decreases.
3. *Asset exchange transactions:* One asset account increases, and another asset account decreases.
4. *Claims exchange transactions:* One claims account increases, and another claims account decreases.

Also, the definitions of revenue and expense have been expanded. The complete definitions of these two elements are as follows.

1. **Revenue:** Revenue is the *economic benefit* derived from operating the business. Its recognition is accompanied by an increase in assets or a decrease in liabilities resulting from providing products or services to customers.
2. **Expense:** An expense is an *economic sacrifice* incurred in the process of generating revenue. Its recognition is accompanied by a decrease in assets or an increase in liabilities resulting from consuming assets and services in an effort to produce revenue.

<< A Look Back

This chapter introduced accrual accounting. Accrual accounting distinguishes between *recognition* and *realization.* Recognition means reporting an economic item or event in the financial statements. In contrast, realization refers to collecting cash from the sale of assets or services. Recognition and realization can occur in different accounting periods. In addition, cash payments for expenses often occur in different accounting periods from when a company recognizes the expenses. Accrual accounting uses both *accruals* and *deferrals.*

■ The term *accrual* applies to a revenue or an expense event that are recognized before cash is exchanged. Recognizing revenue on account or accrued salaries expense are examples of accruals.

■ The term *deferral* applies to a revenue or an expense event that are recognized after cash has been exchanged. Supplies, prepaid items, and unearned revenue are examples of deferrals.

Virtually all major companies operating in the United States use accrual accounting.

A Look Forward

Chapters 1 and 2 focused on businesses that generate revenue by providing services to their customers. Examples of these types of businesses include consulting, real estate sales, medical services, and legal services. The next chapter introduces accounting practices for businesses that generate revenue by selling goods. Examples of these companies include Wal-Mart, Circuit City, Office Depot, and Lowes.

A step-by-step audio-narrated series of slides is provided on the text website at www.mhhe.com/edmondssurvey3e

SELF-STUDY REVIEW PROBLEM

Gifford Company experienced the following accounting events during 2012.

1. Started operations on January 1 when it acquired $20,000 cash by issuing common stock.
2. Earned $18,000 of revenue on account.
3. On March 1 collected $36,000 cash as an advance for services to be performed in the future.
4. Paid cash operating expenses of $17,000.
5. Paid a $2,700 cash dividend to stockholders.
6. On December 31, 2012, adjusted the books to recognize the revenue earned by providing services related to the advance described in Event 3. The contract required Gifford to provide services for a one-year period starting March 1.
7. Collected $15,000 cash from accounts receivable.

Gifford Company experienced the following accounting events during 2013.

1. Earned $38,000 of cash revenue.
2. On April 1 paid $12,000 cash for an insurance policy that provides coverage for one year beginning immediately.
3. Collected $2,000 cash from accounts receivable.
4. Paid cash operating expenses of $21,000.
5. Paid a $5,000 cash dividend to stockholders.
6. On December 31, 2013, adjusted the books to recognize the remaining revenue earned by providing services related to the advance described in Event 3 of 2012.
7. On December 31, 2013, Gifford adjusted the books to recognize the amount of the insurance policy used during 2013.

Required

a. Record the events in a financial statements model like the following one. The first event is recorded as an example.

Event No.	Assets			=	Liab.	+	Stockholders' Equity							
	Cash +	Accts. Rec. −	Prep. Ins.	=	Unearn. Rev.	+	Com. Stk. +	Ret. Earn.	Rev. −	Exp. =	Net Inc.	Cash Flow		
1	20,000 +	NA −	NA	=	NA	+	20,000 +	NA	NA −	NA =	NA	20,000 FA		

b. What amount of revenue would Gifford report on the 2012 income statement?
c. What amount of cash flow from customers would Gifford report on the 2012 statement of cash flows?
d. What amount of unearned revenue would Gifford report on the 2012 and 2013 year-end balance sheets?
e. What are the 2013 opening balances for the revenue and expense accounts?

f. What amount of total assets would Gifford report on the December 31, 2012, balance sheet?

g. What claims on assets would Gifford report on the December 31, 2013, balance sheet?

Solution to Requirement a

The financial statements model follows.

Event No.	Assets				=	Liab.	+	Stockholders' Equity					Rev.	−	Exp.	=	Net Inc.		Cash Flow
	Cash	+	Accts. Rec.	+	Prep. Ins.	=	Unearn. Rev.	+	Com. Stk.	+	Ret. Earn.		Rev.	−	Exp.	=	Net Inc.		Cash Flow
2012																			
1	20,000	+	NA	+	NA	=	NA	+	20,000	+	NA		NA	−	NA	=	NA		20,000 FA
2	NA	+	18,000	+	NA	=	NA	+	NA	+	18,000		18,000	−	NA	=	18,000		NA
3	36,000	+	NA	+	NA	=	36,000	+	NA	+	NA		NA	−	NA	=	NA		36,000 OA
4	(17,000)	+	NA	+	NA	=	NA	+	NA	+	(17,000)		NA	−	17,000	=	(17,000)		(17,000) OA
5	(2,700)	+	NA	+	NA	=	NA	+	NA	+	(2,700)		NA	−	NA	=	NA		(2,700) FA
6*	NA	+	NA	+	NA	=	(30,000)	+	NA	+	30,000		30,000	−	NA	=	30,000		NA
7	15,000	+	(15,000)	+	NA	=	NA	+	NA	+	NA		NA	−	NA	=	NA		15,000 OA
Bal.	51,300	+	3,000	+	NA	=	6,000	+	20,000	+	28,300		48,000	−	17,000	=	31,000		51,300 NC
	Asset, liability, and equity account balances carry forward												Rev. & exp. accts. are closed						
2013																			
Bal.	51,300	+	3,000	+	NA	=	6,000	+	20,000	+	28,300		NA	−	NA	=	NA		NA
1	38,000	+	NA	+	NA	=	NA	+	NA	+	38,000		38,000	−	NA	=	38,000		38,000 OA
2	(12,000)	+	NA	+	12,000	=	NA	+	NA	+	NA		NA	−	NA	=	NA		(12,000) OA
3	2,000	+	(2,000)	+	NA	=	NA	+	NA	+	NA		NA	−	NA	=	NA		2,000 OA
4	(21,000)	+	NA	+	NA	=	NA	+	NA	+	(21,000)		NA	−	21,000	=	(21,000)		(21,000) OA
5	(5,000)	+	NA	+	NA	=	NA	+	NA	+	(5,000)		NA	−	NA	=	NA		(5,000) FA
6*	NA	+	NA	+	NA	=	(6,000)	+	NA	+	6,000		6,000	−	NA	=	6,000		NA
7†	NA	+	NA	+	(9,000)	=	NA	+	NA	+	(9,000)		NA	−	9,000	=	(9,000)		NA
Bal.	53,300	+	1,000	+	3,000	=	0	+	20,000	+	37,300		44,000	−	30,000	=	14,000		2,000 NC

*Revenue is earned at the rate of $3,000 ($36,000 ÷ 12 months) per month. Revenue recognized in 2012 is $30,000 ($3,000 × 10 months). Revenue recognized in 2013 is $6,000 ($3,000 × 2 months).

†Insurance expense is incurred at the rate of $1,000 ($12,000 ÷ 12 months) per month. Insurance expense recognized in 2013 is $9,000 ($1,000 × 9 months).

Solutions to Requirements b–g

b. Gifford would report $48,000 of revenue in 2012 ($18,000 revenue on account plus $30,000 of the $36,000 of unearned revenue).

c. The cash inflow from customers is $51,000 ($36,000 when the unearned revenue was received plus $15,000 collection of accounts receivable).

d. The December 31, 2012, balance sheet will report $6,000 of unearned revenue, which is the amount of the cash advance less the amount of revenue recognized in 2012 ($36,000 − $30,000). The December 31, 2013, unearned revenue balance is zero.

e. Since revenue and expense accounts are closed at the end of each accounting period, the beginning balances in these accounts are always zero.

f. Assets on the December 31, 2012, balance sheet are $54,300 [Gifford's cash at year end plus the balance in accounts receivable ($51,300 + $3,000)].

g. Since all unearned revenue would be recognized before the financial statements were prepared at the end of 2013, there would be no liabilities on the 2013 balance sheet. Common stock and retained earnings would be the only claims as of December 31, 2013, for a claims total of $57,300 ($20,000 + $37,300).

KEY TERMS

Accounts Receivable 46	Accrued expenses 48	Asset source
Accrual 45	Adjusting entry 48	transaction 46
Accrual accounting 45	Asset exchange transaction 46	Asset use transaction 47

Claims exchange
    transaction 48
Conservatism 53
Deferral 45

Matching concept 53
Period costs 53
Prepaid items 54
Realization 44

Recognition 44
Salaries Payable 46
Unearned revenue 55
Vertical statements model 62

QUESTIONS

1. What does accrual accounting attempt to accomplish?

2. Define *recognition*. How is it independent of collecting or paying cash?

3. What does the term *deferral* mean?

4. If cash is collected in advance of performing services, when is the associated revenue recognized?

5. What does the term *asset source transaction* mean?

6. What effect does the issue of common stock have on the accounting equation?

7. How does the recognition of revenue on account (accounts receivable) affect the income statement compared to its effect on the statement of cash flows?

8. Give an example of an asset source transaction. What is the effect of this transaction on the accounting equation?

9. When is revenue recognized under accrual accounting?

10. Give an example of an asset exchange transaction. What is the effect of this transaction on the accounting equation?

11. What is the effect on the claims side of the accounting equation when cash is collected in advance of performing services?

12. What does the term *unearned revenue* mean?

13. What effect does expense recognition have on the accounting equation?

14. What does the term *claims exchange transaction* mean?

15. What type of transaction is a cash payment to creditors? How does this type of transaction affect the accounting equation?

16. When are expenses recognized under accrual accounting?

17. Why may net cash flow from operating activities on the cash flow statement be different from the amount of net income reported on the income statement?

18. What is the relationship between the income statement and changes in assets and liabilities?

19. How does net income affect the stockholders' claims on the business's assets?

20. What is the difference between a cost and an expense?

21. When does a cost become an expense? Do all costs become expenses?

22. How and when is the cost of the *supplies used* recognized in an accounting period?

23. What does the term *expense* mean?

24. What does the term *revenue* mean?

25. What is the purpose of the statement of changes in stockholders' equity?

26. What is the main purpose of the balance sheet?

27. Why is the balance sheet dated *as of* a specific date when the income statement, statement of changes in stockholders' equity, and statement of cash flows are dated with the phrase *for the period ended?*

28. In what order are assets listed on the balance sheet?

29. What does the statement of cash flows explain?

30. What does the term *adjusting entry* mean? Give an example.

31. What types of accounts are closed at the end of the accounting period? Why is it necessary to close these accounts?

32. Give several examples of period costs.

33. Give an example of a cost that can be directly matched with the revenue produced by an accounting firm from preparing a tax return.

34. List and describe the four stages of the accounting cycle discussed in Chapter 2.

 MULTIPLE-CHOICE QUESTIONS

Multiple-choice questions are provided on the text website at www.mhhe.com/edmondssurvey3e.

EXERCISES

All applicable Exercises are available with McGraw-Hill's
Connect Accounting.

Where applicable in all exercises, round computations to the nearest dollar.

LO 2, 3

Exercise 2-1 *Effect of accruals on the financial statements*

Valmont, Inc., experienced the following events in 2012, in its first year of operation.

1. Received $20,000 cash from the issue of common stock.
2. Performed services on account for $50,000.
3. Paid the utility expense of $12,500.
4. Collected $39,000 of the accounts receivable.
5. Recorded $9,000 of accrued salaries at the end of the year.
6. Paid a $5,000 cash dividend to the shareholders.

Required

a. Record the events in general ledger accounts under an accounting equation. In the last column of the table, provide appropriate account titles for the Retained Earnings amounts. The first transaction has been recorded as an example.

VALMONT, INC.							
General Ledger Accounts							
Event	Assets		=	Liabilities	+	Stockholders' Equity		Acct. Titles for RE
	Cash	Accounts Receivable		Salaries Payable		Common Stock	Retained Earnings	
1.	20,000					20,000		

b. Prepare the income statement, statement of changes in stockholders' equity, balance sheet, and statement of cash flows for the 2012 accounting period.
c. Why is the amount of net income different from the amount of net cash flow from operating activities?

LO 2, 3

Exercise 2-2 *Effect of collecting accounts receivable on the accounting equation and financial statements*

Schroder Company earned $14,000 of service revenue on account during 2012. The company collected $11,500 cash from accounts receivable during 2012.

Required

Based on this information alone, determine the following. (*Hint:* Record the events in general ledger accounts under an accounting equation before satisfying the requirements.)

a. The balance of the accounts receivable that Schroder would report on the December 31, 2012, balance sheet.
b. The amount of net income that Schroder would report on the 2012 income statement.
c. The amount of net cash flow from operating activities that Schroder would report on the 2012 statement of cash flows.
d. The amount of retained earnings that Schroder would report on the 2012 balance sheet.
e. Why are the answers to Requirements *b* and *c* different?

LO 2, 3

Exercise 2-3 *Effect of prepaid rent on the accounting equation and financial statements*

The following events apply to 2012, the first year of operations of Sentry Services.

1. Acquired $45,000 cash from the issue of common stock.
2. Paid $18,000 cash in advance for one-year rental contract for office space.

3. Provided services for $36,000 cash.
4. Adjusted the records to recognize the use of the office space. The one-year contract started on May 1, 2012. The adjustment was made as of December 31, 2012.

Required

a. Write an accounting equation and record the effects of each accounting event under the appropriate general ledger account headings.
b. Prepare an income statement and statement of cash flows for the 2012 accounting period.
c. Explain the difference between the amount of net income and amount of net cash flow from operating activities.

Exercise 2-4   *Effect of supplies on the financial statements*

LO 1, 3

Green Copy Service, Inc., started the 2012 accounting period with $16,000 cash, $10,000 of common stock, and $6,000 of retained earnings. Green Copy Service was affected by the following accounting events during 2012.

1. Purchased $9,600 of paper and other supplies on account.
2. Earned and collected $39,000 of cash revenue.
3. Paid $7,000 cash on accounts payable.
4. Adjusted the records to reflect the use of supplies. A physical count indicated that $2,200 of supplies was still on hand on December 31, 2012.

Required

a. Show the effects of the events on the financial statements using a horizontal statements model like the following one. In the Cash Flows column, use OA to designate operating activity, IA for investing activity, FA for financing activity, and NC for net change in cash. Use NA to indicate accounts not affected by the event. The beginning balances are entered in the following example.

Event No.	Assets			=	Liab.	+	Stockholders' Equity			Rev.	–	Exp.	=	Net Inc.	Cash Flows
	Cash	+	Supplies	=	Accts. Pay	+	C. Stock	+	Ret. Earn.						
Beg. Bal.	16,000	+	0	=	0	+	10,000	+	6,000	0	–	0	=	0	0

b. Explain the difference between the amount of net income and amount of net cash flow from operating activities.

Exercise 2-5   *Effect of unearned revenue on financial statements*

LO 1, 3, 5

Michael Stone started a personal financial planning business when he accepted $120,000 cash as advance payment for managing the financial assets of a large estate. Stone agreed to manage the estate for a one-year period, beginning April 1, 2012.

Required

a. Show the effects of the advance payment and revenue recognition on the 2012 financial statements using a horizontal statements model like the following one. In the Cash Flows column, use OA to designate operating activity, IA for investing activity, FA for financing activity, and NC for net change in cash. Use NA if the account is not affected.

Event No.	Assets	=	Liab.	+	Stockholders' Equity	Rev.	–	Exp.	=	Net Inc.	Cash Flows
	Cash	=	Unearn. Rev.	+	Ret. Earn.						

b. How much revenue would Stone recognize on the 2013 income statement?
c. What is the amount of cash flow from operating activities in 2013?

Exercise 2-6   *Unearned revenue defined as a liability*

LO 3

Harry Baldwin received $500 in advance for tutoring fees when he agreed to help Joseph Jones with his introductory accounting course. Upon receiving the cash, Harry mentioned that he would have to record the transaction as a liability on his books. Jones asked, "Why a liability? You don't owe me any money, do you?"

Required

Respond to Jones' question regarding Baldwin's liability.

LO 3

Exercise 2-7 *Distinguishing between an expense and a cost*

Eddie Kirn tells you that the accountants where he works are real hair splitters. For example, they make a big issue over the difference between a cost and an expense. He says the two terms mean the same thing to him.

Required

a. Explain to Eddie the difference between a cost and an expense from an accountant's perspective.

b. Indicate whether each of the following events produces an asset or an expense.

   (1) Recognized accrued salaries.

   (2) Paid in advance for insurance on the building.

   (3) Used supplies on hand to produce revenue.

   (4) Purchased supplies on account.

   (5) Purchased a building for cash.

LO 3

Exercise 2-8 *Revenue and expense recognition*

Required

a. Describe an expense recognition event that results in a decrease in assets.

b. Describe an expense recognition event that results in an increase in liabilities.

c. Describe a revenue recognition event that results in an increase in assets.

d. Describe a revenue recognition event that results in a decrease in liabilities.

LO 3

Exercise 2-9 *Transactions that affect the elements of financial statements*

Required

Give an example of a transaction that will

a. Increase a liability and decrease equity (claims exchange event).

b. Increase an asset and increase equity (asset source event).

c. Decrease a liability and increase equity (claims exchange event).

d. Increase an asset and decrease another asset (asset exchange event).

e. Increase an asset and increase a liability (asset source event).

f. Decrease an asset and decrease a liability (asset use event).

g. Decrease an asset and decrease equity (asset use event).

LO 3

Exercise 2-10 *Identifying deferral and accrual events*

Required

Identify each of the following events as an accrual, deferral, or neither.

a. Provided services on account.

b. Collected accounts receivable.

c. Paid one year's rent in advance.

d. Paid cash for utilities expense.

e. Collected $2,400 in advance for services to be performed over the next 12 months.

f. Incurred other operating expenses on account.

g. Recorded expense for salaries owed to employees at the end of the accounting period.

h. Paid a cash dividend to the stockholders.

i. Paid cash to purchase supplies to be used over the next several months.

j. Purchased land with cash.

Exercise 2-11   *Prepaid and unearned rent*   LO 2

On August 1, 2012, Woodworks paid Warehouse Rentals $54,000 for a 12-month lease on ware-house space.

Required

a. Record the deferral and the related December 31, 2012, adjustment for Woodworks in the accounting equation.

b. Record the deferral and the related December 31, 2012, adjustment for Warehouse Rentals in the accounting equation.

Exercise 2-12   *Classifying events on the statement of cash flows*   LO 3

The following transactions pertain to the operations of Fleming Company for 2012.

1. Acquired $40,000 cash from the issue of common stock.
2. Performed services for $12,000 cash.
3. Provided $55,000 of services on account.
4. Received $36,000 cash in advance for services to be performed over the next two years.
5. Incurred $30,000 of other operating expenses on account.
6. Collected $45,000 cash from accounts receivable.
7. Paid $4,000 cash for rent expense.
8. Paid $12,000 for one year's prepaid insurance.
9. Paid a $5,000 cash dividend to the stockholders.
10. Paid $22,000 cash on accounts payable.

Required

a. Classify the cash flows from these transactions as operating activities (OA), investing activities (IA), or financing activities (FA). Use NA for transactions that do not affect the statement of cash flows.

b. Prepare a statement of cash flows. (There is no beginning cash balance.)

Exercise 2-13   *Effect of accounting events on the income statement and statement*   LO 3
                   of cash flows

Required

Explain how each of the following events and the related adjusting entry will affect the amount of *net income* and the amount of *cash flow from operating activities* reported on the year-end financial statements. Identify the direction of change (increase, decrease, or NA) and the amount of the change. Organize your answers according to the following table. The first event is recorded as an example. If an event does not have a related adjusting entry, record only the effects of the event. All adjustments are made on December 31.

	Net Income		Cash Flows from Operating Activities	
Event No.	Direction of Change	Amount of Change	Direction of Change	Amount of Change
a	NA	NA	NA	NA

a. Acquired $50,000 cash from the issue of common stock.

b. Paid $4,800 cash on October 1 to purchase a one-year insurance policy.

c. Collected $18,000 in advance for services to be performed in the future. The contract called for services to start on September 1 and to continue for one year.

d. Earned $22,000 of revenue on account. Collected $18,000 cash from accounts receivable.

e. Sold land that had cost $10,000 for $10,000.

f. Accrued salaries amounting to $8,000.

g. Provided services for $12,000 cash.

h. Paid cash for other operating expenses of $3,500.

i. Purchased $1,800 of supplies on account. Paid $1,500 cash on accounts payable. The ending balance in the Supplies account, after adjustment, was $600.

LO 1, 6

Exercise 2-14 *Identifying transaction type and effect on the financial statements*

Required

Identify whether each of the following transactions is an asset source (AS), asset use (AU), asset exchange (AE), or claims exchange (CE). Also show the effects of the events on the financial statements using the horizontal statements model. Indicate whether the event increases (I), decreases (D), or does not affect (NA) each element of the financial statements. In the Cash Flows column, designate the cash flows as operating activities (OA), investing activities (IA), or financing activities (FA). The first two transactions have been recorded as examples.

Event No.	Type of Event	Assets	=	Liabilities	+	Stockholders' Equity Common Stock	+	Stockholders' Equity Retained Earnings	Rev.	−	Exp.	=	Net Inc.	Cash Flows	
a	AS	I		NA		I		NA	NA		NA		NA	I	FA
b	AE	I/D		NA		NA		NA	NA		NA		NA	D	IA

a. Acquired cash from the issue of common stock.

b. Purchased land for cash.

c. Paid cash advance for rent on office space.

d. Collected cash from accounts receivable.

e. Performed services for cash.

f. Purchased a building with part cash *and* issued a note payable for the balance.

g. Paid cash for operating expenses.

h. Paid cash for supplies.

i. Paid a cash dividend to the stockholders.

j. Incurred operating expenses on account.

k. Paid cash on accounts payable.

l. Received cash advance for services to be provided in the future.

m. Recorded accrued salaries.

n. Performed services on account.

o. Adjusted books to reflect the amount of prepaid rent expired during the period.

p. Paid cash for salaries accrued at the end of a prior period.

LO 1

Exercise 2-15 *Effect of accruals and deferrals on financial statements: the horizontal statements model*

K. Little, Attorney at Law, experienced the following transactions in 2012, the first year of operations.

1. Purchased $2,800 of office supplies on account.

2. Accepted $30,000 on February 1, 2012, as a retainer for services to be performed evenly over the next 12 months.

3. Performed legal services for cash of $87,000.

4. Paid cash for salaries expense of $38,500.

5. Paid a cash dividend of $10,000 to the stockholders.

6. Paid $1,800 of the amount due on accounts payable.
7. Determined that at the end of the accounting period, $300 of office supplies remained on hand.
8. On December 31, 2012, recognized the revenue that had been earned for services performed in accordance with Transaction 2.

Required

Show the effects of the events on the financial statements using a horizontal statements model like the following one. In the Cash Flow column, use the initials OA to designate operating activity, IA for investing activity, FA for financing activity, and NC for net change in cash. Use NA to indicate accounts not affected by the event. The first event has been recorded as an example.

Event No.	Assets		=	Liabilities			+	Stk. Equity	Rev.	−	Exp.	=	Net Inc.	Cash Flow
	Cash	+ Supp.	=	Accts. Pay.	+	Unearn. Rev.	+	Ret. Earn.						
1	NA	+ 2,800	=	2,800	+	NA	+	NA	NA	−	NA	=	NA	NA

Exercise 2-16 *Effect of an error on financial statements*

LO 2, 3

On May 1, 2012, Virginia Corporation paid $18,000 cash in advance for a one-year lease on an office building. Assume that Virginia records the prepaid rent and that the books are closed on December 31.

Required

a. Show the payment for the one-year lease and the related adjusting entry to rent expense in the accounting equation.
b. Assume that Virginia Corporation failed to record the adjusting entry to reflect using the office building. How would the error affect the company's 2012 income statement and balance sheet?

Exercise 2-17 *Net income versus changes in cash*

LO 2, 3

In 2012, Cherry Design billed its customers $58,000 for services performed. The company collected $46,000 of the amount billed. Cherry Design incurred $41,000 of other operating expenses on acount. Cherry Design paid $30,000 of the accounts payable. Cherry Design acquired $40,000 cash from the issue of common stock. The company invested $20,000 cash in the purchase of land.

Required

Use the preceding information to answer the following questions. (*Hint:* Identify the six events described in the paragraph and record them in general ledger accounts under an accounting equation before attempting to answer the questions.)

a. What amount of revenue will Cherry Design report on the 2012 income statement?
b. What amount of cash flow from revenue will Cherry Design report on the statement of cash flows?
c. What is the net income for the period?
d. What is the net cash flow from operating activities for the period?
e. Why is the amount of net income different from the net cash flow from operating activities for the period?
f. What is the amount of net cash flow from investing activities?
g. What is the amount of net cash flow from financing activities?
h. What amounts of total assets, liabilities, and equity will Cherry Design report on the year-end balance sheet?

LO 3

Exercise 2-18 *Adjusting the accounts*

Keystore Systems experienced the following accounting events during its 2012 accounting period.

1. Paid cash to purchase land.
2. Recognized revenue on account.
3. Issued common stock.
4. Paid cash to purchase supplies.
5. Collected a cash advance for services that will be provided during the coming year.
6. Paid a cash dividend to the stockholders.
7. Paid cash for an insurance policy that provides coverage during the next year.
8. Collected cash from accounts receivable.
9. Paid cash for operating expenses.
10. Paid cash to settle an account payable.

Required

a. Identify the events that would require a year-end adjusting entry.
b. Explain why adjusting entries are made at the end of the accounting period.

LO 4, 5

Exercise 2-19 *Closing the accounts*

The following information was drawn from the accounting records of Kwon Company as of December 31, 2012, before the temporary accounts had been closed. The Cash balance was $4,000, and Notes Payable amounted to $2,000. The company had revenues of $6,000 and expenses of $3,500. The company's Land account had a $9,000 balance. Dividends amounted to $500. There was $6,000 of common stock issued.

Required

a. Identify which accounts would be classified as permanent and which accounts would be classified as temporary.
b. Assuming that Kwon's beginning balance (as of January 1, 2012) in the Retained Earnings account was $2,600, determine its balance after the nominal accounts were closed at the end of 2012.
c. What amount of net income would Kwon Company report on its 2012 income statement?
d. Explain why the amount of net income differs from the amount of the ending Retained Earnings balance.
e. What are the balances in the revenue, expense, and dividend accounts on January 1, 2013?

LO 4

Exercise 2-20 *Closing accounts and the accounting cycle*

Required

a. Identify which of the following accounts are temporary (will be closed to Retained Earnings at the end of the year) and which are permanent.
   (1) Land
   (2) Salaries Expense
   (3) Retained Earnings
   (4) Prepaid Rent
   (5) Supplies Expense
   (6) Common Stock
   (7) Notes Payable
   (8) Cash
   (9) Service Revenue
   (10) Dividends
b. List and explain the four stages of the accounting cycle. Which stage must be first? Which stage is last?

Exercise 2-21 *Closing entries*

Required

Which of the following accounts are closed at the end of the accounting period?

a. Accounts Payable
b. Unearned Revenue
c. Prepaid Rent
d. Rent Expense
e. Service Revenue
f. Advertising Expense
g. Dividends
h. Retained Earnings
i. Utilities Expense
j. Salaries Payable
k. Salaries Expense
l. Operating Expenses

Exercise 2-22 *Matching concept*

Companies make sacrifices known as *expenses* to obtain benefits called *revenues*. The accurate measurement of net income requires that expenses be matched with revenues. In some circumstances matching a particular expense directly with revenue is difficult or impossible. In these circumstances, the expense is matched with the period in which it is incurred.

Required

Distinguish the following items that could be matched directly with revenues from the items that would be classified as period expenses.

a. Sales commissions paid to employees.
b. Utilities expense.
c. Rent expense.
d. The cost of land that has been sold.

Exercise 2-23 *Identifying source, use, and exchange transactions*

Required

Indicate whether each of the following transactions is an asset source (AS), asset use (AU), asset exchange (AE), or claims exchange (CE) transaction.

a. Acquired cash from the issue of stock.
b. Paid a cash dividend to the stockholders.
c. Paid cash on accounts payable.
d. Incurred other operating expenses on account.
e. Paid cash for rent expense.
f. Performed services for cash.
g. Performed services for clients on account.
h. Collected cash from accounts receivable.
i. Invested cash in a certificate of deposit.
j. Purchased land with cash.

Exercise 2-24 *Identifying asset source, use, and exchange transactions*

Required

a. Name an asset exchange transaction that will *not* affect the statement of cash flows.
b. Name an asset exchange transaction that will affect the statement of cash flows.
c. Name an asset source transaction that will *not* affect the income statement.
d. Name an asset use transaction that will affect the income statement.
e. Name an asset use transaction that will *not* affect the income statement.

LO 3

Exercise 2-25   *Relation of elements to financial statements*

Required

Identify whether each of the following items would appear on the income statement (IS), statement of changes in stockholders' equity (SE), balance sheet (BS), or statement of cash flows (CF). Some items may appear on more than one statement; if so, identify all applicable statements. If an item would not appear on any financial statement, label it NA.

a. Prepaid rent

b. Net income

c. Utilities expense

d. Supplies

e. Cash flow from operating activities

f. Service revenue

g. Auditor's opinion

h. Accounts receivable

i. Accounts payable

j. Unearned revenue

k. Dividends

l. Beginning cash balance

m. Ending retained earnings

n. Rent expense

o. Ending cash balance

Exercise 2-26   *Analyzing the cash flow effects of different types of expenses*

The following income statements are available for Hopi, Inc., and Zuni, Inc., for 2012.

	Hopi, Inc.	Zuni, Inc.
Revenue	$100,000	$100,000
Wages expense	70,000	55,000
Depreciation expense	10,000	25,000
Net earnings	$ 20,000	$ 20,000

Required

Assume that neither company had beginning or ending balances in its Accounts Receivable or wages Payable accounts. Explain which company would have the lowest *net cash flows from operating activities* for 2012.

PROBLEMS

connect
|ACCOUNTING

All applicable Problems are available with McGraw-Hill's
Connect Accounting.

LO 1

CHECK FIGURES
Net Income: $15,300
Ending Cash Balance: $33,200

Problem 2-27   *Recording events in a horizontal statements model*

The following events pertain to King Company.

1. Acquired $25,000 cash from the issue of common stock.

2. Provided services for $5,000.

3. Provided $18,000 of services on account.

4. Collected $11,000 cash from the account receivable created in Event 3.

5. Paid $1,400 cash to purchase supplies.

6. Had $300 of supplies on hand at the end of the accounting period.

7. Received $3,600 cash in advance for services to be performed in the future.

8. Performed one-half of the services agreed to in Event 7.

9. Paid $6,000 for salaries expense.

10. Incurred $2,400 of other operating expenses on account.

11. Paid $2,000 cash on the account payable created in Event 10.

12. Paid a $2,000 cash dividend to the stockholders.

Required

Show the effects of the events on the financial statements using a horizontal statements model like the following one. In the Cash Flows column, use the letters OA to designate operating activity, IA for investing activity, FA for financing activity, and NC for net change in cash. Use NA to indicate accounts not affected by the event. The first event is recorded as an example.

Event No.	Assets			=	Liabilities			+	Stockholders' Equity			Rev.	−	Exp.	=	Net Inc.	Cash Flows
	Cash	+	Accts. Rec.	+ Supp. =	Accts. Pay.	+	Unearn. Rev.	+	Com. Stk.	+	Ret. Earn.						
1	25,000	+ NA	+ NA	= NA	+	NA	+ 25,000	+	NA			NA	− NA	=		NA	25,000 FA

Problem 2-28   *Effect of deferrals on financial statements: three separate single-cycle examples*

e**X**cel

Required

a. On February 1, 2012, Heider, Inc., was formed when it received $80,000 cash from the issue of common stock. On May 1, 2012, the company paid $60,000 cash in advance to rent office space for the coming year. The office space was used as a place to consult with clients. The consulting activity generated $120,000 of cash revenue during 2012. Based on this information alone, record the events and related adjusting entry in the general ledger accounts under the accounting equation. Determine the amount of net income and cash flows from operating activities for 2012.

b. On January 1, 2012, the accounting firm of Bonds & Associates was formed. On August 1, 2012, the company received a retainer fee (was paid in advance) of $30,000 for services to be performed monthly during the next 12 months. Assuming that this was the only transaction completed in 2012, prepare an income statement, statement of changes in stockholders' equity, balance sheet, and statement of cash flows for 2012.

c. Edge Company had $2,200 of supplies on hand on January 1, 2012. Edge purchased $7,200 of supplies on account during 2012. A physical count of supplies revealed that $900 of supplies was on hand as of December 31, 2012. Determine the amount of supplies expense that should be recognized in the December 31, 2012 adjusting entry. Use a financial statements model to show how the adjusting entry would affect the balance sheet, income statement, and statement of cash flows.

CHECK FIGURES
a. Net Income: $80,000
b. Net Income: $12,500

Problem 2-29   *Effect of adjusting entries on the accounting equation*

LO 2

Required

Each of the following independent events requires a year-end adjusting entry. Show how each event and its related adjusting entry affect the accounting equation. Assume a December 31 closing date. The first event is recorded as an example.

CHECK FIGURE
b. adjustment amount: $1,250

Event/ Adjustment	Total Assets						Stockholders' Equity		
	Cash	+	Other Assets	=	Liabilities	+	Common Stock	+	Retained Earnings
a	−7,200	+	+7,200	=	NA	+	NA	+	NA
Adj.	NA		−5,400		NA		NA		−5,400

a. Paid $7,200 cash in advance on April 1 for a one-year insurance policy.
b. Purchased $1,400 of supplies on account. At year's end, $150 of supplies remained on hand.
c. Paid $8,400 cash in advance on March 1 for a one-year lease on office space.
d. Received a $18,000 cash advance for a contract to provide services in the future. The contract required a one-year commitment starting September 1 to be provided evenly over the year.
e. Paid $24,000 cash in advance on October 1 for a one-year lease on office space.

LO 3, 5, 6

e**X**cel

CHECK FIGURES
b. Net Income, 2012: $19,300
b. Net Income, 2013: $84,650

Problem 2-30 *Events for two complete accounting cycles*

Energy Consulting Company was formed on Junuary 1, 2012.

Events Affecting the 2012 Accounting Period

1. Acquired cash of $80,000 from the issue of common stock.
2. Purchased $4,200 of suplies on account.
3. Purchased land that cost $30,000 cash.
4. Paid $4,200 cash to settle accounts payable created in Event 2.
5. Recognized revenue on account of $75,000.
6. Paid $46,000 cash for other operating expenses.
7. Collected $68,000 cash from accounts receivable.

Information for 2012 Adjusting Entries

8. Recognized accrued salaries of $5,800 on December 31, 2012.
9. Had $300 of supplies on hand at the end of the accounting period.

Events Affecting the 2013 Accounting Period

1. Acquired an additional $10,000 cash from the issue of common stock.
2. Paid $5,800 cash to settle the salaries payable obligation.
3. Paid $6,000 cash in advance for a lease on office facilities.
4. Sold land that had cost $25,000 for $25,000 cash.
5. Received $8,400 cash in advance for services to be performed in the future.
6. Purchased $1,800 of supplies on account during the year.
7. Provided services on account of $90,000.
8. Collected $92,000 cash from accounts receivable.
9. Paid a cash dividend of $10,000 to the stockholders.

Information for 2013 Adjusting Entries

10. The advance payment for rental of the office facilities (see Event 3) was made on September 1 for a one-year lease term.
11. The cash advance for services to be provided in the future was collected on June 1 (see Event 5). The one-year contract started June 1.
12. Had $350 of supplies on hand at the end of the period.
13. Recognized accrued salaries of $6,500 at the end of the accounting period.

Required

a. Identify each event affecting the 2012 and 2013 accounting periods as asset source (AS), asset use (AU), asset exchange (AE), or claims exchange (CE). Record the effects of each event under the appropriate general ledger account headings of the accounting equation.
b. Prepare an income statement, statement of changes in stockholders' equity, balance sheet, and statement of cash flows for 2012 and 2013, using the vertical statements model.

LO 2, 3

CHECK FIGURES
b. $33,000
h. ($3,000)

Problem 2-31 *Effect of events on financial statements*

Reed Company had the following balances in its accounting records as of December 31, 2012.

Assets		Claims	
Cash	$ 75,000	Accounts Payable	$ 32,000
Accounts Receivable	45,000	Common Stock	90,000
Land	30,000	Retained Earnings	28,000
Totals	$150,000		$150,000

The following accounting events apply to Reed's 2012 fiscal year:

Jan.	1	Acquired an additional $50,000 cash from the issue of common stock.
April	1	Paid $8,400 cash in advance for a one-year lease for office space.
June	1	Paid a $4,000 cash dividend to the stockholders.
July	1	Purchased additional land that cost $15,000 cash.
Aug.	1	Made a cash payment on accounts payable of $28,000.
Sept.	1	Received $9,600 cash in advance as a retainer for services to be performed monthly during the next eight months.
Sept.	30	Sold land for $12,000 cash that had originally cost $12,000.
Oct.	1	Purchased $1,500 of supplies on account.
Dec.	31	Earned $75,000 of service revenue on account during the year.
	31	Received $70,000 cash collections from accounts receivable.
	31	Incurred $24,000 other operating expenses on account during the year.
	31	Recognized accrued salaries expense of $8,000.
	31	Had $400 of supplies on hand at the end of the period.
	31	The land purchased on July 1 had a market value of $21,000.

Required

Based on the preceding information, answer the following questions. All questions pertain to the 2012 financial statements. (*Hint:* Record the events in general ledger accounts under an accounting equation before answering the questions.)

a. What two transactions need additional adjusting entries at the end of the year?
b. What amount would be reported for land on the balance sheet?
c. What amount of net cash flow from operating activities would Reed report on the statement of cash flows?
d. What amount of rent expense would be reported in the income statement?
e. What amount of total liabilities would be reported on the balance sheet?
f. What amount of supplies expense would be reported on the income statement?
g. What amount of unearned revenue would be reported on the balance sheet?
h. What amount of net cash flow from investing activities would be reported on the statement of cash flows?
i. What amount of total expenses would be reported on the income statement?
j. What total amount of service revenues would be reported on the income statement?
k. What amount of cash flows from financing activities would be reported on the statement of cash flows?
l. What amount of net income would be reported on the income statement?
m. What amount of retained earnings would be reported on the balance sheet?

Problem 2-32   *Identifying and arranging elements on financial statements*

The following information was drawn from the records of Paso & Associates at December 31, 2012.

Supplies	$ 2,500	Unearned revenue	$ 5,400
Consulting revenue	120,000	Notes payable	40,000
Land	70,000	Salaries payable	9,000
Dividends	10,000	Salary expense	58,000
Cash flow from fin. activities	30,000	Common stock issued	30,000
Interest revenue	6,000	Beginning common stock	40,000
Ending retained earnings	50,100	Accounts receivable	32,000
Cash	66,000	Cash flow from inv. activities	(21,000)
Interest payable	4,000	Cash flow from oper. activities	18,000
Interest expense	9,000	Prepaid rent	8,000

LO 3

CHECK FIGURES
2012 Net Income: $59,000
2012 Total Assets: $178,500

Required

Use the preceding information to construct an income statement, statement of changes in stockholders' equity, balance sheet, and statement of cash flows. (Show only totals for each activity on the statement of cash flows.)

LO 3

Problem 2-33 *Relationship of accounts to financial statements*

Required

Identify whether each of the following items would appear on the income statement (IS), statement of changes in stockholders' equity (SE), balance sheet (BS), or statement of cash flows (CF). Some items may appear on more than one statement; if so, identify all applicable statements. If an item would not appear on any financial statement, label it NA.

a. Accumulated depreciation
b. Salary expense
c. Prepaid insurance
d. Beginning common stock
e. Beginning retained earnings
f. Supplies expense
g. Operating expenses
h. Cash flow from operating activities
i. Debt to assets ratio
j. Total liabilities
k. Ending common stock
l. Interest expense
m. Consulting revenue
n. Cash flow from investing activities
o. Service revenue
p. Unearned revenue
q. Certificate of deposit
r. Interest receivable
s. Depreciation expense

t. Accounts receivable
u. Notes payable
v. Insurance expense
w. Salaries payable
x. Total assets
y. Accounts payable
z. Notes receivable
aa. Cash
bb. Supplies
cc. Cash flow from financing activities
dd. Interest revenue
ee. Ending retained earnings
ff. Net income
gg. Dividends
hh. Office equipment
ii. Debt to equity ratio
jj. Land
kk. Interest payable
ll. Rent expense

LO 3, 5

Problem 2-34 *Missing information in financial statements*

Required

Fill in the blank (as indicated by the alphabetic letters in parentheses) in the following financial statements. Assume the company started operations January 1, 2010, and that all transactions involve cash.

	For the Years		
	2010	2011	2012
Income Statements			
Revenue	$ 700	$ 1,300	$ 2,000
Expense	(a)	(700)	(1,300)
Net income	$ 200	$ (m)	$ 700
Statement of Changes in Stockholders' Equity			
Beginning common stock	$ 0	$ (n)	$ 6,000
Plus: Common stock issued	5,000	1,000	2,000
Ending common stock	5,000	6,000	(t)
Beginning retained earnings	0	100	200
Plus: Net income	(b)	(o)	700
Less: Dividends	(c)	(500)	(300)
Ending retained earnings	100	(p)	600
Total stockholders' equity	$ (d)	$ 6,200	$ 8,600

continued

Balance Sheets

Assets			
Cash	$ (e)	$ (q)	$ (u)
Land	0	(r)	8,000
Total assets	$ (f)	$11,200	$10,600
Liabilities	$ (g)	$ 5,000	$ 2,000
Stockholders' equity			
Common stock	(h)	(s)	8,000
Retained earnings	(i)	200	600
Total stockholders' equity	(j)	6,200	8,600
Total liabilities and stockholders' equity	$8,100	$11,200	$10,600

Statements of Cash Flows

Cash flows from operating activities			
Cash receipts from revenue	$ (k)	$ 1,300	$ (v)
Cash payments for expenses	(l)	(700)	(w)
Net cash flows from operating activities	200	600	700
Cash flows from investing activities			
Cash payments for land	0	(8,000)	0
Cash flows from financing activities			
Cash receipts from loan	3,000	3,000	0
Cash payments to reduce debt	0	(1,000)	(x)
Cash receipts from stock issue	5,000	1,000	(y)
Cash payments for dividends	(100)	(500)	(z)
Net cash flows from financing activities	7,900	2,500	(1,300)
Net change in cash	8,100	(4,900)	(600)
Plus: Beginning cash balance	0	8,100	3,200
Ending cash balance	$8,100	$ 3,200	$ 2,600

ANALYZE, THINK, COMMUNICATE

ATC 2-1 Business Applications Case *Understanding real-world annual reports*

Required

Use the Target Corporation's annual report in Appendix B to answer the following questions. Note that net income and net earnings are synonymous terms.

Target Corporation

a. Which accounts on Target's balance sheet are accural type accounts?

b. Which accounts on Target's balance sheet are deferral type accounts?

c. Compare Target's 2009 *net earnings* to its 2009 *cash provided by operating activities*. Which is larger?

d. First, compare Target's 2008 net earnings to its 2009 net earnings. Next, compare Target's 2008 cash provided by operating activities to its 2009 cash provided by operating activities. Which changed the most from 2008 to 2009, net earnings or cash provided by operating activities?

ATC 2-2 Group Assignment *Financial reporting and market valuation*

The following financial highlights were drawn from the 2009 annual reports of Microsoft Corporation and Apple Inc.

	Microsoft	Apple
Revenue	$58.4 Billion	$42.9 Billion
Net income	$14.6 Billion	$ 5.7 Billion
Cash and short-term investments	$39.7 Billion	$23.1 Billion

Even so, as of May 26, 2010, Wall Street valued Microsoft at $219.19 billion and Apple at $222.12.

Divide the class into groups of four or five students.

Required

Have the members of each group reach a consensus response for each of the following tasks. Each group should elect a spokes person to represent the group.

Group Tasks

(1) Determine the amount of expenses incurred by each company.

(2) Comment on how the concept of conservatism applies to the financial information presented in this case.

(3) Speculate as to why investors would be willing to pay more for Apple than Microsoft.

Class Discussion

Randomly call on the spokes persons to compare their responses for each of the group tasks.

ATC 2-3 Research Assignment *Investigating nonfinancial information in Nike's annual report*

Although most of this course is concerned with the financial statements themselves, all sections of a company's annual report are important. A company must file various reports with the SEC, and one of these, Form 10-K, is essentially the company's annual report. The requirements below ask you to investigate sections of Nike's annual report that explain various nonfinancial aspects of its business operations.

To obtain the Form 10-K you can use either the EDGAR system following the instructions in Appendix A or the company's website.

Required

a. In what year did Nike begin operations?

b. Other than athletic shoes, what products does Nike sell?

c. Does Nike operate businesses under names other than Nike? If so, what are they?

d. How many employees does Nike have?

e. In how many countries other than the United States does Nike sell its products?

ATC 2-4 Writing Assignment *Conservatism and Matching*

Glenn's Cleaning Services Company is experiencing cash flow problems and needs a loan. Glenn has a friend who is willing to lend him the money he needs provided she can be convinced that he will be able to repay the debt. Glenn has assured his friend that his business is viable, but his friend has asked to see the company's financial statements. Glenn's accountant produced the following financial statements.

Income Statement		Balance Sheet	
Service Revenue	$ 38,000	Assets	$85,000
Operating Expenses	(70,000)	Liabilities	$35,000
Net Loss	$(32,000)	Stockholders' Equity	
		Common Stock	82,000
		Retained Earnings	(32,000)
		Total Liabilities and	
		Stockholders' Equity	$85,000

Glenn made the following adjustments to these statements before showing them to his friend. He recorded $82,000 of revenue on account from Barrymore Manufacturing Company for a contract to clean its headquarters office building that was still being negotiated for the next month. Barrymore had scheduled a meeting to sign a contract the following week, so Glenn was sure that he would get the job. Barrymore was a reputable company, and Glenn was confident that he could ultimately collect the $82,000. Also, he subtracted $30,000 of accrued salaries expense and the corresponding liability. He reasoned that since he had not paid the employees, he had not incurred any expense.

Required

a. Reconstruct the income statement and balance sheet as they would appear after Glenn's adjustments.

b. Write a brief memo explaining how Glenn's treatment of the expected revenue from Barrymore violated the conservatism concept.

c. Write a brief memo explaining how Glenn's treatment of the accrued salaries expense violates the matching concept.

CHAPTER 3

Accounting for Merchandising Businesses

LEARNING OBJECTIVES

After you have mastered the material in this chapter, you will be able to:

1 Identify and explain the primary features of the perpetual inventory system.

2 Show the effects of inventory transactions on financial statements.

3 Explain the meaning of terms used to describe transportation costs, cash discounts, returns or allowances, and financing costs.

4 Explain how gains and losses differ from revenues and expenses.

5 Compare and contrast single and multistep income statements.

6 Show the effect of lost, damaged, or stolen inventory on financial statements.

7 Use common size financial statements to evaluate managerial performance.

8 Identify the primary features of the periodic inventory system. (Appendix)

CHAPTER OPENING

Previous chapters have discussed accounting for service businesses. These businesses obtain revenue by providing some kind of service such as medical or legal advice to their customers. Other examples of service companies include dry cleaning companies, maid service companies, and car washes. This chapter introduces accounting practices for merchandising businesses. **Merchandising businesses** generate revenue by selling goods. They buy the merchandise they sell from companies called suppliers. The goods purchased for resale are called **merchandise inventory.** Merchandising businesses include **retail companies** (companies that sell goods to the final consumer) and **wholesale companies** (companies that sell to other businesses). Sears, JCPenney, Target, and Sam's Club are real-world merchandising businesses.

The Curious Accountant

Janice recently purchased a gold necklace for $250 from her local **Zales** jewelry store. The next day she learned that Zoe bought the same necklace on-line from **Blue Nile** for only $200. Janice questioned how Blue Nile could sell the necklace for so much less than Zales. Zoe suggested that even though both jewelry sellers purchase their products from the same producers at about the same price, Blue Nile can charge lower prices because it does not have to operate expensive bricks-and-mortar stores, and thus has lower operating costs. Janice disagrees. She thinks the cost of operating large distribution centers and Internet server centers will offset any cost savings Blue Nile enjoys from not owning retail jewelry stores.

Exhibit 3.1 presents the income statements for Zales and Blue Nile. Based on these income statements, do you think Janice or Zoe is correct? (Answer on page 104.)

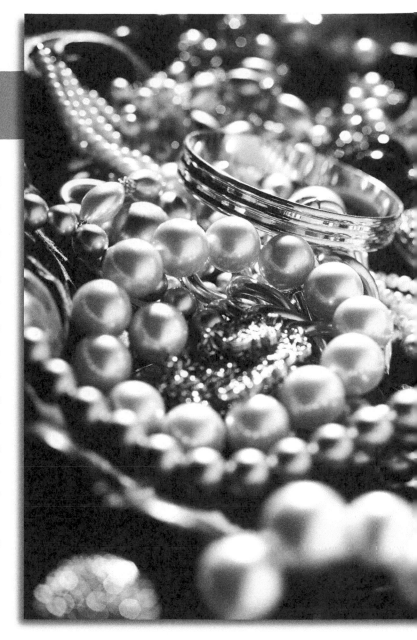

EXHIBIT 3.1   Comparative Income Statements

BLUE NILE, INC.
Consolidated Statements of Operations
(in thousands, except per share data)

	Year Ended	
	January 3, 2010	January 4, 2009
Net sales	$302,134	$295,329
Cost of sales	236,790	235,333
Gross profit	65,344	59,996
Selling, general and administrative expenses	45,997	44,005
Operating income	19,347	15,991
Other income, net:		
Interest income, net	122	1,420
Other income, net	209	445
Total other income, net	331	1,865
Income before income taxes	19,678	17,856
Income tax expense	6,878	6,226
Net income	$ 12,800	$ 11,630

ZALE CORPORATION AND SUBSIDIARIES
Consolidated Statements of Operations
(in thousands, except per share amounts)

	Year Ended July 31,	
	2009	2008 As Restated
Revenues	$1,779,744	$2,138,041
Cost and expenses:		
Cost of sales	948,572	1,089,553
Selling, general and administrative	927,249	985,028
Cost of insurance operations	7,000	6,744
Depreciation and amortization	58,947	60,244
Other charges and gains	70,095	(10,700)
Operating (loss) earnings	(232,119)	7,172
Interest expense	10,399	12,364
Other income	—	(3,500)
Loss before income taxes	(242,518)	(1,692)
Income tax (benefit) expense	(53,015)	4,761
Loss from continuing operations	(189,503)	(6,453)
Earnings from discontinued operations, net of taxes	—	7,084
Net (loss) earnings	$ (189,503)	$ 631

PRODUCT COSTS VERSUS SELLING AND ADMINISTRATIVE COSTS

Identify and explain the primary features of the perpetual inventory system.

Companies report inventory costs on the balance sheet in the asset account Merchandise Inventory. All costs incurred to acquire merchandise and ready it for sale are included in the inventory account. Examples of inventory costs include the price of goods purchased, shipping and handling costs, transit insurance, and storage costs.

Since inventory items are referred to as products, inventory costs are frequently called **product costs.**

Costs that are not included in inventory are usually called **selling and administrative costs.** Examples of selling and administrative costs include advertising, administrative salaries, sales commissions, insurance, and interest. Since selling and administrative costs are usually recognized as expenses *in the period* in which they are incurred, they are sometimes called **period costs.** In contrast, product costs are expensed when inventory is sold regardless of when it was purchased. In other words, product costs are matched directly with sales revenue, while selling and administrative costs are matched with the period in which they are incurred.

ALLOCATING INVENTORY COST BETWEEN ASSET AND EXPENSE ACCOUNTS

The cost of inventory that is available for sale during a specific accounting period is determined as follows.

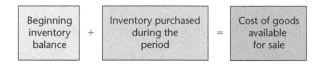

The **cost of goods available for sale** is allocated between the asset account Merchandise Inventory and an expense account called **Cost of Goods Sold.** The cost of inventory items that have not been sold (Merchandise Inventory) is reported as an asset on the balance sheet, and the cost of the items sold (Cost of Goods Sold) is expensed on the income statement. This allocation is depicted graphically as follows.

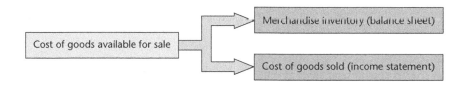

The difference between the sales revenue and the cost of goods sold is called **gross margin** or **gross profit.** The selling and administrative expenses (period costs) are subtracted from gross margin to obtain the net income.

Exhibit 3.1 displays income statements from the annual reports of Blue Nile and Zales. For each company, review the most current income statement and determine the amount of gross margin. You should find a gross profit of $65,344 for Blue Nile and a gross margin of $831,172 ($1,779,744 − $948,572) for Zales.

PERPETUAL INVENTORY SYSTEM

Most modern companies maintain their inventory records using the **perpetual inventory system,** so-called because the inventory account is adjusted perpetually (continually) throughout the accounting period. Each time merchandise is purchased, the inventory account is increased; each time it is sold, the inventory account is decreased. The following illustration demonstrates the basic features of the perpetual inventory system.

Show the effects of inventory transactions on financial statements.

June Gardener loved plants and grew them with such remarkable success that she decided to open a small retail plant store. She started June's Plant Shop (JPS) on January 1, 2012. The following discussion explains and illustrates the effects of the five events the company experienced during its first year of operation.

Effects of 2012 Events on Financial Statements

EVENT 1   JPS acquired $15,000 cash by issuing common stock.

This event is an asset source transaction. It increases both assets (cash) and stockholders' equity (common stock). The income statement is not affected. The statement of cash flows reflects an inflow from financing activities. These effects are shown here.

Assets				=	Liab.	+	Stockholders' Equity							
Cash	+	Inventory	+	Land	=	Accts. Pay.	+	Com. Stk.	+	Ret. Earn.	Rev.	−	Exp.	=	Net Inc.	Cash Flow
15,000	+	NA	+	NA	=	NA	+	15,000	+	NA	NA	−	NA	=	NA	15,000 FA

EVENT 2   JPS purchased merchandise inventory for $14,000 cash.

This event is an asset exchange transaction. One asset, cash, decreases and another asset, merchandise inventory, increases; total assets remain unchanged. Because product costs are expensed when inventory is sold, not when it is purchased, the event does not affect the income statement. The cash outflow, however, is reported in the operating activities section of the statement of cash flows. These effects are illustrated below.

Assets				=	Liab.	+	Stockholders' Equity							
Cash	+	Inventory	+	Land	=	Accts. Pay.	+	Com. Stk.	+	Ret. Earn.	Rev.	−	Exp.	=	Net Inc.	Cash Flow
(14,000)	+	14,000	+	NA	=	NA	+	NA	+	NA	NA	−	NA	=	NA	(14,000) OA

EVENT 3A   JPS recognized sales revenue from selling inventory for $12,000 cash.

The revenue recognition is the first part of a two-part transaction. The *sales part* represents a source of assets (cash increases from earning sales revenue). Both assets (cash) and stockholders' equity (retained earnings) increase. Sales revenue on the income statement increases. The $12,000 cash inflow is reported in the operating activities section of the statement of cash flows. These effects are shown in the following financial statements model.

Assets				=	Liab.	+	Stockholders' Equity							
Cash	+	Inventory	+	Land	=	Accts. Pay.	+	Com. Stk.	+	Ret. Earn.	Rev.	−	Exp.	=	Net Inc.	Cash Flow
12,000	+	NA	+	NA	=	NA	+	NA	+	12,000	12,000	−	NA	=	12,000	12,000 OA

EVENT 3B   JPS recognized $8,000 of cost of goods sold.

The expense recognition is the second part of the two-part transaction. The *expense part* represents a use of assets. Both assets (merchandise inventory) and stockholders' equity (retained earnings) decrease. An expense account, Cost of Goods Sold, is reported on the income statement. This part of the transaction does not affect the statement of cash flows. A cash outflow occurred when the goods were bought, not when they were sold. These effects are shown here.

Assets			=	Liab.	+	Stockholders' Equity							
Cash	+	Inventory	+	Land	=	Accts. Pay.	+	Com. Stk.	+	Ret. Earn.	Rev.	−	Exp.	=	Net Inc.	Cash Flow
NA	+	(8,000)	+	NA	=	NA	+	NA	+	(8,000)	NA	−	8,000	=	(8,000)	NA

EVENT 4   JPS paid $1,000 cash for selling and administrative expenses.

This event is an asset use transaction. The payment decreases both assets (cash) and stockholders' equity (retained earnings). The increase in selling and administrative expenses decreases net income. The $1,000 cash payment is reported in the operating activities section of the statement of cash flows. These effects are illustrated below.

Assets			=	Liab.	+	Stockholders' Equity							
Cash	+	Inventory	+	Land	=	Accts. Pay.	+	Com. Stk.	+	Ret. Earn.	Rev.	−	Exp.	=	Net Inc.	Cash Flow
(1,000)	+	NA	+	NA	=	NA	+	NA	+	(1,000)	NA	−	1,000	=	(1,000)	(1,000) OA

EVENT 5   JPS paid $5,500 cash to purchase land for a place to locate a future store.

Buying the land increases the Land account and decreases the Cash account on the balance sheet. The income statement is not affected. The statement of cash flow shows a cash outflow to purchase land in the investing activities section of the statement of cash flows. These effects are shown below.

Assets			=	Liab.	+	Stockholders' Equity							
Cash	+	Inventory	+	Land	=	Accts. Pay.	+	Com. Stk.	+	Ret. Earn.	Rev.	−	Exp.	=	Net Inc.	Cash Flow
(5,500)	+	NA	+	5,500	=	NA	+	NA	+	NA	NA	−	NA	=	NA	(5,500) IA

Financial Statements for 2012

JPS's financial statements for 2012 are shown in Exhibit 3.2. JPS had no beginning inventory in its first year, so the cost of merchandise inventory available for sale was $14,000 (the amount of inventory purchased during the period). Recall that JPS must allocate the *Cost of Goods (Inventory) Available for Sale* between the *Cost of Goods Sold* ($8,000) and the ending balance ($6,000) in the *Merchandise Inventory* account. The cost of goods sold is reported as an expense on the income statement and the ending balance of merchandise inventory is reported as an asset on the balance sheet. The difference between the sales revenue ($12,000) and the cost of goods sold ($8,000) is labeled *gross margin* ($4,000) on the income statement.

EXHIBIT 3.2

Financial Statements

2012 Income Statement		
Sales revenue		$12,000
Cost of goods sold		(8,000)
Gross margin		4,000
Less: Operating exp.		
Selling and admin. exp.		(1,000)
Net income		$ 3,000

12/31/12 Balance Sheet		
Assets		
Cash	$ 6,500	
Merchandise inventory	6,000	
Land	5,500	
Total assets		$18,000
Liabilities		$ 0
Stockholders' equity		
Common stock	$15,000	
Retained earnings	3,000	
Total stockholders' equity		18,000
Total liab. and stk. equity		$18,000

2012 Statement of Cash Flows		
Operating activities		
Inflow from customers	$12,000	
Outflow for inventory	(14,000)	
Outflow for selling & admin. exp.	(1,000)	
Net cash outflow for operating activities		$ (3,000)
Investing activities		
Outflow to purchase land		(5,500)
Financing activities		
Inflow from stock issue		15,000
Net change in cash		6,500
Plus: Beginning cash balance		0
Ending cash balance		$ 6,500

✓ CHECK YOURSELF 3.1

Phambroom Company began 2012 with $35,600 in its Inventory account. During the year, it purchased inventory costing $356,800 and sold inventory that had cost $360,000 for $520,000. Based on this information alone, determine (1) the inventory balance as of December 31, 2012, and (2) the amount of gross margin Phambroom would report on its 2012 income statement.

Answer

1. $35,600 Beginning inventory + $356,800 Purchases = $392,400 Goods available for sale

   $392,400 Goods available for sale − $360,000 Cost of goods sold = $32,400 Ending inventory

2. Sales revenue − Cost of goods sold = Gross margin

   $520,000 − $360,000 = $160,000

Transportation Cost, Purchase Returns and Allowances, and Cash Discounts Related to Inventory Purchases

Purchasing inventory often involves: (1) incurring transportation costs, (2) returning inventory or receiving purchase allowances (cost reductions), and (3) taking cash discounts (also cost reductions). During its second accounting cycle, JPS encountered these kinds of events. The final account balances at the end of the 2012 fiscal year become the beginning balances for 2013: Cash, $6,500; Merchandise Inventory, $6,000; Land, 5,500; Common Stock, $15,000; and Retained Earnings, $3,000.

Effects of 2013 Events on Financial Statements

JPS experienced the following events during its 2013 accounting period. The effects of each of these events are explained and illustrated in the following discussion.

LO 3

Explain the meaning of terms used to describe transportation costs, cash discounts, returns or allowances, and financing costs.

EVENT 1   JPS borrowed $4,000 cash by issuing a note payable.

JPS borrowed the money to enable it to purchase a plot of land for a site for a store it planned to build in the near future. Borrowing the money increases the Cash account and the Note Payable account on the balance sheet. The income statement is not affected. The statement of cash flow shows a cash flow from financing activities. These effects are shown below.

Assets				=	Liabilities		+	Stockholders' Equity							
Cash	+	Accts. Rec.	+ Inventory + Land	=	Accts. Pay.	+ Notes Pay.	+	Com. Stk.	+ Ret. Earn.		Rev.	− Exp.	= Net Inc.		Cash Flow
4,000	+	NA	+ NA + NA	=	NA	+ 4,000	+	NA	+ NA		NA	− NA	= NA		4,000 FA

EVENT 2   JPS purchased on account merchandise inventory with a list price of $11,000.

The inventory purchase increases both assets (merchandise inventory) and liabilities (accounts payable) on the balance sheet. The income statement is not affected until later, when inventory is sold. Since the inventory was purchased on account, there was no cash outflow. These effects are shown here.

Assets				=	Liab.		+	Stockholders' Equity						
Cash	+	Accts. Rec.	+ Inventory + Land	=	Accts. Pay.	+ Notes Pay.	+	Com. Stk.	+ Ret. Earn.		Rev.	− Exp.	= Net Inc.	Cash Flow
NA	+	NA	+ 11,000 + NA	=	11,000	+ NA	+	NA	+ NA		NA	− NA	= NA	NA

Accounting for Purchase Returns and Allowances

EVENT 3   JPS returned some of the inventory purchased in Event 2. The list price of the returned merchandise was $1,000.

To promote customer satisfaction, many businesses allow customers to return goods for reasons such as wrong size, wrong color, wrong design, or even simply because the purchaser changed his mind. The effect of a purchase return is the *opposite* of the original purchase. For JPS the **purchase return** decreases both assets (merchandise inventory) and liabilities (accounts payable). There is no effect on either the income statement or the statement of cash flows. These effects are shown below.

Assets				=	Liab.		+	Stockholders' Equity						
Cash	+	Accts. Rec.	+ Inventory + Land	=	Accts. Pay.	+ Notes Pay.	+	Com. Stk.	+ Ret. Earn.		Rev.	− Exp.	= Net Inc.	Cash Flow
NA	+	NA	+ (1,000) + NA	=	(1,000)	+ NA	+	NA	+ NA		NA	− NA	= NA	NA

Sometimes dissatisfied buyers will agree to keep goods instead of returning them if the seller offers to reduce the price. Such reductions are called allowances. **Purchase allowances** affect the financial statements the same way purchase returns do.

Purchase Discounts

EVENT 4   JPS received a cash discount on goods purchased in Event 2. The credit terms were 2/10, n/30.

To encourage buyers to pay promptly, sellers sometimes offer **cash discounts.** To illustrate, assume JPS purchased the inventory in Event 2 under terms **2/10, n/30** (two-ten, net thirty). These terms mean the seller will allow a 2 percent cash discount if the purchaser pays cash within 10 days from the date of purchase. The amount not paid within the first 10 days is due at the end of 30 days from date of purchase. Recall that JPS returned $1,000 of the inventory purchased in Event 1 leaving a $10,000 balance ($11,000 list price − $1,000 purchase return). If JPS pays for the inventory within 10 days, the amount of the discount is $200 ($10,000 × .02).

When cash discounts are applied to purchases they are called **purchases discounts.** When they are applied to sales, they are called sales discounts. Sales discounts will be discussed later in the chapter. A *purchase discount* reduces the cost of the inventory and the associated account payable on the balance sheet. A purchase discount does not directly affect the income statement or the statement of cash flow. These effects are shown here.

		Assets			=	Liab.		+	Stockholders' Equity						
Cash	+	Accts. Rec.	+ Inventory	+ Land	=	Accts. Pay.	+ Notes Pay.	+	Com. Stk.	+ Ret. Earn.	Rev.	− Exp.	= Net Inc.		Cash Flow
NA	+	NA	+ (200)	+ NA	=	(200)	+ NA	+	NA	+ NA	NA	− NA	= NA		NA

If JPS paid the account payable after 10 days, there would be no purchase discount. In this case the balances in the Inventory and Account Payable accounts would remain at $10,000.

EVENT 5   JPS paid the $9,800 balance due on the account payable.

The remaining balance in the accounts payable is $9,800 ($10,000 list price − $200 purchase discount). Paying cash to settle the liability reduces cash and accounts payable on the balance sheet. The income statement is not affected. The cash outflow is shown in the operating section of the statement of cash flows. These effects are shown below.

		Assets			=	Liab.		+	Stockholders' Equity						
Cash	+	Accts. Rec.	+ Inventory	+ Land	=	Accts. Pay.	+ Notes Pay.	+	Com. Stk.	+ Ret. Earn.	Rev.	− Exp.	= Net Inc.		Cash Flow
(9,800)	+	NA	+ NA	+ NA	=	(9,800)	+ NA	+	NA	+ NA	NA	− NA	= NA		(9,800) OA

The Cost of Financing Inventory

Suppose you buy inventory this month and sell it next month. Where do you get the money to pay for the inventory at the time you buy it? One way to finance the purchase is to buy it on account and withhold payment until the last day of the term for the account payable. For example, suppose you buy inventory under terms 2/10, net/30. Under these circumstances you could delay payment for 30 days after the day of purchase. This way you may be able to collect enough money from the inventory you sell

REALITY BYTES

Many real-world companies have found it more effective to impose a penalty for late payment than to use a cash discount to encourage early payment. The invoice from Arley Water Works is an example of the penalty strategy. Notice that the amount due, if paid by the due date, is $18.14. A $1.88 late charge is imposed if the bill is paid after the due date. The $1.88 late charge is in fact interest. If Arley Water Works collects the payment after the due date, the utility will receive cash of $20.02. The collection will increase cash ($20.02), reduce accounts receivable ($18.14), and increase interest revenue ($1.88).

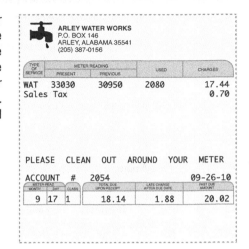

to pay for the inventory you purchased. Refusing the discount allows you the time needed to generate the cash necessary to pay off the liability (account payable). Unfortunately, this is usually a very expensive way to finance the purchase of inventory.

While the amount of a cash discount may appear small, the discount period is short. Consider the terms 2/10, net/30. Since you can pay on the tenth day and still receive the discount, you obtain financing for only 20 days (30-day full credit term − 10-day discount term). In other words, you must forgo a 2 percent discount to obtain a loan with a 20-day term. What is the size of the discount in annual terms? The answer is determined by the following formula.

Annual rate = Discount rate × (365 days ÷ term of the loan)

Annual rate = 2% × (365 ÷ 20)

Annual rate = 36.5%

This means that a 2 percent discount rate for 20 days is equivalent to a 36.5 percent annual rate of interest. So, if you do not have the money to pay the account payable, but can borrow money from a bank at less than 36.5 percent annual interest, you should borrow the money and pay off the account payable within the discount period.

Accounting for Transportation Costs

EVENT 6 **The shipping terms for the inventory purchased in Event 2 were FOB shipping point. JPS paid the freight company $300 cash for delivering the merchandise.**

The terms **FOB shipping point** and **FOB destination** identify whether the buyer or the seller is responsible for transportation costs. If goods are delivered FOB shipping point, the buyer is responsible for the freight cost. If goods are delivered FOB destination, the seller is responsible. When the buyer is responsible, the freight cost is called **transportation-in.** When the seller is responsible, the cost is called **transportation-out.** The following table summarizes freight cost terms.

Responsible Party	Buyer	Seller
Freight terms	FOB shipping point	FOB destination
Account title	Merchandise inventory	Transportation-out

Event 6 indicates the inventory was delivered FOB shipping point, so JPS (the buyer) is responsible for the $300 freight cost. Since incurring transportation-in costs is necessary to obtain inventory, these costs are added to the inventory account. The freight cost increases one asset account (Merchandise Inventory) and decreases another asset account (Cash). The income statement is not affected by this transaction because transportation-in costs are not expensed when they are incurred. Instead they are expensed as part of *cost of goods sold* when the inventory is sold. However, the cash paid for transportation-in costs is reported as an outflow in the operating activities section of the statement of cash flows. The effects of *transportation-in costs* are shown here.

Assets				=	Liab.		+	Stockholders' Equity						
Cash	+	Accts. Rec.	+ Inventory + Land	=	Accts. Pay.	+ Notes Pay.	+	Com. Stk.	+ Ret. Earn.	Rev.	− Exp.	= Net Inc.	Cash Flow	
(300)	+ NA	+	300 + NA	=	NA	+ NA	+	NA	+ NA	NA	− NA	= NA	(300)	OA

EVENT 7A   JPS recognized $24,750 of revenue on the cash sale of merchandise that cost $11,500.

The sale increases assets (cash) and stockholders' equity (retained earnings). The revenue recognition increases net income. The $24,750 cash inflow from the sale is reported in the operating activities section of the statement of cash flows. These effects are shown below.

Assets				=	Liab.		+	Stockholders' Equity						
Cash	+	Accts. Rec.	+ Inventory + Land	=	Accts. Pay.	+ Notes Pay.	+	Com. Stk.	+ Ret. Earn.	Rev.	− Exp.	= Net Inc.	Cash Flow	
24,750	+ NA	+	NA + NA	=	NA	+ NA	+	NA	+ 24,750	24,750	− NA	= 24,750	24,750	OA

EVENT 7B   JPS recognized $11,500 of cost of goods sold.

When goods are sold, the product cost—*including a proportionate share of transportation-in and adjustments for purchase returns and allowances*—is transferred from the Merchandise Inventory account to the expense account, Cost of Goods Sold. Recognizing cost of goods sold decreases both assets (merchandise inventory) and stockholders' equity (retained earnings). The expense recognition for cost of goods sold decreases net income. Cash flow is not affected. These effects are shown here.

Assets				=	Liab.		+	Stockholders' Equity						
Cash	+	Accts. Rec.	+ Inventory + Land	=	Accts. Pay.	+ Notes Pay.	+	Com. Stk.	+ Ret. Earn.	Rev.	− Exp.	= Net Inc.	Cash Flow	
NA	+ NA	+	(11,500) + NA	=	NA	+ NA	+	NA	+ (11,500)	NA	− 11,500	= (11,500)	NA	

EVENT 8   JPS paid $450 cash for freight costs on inventory delivered to customers.

Assume the merchandise sold in Event 7A was shipped FOB destination. Also assume JPS paid the freight cost in cash. FOB destination means the seller is responsible for the freight cost, which is called transportation-out. Transportation-out is reported on the income statement as an operating expense in the section below gross margin. The cost of freight on goods shipped to customers is incurred *after* the goods are sold. It is not part of the costs to obtain goods or ready them for sale. Recognizing the expense of transportation-out reduces assets (cash) and stockholders' equity (retained earnings). Operating expenses increase and net income decreases. The cash outflow is reported in the operating activities section of the statement of cash flows. These effects are shown below.

		Assets			=	Liab.		+	Stockholders' Equity						
Cash	+	Accts. Rec.	+ Inventory	+ Land	=	Accts. Pay.	+ Notes Pay.	+	Com. Stk.	+ Ret. Earn.	Rev.	− Exp.	= Net Inc.	Cash Flow	
(450)	+	NA	+ NA	+ NA	=	NA	+ NA	+	NA	+ (450)	NA	− 450	= (450)	(450)	OA

If the terms had been FOB shipping point, the customer would have been responsible for the transportation cost and JPS would not have recorded an expense.

EVENT 9   JPS paid $5,000 cash for selling and administrative expenses.

The effect on the balance sheet is to decrease both assets (cash) and stockholders' equity (retained earnings). Recognizing the selling and administrative expenses decreases net income. The $5,000 cash outflow is reported in the operating activities section of the statement of cash flows. These effects are shown below.

		Assets			=	Liab.		+	Stockholders' Equity						
Cash	+	Accts. Rec.	+ Inventory	+ Land	=	Accts. Pay.	+ Notes Pay.	+	Com. Stk.	+ Ret. Earn.	Rev.	− Exp.	= Net Inc.	Cash Flow	
(5,000)	+	NA	+ NA	+ NA	=	NA	+ NA	+	NA	+ (5,000)	NA	− 5,000	= (5,000)	(5,000)	OA

EVENT 10   JPS paid $360 cash for interest expense on the note described in Event 1.

The effect on the balance sheet is to decrease both assets (cash) and stockholders' equity (retained earnings). Recognizing the interest expense decreases net income. The $360 cash outflow is reported in the operating activities section of the statement of cash flows. These effects are shown below.

		Assets			=	Liab.		+	Stockholders' Equity						
Cash	+	Accts. Rec.	+ Inventory	+ Land	=	Accts. Pay.	+ Notes Pay.	+	Com. Stk.	+ Ret. Earn.	Rev.	− Exp.	= Net Inc.	Cash Flow	
(360)	+	NA	+ NA	+ NA	=	NA	+ NA	+	NA	+ (360)	NA	− 360	= (360)	(360)	OA

RECOGNIZING GAINS AND LOSSES

EVENT 11   JPS sold the land that had cost $5,500 for $6,200 cash.

When JPS sells merchandise inventory for more than it cost, the difference between the sales revenue and the cost of the goods sold is called the *gross margin*. In contrast, when JPS sells land for more than it cost, the difference between the sales price and the cost of the land is called a **gain**. Why is one called *gross margin* and the other a *gain*? The terms are used to alert financial statement users to the fact that the nature of the underlying transactions is different.

JPS' primary business is selling inventory, not land. The term *gain* indicates profit resulting from transactions that are not likely to regularly recur. Similarly, had the land sold for less than cost the difference would have been labeled **loss** rather than expense. This term also indicates the underlying transaction is not from normal, recurring operating activities. Gains and losses are shown separately on the income statement to communicate the expectation that they are nonrecurring.

The presentation of gains and losses in the income statement is discussed in more detail in a later section of the chapter. At this point note that the sale increases cash, decreases land, and increases retained earnings on the balance sheet. The income statement shows a gain on the sale of land and net income increases. The $6,200 cash inflow is shown as an investing activity on the statement of cash flows. These effects are shown below:

Assets				=	Liab.		+	Stockholders' Equity						
Cash	+ Accts. Rec.	+ Inventory	+ Land	=	Accts. Pay.	+ Notes Pay.	+	Com. Stk.	+ Ret. Earn.	Gain	− Exp.	= Net Inc.	Cash Flow	
6,200	+ NA	+ NA	+ (5,500)	=	NA	+ NA	+	NA	+ 700	700	− NA	= 700	6,200	IA

✓ CHECK YOURSELF 3.2

Tsang Company purchased $32,000 of inventory on account with payment terms of 2/10, n/30 and freight terms FOB shipping point. Freight costs were $1,100. Tsang obtained a $2,000 purchase allowance because the inventory was damaged upon arrival. Tsang paid for the inventory within the discount period. Based on this information alone, determine the balance in the inventory account.

Answer

List price of inventory	$32,000
Plus: Transportation-in costs	1,100
Less: Purchase returns and allowances	(2,000)
Less: Purchase discount [($32,000 − $2,000) × .02]	(600)
Balance in inventory account	$30,500

MULTISTEP INCOME STATEMENT

JPS' 2013 income statement is shown in Exhibit 3.3. Observe the form of this statement carefully. It is more informative than one which simply subtracts expenses from revenues. First, it compares sales revenue with the cost of the goods that were sold to produce that revenue. The difference between the sales revenue and the cost of goods sold is called *gross margin*. Next, the operating expenses are subtracted from the gross margin to determine the *operating income*. **Operating income** is the amount of income that is generated from the normal recurring operations of a business. Items that are not expected to recur on a regular basis are subtracted from the operating income to determine the amount of *net income*.[1]

EXHIBIT 3.3

JUNE'S PLANT SHOP Income Statement For the Period Ended December 31, 2013	
Sales revenue	$ 24,750
Cost of goods sold	(11,500)
Gross margin	13,250
Less: Operating expenses	
Selling and administrative expense	(5,000)
Transportation-out	(450)
Operating income	7,800
Nonoperating items	
Interest expense	(360)
Gain on the sale of land	700
Net income	$ 8,140

EXHIBIT 3.4

Income Statement Format Used by U.S. Companies

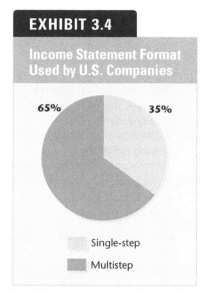

- 65% — Single-step
- 35% — Multistep

Data Source: AICPA, *Accounting Trends and Techniques.*

EXHIBIT 3.5

JUNE'S PLANT SHOP Balance Sheet As of December 31, 2013		
Assets		
Cash	$25,540	
Merchandise inventory	4,600	
Total assets		$30,140
Liabilities		
Notes payable		$ 4,000
Stockholders' equity		
Common stock	$15,000	
Retained earnings	11,140	
Total stockholders' equity		26,140
Total liabilities and stockholders' equity		$30,140

Income statements that show these additional relationships are called **multistep income statements.** Income statements that display a single comparison of all revenues minus all expenses are called **single-step income statements.** To this point in the text we have shown only single-step income statements to promote simplicity. However, the multistep form is used more frequently in practice. Exhibit 3.4 shows the percentage of companies that use the multistep versus the single-step format. Go to Exhibit 3.1 and identify the company that presents its income statement in the multistep format. You should have identified Blue Nile as the company using the multistep format. Zale's statement is shown in the single-step format.

---

[1]Revenue and expense items with special characteristics may be classified as discontinued or extraordinary items. These items are shown separately just above net income regardless of whether a company uses a single-step or multistep format. Further discussion of these items is beyond the scope of this text.

EXHIBIT 3.6

JUNE'S PLANT SHOP
Statement of Cash Flows
For the Period Ended December 31, 2013

Operating activities		
Inflow from customers	$ 24,750	
Outflow for inventory*	(10,100)	
Outflow for transportation-out	(450)	
Outflow for selling and administrative expense	(5,000)	
Outflow for interest expense	(360)	
Net cash outflow for operating activities		$ 8,840
Investing activities		
Inflow from sale of land		6,200
Financing activities		
Inflow from issue of note payable		4,000
Net change in cash		19,040
Plus beginning cash balance		6,500
Ending cash balance		$25,540

*Net cost on inventory $9,800 + transportation-in $300 = $10,100

Note that interest is reported as a *nonoperating* item on the income statement in Exhibit 3.3. In contrast, it is shown in the *operating* activities section of the statement of cash flows in Exhibit 3.6. When the FASB issued Statement of Financial Accounting Standard (SFAS) 95, it required interest to be reported in the operating activities section of the statement of cash flows. There was no corresponding requirement for the treatment of interest on the income statement. Prior to SFAS 95, interest was considered to be a nonoperating item. Most companies continued to report interest as a nonoperating item on their income statements even though they were required to change how it was reported on the statement of cash flows. As a result, there is frequent inconsistency in the way interest is reported on the two financial statements.

Also note that while the gain on the sale of land is shown on the income statement, it is not included in the operating activities section of the statement of cash flows. Since the gain is a nonoperating item, it is included in the cash inflow from the sale of land shown in the investing activities section. In this case the full cash inflow from the sale of land ($6,200) is shown in the investing activities section of the statement of cash flows in Exhibit 3.6.

LOST, DAMAGED, OR STOLEN INVENTORY

Show the effect of lost, damaged, or stolen inventory on financial statements.

Most merchandising companies experience some level of inventory **shrinkage,** a term that reflects decreases in inventory for reasons other than sales to customers. Inventory may be stolen by shoplifters, damaged by customers or employees, or even simply lost or misplaced. Since the *perpetual* inventory system is designed to record purchases and sales of inventory as they occur, the balance in the merchandise inventory account represents the amount of inventory that *should* be on hand at any given time. By taking a physical count of the merchandise inventory at the end of the accounting period and comparing that amount with the book balance in the Merchandise Inventory account, managers can determine the amount of any inventory shrinkage. If goods have been lost, damaged, or stolen, the book balance will be higher than the actual amount of inventory on hand and an adjusting entry is required to reduce assets and equity. The Merchandise Inventory account is reduced, and an expense for the amount of the lost, damaged, or stolen inventory is recognized.

REALITY BYTES

"Closed for Inventory Count" is a sign you frequently see on retail stores sometime during the month of January. Even if companies use a perpetual inventory system, the amount of inventory on hand may be unknown because of lost, damaged, or stolen goods. The only way to determine the amount of inventory on hand is to count it. Why count it in January? Christmas shoppers and many after-Christmas sales shoppers are satiated by mid-January, leaving the stores low on both merchandise and customers. Accordingly, stores have less merchandise to count and "lost sales" are minimized during January. Companies that do not depend on seasonal sales (e.g., a plumbing supplies wholesale business) may choose to count inventory at some other time during the year. Counting inventory is not a revenue-generating activity; it is a necessary evil that should be conducted when it least disrupts operations.

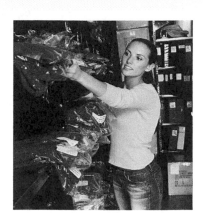

Adjustment for Lost, Damaged, or Stolen Inventory

To illustrate, assume that Midwest Merchandising Company maintains perpetual inventory records. Midwest determined, through a physical count, that it had $23,500 of merchandise inventory on hand at the end of the accounting period. The balance in the Inventory account was $24,000. Midwest must make an adjusting entry to write down the Inventory account so the amount reported on the financial statements agrees with the amount actually on hand at the end of the period. The write-down decreases both assets (inventory) and stockholders' equity (retained earnings). The write-down increases expenses and decreases net income. Cash flow is not affected. The effects on the statements are as follows.

Assets	=	Liab.	+	Equity	Rev.	−	Exp.	=	Net Inc.	Cash Flow
(500)	=	NA	+	(500)	NA	−	500	=	(500)	NA

Theoretically, inventory losses are operating expenses. However, because such losses are normally immaterial in amount, they are usually added to cost of goods sold for external reporting purposes.

EVENTS AFFECTING SALES

To this point we assumed JPS did not offer cash discounts to its customers. However, sales, as well as purchases of inventory, can be affected by returns, allowances, and discounts. **Sales discounts** are price reductions offered by sellers to encourage buyers to pay promptly. To illustrate, assume JPS engaged in the following selected events during January 2014.

EVENT 1A JPS sold on account merchandise with a list price of $8,500. Payment terms were 1/10, n/30. The merchandise had cost JPS $4,000.

The sale increases both assets (accounts receivable) and shareholders' equity (retained earnings). Recognizing revenue increases net income. The statement of cash flows is not affected. The effects on the financial statements follow.

Assets			=	Liab.	+	Stockholders' Equity			Rev.	−	Exp.	=	Net Inc.	Cash Flow
Cash	+	Accts. Rec.	+	Inventory	=	Note Pay.	+	Com. Stk.	+	Retained Earnings					
NA	+	8,500	+	NA	=	NA	+	NA	+	8,500	8,500	−	NA	=	8,500	NA

EVENT 1B   JPS recognized $4,000 of cost of goods sold.

Recognizing the expense decreases assets (merchandise inventory) and stockholders' equity (retained earnings). Cost of goods sold increases and net income decreases. Cash flow is not affected. The effects on the financial statements follow.

Assets			=	Liab.	+	Stockholders' Equity			Rev.	−	Exp.	=	Net Inc.	Cash Flow
Cash	+	Accts. Rec.	+	Inventory	=	Note Pay.	+	Com. Stk.	+	Retained Earnings				
NA	+	NA	+	(4,000)	=	NA	+	NA	+	(4,000)	NA	−	4,000	=	(4,000)	NA

Accounting for Sales Returns and Allowances

EVENT 2A   A customer from Event 1A returned inventory with a $1,000 list price. The merchandise had cost JPS $450.

The sales return decreases both assets (accounts receivable) and stockholders' equity (retained earnings) on the balance sheet. Sales and net income decrease. Cash flow is not affected. The effects on the financial statements follow.

Assets			=	Liab.	+	Stockholders' Equity			Rev.	−	Exp.	=	Net Inc.	Cash Flow
Cash	+	Accts. Rec.	+	Inventory	=	Note Pay.	+	Com. Stk.	+	Retained Earnings				
NA	+	(1,000)	+	NA	=	NA	+	NA	+	(1,000)	(1,000)	−	NA	=	(1,000)	NA

EVENT 2B   The cost of the goods ($450) is returned to the inventory account.

Since JPS got the inventory back, the sales return increases both assets (merchandise inventory) and stockholders' equity (retained earnings). The expense (cost of goods sold) decreases and net income increases. Cash flow is not affected. The effects on the financial statements follow.

Assets			=	Liab.	+	Stockholders' Equity			Rev.	−	Exp.	=	Net Inc.	Cash Flow
Cash	+	Accts. Rec.	+	Inventory	=	Note Pay.	+	Com. Stk.	+	Retained Earnings				
NA	+	NA	+	450	=	NA	+	NA	+	450	NA	−	(450)	=	450	NA

Accounting for Sales Discounts

EVENT 3   JPS collected the balance of the accounts receivable generated in Event 1A. Recall the goods were sold under terms 1/10, net/30.

ALTERNATIVE 1   The collection occurs before the discount period has expired (within 10 days from the date of the sale).

JPS would give the buyer a 1 percent discount. Given the original sales amount of $8,500 and a sales return of $1,000, the amount of the discount is $75 [($8,500 − $1,000) × .01]. The sales discount reduces the amount of accounts receivable and retained earnings on the balance sheet. It also reduces the amount of revenue and the net income shown on the balance sheet. It does not affect the statement of cash flows. The effects on the financial statements follow.

Assets				=	Liab.	+	Stockholders' Equity			Rev.	–	Exp.	=	Net Inc.	Cash Flow
Cash	+	Accts. Rec.	+	Inventory	=	Note Pay.	+	Com. Stk.	+	Retained Earnings					
NA	+	(75)	+	NA	=	NA	+	NA	+	(75)	(75)	–	NA	=	(75)	NA

The balance due on the account receivable is $7,425 ($8,500 original sales − $1,000 sales return − $75 discount). The collection increases the Cash account and decreases the Accounts Receivable account. The income statement is not affected. The cash inflow is shown in the operating activities section of the statement of cash flows. The effects on the financial statements follow.

Assets				=	Liab.	+	Stockholders' Equity			Rev.	–	Exp.	=	Net Inc.	Cash Flow
Cash	+	Accts. Rec.	+	Inventory	=	Accts. Pay.	+	Com. Stk.	+	Retained Earnings					
7,425	+	(7,425)	+	NA	=	NA	+	NA	+	NA	NA	–	NA	=	NA	7,425 OA

Net Sales

The gross amount of sales minus **sales returns and allowance** and sales discounts is commonly called **net sales.** Companies are not required by GAAP to show sales returns and allowance and sales discount on their income statement. Indeed, most companies show only the amount of *net sales* on the income statement. In this case the net sales amount to $7,425 ($8,500 original sales − $1,000 sales return − $75 discount).

ALTERNATIVE 2   The collection occurs after the discount period has expired (after 10 days from the date of the sale).

Under these circumstances there is no sales discount. The amount collected is $7,500 ($8,500 original sale − $1,000 sales return). Net sales shown on the income statement would also be $7,500.

COMMON SIZE FINANCIAL STATEMENTS

How good is a $1,000,000 increase in net income? The answer is not clear because there is no indication as to the size of the company. A million dollar increase may be excellent for a small company but would be virtually meaningless for a company the size of Exxon. To enable meaningful comparisons analysts prepare **common size financial statements.** Common size statements display information in percentages as well as absolute dollar amounts.

To illustrate, we expand the income statements for JPS to include percentages. The results are shown in Exhibit 3.7. The percentage data are computed by defining net sales as the base figure, or 100 percent. The other amounts on the statements are then

Use common sizes financial statements to evaluate managerial performance.

The income statement data show that compared to Zales, Blue Nile does save money by not operating bricks-and-mortar stores. This can be determined by comparing each company's net income to its sales. For Blue Nile this percentage is 4.2% ($12,800 ÷ $302,134), which means that while 4.2% of each dollar of revenue goes to profit, 95.8% goes to pay for expenses. For Zales this percentage is a *negative* 10.6% [($189,503) ÷ 1,779,744]. Clearly, Blue Nile did better than Zales. This result is despite the fact that compared to Blue Nile, Zales charges a higher price for the jewelry it sells. Compare each company's gross margin to its sales. Blue Nile's gross margin is 21.6% of its sales ($65,344 ÷ $302,134), which means that 78.4% of each dollar of revenue goes to pay for the product that was sold. For Zales these percentages are 46.7% for the gross margin [(1,779,744 − $948,572) ÷ 1,779,744] and 53.3% for cost of goods sold. This shows that while Blue Nile charges less for its products, it makes up for the lower gross margin with lower operating expenses.

shown as a percentage of net sales. For example, the *cost of goods sold percentage* is the dollar amount of *cost of goods sold* divided by the dollar amount of *net sales,* which produces a percentage of 66.7 percent ($8,000 ÷ $12,000) for 2012 and 46.5 percent ($11,500 ÷ $24,750) for 2013. Other income statement items are computed using the same approach.

These common size statements provide insight into the company's operating strategy. For example, assume JPS relocated its store in an upscale mall in early 2013.

EXHIBIT 3.7   Common Size Financial Statements

JUNE'S PLANT SHOP
Income Statement
For the Period Ended

	2012		2013	
Net sales*	$12,000	100.0%	$24,750	100.0%
Cost of goods sold	(8,000)	66.7	(11,500)	46.5
Gross margin	4,000	33.3	13,250	53.5
Less: Operating expenses				
Selling and administrative expense	(1,000)	8.3	(5,000)	20.2
Transportation-out			(450)	1.8
Operating income	3,000	25.0	7,800	31.5
Nonoperating items				
Interest expense			(360)	(1.5)
Gain on the sale of land			700	2.8
Net income	$3,000	25.0	$8,140	32.9

*Since JPS did not offer sales discounts or have sales returns and allowances during 2012 or 2013, the amount of sales revenue is equal to the amount of net sales. We use the term *net sales* here because it is more commonly used in business practice. Percentages do not add exactly because they have been rounded.

Management realized that the company would have to pay more for operating expenses but believed those expenses could be offset by charging significantly higher prices. The common size income statement confirms that the company's goals were accomplished. Note that the gross margin increased from 33.3 percent of sales to 53.5 percent, confirming that the company was able to increase prices. Also, note that operating expenses increased. Selling and administrative expense increased from 8.3 percent of sales to 20.2 percent. Also, the company experienced a new expense, transportation out, for delivering merchandise to its customers. These increases in expenses confirm the fact that JPS is paying more for rental space and providing additional services to its customers. The common size statements, therefore, support the conclusion that JPS's increase in net income from $3,000 to $8,140 was a result of management's new operating strategy. As a side note, the new operating strategy may also explain why JPS sold its land in late 2013. Considering the success the company experienced at the new location, there was no motive to build a store on the land.

A Look Back

Merchandising companies earn profits by selling inventory at prices that are higher than the cost paid for the goods. Merchandising companies include *retail companies* (companies that sell goods to the final consumer) and *wholesale companies* (companies that sell to other merchandising companies). The products sold by merchandising companies are called *inventory.* The costs to purchase inventory, to receive it, and to ready it for sale are *product costs,* which are first accumulated in an inventory account (balance sheet asset account) and then recognized as cost of goods sold (income statement expense account) in the period in which goods are sold. Purchases and sales of inventory can be recorded continually as goods are bought and sold (perpetual system) or at the end of the accounting period (periodic system, discussed in the chapter appendix).

Accounting for inventory includes the treatment of cash discounts, transportation costs, and returns and allowances. The cost of inventory is the list price less any purchase returns and allowances and purchase discounts, plus transportation in costs. The cost of freight paid to acquire inventory (*transportation-in*) is considered a product cost. The cost of freight paid to deliver inventory to customers (*transportation-out*) is a selling expense. *Sales returns and allowances* and *sales discounts* are subtracted from sales revenue to determine the amount of *net sales* reported on the income statement. Purchase returns and allowances reduce product cost. Theoretically, the cost of lost, damaged, or stolen inventory is an operating expense. However, because these costs are usually immaterial in amount they are typically included as part of cost of goods sold on the income statement.

Some companies use a *multistep income statement* which reports product costs separately from selling and administrative costs. Cost of goods sold is subtracted from sales revenue to determine *gross margin.* Selling and administrative expenses are subtracted from gross margin to determine income from operations. Other companies report income using a *single-step format* in which the cost of goods sold is listed along with selling and administrative items in a single expense category that is subtracted in total from revenue to determine income from operations.

Managers of merchandising businesses operate in a highly competitive environment. They must manage company operations carefully to remain profitable. *Common size financial statements* (statements presented on a percentage basis) and ratio analysis are useful monitoring tools. Common size financial statements permit ready comparisons among different-size companies. Although a $1 million increase in sales may be good for a small company and bad for a large company, a 10 percent increase can apply to any size company.

>> A Look Forward

To this point, the text has explained the basic accounting cycle for service and merchandising businesses. Future chapters more closely address specific accounting issues. For example, in Chapter 5 you will learn how to deal with inventory items that are purchased at differing prices. Other chapters will discuss a variety of specific practices that are widely used by real-world companies.

APPENDIX

LO 8

Identify the primary features of the periodic inventory system.

Periodic Inventory System

Under certain conditions, it is impractical to record inventory sales transactions as they occur. Consider the operations of a fast-food restaurant. To maintain perpetual inventory records, the restaurant would have to transfer from the Inventory account to the Cost of Goods Sold account the *cost* of each hamburger, order of fries, soft drink, or other food items as they were sold. Obviously, recording the cost of each item at the point of sale would be impractical without using highly sophisticated computer equipment (recording the selling price the customer pays is captured by cash registers; the difficulty lies in capturing inventory cost).

The **periodic inventory system** offers a practical solution for recording inventory transactions in a low-technology, high-volume environment. Inventory costs are recorded in a Purchases account at the time of purchase. Purchase returns and allowances and transportation-in are recorded in separate accounts. No entries for the cost of merchandise purchases or sales are recorded in the Inventory account during the period. The cost of goods sold is determined at the end of the period as shown in Exhibit 3.8.

EXHIBIT 3.8

Schedule of Cost of Goods Sold for 2013	
Beginning inventory	$ 6,000
Purchases	11,000
Purchase returns and allowances	(1,000)
Purchase discounts	(200)
Transportation-in	300
Cost of goods available for sale	16,100
Ending inventory	4,600
Cost of goods sold	$11,500

The perpetual and periodic inventory systems represent alternative procedures for recording the same information. The amounts of cost of goods sold and ending inventory reported in the financial statements will be the same regardless of the method used.

The **schedule of cost of goods sold** presented in Exhibit 3.8 is used for internal reporting purposes. It is normally not shown in published financial statements. The amount of cost of goods sold is reported as a single line item on the income statement. The income statement in Exhibit 3.3 will be the same whether JPS maintains perpetual or periodic inventory records.

Advantages and Disadvantages of the Periodic System versus the Perpetual System

The chief advantage of the periodic method is recording efficiency. Recording inventory transactions occasionally (periodically) requires less effort than recording them continually (perpetually). Historically, practical limitations offered businesses like fast-food restaurants or grocery stores no alternative to using the periodic system. The sheer volume of transactions made recording individual decreases to the Inventory account balance as each item was sold impossible. Imagine the number of transactions a grocery store would have to record every business day to maintain perpetual records.

Although the periodic system provides a recordkeeping advantage over the perpetual system, perpetual inventory records provide significant control advantages over periodic records. With perpetual records, the book balance in the Inventory account should agree with the amount of inventory in stock at any given time. By comparing that book balance with the results of a physical inventory count, management can determine the amount of lost, damaged, destroyed, or stolen inventory. Perpetual records also permit more timely and accurate reorder decisions and profitability assessments.

When a company uses the *periodic* inventory system, lost, damaged, or stolen merchandise is automatically included in cost of goods sold. Because such goods are not included in the year-end physical count, they are treated as sold regardless of the reason for their absence. Since the periodic system does not separate the cost of lost, damaged, or stolen merchandise from the cost of goods sold, the amount of any inventory shrinkage is unknown. This feature is a major disadvantage of the periodic system. Without knowing the amount of inventory losses, management cannot weigh the costs of various security systems against the potential benefits.

Advances in such technology as electronic bar code scanning and increased computing power have eliminated most of the practical constraints that once prevented merchandisers with high-volume, low dollar-value inventories from recording inventory transactions on a continual basis. As a result, use of the perpetual inventory system has expanded rapidly in recent years and continued growth can be expected. This text, therefore, concentrates on the perpetual inventory system.

A step-by-step audio-narrated series of slides is provided on the text website at www.mhhe.com/edmondssurvey3e.

SELF-STUDY REVIEW PROBLEM

Academy Sales Company (ASC) started the 2012 accounting period with the balances given in the financial statements model shown below. During 2012 ASC experienced the following business events.

1. Purchased $16,000 of merchandise inventory on account, terms 2/10, n/30.
2. The goods that were purchased in Event 1 were delivered FOB shipping point. Freight costs of $600 were paid in cash by the responsible party.
3. Returned $500 of goods purchased in Event 1.
4a. Recorded the cash discount on the goods purchased in Event 1.
4b. Paid the balance due on the account payable within the discount period.
5a. Recognized $21,000 of cash revenue from the sale of merchandise.
5b. Recognized $15,000 of cost of goods sold.
6. The merchandise in Event 5a was sold to customers FOB destination. Freight costs of $950 were paid in cash by the responsible party.
7. Paid cash of $4,000 for selling and administrative expenses.
8. Sold the land for $5,600 cash.

Required

a. Record the above transactions in a financial statements model like the one shown below.

Event No.	Cash	+	Inventory	+	Land	=	Accts. Pay.	+	Com. Stk.	+	Ret. Earn.	Rev./ Gain	−	Exp.	=	Net Inc.	Cash Flow
Bal.	25,000	+	3,000	+	5,000	=	–0–	+	18,000	+	15,000	NA	−	NA	=	NA	NA

b. Prepare a schedule of cost of goods sold. (Appendix)
c. Prepare a multistep income statement. Include common size percentages on the income statement.
d. ASC's gross margin percentage in 2011 was 22%. Based on the common size data in the income statement, did ASC raise or lower its prices in 2012? (Appendix)
e. Assuming a 10 percent rate of growth, what is the amount of net income expected for 2013?

Solution

a.

Event No.	Cash	+	Inventory	+	Land	=	Accts. Pay.	+	Com. Stk.	+	Ret. Earn.	Rev./ Gain	−	Exp.	=	Net Inc.	Cash Flow
Bal.	25,000	+	3,000	+	5,000	=	−0−	+	18,000	+	15,000	NA	−	NA	=	NA	NA
1		+	16,000			=	16,000	+		+			−		=		
2	(600)	+	600			=		+		+			−		=		(600) OA
3		+	(500)			=	(500)	+		+			−		=		
4a		+	(310)			=	(310)	+		+			−		=		
4b	(15,190)	+				=	(15,190)	+		+			−		=		(15,190) OA
5a	21,000	+				=		+		+	21,000	21,000	−		=	21,000	21,000 OA
5b		+	(15,000)			=		+		+	(15,000)		−	15,000	=	(15,000)	
6	(950)	+				=		+		+	(950)		−	950	=	(950)	(950) OA
7	(4,000)	+				=		+		+	(4,000)		−	4,000	=	(4,000)	(4,000) OA
8	5,600	+			(5,000)	=		+		+	600	600	−		=	600	5,600 IA
Bal.	30,860	+	3,790		−0−	=	−0−	+	18,000	+	16,650	21,600	−	19,950	=	1,650	5,860 NC

b.

ACADEMY SALES COMPANY
Schedule of Cost of Goods Sold
For the Period Ended December 31, 2012

Beginning inventory	$ 3,000
Plus purchases	16,000
Less: Purchase returns and allowances	(500)
Less: Purchases discounts	(310)
Plus: Transportation-in	600
Goods available for sale	18,790
Less: Ending inventory	3,790
Cost of goods sold	$(15,000)

c.

ACADEMY SALES COMPANY
Income Statement*
For the Period Ended December 31, 2012

Net sales	$21,000	100.0%
Cost of goods sold	(15,000)	71.4
Gross margin	6,000	28.6
Less: Operating expenses		
Selling and administrative expense	(4,000)	19.0
Transportation-out	(950)	4.5
Operating income	1,050	5.0
Nonoperating items		
Gain on the sale of land	600	2.9
Net income	$ 1,650	7.9

*Percentages do not add exactly because they have been rounded.

d. All other things being equal, the higher the gross margin percentage, the higher the sales prices. Since the gross margin percentage increased from 22% to 28.6%, the data suggest that Academy raised its sales prices.

e. $1,155 [$1,050 + (.10 × $1,050)]. Note that the gain is not expected to recur.

KEY TERMS

Cash discount 94	Merchandising businesses 86	Sales returns and
Common size financial	Multistep income	allowances 103
statements 103	statement 99	Schedule of cost of goods
Cost of goods available for	Net sales 103	sold 106
sale 89	Operating income (or loss) 99	Selling and administrative
Cost of Goods Sold 89	Period costs 89	costs 89
FOB (free on board)	Periodic inventory system 106	Shrinkage 100
destination 95	Perpetual inventory	Single-step income
FOB (free on board) shipping	system 89	statement 99
point 95	Product costs 89	Transportation-in
Gain 98	Purchase discount 94	(freight-in) 95
Gross margin 89	Purchase returns and	Transportation-out
Gross profit 89	allowances 93	(freight-out) 95
Loss 98	Retail companies 86	2/10, n/30 94
Merchandise inventory 86	Sales discounts 101	Wholesale companies 86

QUESTIONS

1. Define *merchandise inventory*. What types of costs are included in the Merchandise Inventory account?

2. What is the difference between a product cost and a selling and administrative cost?

3. How is the cost of goods available for sale determined?

4. What portion of cost of goods available for sale is shown on the balance sheet? What portion is shown on the income statement?

5. When are period costs expensed? When are product costs expensed?

6. If PetCo had net sales of $600,000, goods available for sale of $450,000, and cost of goods sold of $375,000, what is its gross margin? What amount of inventory will be shown on its balance sheet?

7. Describe how the perpetual inventory system works. What are some advantages of using the perpetual inventory system? Is it necessary to take a physical inventory when using the perpetual inventory system?

8. What are the effects of the following types of transactions on the accounting equation? Also identify the financial statements that are affected. (Assume that the perpetual inventory system is used.)
   a. Acquisition of cash from the issue of common stock.
   b. Contribution of inventory by an owner of a company.
   c. Purchase of inventory with cash by a company.
   d. Sale of inventory for cash.

9. Northern Merchandising Company sold inventory that cost $12,000 for $20,000 cash. How does this event affect the accounting equation? What financial statements and

accounts are affected? (Assume that the perpetual inventory system is used.)

10. If goods are shipped FOB shipping point, which party (buyer or seller) is responsible for the shipping costs?

11. Define *transportation-in*. Is it a product or a period cost?

12. Quality Cellular Co. paid $80 for freight on merchandise that it had purchased for resale to customers (transportation-in) and paid $135 for freight on merchandise delivered to customers (transportation-out). The $80 payment is added to what account? The $135 payment is added to what account?

13. Why would a seller grant an allowance to a buyer of the his merchandise?

14. Dyer Department Store purchased goods with the terms 2/10, n/30. What do these terms mean?

15. Eastern Discount Stores incurred a $5,000 cash cost. How does the accounting for this cost differ if the cash were paid for inventory versus commissions to sales personnel?

16. What is the purpose of giving a cash discount to charge customers?

17. Define *transportation-out*. Is it a product cost or a period cost for the seller?

18. Ball Co. purchased inventory with a list price of $4,000 with the terms 2/10, n/30. What amount will be added to the Merchandise Inventory account?

19. Explain the difference between purchase returns and sales returns. How do purchase returns affect the financial statements of both buyer and seller? How do sales returns affect the financial statements of both buyer and seller?

20. Explain the difference between gross margin and a gain.
21. What is the difference between a multistep income statement and a single-step income statement?
22. What is the advantage of using common size income statements to present financial information for several accounting periods?
23. What is the purpose of preparing a schedule of cost of goods sold?

24. Explain how the periodic inventory system works. What are some advantages of using the periodic inventory system? What are some disadvantages of using the periodic inventory system? Is it necessary to take a physical inventory when using the periodic inventory system?
25. Why does the periodic inventory system impose a major disadvantage for management in accounting for lost, stolen, or damaged goods?

 MULTIPLE-CHOICE QUESTIONS

Multiple-choice questions are provided on the text website at www.mhhe.com/edmondssurvey3e.

EXERCISES

All applicable Exercises are available with McGraw-Hill's *Connect Accounting*.

When the instructions for *any* exercise or problem call for the preparation of an income statement, use the *multistep format* unless otherwise indicated.

LO 1, 2

Exercise 3-1 *Comparing a merchandising company with a service company*

The following information is available for two different types of businesses for the 2012 accounting period. Eady CPAs is a service business that provides accounting services to small businesses. Campus Clothing is a merchandising business that sells sports clothing to college students.

Data for Eady CPAs

1. Borrowed $40,000 from the bank to start the business.
2. Provided $30,000 of services to customers and collected $30,000 cash.
3. Paid salary expense of $20,000.

Data for Campus Clothing

1. Borrowed $40,000 from the bank to start the business.
2. Purchased $25,000 inventory for cash.
3. Inventory costing $16,400 was sold for $30,000 cash.
4. Paid $3,600 cash for operating expenses.

Required

a. Prepare an income statement, a balance sheet, and a statement of cash flows for each of the companies.
b. Which of the two businesses would have product costs? Why?
c. Why does Eady CPAs not compute gross margin on its income statement?
d. Compare the assets of both companies. What assets do they have in common? What assets are different? Why?

LO 2

Exercise 3-2 *Effect of inventory transactions on financial statements: perpetual system*

Mark Dixon started a small merchandising business in 2012. The business experienced the following events during its first year of operation. Assume that Dixon uses the perpetual inventory system.

1. Acquired $40,000 cash from the issue of common stock.
2. Purchased inventory for $30,000 cash.
3. Sold inventory costing $20,000 for $32,000 cash.

Required

a. Record the events in a statements model like the one shown below.

Assets			=	Equity			Rev.	−	Exp.	=	Net Inc.	Cash Flow
Cash	+	Inv.	=	Com. Stk.	+	Ret. Earn.						

b. Prepare an income statement for 2012 (use the multistep format).
c. What is the amount of total assets at the end of the period?

Exercise 3-3   *Effect of inventory transactions on the income statement and statement of cash flows: Perpetual system*   LO 2

During 2012, Knight Merchandising Company purchased $15,000 of inventory on account. Knight sold inventory on account that cost $12,500 for $17,500. Cash payments on accounts payable were $10,000. There was $11,000 cash collected from accounts receivable. Knight also paid $3,500 cash for operating expenses. Assume that Knight started the accounting period with $14,000 in both cash and common stock.

Required

a. Identify the events described in the preceding paragraph and record them in a horizontal statements model like the following one:

Assets						=	Liab.	+	Equity				Rev.	−	Exp.	=	Net inc.	Cash Flow
Cash	+	Accts. Rec.	+	Inv.		=	Accts. Pay.	+	Com. Stk.	+	Ret. Earn.							
14,000	+	NA	+	NA	−		NA	⊢	14,000	+	NA		NA	−	NA	=	NA	NA

b. What is the balance of accounts receivable at the end of 2012?
c. What is the balance of accounts payable at the end of 2012?
d. What are the amounts of gross margin and net income for 2012?
e. Determine the amount of net cash flow from operating activities.
f. Explain why net income and retained earnings are the same for Knight. Normally would these amounts be the same? Why or why not?

Exercise 3-4   *Recording inventory transactions in a financial statements model*   LO 2

Kona Clothing experienced the following events during 2012, its first year of operation:

1. Acquired $14,000 cash from the issue of common stock.
2. Purchased inventory for $8,000 cash.
3. Sold inventory costing $6,000 for $9,000 cash.
4. Paid $800 for advertising expense.

Required

Record the events in a statements model like the one shown below.

Assets			=	Equity			Rev.	−	Exp.	=	Net Inc.	Cash Flow
Cash	+	Inv.	=	Com. Stk.	+	Ret. Earn.						

Exercise 3-5   *Understanding the freight terms FOB shipping point and FOB destination*

Required

Determine which party, buyer or seller, is responsible for freight charges in each of the following situations:

a. Sold merchandise, freight terms, FOB destination.
b. Sold merchandise, freight terms, FOB shipping point.
c. Purchased merchandise, freight terms, FOB destination.
d. Purchased merchandise, freight terms, FOB shipping point.

LO 2, 3

Exercise 3-6   *Effect of purchase returns and allowances and freight costs on the financial statements: perpetual system*

The beginning account balances for Jerry's Auto Shop as of January 1, 2012 follows:

Account Titles	Beginning Balances
Cash	$28,000
Inventory	14,000
Common stock	36,000
Retained earnings	6,000
Total	$42,000

The following events affected the company during the 2012 accounting period:

1. Purchased merchandise on account that cost $18,000.
2. The goods in Event 1 were purchased FOB shipping point with freight cost of $1,000 cash.
3. Returned $3,600 of damaged merchandise for credit on account.
4. Agreed to keep other damaged merchandise for which the company received a $1,400 allowance.
5. Sold merchandise that cost $16,000 for $34,000 cash.
6. Delivered merchandise to customers in Event 5 under terms FOB destination with freight costs amounting to $800 cash.
7. Paid $12,000 on the merchandise purchased in Event 1.

Required

a. Organize appropriate ledger accounts under an accounting equation. Record the beginning balances and the transaction data in the accounts.
b. Prepare an income statement and a statement of cash flows for 2012.
c. Explain why a difference does or does not exist between net income and net cash flow from operating activities.

LO 2, 3

Exercise 3-7   *Accounting for product costs: Perpetual inventory system*

Which of the following would be *added* to the Inventory account for a merchandising business using the perpetual inventory system?

Required

a. Transportation-out.
b. Purchase discount.
c. Transportation-in.
d. Purchase of a new computer to be used by the business.
e. Purchase of inventory.
f. Allowance received for damaged inventory.

Exercise 3-8 *Effect of product cost and period cost: horizontal statements model*

LO 1, 2, 3

The Toy Store experienced the following events for the 2012 accounting period:

1. Acquired $20,000 cash from the issue of common stock.
2. Purchased $56,000 of inventory on account.
3. Received goods purchased in Event 2 FOB shipping point; freight cost of $600 paid in cash.
4. Sold inventory on account that cost $35,000 for $57,400.
5. Freight cost on the goods sold in Event 4 was $420. The goods were shipped FOB destination. Cash was paid for the freight cost.
6. Customer in Event 4 returned $4,000 worth of goods that had a cost of $2,400.
7. Collected $47,000 cash from accounts receivable.
8. Paid $44,000 cash on accounts payable.
9. Paid $1,100 for advertising expense.
10. Paid $1,000 cash for insurance expense.

Required

a. Which of these events affect period (selling and administrative) costs? Which result in product costs? If neither, label the transaction NA.
b. Record each event in a horizontal statements model like the following one. The first event is recorded as an example.

Assets			=	Liab.	+	Equity			Rev.	−	Exp.	=	Net Inc.	Cash Flow
Cash	+ Accts. Rec.	+ Inv.	=	Accts. Pay.	+	C. Stk.	+	Ret. Earn.						
20,000	+ NA	+ NA =		NA	+	20,000	+	NA	NA	−	NA	=	NA	20,000 FA

Exercise 3-9 *Cash discounts and purchase returns*

LO 3

On April 6, 2012, Taylor Furnishings purchased $12,400 of merchandise from Bergin's Imports, terms 2/10 n/45. On April 8, Taylor returned $1,200 of the merchandise to Bergin's Imports for credit. Taylor paid cash for the merchandise on April 15, 2012.

Required

a. What is the amount that Taylor must pay Bergin's Imports on April 15?
b. Record the events in a horizontal statements model like the following one.

Assets		=	Liab.	+	Equity			Rev.	−	Exp.	=	Net Inc.	Cash Flow
Cash	+ Inv.	=	Accts. Pay.	+	C. Stock.	+	Ret. Earn.						

c. How much must Taylor pay for the merchandise purchased if the payment is not made until April 20, 2012?
d. Record the payment in event (c) in a horizontal statements model like the one above.
e. Why would Taylor want to pay for the merchandise by April 15?

Exercise 3-10 *Effect of sales returns and allowances and freight costs on the financial statements: perpetual system*

LO 2, 3

Stash Company began the 2012 accounting period with $10,000 cash, $38,000 inventory, $25,000 common stock, and $23,000 retained earnings. During the 2012 accounting period, Stash experienced the following events.

1. Sold merchandise costing $28,000 for $46,000 on account to Jack's Furniture Store.
2. Delivered the goods to Jack's under terms FOB destination. Freight costs were $500 cash.

3. Received returned goods from Jack's. The goods cost Stash $2,000 and were sold to Jack's for $3,000.
4. Granted Jack's $2,000 allowance for damaged goods that Jack's agreed to keep.
5. Collected partial payment of $25,000 cash from accounts receivable.

Required

a. Record the events in a statements model like the one shown below.

Assets			=	Equity			Rev.	−	Exp.	=	Net Inc.	Cash Flow
Cash	+ Accts. Rec.	+ Inv.	=	Com. Stk.	+	Ret. Earn.						

b. Prepare an income statement, a balance sheet, and a statement of cash flows.
c. Why would Stash grant the $2,000 allowance to Jack's? Who benefits more?

LO 2, 3

Exercise 3-11   *Effect of cash discounts on financial statements: perpetual system*

Campus Computers was started in 2012. The company experienced the following accounting events during its first year of operation.

1. Started business when it acquired $50,000 cash from the issue of common stock.
2. Purchased merchandise with a list price of $46,000 on account, terms 2/10, n/30.
3. Paid off one-half of the accounts payable balance within the discount period.
4. Sold merchandise on account that had a list price of $48,000. Credit terms were 1/20, n/30. The merchandise had cost Campus Computers $28,000.
5. Collected cash from the account receivable within the discount period.
6. Paid $7,200 cash for operating expenses.
7. Paid the balance due on accounts payable. The payment was not made within the discount period.

Required

a. Record the events in a horizontal statements model like the following one.

Assets			=	Liab.	+	Equity			Rev.	−	Exp.	=	Net Inc.	Cash Flow
Cash	+ Accts. Rec.	+ Inv.	=	Accts. Pay.	+	Com. Stk.	+	Ret. Earn.						

b. What is the amount of gross margin for the period? What is the net income for the period?
c. Why would Campus Computers sell merchandise with the terms 1/20, n/30?
d. What do the terms 2/10, n/30 in Event 2 mean to Campus Computers?

LO 2, 3

Exercise 3-12   *Comparing gross margin and gain on sale of land*

Usrey Sales Company had the following balances in its accounts on January 1, 2012.

Cash	$ 70,000
Merchandise Inventory	50,000
Land	120,000
Common Stock	100,000
Retained Earnings	140,000

Usrey experienced the following events during 2012.

1. Sold merchandise inventory that cost $40,000 for $75,000.
2. Sold land that cost $50,000 for $80,000.

Required

a. Determine the amount of gross margin recognized by Usrey.

b. Determine the amount of the gain on the sale of land recognized by Usrey.

c. Comment on how the gross margin versus the gain will be recognized on the income statement.

d. Comment on how the gross margin versus the gain will be recognized on the statement of cash flows.

Exercise 3-13 *Effect of inventory losses: perpetual system*

LO 2, 6

Reeves Design experienced the following events during 2012, its first year of operation.

1. Started the business when it acquired $40,000 cash from the issue of common stock.
2. Paid $28,000 cash to purchase inventory.
3. Sold inventory costing $21,500 for $34,200 cash.
4. Physically counted inventory showing $5,800 inventory was on hand at the end of the accounting period.

Required

a. Determine the amount of the difference between book balance and the actual amount of inventory as determined by the physical count.

b. Explain how differences between the book balance and the physical count of inventory could arise. Why is being able to determine whether differences exist useful to management?

Exercise 3-14 *Determining the effect of inventory transactions on the horizontal statements model: perpetual system*

LO 2

Causey Sales Company experienced the following events:

1. Purchased merchandise inventory for cash.
2. Purchased merchandise inventory on account.
3. Sold merchandise inventory for cash. Label the revenue recognition 3a and the expense recognition 3b.
4. Sold merchandise inventory on account. Label the revenue recognition 4a and the expense recognition 4b.
5. Returned merchandise purchased on account.
6. Paid cash for selling and administrative expenses.
7. Paid cash on accounts payable not within the discount period.
8. Paid cash for transportation-in.
9. Collected cash from accounts receivable.
10. Paid cash for transportation-out.

Required

Identify each event as asset source (AS), asset use (AU), asset exchange (AE), or claims exchange (CE). Also explain how each event affects the financial statements by placing a + for increase, − for decrease, or NA for not affected under each of the components in the following statements model. Assume the company uses the perpetual inventory system. The first event is recorded as an example.

Event No.	Event Type	Assets	=	Liab.	+	Equity	Rev.	−	Exp.	=	Net Inc.	Cash Flow
1	AE	+ −	=	NA	+	NA	NA	−	NA	=	NA	− OA

LO 4

Exercise 3-15   *Single-step and multistep income statements*

The following information was taken from the accounts of Healthy Foods Market, a small grocery store at December 31, 2012. The accounts are listed in alphabetical order, and all have normal balances.

Accounts payable	$ 300
Accounts receivable	1,040
Advertising expense	200
Cash	820
Common stock	600
Cost of goods sold	900
Interest expense	140
Merchandise inventory	500
Prepaid rent	280
Retained earnings	1,050
Sales revenue	2,400
Salaries expense	260
Supplies expense	210
Gain on sale of land	75

Required

First, prepare an income statement for the year using the single-step approach. Then prepare another income statement using the multistep approach.

LO 2

Exercise 3-16   *Determining the cost of financing inventory*

On January 1, 2012, Fran started a small flower merchandising business that she named Fran's Flowers. The company experienced the following events during the first year of operation.

1. Started the business by issuing common stock for $20,000 cash.
2. Paid $28,000 cash to purchase inventory.
3. Sold merchandise that cost $16,000 for $36,000 on account.
4. Collected $30,000 cash from accounts receivable.
5. Paid $7,500 for operating expenses.

Required

a. Organize ledger accounts under an accounting equation and record the events in the accounts.
b. Prepare an income statement, a balance sheet, and a statement of cash flows.
c. Since Fran sold inventory for $36,000, she will be able to recover more than half of the $40,000 she invested in the stock. Do you agree with this statement? Why or why not?

LO 3

Exercise 3-17   *Inventory financing costs*

Joan Sweatt comes to you for advice. She has just purchased a large amount of inventory with the terms 2/10, n/30. The amount of the invoice is $540,000. She is currently short of cash but has decent credit. She can borrow the money needed to settle the account payable at an annual interest rate of 7%. Joan is sure she will have the necessary cash by the due date of the invoice but not by the last day of the discount period.

Required

a. Convert the discount rate into an annual interest rate.
b. Make a recommendation regarding whether Sweatt should borrow the money and pay off the account payable within the discount period.

LO 8

Exercise 3-18   *Effect of inventory transactions on the income statement and balance sheet: periodic system (Appendix)*

Joe Dodd owns Joe's Sporting Goods. At the beginning of the year, Joe's had $8,400 in inventory. During the year, Joe's purchased inventory that cost $42,000. At the end of the year, inventory on hand amounted to $17,600.

Required

Calculate the following:

a. Cost of goods available for sale during the year.

b. Cost of goods sold for the year.

c. Amount of inventory Joe's would report on the year-end balance sheet.

Exercise 3-19 *Determining cost of goods sold: periodic system (Appendix)*

LO 8

Lane Antiques uses the periodic inventory system to account for its inventory transactions. The following account titles and balances were drawn from Lane's records: beginning balance in inventory, $24,000; purchases, $150,000; purchase returns and allowances, $10,000; sales, $400,000; sales returns and allowances, $2,500; freight-in, $750; and operating expenses, $26,000. A physical count indicated that $18,000 of merchandise was on hand at the end of the accounting period.

Required

a. Prepare a schedule of cost of goods sold.

b. Prepare a multistep income statement.

Exercise 3-20 *Using common size statements and ratios to make comparisons*

LO 7

At the end of 2012, the following information is available for Chicago and St. Louis companies:

	Chicago	St. Louis
Sales	$3,000,000	$3,000
Cost of goods sold	1,800,000	2,100
Selling and administrative expenses	960,000	780
Total assets	3,750,000	3,750
Stockholders' equity	1,000,000	1,200

Required

a. Prepare common size income statements for each company.

b. One company is a high-end retailer, and the other operates a discount store. Which is the discounter? Support your selection by referring to the common size statements.

PROBLEMS

All applicable Problems are available with McGraw-Hill's
Connect Accounting.

≡ connect
|ACCOUNTING

Problem 3-21 *Basic transactions for three accounting cycles: perpetual system*

LO 2

Ginger's Flower Company was started in 2012 when it acquired $80,000 cash from the issue of common stock. The following data summarize the company's first three years' operating activities. Assume that all transactions were cash transactions.

CHECK FIGURES
2012 Net Income: $8,000
2014 Total Assets: $112,000

	2012	2013	2014
Purchases of inventory	$ 60,000	$ 90,000	$ 130,000
Sales	102,000	146,000	220,000
Cost of goods sold	54,000	78,000	140,000
Selling and administrative expenses	40,000	52,000	72,000

Required

Prepare an income statement (use multistep format) and balance sheet for each fiscal year. (*Hint:* Record the transaction data for each accounting period in the accounting equation before preparing the statements for that year.)

Problem 3-22 *Identifying product and period costs*

Required

Indicate whether each of the following costs is a product cost or a period (selling and administrative) cost.

a. Advertising expense.
b. Insurance on vans used to deliver goods to customers.
c. Salaries of sales supervisors.
d. Monthly maintenance expense for a copier.
e. Goods purchased for resale.
f. Cleaning supplies for the office.
g. Freight on goods purchased for resale.
h. Salary of the marketing director.
i. Freight on goods sold to customer with terms FOB destination.
j. Utilities expense incurred for office building.

Problem 3-23 *Identifying freight costs*

Required

For each of the following events, determine the amount of freight paid by The Dive Shop. Also indicate whether the freight cost would be classified as a product or period (selling and administrative) cost.

a. Purchased merchandise inventory with freight costs of $1,400. The merchandise was shipped FOB destination.
b. Shipped merchandise to customers, freight terms FOB destination. The freight costs were $300.
c. Purchased inventory with freight costs of $500. The goods were shipped FOB shipping point.
d. Sold merchandise to a customer. Freight costs were $800. The goods were shipped FOB shipping point.

Problem 3-24 *Effect of purchase returns and allowances and purchase discounts on the financial statements: perpetual system*

The following events were completed by Chan's Imports in September 2012.

Sept. 1 Acquired $60,000 cash from the issue of common stock.
       1 Purchased $36,000 of merchandise on account with terms 2/10, n/30.
       5 Paid $800 cash for freight to obtain merchandise purchased on September 1.
       8 Sold merchandise that cost $20,000 to customers for $38,000 on account, with terms 2/10, n/30.
       8 Returned $1,500 of defective merchandise from the September 1 purchase to the supplier.
      10 Paid cash for the balance due on the merchandise purchased on September 1.
      20 Received cash from customers of September 8 sale in settlement of the account balances, but not within the discount period.
      30 Paid $4,900 cash for selling expenses.

Required

a. Record each event in a statements model like the following one. The first event is recorded as an example.

Assets			=	Liab.	+	Equity			Rev.	−	Exp.	=	Net Inc.	Cash Flow
Cash	+ Accts. Rec.	+ Inv.	=	Accts. Pay.	+	Com. Stk.	+	Ret. Earn.						
60,000	+ NA	+ NA	=	NA	+	60,000	+	NA	NA	− NA	=	NA		60,000 FA

b. Prepare an income statement for the month ending September 30.

c. Prepare a statement of cash flows for the month ending September 30.

d. Explain why there is a difference between net income and cash flow from operating activities.

Problem 3-25 *Comprehensive cycle problem: Perpetual system*

LO 2, 3, 5, 6

At the beginning of 2012, the Jeater Company had the following balances in its accounts:

CHECK FIGURES
c. Net Income: $1,500
Total Assets: $14,800

Cash	$ 4,300
Inventory	9,000
Common stock	10,000
Retained earnings	3,300

During 2012, the company experienced the following events.

1. Purchased inventory that cost $2,200 on account from Blue Company under terms 1/10, n/30. The merchandise was delivered FOB shipping point. Freight costs of $110 were paid in cash.

2. Returned $200 of the inventory that it had purchased because the inventory was damaged in transit. The freight company agreed to pay the return freight cost.

3. Paid the amount due on its account payable to Blue Company within the cash discount period.

4. Sold inventory that had cost $3,000 for $5,500 on account, under terms 2/10, n/45.

5. Received merchandise returned from a customer. The merchandise originally cost $400 and was sold to the customer for $710 cash during the previous accounting period. The customer was paid $710 cash for the returned merchandise.

6. Delivered goods FOB destination in Event 4. Freight costs of $60 were paid in cash.

7. Collected the amount due on the account receivable within the discount period.

8. Took a physical count indicating that $7,970 of inventory was on hand at the end of the accounting period.

Required

a. Identify these events as asset source (AS), asset use (AU), asset exchange (AE), or claims exchange (CE).

b. Record each event in a statements model like the following one.

	Balance Sheet							Income Statement				
Event	**Assets**			=	**Liab.**	=	**Equity**	**Rev.**	−	**Exp.**	=	**Net Inc.**	**Statement of Cash Flows**
	Cash	+ Accts. Rec.	+ Mdse. Inv.	=	Accts. Pay.	+	Ret. Earn.						

c. Prepare an income statement, a statement of changes in stockholders' equity, a balance sheet, and a statement of cash flows.

Problem 3-26 *Using common size income statements to make comparisons*

LO 7

The following income statements were drawn from the annual reports of Pierro Sales Company.

	2012*	2013*
Net sales	$520,600	$580,500
Cost of goods sold	(369,600)	(401,500)
Gross margin	151,000	179,000
Less: Operating expense		
Selling and administrative expenses	(64,800)	(81,300)
Net income	$ 86,200	$ 97,700

*All dollar amounts are reported in thousands.

The president's message in the company's annual report stated that the company had implemented a strategy to increase market share by spending more on advertising. The president indicated that prices held steady and sales grew as expected. Write a memo indicating whether you agree with the president's statements. How has the strategy affected profitability? Support your answer by measuring growth in sales and selling expenses. Also prepare common size income statements and make appropriate references to the differences between 2012 and 2013.

LO 5, 8

Problem 3-27 *Preparing a schedule of cost of goods sold and multistep and single-step income statements: Periodic system (Appendix)*

The following account titles and balances were taken from the adjusted trial balance of Brisco Farm Co. for 2012. The company uses the periodic inventory system.

CHECK FIGURES
a. Cost of Goods Available for Sale: $48,675
b. Net Income: $55,000

Account Title	Balance
Sales returns and allowances	$ 3,250
Miscellaneous expense	400
Transportation-out	700
Sales	69,750
Advertising expense	2,750
Salaries expense	8,500
Transportation-in	1,725
Purchases	42,000
Interest expense	360
Merchandise inventory, January 1	6,200
Rent expense	5,000
Merchandise inventory, December 31	4,050
Purchase returns and allowances	1,250
Loss on sale of land	3,400
Utilities expense	710

Required

a. Prepare a schedule to determine the amount of cost of goods sold.
b. Prepare a multistep income statement.
c. Prepare a single-step income statement.

LO 8

Problem 3-28 *Comprehensive cycle problem: Periodic system (Appendix)*

The following trial balance pertains to Nate's Grocery as of January 1, 2012:

CHECK FIGURES
a. Ending Cash: $70,524
b. Cost of Goods Sold: $94,876

Account Title	Beginning Balances
Cash	$26,000
Accounts receivable	4,000
Merchandise inventory	50,000
Accounts payable	4,000
Common stock	43,000
Retained earnings	33,000
Totals	$80,000

The following events occurred in 2012. Assume that Nate's uses the periodic inventory method.

1. Purchased land for $9,000 cash.
2. Purchased merchandise on account for $96,000, terms 1/10 n/45.
3. Paid freight of $1,000 cash on merchandise purchased FOB shipping point.
4. Returned $3,600 of defective merchandise purchased in Event 2.
5. Sold merchandise for $86,000 cash.
6. Sold merchandise on account for $90,000, terms 2/10 n/30.
7. Paid cash within the discount period on accounts payable due on merchandise purchased in Event 2.

8. Paid $11,600 cash for selling expenses.
9. Collected $50,000 of the accounts receivable from Event 6 within the discount period.
10. Collected $40,000 of the accounts receivable but not within the discount period.
11. Paid $6,400 of other operating expenses.
12. A physical count indicated that $47,600 of inventory was on hand at the end of the accounting period.

Required

a. Record the above transactions in a horizontal statements model like the following one.

Event	Balance Sheet										Income Statement				Statement of Cash Flows
	Assets				=	Equity					Rev.	− Exp.	= Net Inc.		
	Cash +	Accts. Rec. +	Mdse. Inv. +	Land =		Accts. Pay. +	Com. Stock +	Ret. Earn.							

b. Prepare a schedule of cost of goods sold and an income statement.

ANALYZE, THINK, COMMUNICATE

ATC 3-1 Business Application Case *Understanding real world annual reports*

Use the Target Corporation's annual report in Appendix B to answer the following questions related to Target's 2009 fiscal year.

Target Corporation

Required

a. What percentage of Target's *total revenues* end up as net earnings?
b. What percentage of Target's *sales* go to pay for the costs of the goods being sold?
c. What costs does Target include in its Cost of Sales account?
d. When does Target recognize revenue from the sale of gift cards?

ATC 3-2 Group Exercise *Multistep income statement*

The following quarterly information is given for Raybon for the year ended 2012 (amounts shown are in millions).

	First Quarter	Second Quarter	Third Quarter	Fourth Quarter
Net Sales	$736.0	$717.4	$815.2	$620.1
Gross Margin	461.9	440.3	525.3	252.3
Net Income	37.1	24.6	38.6	31.4

Required

a. Divide the class into groups and organize the groups into four sections. Assign each section financial information for one of the quarters.
  (1) Each group should compute the cost of goods sold and operating expenses for the specific quarter assigned to its section and prepare a multistep income statement for the quarter.
  (2) Each group should compute the gross margin percentage and cost of goods sold percentage for its specific quarter.
  (3) Have a representative of each group put that quarter's sales, cost of goods sold percentage, and gross margin percentage on the board.

Class Discussion

b. Have the class discuss the change in each of these items from quarter to quarter and explain why the change might have occurred. Which was the best quarter and why?

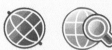

ATC 3-3   Research Assignment   *Analyzing Amazon.com's income statement*

Complete the requirements below using the most recent financial statements available [20xx] on Amazon.com's corporate website. Obtain the statements on the internet by following the steps below. (Be aware that the formatting of the company's website may have changed since these instructions were written.)

- Go to www.amazon.com.
- At the bottom of the screen, under "Get to Know Us," click on "Investor Relations."
- Annual Reports and Proxies.
- Click on "20xx Annual Report" (the most recent year).

Read the following sections of the annual report:

- The income statement, which Amazon.com calls the "Consolidated Statement of Operations."
- In the footnotes section, "Note 1—Description of Business and Accounting Policies," read the subsections titled "*Revenues,*" "*Shipping Activities,*" and "*Cost of Sales.*"

Required

a. What percentage of Amazon's sales end up as net income?

b. What percentage of Amazon's sales go to pay for the costs of the goods being sold?

c. What specific criteria are necessary before Amazon will recognize a sale as having been completed and record the related revenue?

d. How does Amazon account for (report on its income statement) the shipping costs it incurs to ship goods to its customers?

ATC 3-4   Written Assignment, Critical Thinking   *Effect of sales returns on financial statements*

Bell Farm and Garden Equipment reported the following information for 2012:

Net Sales of Equipment	$2,450,567
Other Income	6,786
Cost of Goods Sold	1,425,990
Selling, General, and Administrative Expense	325,965
Net Operating Income	$ 705,398

Selected information from the balance sheet as of December 31, 2012, follows.

Cash and Marketable Securities	$113,545
Inventory	248,600
Accounts Receivable	82,462
Property, Plant, and Equipment—Net	335,890
Other Assets	5,410
Total Assets	$785,907

Assume that a major customer returned a large order to Bell on December 31, 2012. The amount of the sale had been $146,800 with a cost of sales of $94,623. The return was recorded in the books on January 1, 2013. The company president does not want to correct the books. He argues that it makes no difference as to whether the return is recorded in 2012 or 2013. Either way, the return has been duly recognized.

Required

a. Assume that you are the CFO for Bell Farm and Garden Equipment Co. Write a memo to the president explaining how omitting the entry on December 31, 2012, could cause the financial statements to be misleading to investors and creditors. Explain how omitting the return from the customer would affect net income and the balance sheet.

b. Why might the president want to record the return on January 1, 2013, instead of December 31, 2012?

CHAPTER 4

Internal Controls, Accounting for Cash, and Ethics

LEARNING OBJECTIVES

LEARNING OBJECTIVES

After you have mastered the material in this chapter, you will be able to:

1 Identify the key elements of a strong system of internal control.

2 Prepare a bank reconciliation.

3 Discuss the role of ethics in the accounting profession.

4 Describe the auditor's role in financial reporting.

CHAPTER OPENING

In the first three chapters, we covered the basics of the accounting system. By now you should understand how basic business events affect financial statements and how the accounting cycle works. Accounting is an elegant system that when implemented correctly provides meaningful information to investors and other stakeholders. However, without effective control, the accounting system can be manipulated in ways that may overstate business performance. This can lead investors to make bad decisions, which can result in huge losses when the true performance is revealed. This chapter discusses the importance of internal control systems. The chapter also discuses accounting for cash, an area where good internal controls are critical. The chapter concludes with a discussion on the importance of ethical conduct in the accounting profession.

The Curious Accountant

On December 11, 2008, Bernard Madoff was arrested on suspicion of having defrauded the clients of his investment company, Bernard L. Madoff Investments (BMI), of $50 billion. Later estimates would put the losses at over $60 billion. Although his clients believed the money they sent to BMI was being invested in the stock market, it was actually just being deposited into bank accounts.

Mr. Madoff was accused of operating the largest Ponzi scheme in history. Clients were sent monthly statements falsely showing that their investments were earning income and growing at a steady rate, even when the overall stock market was falling. When individual investors asked to withdraw their funds, they were simply given money that had been deposited by other investors.

This fraudulent system works as long as more new money is being deposited than is being withdrawn. Unfortunately for BMI, with the severe stock-market decline of 2008 too many clients got nervous and asked to withdraw their money, including the gains they believed they had earned over the years. At this point the Ponzi scheme failed.

How could such a pervasive fraud go undetected for so long? (Answer on page 136.)

KEY FEATURES OF INTERNAL CONTROL SYSTEMS

Identify the key elements of a strong system of internal control.

During the early 2000s a number of accounting related scandals cost investors billions. In 2001, Enron's share price went from $85 to $0.30 after it was revealed that the company had billions of dollars in losses that were not reported on the financial statements. Several months later, WorldCom reported an $11 billion accounting fraud, which included hundreds of millions in personal loans to then CEO, Bernie Ebbers.

The Enron and WorldCom accounting scandals had such devastating effects that they led congress to pass the Sarbanes-Oxley Act of 2002 (SOX). SOX requires public companies to evaluate their *internal control* and to publish those findings with their SEC filings. **Internal control** is the process designed to ensure reliable financial reporting, effective and efficient operations, and compliance with applicable laws and regulations. Safeguarding assets against theft and unauthorized use, acquisition, or disposal is also part of internal control.

Section 404 of Sarbanes-Oxley requires a statement of management's responsibility for establishing and maintaining adequate internal control over financial reporting by public companies. This section includes an assessment of the controls and the identification of the framework used for the assessment. The framework established by The Committee of Sponsoring Organizations of the Treadway Commission (COSO) in 1992 is the de facto standard by which SOX compliance is judged. COSO's framework titled *Internal Control—An Integrated Framework* recognizes five interrelated components including:

1. *Control Environment.* The integrity and ethical values of the company, including its code of conduct, involvement of the board of directors, and other actions that set the tone of the organization.

2. *Risk Assessment.* Management's process of identifying potential risks that could result in misstated financial statements and developing actions to address those risks.

3. *Control Activities.* These are the activities usually thought of as "the internal controls." They include such things as segregation of duties, account reconciliations, and information processing controls that are designed to safeguard assets and enable an organization to timely prepare reliable financial statements.

4. *Information and Communication.* The internal and external reporting process, and includes an assessment of the technology environment.

5. *Monitoring.* Assessing the quality of a company's internal control over time and taking actions as necessary to ensure it continues to address the risks of the organization.

In 2004 COSO updated the framework to help entities design and implement effective enterprise-wide approaches to risk management. The updated document is titled *Enterprise Risk Management (ERM)—An Integrated Framework.* The ERM framework introduces an enterprise-wide approach to risk management as well as concepts such as risk appetite, risk tolerance, and portfolio view. While SOX applies only to U.S. public companies, the ERM framework has been adopted by both public and private organizations around the world.

The ERM framework does not replace the internal control framework. Instead, it incorporates the internal control framework within it. Accordingly, companies may decide to look to the ERM framework both to satisfy their internal control needs and to move toward a fuller risk management process.

While a detailed discussion of the COSO documents is beyond the scope of this text, the following overview of the more common *control activities* of the internal control framework is insightful.

Separation of Duties

The likelihood of fraud or theft is reduced if collusion is required to accomplish it. Clear **separation of duties** is frequently used as a deterrent to corruption. When duties are separated, the work of one employee can act as a check on the work of another employee. For example, a person selling seats to a movie may be tempted to steal money received from customers who enter the theater. This temptation is reduced if the person staffing the box office is required to issue tickets that a second employee collects as people enter the theater. If ticket stubs collected by the second employee are compared with the cash receipts from ticket sales, any cash shortages would become apparent. Furthermore, friends and relatives of the ticket agent could not easily enter the theater without paying. Theft or unauthorized entry would require collusion between the ticket agent and the usher who collects the tickets. Both individuals would have to be dishonest enough to steal, yet trustworthy enough to convince each other they would keep the embezzlement secret. Whenever possible, the functions of *authorization, recording,* and *custody of assets,* should be performed by separate individuals.

Quality of Employees

A business is only as good as the people it employs. Cheap labor is not a bargain if the employees are incompetent. Employees should be properly trained. In fact, they should be trained to perform a variety of tasks. The ability of employees to substitute for one another prevents disruptions when co-workers are absent because of illnesses, vacations, or other commitments. The capacity to rotate jobs also relieves boredom and increases respect for the contributions of other employees. Every business should strive to maximize the productivity of every employee. Ongoing training programs are essential to a strong system of internal control.

Bonded Employees

The best way to ensure employee honesty is to hire individuals with *high levels of personal integrity.* Employers should screen job applicants using interviews, background checks, and recommendations from prior employers or educators. Even so, screening programs may fail to identify character weaknesses. Further, unusual circumstances may cause honest employees to go astray. Therefore, employees in positions of trust should be bonded. A **fidelity bond** provides insurance that protects a company from losses caused by employee dishonesty.

Required Absences

Employees should be required to take regular vacations and their duties should be rotated periodically. Employees may be able to cover up fraudulent activities if they are always present at work. Consider the case of a parking meter collection agent who covered the same route for several years with no vacation. When the agent became sick, a substitute collected more money each day than the regular reader usually reported. Management checked past records and found that the ill meter reader had been understating the cash receipts and pocketing the difference. If management had required vacations or rotated the routes, the embezzlement would have been discovered much earlier.

Procedures Manual

Appropriate accounting procedures should be documented in a **procedures manual.** The manual should be routinely updated. Periodic reviews should be conducted to ensure that employees are following the procedures outlined in the manual.

Authority and Responsibility

Employees are motivated by clear lines of authority and responsibility. They work harder when they have the authority to use their own judgment and they exercise reasonable caution when they are held responsible for their actions. Businesses should prepare an **authority manual** that establishes a definitive *chain of command.* The authority manual should guide both specific and general authorizations. **Specific authorizations** apply to specific positions within the organization. For example, investment decisions are authorized at the division level while hiring decisions are authorized at the departmental level. In contrast, **general authority** applies across different levels of management. For example, employees at all levels may be required to fly coach or to make purchases from specific vendors.

Prenumbered Documents

How would you know if a check were stolen from your check book? If you keep a record of your check numbers, the missing number would tip you off immediately. Businesses also use prenumbered checks to avoid the unauthorized use of their bank accounts. In fact, prenumbered forms are used for all important documents such as purchase orders, receiving reports, invoices, and checks. To reduce errors, prenumbered forms should be as simple and easy to use as possible. Also, the documents should allow for authorized signatures. For example, credit sales slips should be signed by the customer to clearly establish who made the purchase, reducing the likelihood of unauthorized transactions.

Physical Control

Employees walk away with billions of dollars of business assets each year. To limit losses, companies should establish adequate physical control over valuable assets. For example, inventory should be kept in a storeroom and not released without proper authorization. Serial numbers on equipment should be recorded along with the name of the individual who is responsible for the equipment. Unannounced physical counts should be conducted randomly to verify the presence of company-owned equipment. Certificates of deposit and marketable securities should be kept in fireproof vaults. Access to these vaults should be limited to authorized personnel. These procedures protect the documents from fire and limit access to only those individuals who have the appropriate security clearance to handle the documents.

In addition to safeguarding assets, there should be physical control over the accounting records. The accounting journals, ledgers, and supporting documents should be kept in a fireproof safe. Only personnel responsible for recording transactions in the journals should have access to them. With limited access, there is less chance that someone will change the records to conceal fraud or embezzlement.

Performance Evaluations

Because few people can evaluate their own performance objectively, internal controls should include independent verification of employee performance. For example, someone other than the person who has control over inventory should take a physical count of inventory. Internal and external audits serve as independent verification of performance. Auditors should evaluate the effectiveness of the internal control system as well as verify the accuracy of the accounting records. In addition, the external auditors attest to the company's use of generally accepted accounting principles in the financial statements.

Limitations

A system of internal controls is designed to prevent or detect errors and fraud. However, no control system is foolproof. Internal controls can be circumvented by collusion among employees. Two or more employees working together can hide embezzlement by covering for each other. For example, if an embezzler goes on vacation, fraud will not be reported by a replacement who is in collusion with the embezzler. No system can prevent all fraud. However, a good system of internal controls minimizes illegal or unethical activities by reducing temptation and increasing the likelihood of early detection.

✓ CHECK YOURSELF 4.1

What are nine features of an internal control system?

Answer

The nine features follow.

1. Separating duties so that fraud or theft requires collusion.
2. Hiring and training competent employees.
3. Bonding employees to recover losses through insurance.

4. Requiring employees to be absent from their jobs so that their replacements can discover errors or fraudulent activity that might have occurred.
5. Establishing proper procedures for processing transactions.
6. Establishing clear lines of authority and responsibility.
7. Using prenumbered documents.
8. Implementing physical controls such as locking cash in a safe.
9. Conducting performance evaluations through independent internal and external audits.

ACCOUNTING FOR CASH

For financial reporting purposes, **cash** generally includes currency and other items that are payable *on demand,* such as checks, money orders, bank drafts, and certain savings accounts. Savings accounts that impose substantial penalties for early withdrawal should be classified as *investments* rather than cash. Postdated checks or IOUs represent *receivables* and should not be included in cash. As illustrated in Exhibit 4.1, most companies combine currency and other payable on demand items in a single balance sheet account with varying titles.

Companies must maintain a sufficient amount of cash to pay employees, suppliers, and other creditors. When a company fails to pay its legal obligations, its creditors can force the company into bankruptcy. Even so, management should avoid accumulating more cash than is needed. The failure to invest excess cash in earning assets reduces profitability. Cash inflows and outflows must be managed to prevent a shortage or surplus of cash.

Controlling Cash

Controlling cash, more than any other asset, requires strict adherence to internal control procedures. Cash has universal appeal. A relatively small suitcase filled with high-denomination currency can represent significant value. Furthermore, the rightful owner of currency is difficult to prove. In most cases, possession constitutes ownership. As a result, cash is highly susceptible to theft and must be carefully protected. Cash is most susceptible to embezzlement when it is received or disbursed. The following controls should be employed to reduce the likelihood of theft.

Cash Receipts

A record of all cash collections should be prepared immediately upon receipt. The amount of cash on hand should be counted regularly. Missing amounts of money can be detected by comparing the actual cash on hand with the book balance. Employees who receive cash should give customers a copy of a written receipt. Customers usually review their receipts to ensure they have gotten credit for the amount paid and call any errors to the receipts clerk's attention. This not only reduces errors but also provides a control on the clerk's honesty. Cash receipts should be deposited in a bank on a timely basis. Cash collected late in the day should be deposited in a night depository. Every effort should be made to minimize the amount of cash on hand. Keeping large amounts of cash on hand not only increases the risk of loss from theft but also places employees in danger of being harmed by criminals who may be tempted to rob the company.

Cash Payments

To effectively control cash, a company should make all disbursements using checks, thereby providing a record of cash payments. All checks should be prenumbered, and unused checks should be locked up. Using prenumbered checks allows companies to easily identify lost or stolen checks by comparing the numbers on unused and canceled checks with the numbers used for legitimate disbursements.

EXHIBIT 4.1

Balance Sheet Classifications That Include the Word Cash

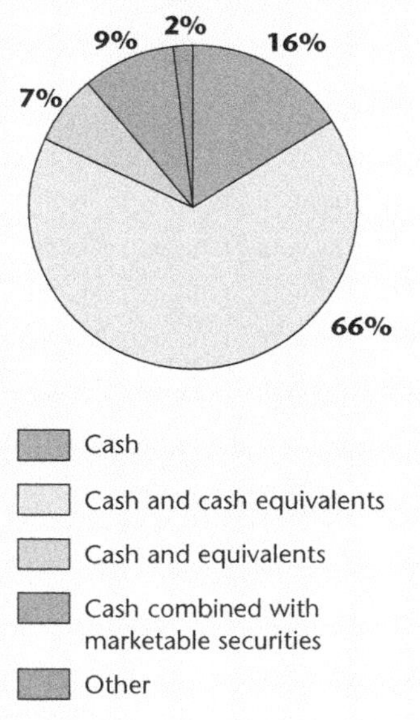
9%
2%
16%
7%
66%
Cash
Cash and cash equivalents
Cash and equivalents
Cash combined with marketable securities
Other

Data Source: AICPA, *Accounting Trends and Techniques.*

REALITY BYTES

Could you afford to buy a safe like the one shown here? The vault is only one of many expensive security devices used by banks to safeguard cash. By using checking accounts, companies are able to avoid many of the costs associated with keeping cash safe. In addition to providing physical control, checking accounts enable companies to maintain a written audit trail of cash receipts and payments. Checking accounts represent the most widely used internal control device in modern society. It is difficult to imagine a business operating without the use of checking accounts.

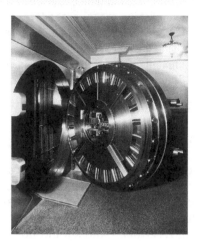

The duties of approving disbursements, signing checks, and recording transactions should be separated. If one person is authorized to approve, sign, and record checks, he or she could falsify supporting documents, write an unauthorized check, and record a cover-up transaction in the accounting records. By separating these duties, the check signer reviews the documentation provided by the approving individual before signing the check. Likewise, the recording clerk reviews the work of both the approving person and the check signer when the disbursement is recorded in the accounting records. Thus writing unauthorized checks requires trilevel collusion.

Supporting documents with authorized approval signatures should be required when checks are presented to the check signer. For example, a warehouse receiving order should be matched with a purchase order before a check is approved to pay a bill from a supplier. Before payments are approved, invoice amounts should be checked and payees verified as valid vendors. Matching supporting documents with proper authorization discourages employees from creating phony documents for a disbursement to a friend or fictitious business. Also, the approval process serves as a check on the accuracy of the work of all employees involved.

Supporting documents should be marked *Paid* when the check is signed. If the documents are not indelibly marked, they could be retrieved from the files and resubmitted for a duplicate, unauthorized payment. A payables clerk could collude with the payee to split extra cash paid out by submitting the same supporting documents for a second payment.

All spoiled and voided checks should be defaced and retained. If defaced checks are not retained, an employee could steal a check and then claim that it was written incorrectly and thrown away. The clerk could then use the stolen check to make an unauthorized payment.

Checking Account Documents

The previous section explained the need for businesses to use checking accounts. A description of four main types of forms associated with a bank checking account follows.

Signature Card

A bank **signature card** shows the bank account number and the signatures of the people authorized to sign checks. The card is retained in the bank's files. If a bank employee is unfamiliar with the signature on a check, he or she can refer to the signature card to verify the signature before cashing the check.

Deposit Ticket

Each deposit of cash or checks is accompanied by a **deposit ticket,** which normally identifies the account number and the name of the account. The depositor lists the individual amounts of currency, coins, and checks, as well as the total deposited, on the deposit ticket.

Bank Check

A written check affects three parties: (1) the person or business writing the check (the *payer*); (2) the bank on which the check is drawn; and (3) the person or business to whom the check is payable (the *payee*). Companies often write **checks** using multicopy, prenumbered forms, with the name of the issuing business preprinted on the face of each check. A remittance notice is usually attached to the check forms. This portion of the form provides the issuer space to record what the check is for (e.g., what invoices are being paid), the amount being disbursed, and the date of payment. When signed by the person whose signature is on the signature card, the check authorizes the bank to transfer the face amount of the check from the payer's account to the payee.

Bank Statement

Periodically, the bank sends the depositor a **bank statement.** The bank statement is presented from the bank's point of view. Checking accounts are liabilities to a bank because the bank is obligated to pay back the money that customers have deposited in their accounts. Therefore, in the bank's accounting records a customer's checking account has a *credit* balance. As a result, **bank statement debit memos** describe transactions that reduce the customer's account balance (the bank's liability). **Bank statement credit memos** describe activities that increase the customer's account balance (the bank's liability). Since a checking account is an asset (cash) to the depositor, a *bank statement debit memo* requires a *credit entry* to the cash account on the depositor's books. Likewise, when a bank tells you that it has credited your account, you will debit your cash account in response.

Bank statements normally report (a) the balance of the account at the beginning of the period; (b) additions for customer deposits made during the period; (c) other additions described in credit memos (e.g., for interest earned); (d) subtractions for the payment of checks drawn on the account during the period; (e) other subtractions described in debit memos (e.g., for service charges); (f) a running balance of the account; and (g) the balance of the account at the end of the period. The sample bank statement in Exhibit 4.2 on the next page illustrates these items. Normally, the canceled checks or copies of them are enclosed with the bank statement.

RECONCILING THE BANK ACCOUNT

Usually the ending balance reported on the bank statement differs from the balance in the depositor's cash account as of the same date. The discrepancy is normally attributable to timing differences. For example, a depositor deducts the amount of a check from its cash account when it writes the check. However, the bank does not deduct the amount of the check from the depositor's account until the payee presents it for payment, which may be days, weeks, or even months after the check is written. As a result, the balance on the depositor's books is lower than the balance on the bank's books. Companies prepare a **bank reconciliation** to explain the differences between the cash balance reported on the bank statement and the cash balance recorded in the depositor's accounting records.

Prepare a bank reconciliation.

Determining True Cash Balance

A bank reconciliation normally begins with the cash balance reported by the bank which is called the **unadjusted bank balance.** The adjustments necessary to determine the amount of cash that the depositor actually owns as of the date of the bank statement are then added to and subtracted from the unadjusted bank balance. The final total is the **true cash balance.** The true cash balance is independently reached a second time by making adjustments to the **unadjusted book balance.** The bank account is reconciled when the true cash balance determined from the perspective of the unadjusted

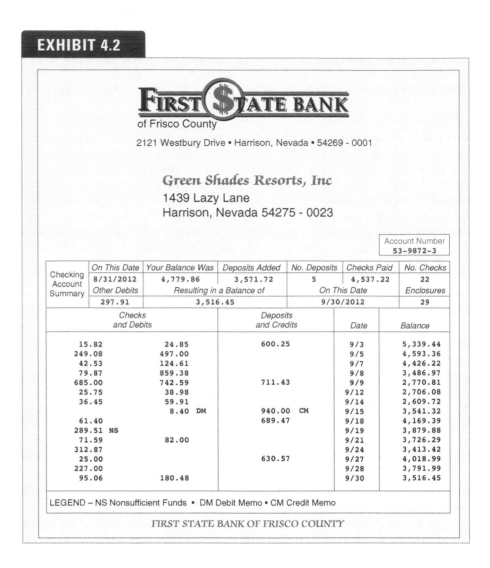

bank balance agrees with the true cash balance determined from the perspective of the unadjusted *book* balance. The procedures a company uses to determine the *true cash balance* from the two different perspectives are outlined here.

Adjustments to the Bank Balance

A typical format for determining the true cash balance beginning with the unadjusted bank balance is

>   Unadjusted bank balance
> \+ Deposits in transit
> − Outstanding checks
> ————————————————
> = True cash balance

Deposits in transit. Companies frequently leave deposits in the bank's night depository or make them on the day following the receipt of cash. Such deposits are called **deposits in transit.** Because these deposits have been recorded in the depositor's accounting records but have not yet been added to the depositor's account by the bank, they must be added to the unadjusted bank balance.

Outstanding checks. These are disbursements that have been properly recorded as cash deductions on the depositor's books. However, the bank has not deducted the amounts from the depositor's bank account because the checks have not yet been presented by the payee to the bank for payment; that is, the checks have not cleared the bank. **Outstanding checks** must be subtracted from the unadjusted bank balance to determine the true cash balance.

Adjustments to the Book Balance

A typical format for determining the true cash balance beginning with the unadjusted book balance is as follows.

```
Unadjusted book balance
+ Accounts receivable collections
+ Interest earned
− Bank service charges
− Non-sufficient-funds (NSF) checks
= True cash balance
```

Accounts receivable collections. To collect cash as quickly as possible, many companies have their customers send payments directly to the bank. The bank adds the collection directly to the depositor's account and notifies the depositor about the collection through a credit memo that is included on the bank statement. The depositor adds the amount of the cash collections to the unadjusted book balance in the process of determining the true cash balance.

Interest earned. Banks pay interest on certain checking accounts. The amount of the interest is added directly to the depositor's bank account. The bank notifies the depositor about the interest through a credit memo that is included on the bank statement. The depositor adds the amount of the interest revenue to the unadjusted book balance in the process of determining the true cash balance.

Service charges. Banks frequently charge depositors fees for services performed. They may also charge a penalty if the depositor fails to maintain a specified minimum cash balance throughout the period. Banks deduct such fees and penalties directly from the depositor's account and advise the depositor of the deduction through a debit memo that is included on the bank statement. The depositor deducts such **service charges** from the unadjusted book balance to determine the true cash balance.

Non-sufficient-funds (NSF) checks. **NSF checks** are checks that a company obtains from its customers and deposits in its checking account. However, when the checks are submitted to the customers' banks for payment, the banks refuse payment because there is insufficient money in the customers' accounts. When such checks are returned, the amounts of the checks are deducted from the company's bank account balance. The company is advised of NSF checks through debit memos that appear on the bank statement. The depositor deducts the amounts of the NSF checks from the unadjusted book balance in the process of determining the true cash balance.

Correction of Errors

In the course of reconciling the bank statement with the cash account, the depositor may discover errors in the bank's records, the depositor's records, or both. If an error is found on the bank statement, an adjustment for it is made to the unadjusted bank balance to determine the true cash balance, and the bank should be notified immediately to correct its records. Errors made by the depositor require adjustments to the book balance to arrive at the true cash balance.

Certified Checks

A **certified check** is guaranteed for payment by a bank. Whereas a regular check is deducted from the customer's account when it is presented for payment, a certified check is deducted from the customer's account when the bank certifies that the check is good.

Certified checks, therefore, *have* been deducted by the bank in determining the unadjusted bank balance, whether they have cleared the bank or remain outstanding as of the date of the bank statement. Since certified checks are deducted both from bank and depositor records immediately, they do not cause differences between the depositor and bank balances. As a result, certified checks are not included in a bank reconciliation.

Illustrating a Bank Reconciliation

The following example illustrates preparing the bank reconciliation for Green Shades Resorts, Inc. (GSRI). The bank statement for GSRI is displayed in Exhibit 4.2. Exhibit 4.3 illustrates the completed bank reconciliation. The items on the reconciliation are described below.

Adjustments to the Bank Balance

As of September 30, 2012, the bank statement showed an unadjusted balance of $3,516.45. A review of the bank statement disclosed three adjustments that had to be made to the unadjusted bank balance to determine GSRI's true cash balance.

1. Comparing the deposits on the bank statement with deposits recorded in GSRI's accounting records indicated there was $724.11 of deposits in transit.

2. An examination of the returned checks disclosed that the bank had erroneously deducted a $25 check written by Green Valley Resorts from GSRI's bank account. This amount must be added back to the unadjusted bank balance to determine the true cash balance.

3. The checks returned with the bank statement were sorted and compared to the cash records. Three checks with amounts totaling $235.25 were outstanding.

After these adjustment are made GSRI's true cash balance is determined to be $4,030.31.

EXHIBIT 4.3

GREEN SHADES RESORTS, INC.
Bank Reconciliation
September 30, 2012

Unadjusted bank balance, September 30, 2012	$3,516.45
Add: Deposits in transit	724.11
Bank error: Check drawn on Green Valley Resorts charged to GSRI	25.00
Less: Outstanding checks	

Check No.	Date	Amount
639	Sept. 18	$ 13.75
646	Sept. 20	29.00
672	Sept. 27	192.50

Total	(235.25)
True cash balance, September 30, 2012	$4,030.31
Unadjusted book balance, September 30, 2012	$3,361.22
Add: Receivable collected by bank	940.00
Error made by accountant (Check no. 633 recorded as $63.45 instead of $36.45)	27.00
Less: Bank service charges	(8.40)
NSF check	(289.51)
True cash balance, September 30, 2012	$4,030.31

Adjustments to the Book Balance

As indicated in Exhibit 4.3, GSRI's unadjusted book balance as of September 30, 2012, was $3,361.22. This balance differs from GSRI's true cash balance because of four unrecorded accounting events:

1. The bank collected a $940 account receivable for GSRI.
2. GSRI's accountant made a $27 recording error.
3. The bank charged GSRI an $8.40 service fee.
4. GSRI had deposited a $289.51 check from a customer who did not have sufficient funds to cover the check.

Two of these four adjustments increase the unadjusted cash balance. The other two decrease the unadjusted cash balance. After the adjustments have been recorded, the cash account reflects the true cash balance of $4,030.31 ($3,361.22 unadjusted cash balance + $940.00 receivable collection + $27.00 recording error − $8.40 service charge − $289.51 NSF check). Because the true balance determined from the perspective of the bank statement agrees with the true balance determined from the perspective of GSRI's books, the bank statement has been successfully reconciled with the accounting records.

Updating GSRI's Accounting Records

Each of the adjustments to the book balance must be recorded in GSRI's financial records. The effects of each adjustment on the financial statements are as follows.

ADJUSTMENT 1 *Recording the $940 receivable collection increases cash and reduces accounts receivable.*

The event is an asset exchange transaction. The effect of the collection on GSRI's financial statements is

Assets			=	Liab.	+	Equity	Rev.	−	Exp.	=	Net Inc.	Cash Flow	
Cash	+	Accts. Rec.											
940	+	(940)	=	NA	+	NA	NA	−	NA	=	NA	940	OA

ADJUSTMENT 2 *Assume the $27 recording error occurred because GSRI's accountant accidentally transposed two numbers when recording check no. 633 for utilities expense.*

The check was written to pay utilities expense of $36.45 but was recorded as a $63.45 disbursement. Since cash payments are overstated by $27.00 ($63.45 − $36.45), this amount must be added back to GSRI's cash balance and deducted from the utilities expense account, which increases net income. The effects on the financial statements are

Assets	=	Liab.	+	Equity	Rev.	−	Exp.	=	Net Inc.	Cash Flow	
Cash	=			Ret. Earn.							
27	−	NA	I	27	NA	−	(27)	−	27	27	OA

ADJUSTMENT 3 *The $8.40 service charge is an expense that reduces assets, stockholders' equity, net income, and cash.*

The effects are

Assets	=	Liab.	+	Equity	Rev.	−	Exp.	=	Net Inc.	Cash Flow	
Cash	=			Ret. Earn.							
(8.40)	=	NA	+	(8.40)	NA	−	8.40	=	(8.40)	(8.40)	OA

ADJUSTMENT 4 *The $289.51 NSF check reduces GSRI's cash balance.*

When it originally accepted the customer's check, GSRI increased its cash account. Because there is not enough money in the customer's bank account to pay the check, GSRI didn't actually receive cash so GSRI must reduce its cash account. GSRI will still try to collect the money from the customer. In the meantime, it will show the amount of the NSF check as an account receivable. The adjusting entry to record the NSF check is an asset exchange transaction. Cash decreases and accounts receivable increases. The effect on GSRI's financial statements is

	Assets		=	Liab.	+	Equity	Rev.	−	Exp.	=	Net Inc.	Cash Flow	
Cash	+	Accts. Rec.											
(289.51)	+	289.51	=	NA	+	NA	NA	−	NA	=	NA	(289.51)	OA

Answers to The Curious Accountant

As this chapter explains, separation of duties is one of the primary features of a good system of internal controls. However, separation of duties is not designed to detect fraud at the very top level of management. Mr. Madoff ran BMI with almost complete control; he had no boss.

Even with a good system of internal controls, there is always some level of trust required in business. Mr. Madoff had an excellent reputation in the investment community. He had even been the president of the NASDAQ. His investors trusted him and assumed they could depend on his independent auditor to detect any major problems with the way BMI was investing, or not investing, their money.

Federal prosecutors believe that BMI's auditor, David Friehling, did very little in the way of properly auditing BMI's books. In fact, on March 18, 2009, he also was arrested and charged with falsely certifying BMI's financial statements. He faces up to 105 years in prison if convicted.

On March 12, 2009, the 70-year-old Mr. Madoff pled guilty to 11 felony charges. On June 29, 2009, he was sentenced to a term of 150 years in prison.

✓ **CHECK YOURSELF 4.2**

The following information was drawn from Reliance Company's October bank statement. The unadjusted bank balance on October 31 was $2,300. The statement showed that the bank had collected a $200 account receivable for Reliance. The statement also included $20 of bank service charges for October and a $100 check payable to Reliance that was returned NSF. A comparison of the bank statement with company accounting records indicates that there was a $500 deposit in transit and $1,800 of checks outstanding at the end of the month. Based on this information, determine the true cash balance on October 31.

Answer   Since the unadjusted book balance is not given, start with the unadjusted bank balance to determine the true cash balance. The collection of the receivable, the bank service charges, and the NSF check are already recognized in the unadjusted bank balance, so these items are not used to determine the true cash balance. Determine the true cash balance by adding the deposit in transit to and subtracting the outstanding checks from the unadjusted bank balance. The true cash balance is $1,000 ($2,300 unadjusted bank balance + $500 deposit in transit − $1,800 outstanding checks).

IMPORTANCE OF ETHICS

The chapter began with a discussion of the importance of internal control systems in preventing accounting scandals. After the Enron and WorldCom scandals and the passage of the Sarbanes-Oxley Act, much more attention has been paid to establishing effective internal control systems. However, despite this increase in legislation and awareness, accounting scandals continue to occur. In 2008, Lehman Brothers declared bankruptcy after it was discovered that the company had kept more than $50 billion in loans off the balance sheet by classifying them as sales. Several months later, Bernie Madoff used a Ponzi scheme to leave his investors with more than $21.2 billion in cash losses. These examples illustrate that legislation alone will not prevent accounting scandals. To prevent a scandal it is necessary to develop a culture that fosters and promotes ethical conduct.

Discuss the role of ethics in the accounting profession.

The accountant's role in society requires trust and credibility. Accounting information is worthless if the accountant is not trustworthy. Similarly, tax and consulting advice is useless if it comes from an incompetent person. The high ethical standards required by the profession state "a certified public accountant assumes an obligation of self-discipline above and beyond requirements of laws and regulations." The **American Institute of Certified Public Accountants** requires its members to comply with the **Code of Professional Conduct.** Section I of the Code includes six articles that are summarized in Exhibit 4.4. The importance of ethical conduct is universally recognized across a broad spectrum of accounting organizations. The Institute of Management Accountants requires its members to follow a set of Standards of Ethical Conduct. The Institute of Internal Auditors also requires its members to subscribe to the organization's Code of Ethics.

Common Features of Criminal and Ethical Misconduct

Unfortunately, it takes more than a code of conduct to stop fraud. People frequently engage in activities that they know are unethical or even criminal. The auditing profession has identified three elements that are typically present when fraud occurs.

1.   The availability of an opportunity.
2.   The existence of some form of pressure leading to an incentive.
3.   The capacity to rationalize.

EXHIBIT 4.4

Articles of AICPA Code of Professional Conduct

Article I Responsibilities
In carrying out their responsibilities as professionals, members should exercise sensitive professional and moral judgments in all their activities.

Article II The Public Interest
Members should accept the obligation to act in a way that will serve the public interest, honor the public trust, and demonstrate commitment to professionalism.

Article III Integrity
To maintain and broaden public confidence, members should perform all professional responsibilities with the highest sense of integrity.

Article IV Objectivity and Independence
A member should maintain objectivity and be free of conflicts of interest in discharging professional responsibilities. A member in public practice should be independent in fact and appearance when providing auditing and other attestation services.

Article V Due Care
A member should observe the profession's technical and ethical standards, strive continually to improve competence and the quality of services, and discharge professional responsibility to the best of the member's ability.

Article VI Scope and Nature of Services
A member in public practice should observe the principles of the Code of Professional Conduct in determining the scope and nature of services to be provided.

The three elements are frequently arranged in the shape of a triangle as shown in Exhibit 4.5.

Opportunity is shown at the head to the triangle because without opportunity fraud could not exist. The most effective way to reduce opportunities for ethical or criminal misconduct is to implement an effective set of internal controls. *Internal controls* are policies and procedures that a business implements to reduce opportunities

EXHIBIT 4.5

The Fraud Triangle

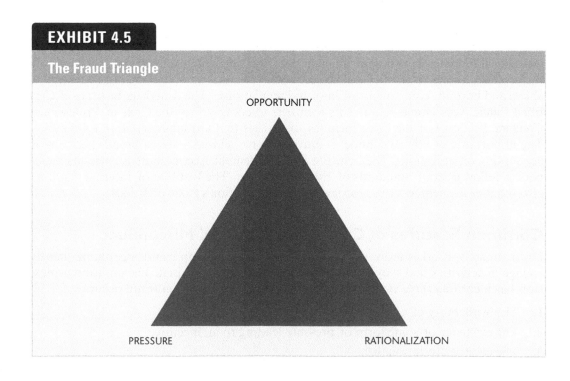

for fraud and to assure that its objectives will be accomplished. Specific controls are tailored to meet the individual needs of particular businesses. For example, banks use elaborate vaults to protect cash and safety deposit boxes, but universities have little use for this type of equipment. Even so, many of the same procedures are used by a wide variety of businesses. The internal control policies and procedures that have gained widespread acceptance are discussed in a subsequent chapter.

Only a few employees turn to the dark side even when internal control is weak and opportunities abound. So, what causes one person to commit fraud and another to remain honest? The second element of the fraud triangle recognizes **pressure** as a key ingredient of misconduct. A manager who is told "either make the numbers or you are fired" is more likely to cheat than one who is told to "tell it like it is." Pressure can come from a variety of sources.

- Personal vices such as drug addiction, gambling, and promiscuity.
- Intimidation from superiors.
- Personal debt from credit cards, consumer and mortgage loans, or poor investments.
- Family expectations to provide a standard of living that is beyond one's capabilities.
- Business failure caused by poor decision making or temporary factors such as a poor economy.
- Loyalty or trying to be agreeable.

The third and final element of the fraud triangle is **rationalization.** Few individuals think of themselves as evil. They develop rationalizations to justify their misconduct. Common rationalizations include the following.

- Everybody does it.
- They are not paying me enough. I'm only taking what I deserve.
- I'm only borrowing the money. I'll pay it back.
- The company can afford it. Look what they are paying the officers.
- I'm taking what my family needs to live like everyone else.

Most people are able to resist pressure and the tendency to rationalize ethical or legal misconduct. However, some people will yield to temptation. What can accountants do to protect themselves and their companies from unscrupulous characters? The answer lies in personal integrity. The best indicator of personal integrity is past performance. Accordingly, companies must exercise due care in performing appropriate background investigations before hiring people to fill positions of trust.

Ethical misconduct is a serious offense in the accounting profession. A single mistake can destroy an accounting career. If you commit a white-collar crime, you normally lose the opportunity to hold a white-collar job. Second chances are rarely granted; it is extremely important that you learn how to recognize and avoid the common features of ethical misconduct. To help you prepare for the real-world situations you are likely to encounter, we include ethical dilemmas in the end-of-chapter materials. When working with these dilemmas, try to identify the (1) opportunity, (2) pressure, and (3) rationalization associated with the particular ethical situation described. If you are not an ethical person, accounting is not the career for you.

ROLE OF THE INDEPENDENT AUDITOR

As previously explained, financial statements are prepared in accordance with certain rules called *generally accepted accounting principles (GAAP)*. Thus, when General Electric publishes its financial statements, it is saying, "here are our financial statements prepared according to GAAP." How can a financial analyst know that a company really did follow GAAP? Analysts and other statement users rely on **audits** conducted by **certified public accountants (CPAs).**

LO 4

Describe the auditor's role in financial reporting.

The primary roles of an independent auditor (CPA) are summarized below:

1. Conducts a financial audit (a detailed examination of a company's financial statements and underlying accounting records).
2. Assumes both legal and professional responsibilities to the public as well as to the company paying the auditor.
3. Determines if financial statements are *materially* correct rather than *absolutely* correct.
4. Presents conclusions in an audit report that includes an opinion as to whether the statements are prepared in conformity with GAAP. In rare cases, the auditor issues a disclaimer.
5. Maintains professional confidentiality of client records. The auditor is not, however, exempt from legal obligations such as testifying in court.

The Financial Statement Audit

What is an audit? There are several types of audits. The type most relevant to this course is a **financial statement audit,** often referred to as simply a financial audit. The financial audit is a detailed examination of a company's financial statements and the documents that support those statements. It also tests the reliability of the accounting system used to produce the financial reports. A financial audit is conducted by an **independent auditor.**

The term *independent auditor* typically refers to a *firm* of certified public accountants. CPAs are licensed by state governments to provide services to the public. They are to be as independent of the companies they audit as is reasonably possible. To help assure independence, CPAs and members of their immediate families may not be employees of the companies they audit. Further, they cannot have investments in the companies they audit. Although CPAs are paid by the companies they audit, the audit fee may not be based on the outcome of the audit.

Although the independent auditors are chosen by, paid by, and can be fired by their client companies, the auditors are primarily responsible to *the public.* In fact, auditors have a legal responsibility to those members of the public who have a financial interest in the company being audited. If investors in a company lose money, they sometimes sue the independent auditors in an attempt to recover their losses, especially if the losses were related to financial failure. A lawsuit against auditors will succeed only if the auditors failed in their professional responsibilities when conducting the audit. Auditors are not responsible for the success or failure of a company. Instead, they are responsible for the appropriate reporting of that success or failure. While recent debacles such as Bernard Madoff Investments produce spectacular headlines, auditors are actually not sued very often, considering the number of audits they perform.

Materiality and Financial Audits

Auditors do not guarantee that financial statements are absolutely correct—only that they are free from *material* misstatements. This is where things get a little fuzzy. What is a *material misstatement?* The concept of materiality is very subjective. If ExxonMobil inadvertently overstated its sales by $1 million, would this be material? In 2009, ExxonMobil had approximately $311 billion of sales! A $1 million error in computing sales at ExxonMobil is like a $1 error in computing the pay of a person who makes $311,000 per year—not material at all! An error, or other reporting problem, is **material** if knowing about it would influence the decisions of an *average prudent investor.*

Financial audits are not directed toward the discovery of fraud. Auditors are, however, responsible for providing *reasonable assurance* that statements are free from material misstatements, whether caused by errors or fraud. Also, auditors are responsible for evaluating whether internal control procedures are in place to help prevent material misstatements due to fraud. If fraud is widespread in a company, normal audit procedures should detect it.

Accounting majors take at least one and often two or more courses in auditing to understand how to conduct an audit. An explanation of auditing techniques is beyond the scope of this course, but at least be aware that auditors do not review how the company accounted for every transaction. Along with other methods, auditors use statistics to choose representative samples of transactions to examine.

Types of Audit Opinions

Once an audit is complete, the auditors present their conclusions in a report that includes an *audit opinion*. There are three basic types of audit opinions.

An **unqualified opinion,** despite its negative-sounding name, is the most favorable opinion auditors can express. It means the auditor believes the financial statements are in compliance with GAAP without qualification, reservation, or exception. Most audits result in unqualified opinions because companies correct any reporting deficiencies the auditors find before the financial statements are released.

The most negative report an auditor can issue is an **adverse opinion.** An adverse opinion means that one or more departures from GAAP are so material that the financial statements do not present a fair picture of the company's status. The auditor's report explains the unacceptable accounting practice(s) that resulted in the adverse opinion being issued. Adverse opinions are very rare because public companies are required by law to follow GAAP.

A **qualified opinion** falls between an unqualified and an adverse opinion. A qualified opinion means that for the most part, the company's financial statements are in compliance with GAAP, but the auditors have reservations about something in the statements. The auditors' report explains why the opinion is qualified. A qualified opinion usually does not imply a serious accounting problem, but users should read the auditors' report and draw their own conclusions.

If an auditor is unable to perform the audit procedures necessary to determine whether the statements are prepared in accordance with GAAP, the auditor cannot issue an opinion on the financial statements. Instead, the auditor issues a **disclaimer of opinion.** A disclaimer means that the auditor is unable to obtain enough information to confirm compliance with GAAP.

Regardless of the type of report they issue, auditors are only expressing their judgment about whether the financial statements present a fair picture of a company. They do not provide opinions regarding the investment quality of a company.

The ultimate responsibility for financial statements rests with the executives of the reporting company. Just like auditors, managers can be sued by investors who believe they lost money due to improper financial reporting. This is one reason all business persons should understand accounting fundamentals.

Confidentiality

The **confidentiality** rules in the AICPA's code of ethics for CPAs prohibits auditors from *voluntarily disclosing* information they have acquired as a result of their accountant-client relationships. However, accountants may be required to testify in a court of law. In general, federal law does not recognize an accountant-client privilege as it does with attorneys and clergy. Some federal courts have taken exception to this position, especially as it applies to tax cases. State law varies with respect to accountant-client privilege. Furthermore, if auditors terminate a client relationship because of ethical or legal disagreements and they are subsequently contacted by a successor auditor, they are required to inform the successor of the reasons for the termination. In addition, auditors must consider the particular circumstances of a case when assessing the appropriateness of disclosing confidential information. Given the diverse legal positions governing accountant-client confidentiality, auditors should seek legal counsel prior to disclosing any information obtained in an accountant-client relationship.

To illustrate, assume that Joe Smith, CPA, discovers that his client Jane Doe is misrepresenting information reported in her financial statements. Smith tries to convince Doe to correct the misrepresentations, but she refuses to do so. Smith is required by the code of ethics to terminate his relationship with Doe. However, Smith is not permitted to disclose Doe's dishonest reporting practices unless he is called on to testify in a legal hearing or to respond to an inquiry by Doe's successor accountant.

With respect to the discovery of significant fraud, the auditor is required to inform management at least one level above the position of the employee who is engaged in the fraud and to notify the board of directors of the company. Suppose that Joe Smith, CPA, discovers that Jane Doe, employee of Western Company, is embezzling money from Western. Smith is required to inform Doe's supervisor and to notify Western's board of directors. However, Smith is prohibited from publicly disclosing the fraud.

<< A Look Back

The policies and procedures used to provide reasonable assurance that the objectives of an enterprise will be accomplished are called *internal controls*. While the mechanics of internal control systems vary from company to company, the more prevalent features include the following.

1. *Separation of duties.* Whenever possible, the functions of authorization, recording, and custody should be exercised by different individuals.
2. *Quality of employees.* Employees should be qualified to competently perform the duties that are assigned to them. Companies must establish hiring practices to screen out unqualified candidates. Furthermore, procedures should be established to ensure that employees receive appropriate training to maintain their competence.
3. *Bonded employees.* Employees in sensitive positions should be covered by a fidelity bond that provides insurance to reimburse losses due to illegal actions committed by employees.
4. *Required absences.* Employees should be required to take extended absences from their jobs so that they are not always present to hide unscrupulous or illegal activities.
5. *Procedures manual.* To promote compliance, the procedures for processing transactions should be clearly described in a manual.
6. *Authority and responsibility.* To motivate employees and promote effective control, clear lines of authority and responsibility should be established.
7. *Prenumbered documents.* Prenumbered documents minimize the likelihood of missing or duplicate documents. Prenumbered forms should be used for all important documents such as purchase orders, receiving reports, invoices, and checks.
8. *Physical control.* Locks, fences, security personnel, and other physical devices should be employed to safeguard assets.
9. *Performance evaluations.* Because few people can evaluate their own performance objectively, independent performance evaluations should be performed. Substandard performance will likely persist unless employees are encouraged to take corrective action.

Because cash is such an important business asset and because it is tempting to steal, much of the discussion of internal controls in this chapter focused on cash controls. Special procedures should be employed to control the receipts and payments of cash. One of the most common control policies is to use *checking accounts* for all payments except petty cash disbursements.

A *bank reconciliation* should be prepared each month to explain differences between the bank statement and a company's internal accounting records. A common reconciliation format determines the true cash balance based on both bank and book records. Items that typically appear on a bank reconciliation include the following:

Unadjusted bank balance	xxx	Unadjusted book balance	xxx
Add		Add	
Deposits in transit	xxx	Interest revenue	xxx
		Collection of receivables	xxx
Subtract		Subtract	
Outstanding checks	xxx	Bank service charges	xxx
		NSF checks	xxx
True cash balance	xxx	True cash balance	xxx

Agreement of the two true cash balances provides evidence that accounting for cash transactions has been accurate.

The chapter discussed the importance of ethics in the accounting profession. The *American Institute of Public Accountants* requires all of its members to comply with the *Code of Professional Conduct*. Situations where *opportunity, pressure,* and *rationalization* exist can lead employees to conduct unethical acts, which, in cases like Enron, have destroyed the organization. Finally, the chapter discussed the auditor's role in financial reporting, including the materiality concept and the types of audit opinions that may be issued.

A Look Forward

The next chapter focuses on more specific issues related to accounts receivables and inventory. Accounting for receivables and payable was introduced in Chapter 2, using relatively simple illustrations. For example, we assumed that customers who purchased services on account always paid their bills. In real business practice, some customers do not pay their bills. Among other topics, Chapter 5 examines how companies account for uncollectible accounts receivable.

Accounting for inventory was discussed in Chapter 3. However, we assumed that all inventory items were purchased at the same price. This is unrealistic given that the price of goods is constantly changing. Chapter 5 discusses how to account for inventory items that are purchased at different times and different prices.

A step-by-step audio-narrated series of slides is provided on the text website at www.mhhe.com/edmondssurvey3e.

 ## SELF-STUDY REVIEW PROBLEM

The following information pertains to Terry's Pest Control Company (TPCC) for July:

1. The unadjusted bank balance at July 31 was $870.
2. The bank statement included the following items:
    (a) A $60 credit memo for interest earned by TPCC.
    (b) A $200 NSF check made payable to TPCC.
    (c) A $110 debit memo for bank service charges.
3. The unadjusted book balance at July 31 was $1,400.

4. A comparison of the bank statement with company accounting records disclosed the following:

   (a) A $400 deposit in transit at July 31.

   (b) Outstanding checks totaling $120 at the end of the month.

Required

Prepare a bank reconciliation.

Solution

TERRY'S PEST CONTROL COMPANY Bank Reconciliation July 31	
Unadjusted bank balance	$ 870
Add: Deposits in transit	400
Less: Outstanding checks	(120)
True cash balance	$1,150
Unadjusted book balance	$1,400
Add: Interest revenue	60
Less: NSF check	(200)
Less: Bank service charges	(110)
True cash balance	$1,150

KEY TERMS

Adverse opinion 141
American Institute of
  Certified Public
  Accountants 137
Audits 139
Authority manual 127
Bank reconciliation 131
Bank statement 131
Bank statement credit
  memo 131
Bank statement debit memo 131
Cash 129
Certified check 133
Certified public accountants
  (CPAs) 139

Checks 131
Code of Professional
  Conduct 137
Confidentiality 141
Deposit ticket 131
Deposits in transit 132
Disclaimer of opinion 141
Fidelity bond 127
Financial statement audit 140
General authority 127
Independent auditor 140
Internal controls 126
Material 140
Non-sufficient-funds (NSF)
  checks 133

Opportunity 138
Outstanding checks 133
Pressure 139
Procedures manual 127
Qualified opinion 141
Rationalization 139
Separation of duties 126
Service charges 133
Signature card 130
Specific authorizations 127
True cash balance 131
Unadjusted bank balance 131
Unadjusted book
  balance 131
Unqualified opinion 141

QUESTIONS

1. What motivated congress to pass the Sarbanes-Oxley Act (SOX) of 2002?

2. Define the term *internal control*.

3. Explain the relationship between SOX and COSO.

4. Name and briefly define the five components of COSO's internal control framework.

5. Explain how COSO's *Enterprise Risk Management—An Integrated Framework* project relates to COSO's *Internal Control— An Integrated Framework* project.

6. List several control activities of an effective internal control system.

7. What is meant by *separation of duties?* Give an illustration.

8. What are the attributes of a high-quality employee?

9. What is a fidelity bond? Explain its purpose.

10. Why is it important that every employee periodically take a leave of absence or vacation?

11. What are the purpose and importance of a procedures manual?

12. What is the difference between specific and general authorizations?

13. Why should documents (checks, invoices, receipts) be prenumbered?

14. What procedures are important in the physical control of assets and accounting records?

15. What is the purpose of independent verification of performance?

16. What items are considered cash?

17. Why is cash more susceptible to theft or embezzlement than other assets?

18. Giving written copies of receipts to customers can help prevent what type of illegal acts?

19. What procedures can help to protect cash receipts?

20. What procedures can help protect cash disbursements?

21. What effect does a debit memo in a bank statement have on the Cash account? What effect does a credit memo in a bank statement have on the Cash account?

22. What information is normally included in a bank statement?

23. Why might a bank statement reflect a balance that is larger than the balance recorded in the depositor's books? What could cause the bank balance to be smaller than the book balance?

24. What is the purpose of a bank reconciliation?

25. What is an outstanding check?

26. What is a deposit in transit?

27. What is a certified check?

28. How is an NSF check accounted for in the accounting records?

29. Name and comment on the three elements of the fraud triangle.

30. What are the six articles of ethical conduct set out under section I of the AICPA's Code of Professional Conduct?

MULTIPLE-CHOICE QUESTIONS

Multiple-choice questions are provided on the text website at www.mhhe.com/edmondssurvey3e.

EXERCISES

All applicable Exercises are available with McGraw-Hill's *Connect Accounting.*

Exercise 4-1   *SOX and COSO's Internal Control Frameworks*   **LO 1**

Required

a. Explain what the acronym SOX refers to.

b. Define the acronym COSO and explain how it relates to SOX.

c. Name and briefly define the five components of COSO's internal control framework.

d. Define the acronym ERM and explain how it relates to COSO's internal control framework.

Exercise 4-2   *Control activities of a strong internal control system*   **LO 1**

Required

List and describe nine control activities of a strong internal control system discussed in this chapter.

Exercise 4-3   *Internal controls for small businesses*   **LO 1**

Required

Assume you are the owner of a small business that has only two employees.

a. Which of the internal control procedures are most important to you?

b. How can you overcome the limited opportunity to use the separation-of-duties control procedure?

Exercise 4-4   *Internal control for cash*   **LO 1**

Required

a. Why are special controls needed for cash?

b. What is included in the definition of *cash*?

LO 1

Exercise 4-5 *Internal control procedures to prevent deception*

Emergency Care Medical Centers (ECMC) hired a new physician, Ken Major, who was an immediate success. Everyone loved his bedside manner; he could charm the most cantankerous patient. Indeed, he was a master salesman as well as an expert physician. Unfortunately, Major misdiagnosed a case that resulted in serious consequences to the patient. The patient filed suit against ECMC. In preparation for the defense, ECMC's attorneys discovered that Major was indeed an exceptional salesman. He had worked for several years as district marketing manager for a pharmaceutical company. In fact, he was not a physician at all! He had changed professions without going to medical school. He had lied on his application form. His knowledge of medical terminology had enabled him to fool everyone. ECMC was found negligent and lost a $3 million lawsuit.

Required

Identify the relevant internal control procedures that could have prevented the company's losses. Explain how these procedures would have prevented Major's deception.

LO 1

Exercise 4-6 *Internal control procedures to prevent embezzlement*

Bell Gates was in charge of the returns department at The Software Company. She was responsible for evaluating returned merchandise. She sent merchandise that was reusable back to the warehouse, where it was restocked in inventory. Gates was also responsible for taking the merchandise that she determined to be defective to the city dump for disposal. She had agreed to buy a tax planning program for one of her friends at a discount through her contacts at work. That is when the idea came to her. She could simply classify one of the reusable returns as defective and bring it home instead of taking it to the dump. She did so and made a quick $150. She was happy, and her friend was ecstatic; he was able to buy a $400 software package for only $150. He told his friends about the deal, and soon Gates had a regular set of customers. She was caught when a retail store owner complained to the marketing manager that his pricing strategy was being undercut by The Software Company's direct sales to the public. The marketing manager was suspicious because The Software Company had no direct marketing program. When the outside sales were ultimately traced back to Gates, the company discovered that it had lost over $10,000 in sales revenue because of her criminal activity.

Required

Identify an internal control procedure that could have prevented the company's losses. Explain how the procedure would have stopped the embezzlement.

LO 2

Exercise 4-7 *Treatment of NSF check*

Rankin Stationery's bank statement contained a $250 NSF check that one of its customers had written to pay for supplies purchased.

Required

a. Show the effects of recognizing the NSF check on the financial statements by recording the appropriate amounts in a horizontal statements model like the following one:

Assets		= Liab.	+ Equity	Rev.	− Exp.	= Net Inc.	Cash Flow
Cash +	Accts. Rec.						

b. Is the recognition of the NSF check on Rankin's books an asset source, use, or exchange transaction?

c. Suppose the customer redeems the check by giving Rankin $270 cash in exchange for the bad check. The additional $20 was a service fee charged by Rankin. Show the effects on the financial statements in the horizontal statements model in Requirement *a*.

d. Is the receipt of cash referenced in Requirement *c* an asset source, use, or exchange transaction?

Exercise 4-8 *Adjustments to the balance per books* **LO 2**

Required

Identify which of the following items are added to or subtracted from the unadjusted *book balance* to arrive at the true cash balance. Distinguish the additions from the subtractions by placing a + beside the items that are added to the unadjusted book balance and a − beside those that are subtracted from it. The first item is recorded as an example.

Reconciling Items	Book Balance Adjusted?	Added or Subtracted?
Outstanding checks	No	N/A
Interest revenue earned on the account		
Deposits in transit		
Service charge		
Automatic debit for utility bill		
Charge for checks		
NSF check from customer		
ATM fee		

Exercise 4-9 *Adjustments to the balance per bank* **LO 2**

Required

Identify which of the following items are added to or subtracted from the unadjusted *bank balance* to arrive at the true cash balance. Distinguish the additions from the subtractions by placing a + beside the items that are added to the unadjusted bank balance and a − beside those that are subtracted from it. The first item is recorded as an example.

Reconciling Items	Bank Balance Adjusted?	Added or Subtracted?
Bank service charge	No	N/A
Outstanding checks		
Deposits in transit		
Debit memo		
Credit memo		
ATM fee		
Petty cash voucher		
NSF check from customer		
Interest revenue		

Exercise 4-10 *Adjusting the cash account* **LO 2**

As of June 30, 2012, the bank statement showed an ending balance of $13,879.85. The unadjusted Cash account balance was $13,483.75. The following information is available:

1. Deposit in transit, $1,476.30.
2. Credit memo in bank statement for interest earned in June, $35.
3. Outstanding check, $1,843.74.
4. Debit memo for service charge, $6.34.

Required

Determine the true cash balance by preparing a bank reconciliation as of June 30, 2012, using the preceding information.

LO 2

Exercise 4-11   *Determining the true cash balance, starting with the unadjusted bank balance*

The following information is available for Hamby Company for the month of June:

1. The unadjusted balance per the bank statement on June 30 was $68,714.35.
2. Deposits in transit on June 30 were $1,464.95.
3. A debit memo was included with the bank statement for a service charge of $25.38.
4. A $4,745.66 check written in June had not been paid by the bank.
5. The bank statement included a $944 credit memo for the collection of a note. The principal of the note was $859, and the interest collected amounted to $85.

Required

Determine the true cash balance as of June 30 (*Hint:* It is not necessary to use all of the preceding items to determine the true balance.)

LO 2

Exercise 4-12   *Determining the true cash balance, starting with the unadjusted book balance*

Crumbley Company had an unadjusted cash balance of $6,450 as of May 31. The company's bank statement, also dated May 31, included a $38 NSF check written by one of Crumbley's customers. There were $548.60 in outstanding checks and $143.74 in deposits in transit as of May 31. According to the bank statement, service charges were $30, and the bank collected a $450 note receivable for Crumbley. The bank statement also showed $18 of interest revenue earned by Crumbley.

Required

Determine the true cash balance as of May 31. (*Hint:* It is not necessary to use all of the preceding items to determine the true balance.)

LO 3

Exercise 4-13   *AICPA Code of Professional Conduct*

Walter Walker owns and operates Walker Enterprises. Walter's sister, Sarah, is the independent public accountant for Walker Enterprises. Sarah worked for the Walker Enterprises for five years before she started her independent CPA practice. Walter considered hiring a different accounting firm but ultimately decided that no one knew his business as well as his sister.

Required

Use the AICPA Code of Professional Conduct to evaluate the appropriateness of Sarah's client relationship with Walker Enterprises.

LO 3

Exercise 4-14   *AICPA Code of Professional Conduct*

Courtney Simmons owns the fastest growing CPA practice in her local community. She attributes her success to her marketing skills. She makes a special effort to get to know her clients personally. She attends their weddings, anniversary celebrations, and birthday parties on a regular basis. Courtney always brings lavish presents, and her clients reciprocate by showering her with expensive gifts on her special occasions. This social activity consumes a lot of time. Indeed, it has cut into the time she once spent on continuing education. Even so, her practice has grown at the rate of 25 percent per year for the last three years. Courtney could not be happier with her progress.

Required

Use the AICPA Code of Professional Conduct to evaluate the appropriateness of Courtney's marketing strategy.

LO 3

Exercise 4-15   *Fraud triangle*

Bill Perry is a CPA with a secret. His secret is that he gambles on sports. Bill knows that his profession disapproves of gambling, but considers the professional standards to be misguided in his case. Bill really doesn't consider his bets to be gambling because he spends a lot of time studying sports facts. He believes that he is simply making educated decisions based on facts. He argues that using sports, facts to place bets is no different than using accounting information to buy stock.

Required

Use the fraud triangle as a basis to comment on Bill Perry's gambling activities.

Exercise 4-16 *Confidentiality and the auditor*

LO 4

West Aston discovered a significant fraud in the accounting records of a high profile client. The story has been broadcast on national airways. Aston was unable to resolve his remaining concerns with the company's management team and ultimately resigned from the audit engagement. Aston knows that he will be asked by several interested parties, including his friends and relatives, the successor auditor, and prosecuting attorneys in a court of law to tell what he knows. He has asked you for advice.

Required

Write a memo that explains Aston's disclosure responsibilities to each of the interested parties.

Exercise 4-17 *Auditor responsibilities*

LO 4

You have probably heard it is unwise to bite the hand that feeds you. Independent auditors are chosen by, paid by, and can be fired by the companies they audit. What keeps the auditor independent? In other words, what stops an auditor from blindly following the orders of a client?

Required

Write a memo that explains the reporting responsibilities of an independent auditor.

PROBLEMS

All applicable Problems are available with McGraw-Hill's
Connect Accounting.

Problem 4-18 *Using internal control to restrict illegal or unethical behavior*

LO 1

Required

For each of the following fraudulent acts, describe one or more internal control procedures that could have prevented (or helped prevent) the problems.

a. Everyone in the office has noticed what a dedicated employee Jennifer Reidel is. She never misses work, not even for a vacation. Reidel is in charge of the petty cash fund. She transfers funds from the company's bank account to the petty cash account on an as-needed basis. During a surprise audit, the petty cash fund was found to contain fictitious receipts. Over a three-year period, Reidel had used more than $4,000 of petty cash to pay for personal expenses.

b. Bill Bruton was hired as the vice president of the manufacturing division of a corporation. His impressive resume listed a master's degree in business administration from a large state university and numerous collegiate awards and activities, when in fact Bruton had only a high school diploma. In a short time, the company was in poor financial condition because of his inadequate knowledge and bad decisions.

c. Havolene Manufacturing has good internal control over its manufacturing materials inventory. However, office supplies are kept on open shelves in the employee break room. The office supervisor has noticed that he is having to order paper, tape, staplers, and pens with increasing frequency.

Problem 4-19 *Preparing a bank reconciliation*

LO 2

CHECK FIGURE
True Cash Balance, August 31,
2012: $16,260

Bob Carson owns a card shop, Card Talk. The following cash information is available for the month of August, 2012.

As of August 31, the bank statement shows a balance of $17,000. The August 31 unadjusted balance in the Cash account of Card Talk is $16,000. A review of the bank statement revealed the following information:

1. A deposit of $2,260 on August 31, 2012, does not appear on the August bank statement.
2. It was discovered that a check to pay for baseball cards was correctly written and paid by the bank for $4,040 but was recorded on the books as $4,400.

3. When checks written during the month were compared with those paid by the bank, three checks amounting to $3,000 were found to be outstanding.
4. A debit memo for $100 was included in the bank statement for the purchase of a new supply of checks.

Required

Prepare a bank reconciliation at the end of August showing the true cash balance.

LO 2

Problem 4-20   *Missing information in a bank reconciliation*

The following data apply to Superior Auto Supply Inc. for May 2012.

1. Balance per the bank on May 31, $8,000.
2. Deposits in transit not recorded by the bank, $975.
3. Bank error; check written by Allen Auto Supply was charged to Superior Auto Supply's account, $650.
4. The following checks written and recorded by Superior Auto Supply were not included in the bank statement:

3013	$ 385
3054	735
3056	1,900

CHECK FIGURE
Unadjusted Cash Balance,
May 31, 2012: $5,565

5. Note collected by the bank, $500.
6. Service charge for collection of note, $10.
7. The bookkeeper recorded a check written for $188 to pay for the May utilities expense as $888 in the cash disbursements journal.
8. Bank service charge in addition to the note collection fee, $25.
9. Customer checks returned by the bank as NSF, $125.

Required

Determine the amount of the unadjusted cash balance per Superior Auto Supply's books.

LO 2

CHECK FIGURE
b. No book adjustment

Problem 4-21   *Adjustments to the cash account based on the bank reconciliation*

Required

Determine whether the following items included in Yang Company's bank reconciliation will require adjustments or corrections on Yang's books.

a. An $877 deposit was recorded by the bank as $778.
b. Four checks totaling $450 written during the month of January were not included with the January bank statement.
c. A $54 check written to Office Max for office supplies was recorded in the general journal as $45.
d. The bank statement indicated that the bank had collected a $330 note for Yang.
e. Yang recorded $500 of receipts on January 31, which were deposited in the night depository of the bank. These deposits were not included in the bank statement.
f. Service charges of $22 for the month of January were listed on the bank statement.
g. The bank charged a $297 check drawn on Cave Restaurant to Yang's account. The check was included in Yang's bank statement.
h. A check of $31 was returned by the bank because of insufficient funds and was noted on the bank statement. Yang received the check from a customer and thought that it was good when it was deposited into the account.

Problem 4-22 *Bank reconciliation and adjustments to the cash account*   **LO 2**

The following information is available for Cooters Garage for March 2012:

BANK STATEMENT
HAZARD STATE BANK
215 MAIN STREET
HAZARD, GA 30321

Cooters Garage	Account number
629 Main Street	62-00062
Hazard, GA 30321	March 31, 2012

Beginning balance 3/1/2012	$15,000.00
Total deposits and other credits	7,000.00
Total checks and other debits	6,000.00
Ending balance 3/31/2012	16,000.00

Checks and Debits		Deposits and Credits	
Check No.	Amount	Date	Amount
1462	$1,163.00	March 1	$1,000.00
1463	62.00	March 2	1,340.00
1464	1,235.00	March 6	210.00
1465	750.00	March 12	1,940.00
1466	1,111.00	March 17	855.00
1467	964.00	March 22	1,480.00
DM	15.00	CM	175.00
1468	700.00		

The following is a list of checks and deposits recorded on the books of Cooters Garage for March 2012:

Date	Check No.	Amount of Check	Date	Amount of Deposit
March 1	1463	$ 62.00	March 1	$1,340.00
March 5	1464	1,235.00	March 5	210.00
March 6	1465	750.00		
March 9	1466	1,111.00	March 10	1,940.00
March 10	1467	964.00		
March 14	1468	70.00	March 16	855.00
March 19	1469	1,500.00	March 19	1,480.00
March 28	1470	102.00	March 29	2,000.00

Other Information

1. Check no. 1462 was outstanding from February.
2. A credit memo for collection of accounts receivable was included in the bank statement.
3. All checks were paid at the correct amount.
4. The bank statement included a debit memo for service charges.
5. The February 28 bank reconciliation showed a deposit in transit of $1,000.
6. Check no. 1468 was for the purchase of equipment.
7. The unadjusted Cash account balance at March 31 was $16,868.

Required

a. Prepare the bank reconciliation for Cooters Garage at the end of March.
b. Explain how the adjustments described above affect the cash account.

Problem 4-23 *Bank reconciliation and internal control*

Following is a bank reconciliation for Surf Shop for June 30, 2012:

	Cash Account	Bank Statement
Balance as of 6/30/2012	$ 1,618	$ 3,000
Deposit in transit		600
Outstanding checks		(1,507)
Note collected by bank	2,000	
Bank service charge	(25)	
NSF check	(1,500)	
Adjusted cash balance as of 6/30/2012	$ 2,093	$ 2,093

When reviewing the bank reconciliation, Surf's auditor was unable to locate any reference to the NSF check on the bank statement. Furthermore, the clerk who reconciles the bank account and records the adjusting entries could not find the actual NSF check that should have been included in the bank statement. Finally, there was no specific reference in the accounts receivable supporting records identifying a party who had written a bad check.

Required

a. Prepare a corrected bank reconciliation.
b. What is the total amount of cash missing, and how was the difference between the "true cash" per the bank and the "true cash" per the books hidden on the reconciliation prepared by the former employee?
c. What could Surf's Shop do to avoid cash theft in the future?

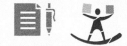

Problem 4-24 *Fraud Triangle*

Pete Chalance is an accountant with a shady past. Suffice it to say that he owes some very unsavory characters a lot of money. Despite his past, Pete works hard at keeping up a strong professional image. He is a manager at Smith and Associates, a fast-growing CPA firm. Pete is highly regarded around the office because he is a strong producer of client revenue. Indeed, on several occasions he exceeded his authority in establishing prices with clients. This is typically a partner's job but who could criticize Pete, who is most certainly bringing in the business. Indeed, Pete is so good that he is able to pull off the following scheme. He bills clients at inflated rates and then reports the ordinary rate to his accounting firm. Say, for example, the normal charge for a job is $2,500. Pete will smooth talk the client, then charge him $3,000. He reports the normal charge of $2,500 to his firm and keeps the extra $500 for himself. He knows it isn't exactly right. Even so, his firm gets its regular charges and the client willingly pays for the services rendered. He thinks to himself, as he pockets his ill-gotten gains, who is getting hurt anyway?

Required

The text discusses three common features (conditions) that motivate ethical misconduct. Identify and explain each of the three features as they appear in the above scenario.

Problem 4-25 *Materiality and the auditor*

Sharon Waters is an auditor. Her work at two companies disclosed inappropriate recognition of revenue. Both cases involved dollar amounts in the $100,000 range. In one case. Waters considered the item material and required her client to restate earnings. In the other case, Waters dismissed the misstatement as being immaterial.

Required

Write a memo that explains how a $100,000 misstatement of revenue is acceptable for one company but unacceptable for a different company.

Problem 4-26   *Types of audit reports*   **LO 4**

Jim Morris is a partner of a regional accounting firm. Mr. Morris was hired by a client to audit the company's books. After extensive work, Mr. Morris determined that he was unable to perform the appropriate audit procedures.

Required

a. Name the type of audit report that Mr. Morris should issue with respect to the work that he did accomplish.

b. If Mr. Morris had been able to perform the necessary audit procedures, there are three types of audit reports that he could have issued depending on the outcome of the audit. Name and describe these three types of audit reports.

ANALYZE, THINK, COMMUNICATE

ATC 4-1   Business Application Case   *Understanding real-world annual reports*

Use the Target Corporation's annual report in Appendix B to answer the following questions.

Required

a. Instead of "Cash," the company's balance sheet uses the account name "Cash and cash equivalents." How does the company define cash equivalents?

b. The annual report has two reports in which management is clearly identified as having responsibility for the company's financial reporting and internal controls. What are the names of these reports and on what pages are they located?

ATC 4-2   Group Assignment   *Bank reconciliations*

The following cash and bank information is available for three companies at June 30, 2012.

Cash and Adjustment Information	Peach Co.	Apple Co.	Pear Co.
Unadjusted cash balance per books, 6/30	$45,620	$32,450	$23,467
Outstanding checks	1,345	2,478	2,540
Service charge	50	75	35
Balance per bank statement, 6/30	48,632	37,176	24,894
Credit memo for collection of notes receivable	4,500	5,600	3,800
NSF check	325	145	90
Deposits in transit	2,500	3,200	4,800
Credit memo for interest earned	42	68	12

Required

a. Organize the class into three sections and divide each section into groups of three to five students. Assign Peach Co. to section 1, Apple Co. to section 2, and Pear Co. to section 3.

Group Tasks

(1) Prepare a bank reconciliation for the company assigned to your group.

(2) Select a representative from a group in each section to put the bank reconciliation on the board.

Class Discussion:

b. Discuss the cause of the difference between the unadjusted cash balance and the ending balance for the bank statement. Also, discuss types of adjustment that are commonly made to the bank balance and types of adjustment that are commonly made to the unadjusted book balance.

ATC 4-3   Research Assignment   *Investigating Cash and Management Issues at Smucker's*

Using the most current Form 10-K available on EDGAR, or the company's website, answer the following questions about the J. M. Smucker Company. Instructions for using EDGAR are in Appendix A. *Note: In some years the financial statements, footnotes, etc., portion of Smucker's annual report have been located at the end of the Form 10-K, in or just after "Item 15."*

Required

a. Instead of "Cash," the company's balance sheet uses the account name "Cash and cash equivalents." How does the company define cash equivalents?

b. The annual report has two reports in which management clearly acknowledges its responsibility for the company's financial reporting and internal controls. What are the names of these reports and on what pages are they located?

ATC 4-4   Writing Assignment   *Internal control procedures*

Sarah Johnson was a trusted employee of Evergreen Trust Bank. She was involved in everything. She worked as a teller, she accounted for the cash at the other teller windows, and she recorded many of the transactions in the accounting records. She was so loyal that she never would take a day off, even when she was really too sick to work. She routinely worked late to see that all the day's work was posted into the accounting records. She would never take even a day's vacation because they might need her at the bank. Adam and Jammie, CPAs, were hired to perform an audit, the first complete audit that had been done in several years. Johnson seemed somewhat upset by the upcoming audit. She said that everything had been properly accounted for and that the audit was a needless expense. When Adam and Jammie examined some of the bank's internal control procedures, it discovered problems. In fact, as the audit progressed, it became apparent that a large amount of cash was missing. Numerous adjustments had been made to customer accounts with credit memorandums, and many of the transactions had been posted several days late. In addition, there were numerous cash payments for "office expenses." When the audit was complete, it was determined that more than $100,000 of funds was missing or improperly accounted for. All fingers pointed to Johnson. The bank's president, who was a close friend of Johnson, was bewildered. How could this type of thing happen at this bank?

Required

Prepare a written memo to the bank president, outlining the procedures that should be followed to prevent this type of problem in the future.

ATC 4-5   Ethical Dilemma   *I need just a little extra money*

John Riley, a certified public accountant, has worked for the past eight years as a payroll clerk for Southeast Industries, a small furniture manufacturing firm in the Northeast. John recently experienced unfortunate circumstances. His teenage son required major surgery and the medical bills not covered by John's insurance have financially strained John's family.

John works hard and is a model employee. Although he received regular performance raises during his first few years with Southeast. John's wages have not increased in three years. John asked his supervisor, Bill Jameson, for a raise. Bill agreed that John deserved a raise, but told him he could not currently approve one because of sluggish sales.

A disappointed John returned to his duties while the financial pressures in his life continued. Two weeks later, Larry Tyler, an assembly worker at Southwest, quit over a dispute with management. John conceived an idea. John's duties included not only processing employee terminations but also approving time cards before paychecks were issued and then distributing the paychecks to firm personnel. John decided to delay processing Mr. Tyler's termination, to forge timecards for Larry Tyler for the next few weeks, and to cash the checks himself. Since he distributed paychecks, no one would find out, and John reasoned that he was really entitled to the extra money anyway. In fact, no one did discover his maneuver and John stopped the practice after three weeks.

Required

a. Does John's scheme affect Southeast's balance sheet? Explain your answer.

b. Review the AICPA's Articles of Professional Conduct and comment on any of the standards that have been violated.

c. Identify the three elements of unethical and criminal conduct recognized in the fraud triangle.

CHAPTER 8

Proprietorships, Partnerships, and Corporations

LEARNING OBJECTIVES

After you have mastered the material in this chapter, you will be able to:

1 Identify the primary characteristics of sole proprietorships, partnerships, and corporations.

2 Analyze financial statements to identify the different types of business organizations.

3 Explain the characteristics of major types of stock issued by corporations.

4 Explain how to account for different types of stock issued by corporations.

5 Show how treasury stock transactions affect a company's financial statements.

6 Explain the effects of declaring and paying cash dividends on a company's financial statements.

7 Explain the effects of stock dividends and stock splits on a company's financial statements.

8 Show how the appropriation of retained earnings affects financial statements.

9 Explain some uses of accounting information in making stock investment decisions.

CHAPTER OPENING

You want to start a business. How should you structure it? Should it be a sole proprietorship, partnership, or corporation? Each form of business structure presents advantages and disadvantages. For example, a sole proprietorship allows maximum independence and control while partnerships and corporations allow individuals to pool resources and talents with other people. This chapter discusses these and other features of the three primary forms of business structure.

The Curious Accountant

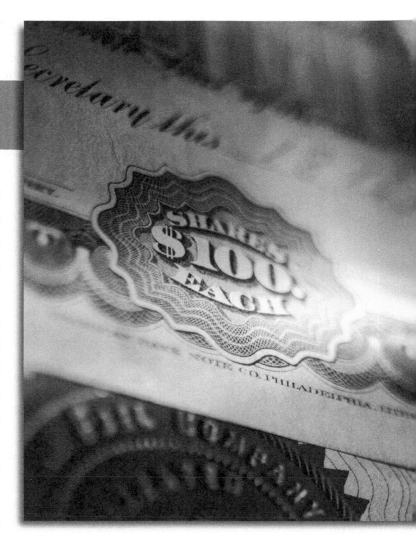

Imagine your rich uncle rewarded you for doing well in your first accounting course by giving you $10,000 to invest in the stock of one company. After reviewing many recent annual reports, you narrowed your choice to two companies with the following characteristics:

Mystery Company A: This company began operations in 2003, but did not begin selling its stock to the public until April 16, 2009. In its first six years of operations it had total earnings of approximately $1.6 million. By the time it went public it was already a leader in its field. At its current price of $23 you could buy approximately 435 shares. A friend told you that a globally minded person like you would be crazy not to buy this stock.

Mystery Company B: This company has been in existence since 1837 and has made a profit most years. In the most recent five years, its net earnings totaled over $51.8 *billion*, and it paid dividends of over $21 *billion*. This stock is selling for about $62 per share, so you can buy 161 shares of it. Your friend said "you would have to be goofy to buy this stock."

The names of the real-world companies described above are disclosed later. Based on the information provided, which company's stock would you buy? (Answer on page 290.)

FORMS OF BUSINESS ORGANIZATIONS

Identify the primary characteristics of sole proprietorships, partnerships, and corporations.

Sole proprietorships are owned by a single individual who is responsible for making business and profit distribution decisions. If you want to be the absolute master of your destiny, you should organize your business as a proprietorship. Establishing a sole proprietorship is usually as simple as obtaining a business license from local government authorities. Usually no legal ownership agreement is required.

Partnerships allow persons to share their talents, capital, and the risks and rewards of business ownership. Because two or more individuals share ownership, partnerships require clear agreements about how authority, risks, and profits will be shared. Prudent partners minimize misunderstandings by hiring attorneys to prepare a **partnership agreement** which defines the responsibilities of each partner and describes how income or losses will be divided. Because the measurement of income affects the distribution of profits, partnerships frequently hire accountants to ensure that records are maintained in accordance with generally accepted accounting principles (GAAP). Partnerships (and sole proprietorships) also may need professional advice to deal with tax issues.

A **corporation** is a separate legal entity created by the authority of a state government. The paperwork to start a corporation is complex. For most laypersons, engaging professional attorneys and accountants to assist with the paperwork is well worth the fees charged.

Each state has separate laws governing establishing corporations. Many states follow the standard provisions of the Model Business Corporation Act. All states require the initial application to provide **articles of incorporation** which normally include the following information: (1) the corporation's name and proposed date of incorporation; (2) the purpose of the corporation; (3) the location of the business and its expected life (which can be *perpetuity,* meaning *endless*); (4) provisions for capital stock; and (5) the names and addresses of the members of the first board of directors, the individuals with the ultimate authority for operating the business. If the articles are in order, the state establishes the legal existence of the corporation by issuing a charter of incorporation. The charter and the articles are public documents.

ADVANTAGES AND DISADVANTAGES OF DIFFERENT FORMS OF BUSINESS ORGANIZATION

Each form of business organization presents a different combination of advantages and disadvantages. Persons wanting to start a business or invest in one should consider the characteristics of each type of business structure.

Regulation

Few laws specifically affect the operations of proprietorships and partnerships. Corporations, however, are usually heavily regulated. The extent of government regulation depends on the size and distribution of a company's ownership interests. Ownership interests in corporations are normally evidenced by **stock certificates.**

Ownership of corporations can be transferred from one individual to another through exchanging stock certificates. As long as the exchanges (buying and selling of shares of stock, often called *trading*) are limited to transactions between individuals, a company is defined as a **closely held corporation.** However, once a corporation reaches a certain size, it may list its stock on a stock exchange such as the New York Stock Exchange or the American Stock Exchange. Trading on a stock exchange is limited to the stockbrokers who are members of the exchange. These brokers represent buyers and sellers who are willing to pay the brokers commissions for exchanging stock certificates on their behalf. Although closely held corporations are relatively free from government regulation, companies whose stock is publicly traded on the exchanges by brokers are subject to extensive regulation.

The extensive regulation of trading on stock exchanges began in the 1930s. The stock market crash of 1929 and the subsequent Great Depression led Congress to pass the **Securities Act of 1933** and the **Securities Exchange Act of 1934** to regulate issuing stock and to govern the exchanges. The 1934 act also created the Securities and Exchange Commission (SEC) to enforce the securities laws. Congress gave the SEC legal authority to establish accounting principles for corporations that are registered on the exchanges. However, the SEC has generally deferred its rule-making authority to private sector accounting bodies such as the Financial Accounting Standards Board (FASB), effectively allowing the accounting profession to regulate itself.

A number of high-profile business failures around the turn of the last century raised questions about the effectiveness of self-regulation and the usefulness of audits to protect the public. The Sarbanes-Oxley Act of 2002 was adopted to address these concerns. The act creates a five-member Public Company Accounting Oversight Board (PCAOB) with the authority to set and enforce auditing, attestation, quality control, and ethics standards for auditors of public companies. The PCAOB is empowered to impose disciplinary and remedial sanctions for violations of its rules, securities laws, and professional auditing and accounting standards. Public corporations operate in a complex regulatory environment that requires the services of attorneys and professional accountants.

Double Taxation

Corporations pay income taxes on their earnings and then owners pay income taxes on distributions (dividends) received from corporations. As a result, distributed corporate profits are taxed twice—first when income is reported on the corporation's income tax return and a second time when distributions are reported on individual owners' tax returns. This phenomenon is commonly called **double taxation** and is a significant disadvantage of the corporate form of business organization.

To illustrate, assume Glide Corporation earns pretax income of $100,000. Glide is in a 30 percent tax bracket. The corporation itself will pay income tax of $30,000 ($100,000 × 0.30). If the corporation distributes the after-tax income of $70,000 ($100,000 − $30,000) to individual stockholders in 15 percent tax brackets,[1] the $70,000 dividend will be reported on the individual tax returns, requiring tax payments of $10,500 ($70,000 × .15). Total income tax of $40,500 ($30,000 + $10,500) is due on $100,000 of earned income. In contrast, consider a proprietorship that is owned by an individual in a 30 percent tax bracket. If the proprietorship earns and distributes $100,000 profit, the total tax would be only $30,000 ($100,000 × .30).

Double taxation can be a burden for small companies. To reduce that burden, tax laws permit small closely held corporations to elect "S Corporation" status. S Corporations are taxed as proprietorships or partnerships. Also, many states have recently enacted laws permitting the formation of **limited liability companies (LLCs)** which offer many of the benefits of corporate ownership yet are in general taxed as partnerships. Because proprietorships and partnerships are not separate legal entities, company earnings are taxable to the owners rather than the company itself.

Limited Liability

Given the disadvantages of increased regulation and double taxation, why would anyone choose the corporate form of business structure over a partnership or proprietorship? A major reason is that the corporate form limits an investor's potential liability as an owner of a business venture. Because a corporation is legally separate from its owners, creditors cannot claim owners' personal assets as payment for the company's debts. Also, plaintiffs

---

[1] As a result of the Jobs and Growth Tax Relief Reconciliation Act (JGTRRA) of 2003, dividends received in tax years after 2002 are taxed at a maximum rate of 15 percent for most taxpayers. Lower income individuals pay a 5 percent tax on dividends received on December 31, 2007, or earlier. This rate falls to zero in 2008. The provisions of JGTRRA are set to expire on December 31, 2008.

must sue the corporation, not its owners. The most that owners of a corporation can lose is the amount they have invested in the company (the value of the company's stock).

Unlike corporate stockholders, the owners of proprietorships and partnerships are *personally liable* for actions they take in the name of their companies. In fact, partners are responsible not only for their own actions but also for those taken by any other partner on behalf of the partnership. The benefit of **limited liability** is one of the most significant reasons the corporate form of business organization is so popular.

Continuity

Unlike partnerships or proprietorships, which terminate with the departure of their owners, a corporation's life continues when a shareholder dies or sells his or her stock. Because of **continuity** of existence, many corporations formed in the 1800s still thrive today.

Transferability of Ownership

The **transferability** of corporate ownership is easy. An investor simply buys or sells stock to acquire or give up an ownership interest in a corporation. Hundreds of millions of shares of stock are bought and sold on the major stock exchanges each day.

Transferring the ownership of proprietorships is much more difficult. To sell an ownership interest in a proprietorship, the proprietor must find someone willing to purchase the entire business. Because most proprietors also run their businesses, transferring ownership also requires transferring management responsibilities. Consider the difference in selling $1 million of Exxon stock versus selling a locally owned gas station. The stock could be sold on the New York Stock Exchange within minutes. In contrast, it could take years to find a buyer who is financially capable of and interested in owning and operating a gas station.

Transferring ownership in partnerships can also be difficult. As with proprietorships, ownership transfers may require a new partner to make a significant investment and accept management responsibilities in the business. Further, a new partner must accept and be accepted by the other partners. Personality conflicts and differences in management style can cause problems in transferring ownership interests in partnerships.

Management Structure

Partnerships and proprietorships are usually managed by their owners. Corporations, in contrast, have three tiers of management authority. The *owners* (**stockholders**) represent the highest level of organizational authority. The stockholders *elect* a **board of directors** to oversee company operations. The directors then *hire* professional executives to manage the company on a daily basis. Because large corporations can offer high salaries and challenging career opportunities, they can often attract superior managerial talent.

While the management structure used by corporations is generally effective, it sometimes complicates dismissing incompetent managers. The chief executive officer (CEO) is usually a member of the board of directors and is frequently influential in choosing other board members. The CEO is also in a position to reward loyal board members. As a result, board members may be reluctant to fire the CEO or other top executives even if the individuals are performing poorly. Corporations operating under such conditions are said to be experiencing **entrenched management.**

Ability to Raise Capital

Because corporations can have millions of owners (shareholders), they have the opportunity to raise huge amounts of capital. Few individuals have the financial means to build and operate a telecommunications network such as AT&T or a marketing distribution system such as Walmart. However, by pooling the resources of millions of owners through public stock and bond offerings, corporations generate the billions of dollars of capital needed for such massive investments. In contrast, the capital resources of proprietorships and partnerships are limited to a relatively small number of private owners. Although proprietorships and partnerships can also obtain resources by borrowing, the amount creditors are willing to lend them is usually limited by the size of the owners' net worth.

APPEARANCE OF CAPITAL STRUCTURE IN FINANCIAL STATEMENTS

The ownership interest (equity) in a business is composed of two elements: (1) owner/investor contributions and (2) retained earnings. The way these two elements are reported in the financial statements differs for each type of business structure (proprietorship, partnership, or corporation).

LO 2

Analyze financial statements to identify the different types of business organizations.

Presentation of Equity in Proprietorships

Owner contributions and retained earnings are combined in a single Capital account on the balance sheets of proprietorships. To illustrate, assume that Worthington Sole Proprietorship was started on January 1, 2012, when it acquired a $5,000 capital contribution from its owner, Phil Worthington. During the first year of operation, the company generated $4,000 of cash revenues, incurred $2,500 of cash expenses, and distributed $1,000 cash to the owner. Exhibit 8.1 displays 2012 financial statements for Worthington's company. Note on the *capital statement* that distributions are called **withdrawals.** Verify that the $5,500 balance in the Capital account on the balance sheet includes the $5,000 owner contribution and the retained earnings of $500 ($1,500 net income − $1,000 withdrawal).

EXHIBIT 8.1

WORTHINGTON SOLE PROPRIETORSHIP
Financial Statements
As of December 31, 2012

Income Statement		Capital Statement		Balance Sheet	
Revenue	$4,000	Beginning capital balance	$ 0	Assets	
Expenses	2,500	Plus: Investment by owner	5,000	Cash	$5,500
Net income	$1,500	Plus: Net income	1,500	Equity	
		Less: Withdrawal by owner	(1,000)	Worthington, capital	$5,500
		Ending capital balance	$5,500		

CHECK YOURSELF 8.1

Weiss Company was started on January 1, 2012, when it acquired $50,000 cash from its owner(s). During 2012 the company earned $72,000 of net income. Explain how the equity section of Weiss's December 31, 2012, balance sheet would differ if the company were a proprietorship versus a corporation.

Answer *Proprietorship* records combine capital acquisitions from the owner and earnings from operating the business in a single capital account. In contrast, *corporation* records separate capital acquisitions from the owners and earnings from operating the business. If Weiss were a proprietorship, the equity section of the year-end balance sheet would report a single capital component of $122,000. If Weiss were a corporation, the equity section would report two separate equity components, most likely common stock of $50,000 and retained earnings of $72,000.

Presentation of Equity in Partnerships

The financial statement format for reporting partnership equity is similar to that used for proprietorships. Contributed capital and retained earnings are combined. However, a separate capital account is maintained for each partner in the business to reflect each partner's ownership interest.

To illustrate, assume that Sara Slater and Jill Johnson formed a partnership on January 1, 2012. The partnership acquired $2,000 of capital from Slater and $4,000 from Johnson. The partnership agreement called for each partner to receive an annual distribution equal to 10 percent of her capital contribution. Any further earnings were to be retained in the business and divided equally between the partners. During 2012, the company earned $5,000 of cash revenue and incurred $3,000 of cash expenses, for net income of $2,000 ($5,000 − $3,000). As specified by the partnership agreement, Slater received a $200 ($2,000 × 0.10) cash withdrawal and Johnson received $400 ($4,000 × 0.10). The remaining $1,400 ($2,000 − $200 − $400) of income was retained in the business and divided equally, adding $700 to each partner's capital account.

Exhibit 8.2 displays financial statements for the Slater and Johnson partnership. Again, note that distributions are called *withdrawals*. Also find on the balance sheet a *separate capital account* for each partner. Each capital account includes the amount of the partner's contributed capital plus her proportionate share of the retained earnings.

EXHIBIT 8.2

SLATER AND JOHNSON PARTNERSHIP
Financial Statements
As of December 31, 2012

Income Statement		Capital Statement		Balance Sheet	
Revenue	$5,000	Beginning capital balance	$ 0	Assets	
Expenses	3,000	Plus: Investment by owners	6,000	Cash	$7,400
Net income	$2,000	Plus: Net income	2,000	Equity	
		Less: Withdrawal by owners	(600)	Slater, capital	$2,700
		Ending capital balance	$7,400	Johnson, capital	4,700
				Total capital	$7,400

Presentation of Equity in Corporations

Corporations have more complex capital structures than proprietorships and partnerships. Explanations of some of the more common features of corporate capital structures and transactions follow.

CHARACTERISTICS OF CAPITAL STOCK

Stock issued by corporations may have a variety of different characteristics. For example, a company may issue different classes of stock that grant owners different rights and privileges. Also, the number of shares a corporation can legally issue may differ from the number it actually has issued. Further, a corporation can even buy back its own stock. Finally, a corporation may assign different values to the stock it issues. Accounting for corporate equity transactions is discussed in the next section of the text.

Explain the characteristics of major types of stock issued by corporations.

Par Value

Many states require assigning a **par value** to stock. Historically, par value represented the maximum liability of the investors. Par value multiplied by the number of shares of stock issued represents the minimum amount of assets that must be retained in the company as protection for creditors. This amount is known as **legal capital.** To ensure that the amount of legal capital is maintained in a corporation, many states require that purchasers pay at least the par value for a share of stock initially purchased from a corporation. To minimize the amount of assets that owners must maintain in the business, many corporations issue stock with very low par values, often $1 or less. Therefore, *legal capital* as defined by par value has come to have very little relevance to investors or creditors. As a result, many states allow corporations to issue no-par stock.

Stated Value

No-par stock may have a stated value. Like par value, **stated value** is an arbitrary amount assigned by the board of directors to the stock. It also has little relevance to investors and creditors. Stock with a par value and stock with a stated value are accounted for exactly the same way. When stock has no par or stated value, accounting for it is slightly different. These accounting differences are illustrated later in this chapter.

Other Valuation Terminology

The price an investor must pay to purchase a share of stock is the **market value.** The sales price of a share of stock may be more or less than the par value. Another term analysts frequently associate with stock is *book value*. **Book value per share** is calculated by dividing total stockholders' equity (assets − liabilities) by the number of shares of stock owned by investors. Book value per share differs from market value per share because equity is measured in historical dollars and market value reflects investors' estimates of a company's current value.

Stock: Authorized, Issued, and Outstanding

As part of the regulatory function, states approve the maximum number of shares of stock corporations are legally permitted to issue. This maximum number is called **authorized stock.** Authorized stock that has been sold to the public is called **issued stock.** When a corporation buys back some of its issued stock from the public, the repurchased stock is called **treasury stock.** Treasury stock is still considered to be issued stock, but it is no longer outstanding. **Outstanding stock** (total issued stock minus treasury stock) is stock owned by investors outside the corporation. For example, assume a company that is authorized to issue 150 shares of stock issues 100 shares to investors, and then buys back 20 shares of treasury stock. There are 150 shares authorized, 100 shares issued, and 80 shares outstanding.

FOCUS ON INTERNATIONAL ISSUES

PICKY, PICKY, PICKY ...

Considering the almost countless number of differences that could exist between U.S. GAAP and IFRS, it is not surprising that some of those that do exist relate to very specific issues. Consider the case of the timing of stock splits.

Assume a company that ends its fiscal year on December 31, 2011, declares a 2-for-1 stock split on January 15, 2012, before it has issued its 2011 annual report. Should the company apply the effects of the stock split retroactively to is 2011 financial statements, or begin showing the effects of the split on its 2012 statements? Under U.S. GAAP the split must be applied retroactively to the 2011 statements since they had not been issued at the time of the split. Under IFRS the 2011 statements would not show the effects of the split, but the 2012 statements would. By the way, an event that occurs between a company's fiscal year-end and the date its annual report is released is called a *subsequent event* by accountants.

Obviously no one can know every GAAP rule, much less all of the differences between GAAP and IFRS. This is why it is important to learn how to find answers to specific accounting questions as well as to develop an understanding of the basic accounting rules. Most important, if you are not sure you know the answer, do not assume you do.

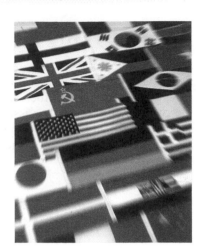

Classes of Stock

The corporate charter defines the number of shares of stock authorized, the par value or stated value (if any), and the classes of stock that a corporation can issue. Most stock issued is either *common* or *preferred*.

Common Stock

All corporations issue **common stock.** Common stockholders bear the highest risk of losing their investment if a company is forced to liquidate. On the other hand, they reap the greatest rewards when a corporation prospers. Common stockholders generally enjoy several rights, including: (1) the right to buy and sell stock, (2) the right to share in the distribution of profits, (3) the right to share in the distribution of corporate assets in the case of liquidation, (4) the right to vote on significant matters that affect the corporate charter, and (5) the right to participate in the election of directors.

Preferred Stock

Many corporations issue **preferred stock** in addition to common stock. Holders of preferred stock receive certain privileges relative to holders of common stock. In exchange for special privileges in some areas, preferred stockholders give up rights in other areas. Preferred stockholders usually have no voting rights and the amount of their dividends is usually limited. Preferences granted to preferred stockholders include the following.

1. *Preference as to assets.* Preferred stock often has a liquidation value. In case of bankruptcy, preferred stockholders must be paid the liquidation value before any assets are distributed to common stockholders. However, preferred stockholder claims still fall behind creditor claims.
2. *Preference as to dividends.* Preferred shareholders are frequently guaranteed the right to receive dividends before common stockholders. The amount of the preferred dividend is normally stated on the stock certificate. It may be stated as a

dollar value (say, $5) per share or as a percentage of the par value. Most preferred stock has **cumulative dividends,** meaning that if a corporation is unable to pay the preferred dividend in any year, the dividend is not lost but begins to accumulate. Cumulative dividends that have not been paid are called **dividends in arrears.** When a company pays dividends, any preferred stock arrearages must be paid before any other dividends are paid. Noncumulative preferred stock is not often issued because preferred stock is much less attractive if missed dividends do not accumulate.

To illustrate the effects of preferred dividends, consider Dillion, Incorporated, which has the following shares of stock outstanding.

> Preferred stock, 4%, $10 par, 10,000 shares
> Common stock, $10 par, 20,000 shares

Assume the preferred stock dividend has not been paid for two years. If Dillion pays $22,000 in dividends, how much will each class of stock receive? It depends on whether the preferred stock is cumulative.

Allocation of Distribution for Cumulative Preferred Stock		
	To Preferred	**To Common**
Dividends in arrears	$ 8,000	$ 0
Current year's dividends	4,000	10,000
Total distribution	$12,000	$10,000

Allocation of Distribution for Noncumulative Preferred Stock		
	To Preferred	**To Common**
Dividends in arrears	$ 0	$ 0
Current year's dividends	4,000	18,000
Total distribution	$4,000	$18,000

The total annual dividend on the preferred stock is $4,000 (0.04 × $10 par × 10,000 shares). If the preferred stock is cumulative, the $8,000 in arrears must be paid first. Then $4,000 for the current year's dividend is paid next. The remaining $10,000 goes to common stockholders. If the preferred stock is noncumulative, the $8,000 of dividends from past periods is ignored. This year's $4,000 preferred dividend is paid first, with the remaining $18,000 going to common.

Other features of preferred stock may include the right to participate in distributions beyond the established amount of the preferred dividend, the right to convert preferred stock to common stock or to bonds, and the potential for having the preferred stock called (repurchased) by the corporation. Detailed discussion of these topics is left to more advanced courses. Exhibit 8.3 indicates that roughly 25 percent of U.S. companies have preferred shares outstanding.

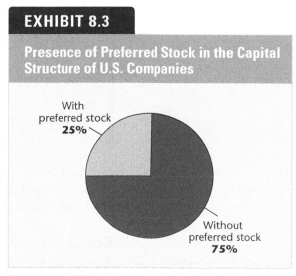

EXHIBIT 8.3

Presence of Preferred Stock in the Capital Structure of U.S. Companies

With preferred stock 25%

Without preferred stock 75%

Data source: AICPA, Accounting Trends and Techniques, 2006.

Explain how to account for different types of stock issued by corporations.

ACCOUNTING FOR STOCK TRANSACTIONS ON THE DAY OF ISSUE

Issuing stock with a par or stated value is accounted for differently from issuing no-par stock. For stock with either a par or stated value, the total amount acquired from the owners is divided between two separate equity accounts. The amount of the par or stated value is recorded in the stock account. Any amount received above the par or stated value is recorded in an account called **Paid-in Capital in Excess of Par** (or **Stated**) **Value.**

Issuing Par Value Stock

To illustrate the issue of common stock with a par value, assume that Nelson Incorporated is authorized to issue 250 shares of common stock. During 2012, Nelson issued 100 shares of $10 par common stock for $22 per share. The event increases assets and stockholders' equity by $2,200 ($22 × 100 shares). The increase in stockholders' equity is divided into two parts, $1,000 of par value ($10 per share × 100 shares) and $1,200 ($2,200 − $1,000) received in excess of par value. The income statement is not affected. The $2,200 cash inflow is reported in the financing activities section of the statement of cash flows. The effects on the financial statements follow.

Assets	=	Liab.	+	Equity			Rev.	−	Exp.	=	Net Inc.	Cash Flow
Cash	=			Com. Stk.	+	PIC in Excess						
2,200	=	NA	+	1,000	+	1,200	NA	−	NA	=	NA	2,200 FA

The *legal capital* of the corporation is $1,000, the total par value of the issued common stock. The number of shares issued can be easily verified by dividing the total amount in the common stock account by the par value ($1,000 ÷ $10 = 100 shares).

Stock Classification

Assume Nelson Incorporated obtains authorization to issue 400 shares of Class B, $20 par value common stock. The company issues 150 shares of this stock at $25 per share. The event increases assets and stockholders' equity by $3,750 ($25 × 150 shares). The increase in stockholders' equity is divided into two parts, $3,000 of par value ($20 per share × 150 shares) and $750 ($3,750 − $3,000) received in excess of par value. The income statement is not affected. The $3,750 cash inflow is reported in the financing activities section of the statement of cash flows. The effects on the financial statements follow.

Assets	=	Liab.	+	Equity			Rev.	−	Exp.	=	Net Inc.	Cash Flow
Cash	=			Com. Stk.	+	PIC in Excess						
3,750	=	NA	+	3,000	+	750	NA	−	NA	=	NA	3,750 FA

As the preceding event suggests, companies can issue numerous classes of common stock. The specific rights and privileges for each class are described in the individual stock certificates.

Stock Issued at Stated Value

Assume Nelson is authorized to issue 300 shares of a third class of stock, 7 percent cumulative preferred stock with a stated value of $10 per share. Nelson issued 100 shares of the preferred stock at a price of $22 per share. The effects on the financial statements are identical to those described for the issue of the $10 par value common stock.

Assets	=	Liab.	+	Equity			Rev.	−	Exp.	=	Net Inc.	Cash Flow
Cash	=			Pfd. Stk.	+	PIC in Excess						
2,200	=	NA	+	1,000	+	1,200	NA	−	NA	=	NA	2,200 FA

Stock Issued with No Par Value

Assume that Nelson Incorporated is authorized to issue 150 shares of a fourth class of stock. This stock is no-par common stock. Nelson issues 100 shares of this no-par stock at $22 per share. The entire amount received ($22 × 100 = $2,200) is recorded in the stock account. The effects on the financial statements follow.

Assets	=	Liab.	+	Equity			Rev.	−	Exp.	=	Net Inc.	Cash Flow
Cash	=			Com. Stk.	+	PIC in Excess						
2,200	=	NA	+	2,200	+	NA	NA	−	NA	=	NA	2,200 FA

Financial Statement Presentation

Exhibit 8.4 displays Nelson Incorporated's balance sheet after the four stock issuances described above. The exhibit assumes that Nelson earned and retained $5,000 of cash income during 2012. The stock accounts are presented first, followed by the paid-in capital in excess of par (or stated) value accounts. A wide variety of reporting formats is used in practice. For example, another popular format is to group accounts by stock class, with the paid-in capital in excess accounts listed with their associated stock accounts. Alternatively, many companies combine the different classes of stock into a single amount and provide the detailed information in footnotes to the financial statements.

EXHIBIT 8.4

NELSON INCORPORATED
Balance Sheet
As of December 31, 2012

Assets	
Cash	$15,350
Stockholders' equity	
Preferred stock, $10 stated value, 7% cumulative, 300 shares authorized, 100 issued and outstanding	$ 1,000
Common stock, $10 par value, 250 shares authorized, 100 issued and outstanding	1,000
Common stock, class B, $20 par value, 400 shares authorized, 150 issued and outstanding	3,000
Common stock, no par, 150 shares authorized, 100 issued and outstanding	2,200
Paid-in capital in excess of stated value—preferred	1,200
Paid-in capital in excess of par value—common	1,200
Paid-in capital in excess of par value—class B common	750
Total paid-in capital	10,350
Retained earnings	5,000
Total stockholders' equity	$15,350

STOCKHOLDERS' EQUITY TRANSACTIONS AFTER THE DAY OF ISSUE

Treasury Stock

LO 5

Show how treasury stock transactions affect a company's financial statements.

When a company buys its own stock, the stock purchased is called *treasury stock*. Why would a company buy its own stock? Common reasons include (1) to have stock available to give employees pursuant to stock option plans, (2) to accumulate stock in preparation for a merger or business combination, (3) to reduce the number of shares outstanding in order to increase earnings per share, (4) to keep the price of the stock high when it appears to be falling, and (5) to avoid a hostile takeover (removing shares from the open market reduces the opportunity for outsiders to obtain enough voting shares to gain control of the company).

Conceptually, purchasing treasury stock is the reverse of issuing stock. When a business issues stock, the assets and equity of the business increase. When a business buys treasury stock, the assets and equity of the business decrease. To illustrate, return to the Nelson Incorporated example. Assume that in 2013 Nelson paid $20 per share to buy back 50 shares of the $10 par value common stock that it originally issued at $22 per share. The purchase of treasury stock is an asset use transaction. Assets and stockholders' equity decrease by the cost of the purchase ($20 × 50 shares = $1,000). The income statement is not affected. The cash outflow is reported in the financing activities section of the statement of cash flows. The effects on the financial statements follow.

Assets	=	Liab.	+	Equity			Rev.	−	Exp.	=	Net Inc.	Cash Flow
Cash	=			Other Equity Accts.	−	Treasury Stk.						
(1,000)	=	NA	+	NA	−	1,000	NA	−	NA	=	NA	(1,000) FA

The Treasury Stock account is a contra equity account. It is deducted from the other equity accounts in determining total stockholders' equity. In this example, the Treasury Stock account contains the full amount paid ($1,000). The original issue price and the par value of the stock have no effect on the Treasury Stock account. Recognizing the full amount paid in the treasury stock account is called the **cost method of accounting for treasury stock** transactions. Although other methods could be used, the cost method is the most common.

Assume Nelson reissues 30 shares of treasury stock at a price of $25 per share. As with any other stock issue, the sale of treasury stock is an asset source transaction. In this case, assets and stockholders' equity increase by $750 ($25 × 30 shares). The income statement is not affected. The cash inflow is reported in the financing activities section of the statement of cash flows. The effects on the financial statements follow.

Assets	=	Liab.	+	Equity					Rev.	−	Exp.	=	Net Inc.	Cash Flow
Cash	=			Other Equity Accounts	−	Treasury Stock	+	PIC from Treasury Stk.						
750	=	NA	+	NA	−	(600)	+	150	NA	−	NA	=	NA	750 FA

The decrease in the Treasury Stock account increases stockholders' equity. The $150 difference between the cost of the treasury stock ($20 per share × 30 shares = $600) and the sales price ($750) is *not* reported as a gain. The sale of treasury stock is a capital acquisition, not a revenue transaction. The $150 is additional paid-in capital. *Corporations do not recognize gains or losses on the sale of treasury stock.*

After selling 30 shares of treasury stock, 20 shares remain in Nelson's possession. These shares cost $20 each, so the balance in the Treasury Stock account is now $400 ($20 × 20 shares). Treasury stock is reported on the balance sheet directly below retained earnings. Although this placement suggests that treasury stock reduces retained earnings, the reduction actually applies to the entire stockholders' equity section. Exhibit 8.5 on page 302 shows the presentation of treasury stock in the balance sheet.

✓ CHECK YOURSELF 8.2

On January 1, 2012, Janell Company's Common Stock account balance was $20,000. On April 1, 2012, Janell paid $12,000 cash to purchase some of its own stock. Janell resold this stock on October 1, 2012, for $14,500. What is the effect on the company's cash and stockholders' equity from both the April 1 purchase and the October 1 resale of the stock?

Answer The April 1 purchase would reduce both cash and stockholders' equity by $12,000. The treasury stock transaction represents a return of invested capital to those owners who sold stock back to the company.

The sale of the treasury stock on October 1 would increase both cash and stockholders' equity by $14,500. The difference between the sales price of the treasury stock and its cost ($14,500 − $12,000) represents additional paid-in capital from treasury stock transactions. The stockholders' equity section of the balance sheet would include Common Stock, $20,000, and Additional Paid-in Capital from Treasury Stock Transactions, $2,500.

Cash Dividend

Cash dividends are affected by three significant dates: *the declaration date, the date of record,* and *the payment date.* Assume that on October 15, 2013, the board of Nelson Incorporated declared a 7% cash dividend on the 100 outstanding shares of its $10 stated value preferred stock. The dividend will be paid to stockholders of record as of November 15, 2013. The cash payment will be made on December 15, 2013.

LO 6

Explain the effects of declaring and paying cash dividends on a company's financial statements.

Declaration Date

Although corporations are not required to declare dividends, they are legally obligated to pay dividends once they have been declared. They must recognize a liability on the **declaration date** (in this case, October 15, 2013). The increase in liabilities is accompanied by a decrease in retained earnings. The income statement and statement of cash flows are not affected. The effects on the financial statements of *declaring* the $70 (0.07 × $10 × 100 shares) dividend follow.

Assets	=	Liab.	+	Equity			Rev.	−	Exp.	=	Net Inc.	Cash Flow
Cash	=	Div. Pay.	+	Com. Stk.	+	Ret. Earn.						
NA	=	70	+	NA	+	(70)	NA	−	NA	=	NA	NA

Date of Record

Cash dividends are paid to investors who owned the preferred stock on the **date of record** (in this case November 15, 2013). Any stock sold after the date of record but

REALITY BYTES

As you have learned, dividends, unlike interest on bonds, do not have to be paid. In fact, a company's board of directors must vote to pay dividends before they can be paid. Even so, once a company establishes a practice of paying a dividend of a given amount each period, usually quarterly, the company is reluctant to not pay the dividend. Furthermore, it is usually a significant news event when a company decides to increase the amount of its regular dividend.

When times are bad, however, dividends are often reduced, or eliminated entirely, as a quick way to conserve the company's cash. This occurred often as a result of the economic downturn of 2008. An article in the Feburary 28, 2009, edition of *The Wall Street Journal* listed ten large companies who had recently reduced or eliminated their common stock dividend. The companies named were: Blackstone Group, CBS, Citigroup, Dow Chemical, General Electric, JP Morgan Chase, Motorola, New York Times, Pfizer, and Textron. The article also noted that for the month of January 2009, dividends paid by companies in the S&P 500 Index were 24 percent lower than they had been in January 2008.

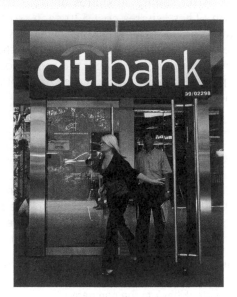

before the payment date (in this case December 15, 2013) is traded **ex-dividend,** meaning the buyer will not receive the upcoming dividend. The date of record is merely a cutoff date. It does not affect the financial statements.

Payment Date

Nelson actually paid the cash dividend on the **payment date.** This event has the same effect as paying any other liability. Assets (cash) and liabilities (dividends payable) both decrease. The income statement is not affected. The cash outflow is reported in the financing activities section of the statement of cash flows. The effects of the cash payment on the financial statements follow.

Assets	=	Liab.	+		Equity			Rev.	−	Exp.	=	Net Inc.	Cash Flow	
Cash	=	Div. Pay.	+	Com. Stk.	+	Ret. Earn.								
(70)	=	(70)	+	NA	+	NA		NA	−	NA	=	NA	(70)	FA

Stock Dividend

LO 7

Explain the effects of stock dividends and stock splits on a company's financial statements.

Dividends are not always paid in cash. Companies sometimes choose to issue **stock dividends,** wherein they distribute additional shares of stock to the stockholders. To illustrate, assume that Nelson Incorporated decided to issue a 10 percent stock dividend on its class B, $20 par value common stock. Because dividends apply to outstanding shares only, Nelson will issue 15 (150 outstanding shares × 0.10) additional shares of class B stock.

Assume the new shares are distributed when the market value of the stock is $30 per share. As a result of the stock dividend, Nelson will transfer $450 ($30 × 15 new shares) from retained earnings to paid-in capital.[2] The stock dividend is an equity exchange

---

[2]The accounting here applies to small stock dividends. Accounting for large stock dividends is explained in a more advanced course.

transaction. The income statement and statement of cash flows are not affected. The effects of the stock dividend on the financial statements follow.

Assets	=	Liab.	+	Equity						Rev.	−	Exp.	=	Net Inc.	Cash Flow
				Com. Stk.	+	PIC in Excess	+	Ret. Earn.							
NA	=	NA	+	300	+	150	+	(450)		NA	−	NA	=	NA	NA

Stock dividends have no effect on assets. They merely increase the number of shares of stock outstanding. Because a greater number of shares represents the same ownership interest in the same amount of assets, the market value per share of a company's stock normally declines when a stock dividend is distributed. A lower market price makes the stock more affordable and may increase demand for the stock, which benefits both the company and its stockholders.

Stock Split

A corporation may also reduce the market price of its stock through a **stock split.** A stock split replaces existing shares with a greater number of new shares. Any par or stated value of the stock is proportionately reduced to reflect the new number of shares outstanding. For example, assume Nelson Incorporated declared a 2-for-1 stock split on the 165 outstanding shares (150 originally issued + 15 shares distributed in a stock dividend) of its $20 par value, class B common stock. Nelson notes in the accounting records that the 165 old $20 par shares are replaced with 330 new $10 par shares. Investors who owned the 165 shares of old common stock would now own 330 shares of the new common stock.

Stock splits have no effect on the dollar amounts of assets, liabilities, and stockholders' equity. They only affect the number of shares of stock outstanding. In Nelson's case, the ownership interest that was previously represented by 165 shares of stock is now represented by 330 shares. Because twice as many shares now represent the same ownership interest, the market value per share should be one-half as much as it was prior to the split. However, as with a stock dividend, the lower market price will probably stimulate demand for the stock. As a result, doubling the number of shares will likely reduce the market price to slightly more than one-half of the pre-split value. For example, if the stock were selling for $30 per share before the 2-for-1 split, it might sell for $15.50 after the split.

Appropriation of Retained Earnings

The board of directors may restrict the amount of retained earnings available to distribute as dividends. The restriction may be required by credit agreements, or it may be discretionary. A retained earnings restriction, often called an *appropriation,* is an equity exchange event. It transfers a portion of existing retained earnings to **Appropriated Retained Earnings.** Total retained earnings remains unchanged. To illustrate, assume that Nelson appropriates $1,000 of retained earnings for future expansion. The income statement and the statement of cash flows are not affected. The effects on the financial statements of appropriating $1,000 of retained earnings follow.

Show how the appropriation of retained earnings affects financial statements.

Assets	=	Liab.	+	Equity						Rev.	−	Exp.	=	Net Inc.	Cash Flow
				Com. Stk.	+	Ret. Earn.	+	App. Ret. Earn.							
NA	=	NA	+	NA	+	(1,000)	+	1,000		NA	−	NA	=	NA	NA

FINANCIAL STATEMENT PRESENTATION

The 2012 and 2013 events for Nelson Incorporated are summarized below. Events 1 through 8 are cash transactions. The results of the 2012 transactions (nos. 1–5) are reflected in Exhibit 8.4. The results of the 2013 transactions (nos. 6–9) are shown in Exhibit 8.5.

1. Issued 100 shares of $10 par value common stock at a market price of $22 per share.
2. Issued 150 shares of class B, $20 par value common stock at a market price of $25 per share.
3. Issued 100 shares of $10 stated value, 7 percent cumulative preferred stock at a market price of $22 per share.
4. Issued 100 shares of no-par common stock at a market price of $22 per share.
5. Earned and retained $5,000 cash from operations.
6. Purchased 50 shares of $10 par value common stock as treasury stock at a market price of $20 per share.
7. Sold 30 shares of treasury stock at a market price of $25 per share.
8. Declared and paid a $70 cash dividend on the preferred stock.
9. Issued a 10 percent stock dividend on the 150 shares of outstanding class B, $20 par value common stock (15 additional shares). The additional shares were issued when the market price of the stock was $30 per share. There are 165 (150 + 15) class B common shares outstanding after the stock dividend.
10. Issued a 2-for-1 stock split on the 165 shares of class B, $20 par value common stock. After this transaction, there are 330 shares outstanding of the class B common stock with a $10 par value.
11. Appropriated $1,000 of retained earnings.

EXHIBIT 8.5

NELSON INCORPORATED
Balance Sheet
As of December 31, 2013

Assets		
Cash		$21,030
Stockholders' equity		
Preferred stock, $10 stated value, 7% cumulative,		
300 shares authorized, 100 issued and outstanding	$1,000	
Common stock, $10 par value, 250 shares authorized,		
100 issued, and 80 outstanding	1,000	
Common stock, class B, $10 par, 800 shares authorized,		
330 issued and outstanding	3,300	
Common stock, no par, 150 shares authorized,		
100 issued and outstanding	2,200	
Paid-in capital in excess of stated value—preferred	1,200	
Paid-in capital in excess of par value—common	1,200	
Paid-in capital in excess of par value—class B common	900	
Paid-in capital in excess of cost of treasury stock	150	
Total paid-in capital		$10,950
Retained earnings		
Appropriated	1,000	
Unappropriated	9,480	
Total retained earnings		10,480
Less: Treasury stock, 20 shares @ $20 per share		(400)
Total stockholders' equity		$21,030

The illustration assumes that Nelson earned net income of $6,000 in 2013. The ending retained earnings balance is determined as follows: Beginning Balance $5,000 − $70 Cash Dividend − $450 Stock Dividend + $6,000 Net Income = $10,480.

INVESTING IN CAPITAL STOCK

Stockholders may benefit in two ways when a company generates earnings. The company may distribute the earnings directly to the stockholders in the form of dividends. Alternatively, the company may retain some or all of the earnings to finance growth and increase its potential for future earnings. If the company retains earnings, the market value of its stock should increase to reflect its greater earnings prospects. How can analysts use financial reporting to help assess the potential for dividend payments or growth in market value?

Explain some uses of accounting information in making stock investment decisions.

Receiving Dividends

Is a company likely to pay dividends in the future? The financial statements can help answer this question. They show if dividends were paid in the past. Companies with a history of paying dividends usually continue to pay dividends. Also, to pay dividends in the future, a company must have sufficient cash and retained earnings. These amounts are reported on the balance sheet and the statement of cash flows.

Increasing the Price of Stock

Is the market value (price) of a company's stock likely to increase? Increases in a company's stock price occur when investors believe the company's earnings will grow. Financial statements provide information that is useful in predicting the prospects for earnings growth. Here also, a company's earnings history is an indicator of its growth potential. However, because published financial statements report historical information, investors must recognize their limitations. Investors want to know about the future. Stock prices are therefore influenced more by forecasts than by history.

For example:

■ On April 15, 2009, Abbott Laboratories, Inc., announced that profits for the first quarter of its 2009 fiscal year were 53 percent higher than profits in the same quarter of 2008. In reaction to this news, the price of Abbott's stock *fell* by almost 5 percent. Why did the stock market respond in this way? Because company's revenues for the quarter were less than had been expected by analysts who follow the company.

■ On May 18, 2009, Lowe's Companies, Inc., announced first quarter earnings were $0.32 per share, which was 22 percent lower than for the same period of the previous year. The stock market's reaction to the news was to *increase* the price of Lowe's stock by 8 percent. The market reacted this way because the analysts were expecting earnings per share for the first quarter to be only $0.25 per share.

In each case, investors reacted to the potential for earnings growth rather than the historical earnings reports. Because investors find forecasted statements more relevant to decision making than historical financial statements, most companies provide forecasts in addition to historical financial statements.

The value of a company's stock is also influenced by nonfinancial information that financial statements cannot provide. For example, suppose ExxonMobil announced in the middle of its fiscal year that it had just discovered substantial oil reserves on property to which it held drilling rights. Consider the following questions:

■ What would happen to the price of ExxonMobil's stock on the day of the announcement?

■ What would happen to ExxonMobil's financial statements on that day?

The price of ExxonMobil's stock would almost certainly increase as soon as the discovery was made public. However, nothing would happen to its financial statements on that day. There would probably be very little effect on its financial statements for that year. Only after the company begins to develop the oil field and sell the oil will its financial statements reflect the discovery. Changes in financial statements tend to lag behind the announcements companies make regarding their earnings potential.

Stock prices are also affected by general economic conditions and consumer confidence as well as the performance measures reported in financial statements. For example, the stock prices of virtually all companies declined sharply immediately after the September 11, 2001, terrorist attacks on the World Trade Center and the Pentagon. Historically based financial statements are of little benefit in predicting general economic conditions or changes in consumer confidence.

Exercising Control through Stock Ownership

The more influence an investor has over the operations of a company, the more the investor can benefit from owning stock in the company. For example, consider a power company that needs coal to produce electricity. The power company may purchase some common stock in a coal mining company to ensure a stable supply of coal. What percentage of the mining company's stock must the power company acquire to exercise significant influence over the mining company? The answer depends on how many investors own stock in the mining company and how the number of shares is distributed among the stockholders.

The greater its number of stockholders, the more *widely held* a company is. If stock ownership is concentrated in the hands of a few persons, a company is *closely held.* Widely held companies can generally be controlled with smaller percentages of ownership than closely held companies. Consider a company in which no existing investor owns more than 1 percent of the voting stock. A new investor who acquires a 5 percent interest would immediately become, by far, the largest shareholder and would likely be able to significantly influence board decisions. In contrast, consider a closely held company in which one current shareholder owns 51 percent of the company's stock. Even if another investor acquired the remaining 49 percent of the company, that investor could not control the company.

Financial statements contain some, but not all, of the information needed to help an investor determine ownership levels necessary to permit control. For example, the financial statements disclose the total number of shares of stock outstanding, but they normally contain little information about the number of shareholders and even less information about any relationships between shareholders. Relationships between shareholders are critically important because related shareholders, whether bound by family or business interests, might exercise control by voting as a block. For publicly traded companies, information about the number of shareholders and the identity of some large shareholders is disclosed in reports filed with the Securities and Exchange Commission.

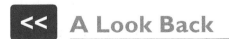 **A Look Back**

Starting a business requires obtaining financing; it takes money to make money. Although some money may be borrowed, lenders are unlikely to make loans to businesses that lack some degree of owner financing. Equity financing is therefore critical to virtually all profit-oriented businesses. This chapter has examined some of the issues related to accounting for equity transactions.

The idea that a business must obtain financing from its owners was one of the first events presented in this textbook. This chapter discussed the advantages and disadvantages of organizing a business as a sole proprietorship versus a partnership versus a corporation. These advantages and disadvantages include the following.

1. *Double taxation*—Income of corporations is subject to double taxation, but that of proprietorships and partnerships is not.

2. *Regulation*—Corporations are subject to more regulation than are proprietorships and partnerships.

3. *Limited liability*—An investor's personal assets are not at risk as a result of owning corporate securities. The investor's liability is limited to the amount of the investment. In general proprietorships and partnerships do not offer limited liability. However, laws in some states permit the formation of limited liability companies which operate like proprietorships and partnerships yet place some limits on the personal liability of their owners.

4. *Continuity*—Proprietorships and partnerships dissolve when one of the owners leaves the business. Corporations are separate legal entities that continue to exist regardless of changes in ownership.

5. *Transferability*—Ownership interests in corporations are easier to transfer than those of proprietorships or partnerships.

6. *Management structure*—Corporations are more likely to have independent professional managers than are proprietorships or partnerships.

7. *Ability to raise capital*—Because they can be owned by millions of investors, corporations have the opportunity to raise more capital than proprietorships or partnerships.

Corporations issue different classes of common stock and preferred stock as evidence of ownership interests. In general, *common stock* provides the widest range of privileges including the right to vote and participate in earnings. *Preferred stockholders* usually give up the right to vote in exchange for preferences such as the right to receive dividends or assets upon liquidation before common stockholders. Stock may have a *par value* or *stated value,* which relates to legal requirements governing the amount of capital that must be maintained in the corporation. Corporations may also issue *no-par stock,* avoiding some of the legal requirements that pertain to par or stated value stock.

Stock that a company issues and then repurchases is called *treasury stock.* Purchasing treasury stock reduces total assets and stockholders' equity. Reselling treasury stock represents a capital acquisition. The difference between the reissue price and the cost of the treasury stock is recorded directly in the equity accounts. Treasury stock transactions do not result in gains or losses on the income statement.

Companies may issue *stock splits* or *stock dividends.* These transactions increase the number of shares of stock without changing the net assets of a company. The per share market value usually drops when a company issues stock splits or dividends.

A Look Forward

Financial statement analysis is so important that Chapter 9 is devoted solely to a detailed discussion of this subject. The chapter covers vertical analysis (analyzing relationships within a specific statement) and horizontal analysis (analyzing relationships across accounting periods). Finally, the chapter discusses limitations associated with financial statement analysis.

A step-by-step audio-narrated series of slides is provided on the text website at www.mhhe.com/edmondssurvey3e.

SELF-STUDY REVIEW PROBLEM

Edwards Inc. experienced the following events:

1. Issued common stock for cash.
2. Declared a cash dividend.
3. Issued noncumulative preferred stock for cash.
4. Appropriated retained earnings.
5. Distributed a stock dividend.
6. Paid cash to purchase treasury stock.
7. Distributed a 2-for-1 stock split.
8. Issued cumulative preferred stock for cash.
9. Paid a cash dividend that had previously been declared.
10. Sold treasury stock for cash at a higher amount than the cost of the treasury stock.

Required

Show the effect of each event on the elements of the financial statements using a horizontal statements model like the one shown here. Use + for increase, − for decrease, and NA for not affected. In the Cash Flow column, indicate whether the item is an operating activity (OA), investing activity (IA), or a financing activity (FA). The first transaction is entered as an example.

Event	Assets	=	Liab.	+	Equity	Rev.	−	Exp.	=	Net Inc.	Cash Flow
1	+		NA		+	NA		NA		NA	+ FA

Solution to Self-Study Review Problem

Event	Assets	=	Liab.	+	Equity	Rev.	−	Exp.	=	Net Inc.	Cash Flow
1	+		NA		+	NA		NA		NA	+ FA
2	NA		+		−	NA		NA		NA	NA
3	+		NA		+	NA		NA		NA	+ FA
4	NA		NA		− +	NA		NA		NA	NA
5	NA		NA		− +	NA		NA		NA	NA
6	−		NA		−	NA		NA		NA	− FA
7	NA		NA		NA	NA		NA		NA	NA
8	+		NA		+	NA		NA		NA	+ FA
9	−		−		NA	NA		NA		NA	− FA
10	+		NA		+	NA		NA		NA	+ FA

KEY TERMS

Appropriated Retained
  Earnings 301
Articles of incorporation 288
Authorized stock 293
Board of directors 290
Book value per share 293

Closely held corporation 288
Common stock 294
Continuity 290
Corporation 288
Cost method of accounting for
  treasury stock 298

Cumulative dividends 295
Date of record 299
Declaration date 299
Dividends in arrears 295
Double taxation 289
Entrenched management 291

Ex-dividend 300
Issued stock 293
Legal capital 293
Limited liability 290
Limited liability companies
    (LLCs) 289
Market value 293
Outstanding stock 293
Paid-in Capital in Excess of
    Par Value 296

Par value 293
Partnerships 288
Partnership
    agreement 288
Payment date 300
Preferred stock 294
Securities Act of 1933 and
    Securities Exchange Act of
    1934 289
Sole proprietorships 288

Stated value 293
Stock certificates 288
Stock dividends 300
Stockholders 290
Stock split 301
Transferability 290
Treasury stock 293
Withdrawals 291

QUESTIONS

1. What are the three major forms of business organizations? Describe each.

2. How are sole proprietorships formed?

3. Discuss the purpose of a partnership agreement. Is such an agreement necessary for partnership formation?

4. What is meant by the phrase *separate legal entity?* To which type of business organization does it apply?

5. What is the purpose of the articles of incorporation? What information do they provide?

6. What is the function of the stock certificate?

7. What prompted Congress to pass the Securities Act of 1933 and the Securities Exchange Act of 1934? What is the purpose of these laws?

8. What are the advantages and disadvantages of the corporate form of business organization?

9. What is a limited liability company? Discuss its advantages and disadvantages.

10. How does the term *double taxation* apply to corporations? Give an example of double taxation.

11. What is the difference between contributed capital and retained earnings for a corporation?

12. What are the similarities and differences in the equity structure of a sole proprietorship, a partnership, and a corporation?

13. Why is it easier for a corporation to raise large amounts of capital than it is for a partnership?

14. What is the meaning of each of the following terms with respect to the corporate form of organization?

    (a) Legal capital

    (b) Par value of stock

    (c) Stated value of stock

    (d) Market value of stock

    (e) Book value of stock

    (f) Authorized shares of stock

    (g) Issued stock

    (h) Outstanding stock

    (i) Treasury stock

    (j) Common stock

    (k) Preferred stock

    (l) Dividends

15. What is the difference between cumulative preferred stock and noncumulative preferred stock?

16. What is no-par stock? How is it recorded in the accounting records?

17. Assume that Best Co. has issued and outstanding 1,000 shares of $100 par value, 10 percent, cumulative preferred stock. What is the dividend per share? If the preferred dividend is two years in arrears, what total amount of dividends must be paid before the common shareholders can receive any dividends?

18. If Best Co. issued 10,000 shares of $20 par value common stock for $30 per share, what amount is added to the Common Stock account? What amount of cash is received?

19. What is the difference between par value stock and stated value stock?

20. Why might a company repurchase its own stock?

21. What effect does the purchase of treasury stock have on the equity of a company?

22. Assume that Day Company repurchased 1,000 of its own shares for $30 per share and sold the shares two weeks later for $35 per share. What is the amount of gain on the sale? How is it reported on the balance sheet? What type of account is treasury stock?

23. What is the importance of the declaration date, record date, and payment date in conjunction with corporate dividends?

24. What is the difference between a stock dividend and a stock split?

25. Why would a company choose to distribute a stock dividend instead of a cash dividend?

26. What is the primary reason that a company would declare a stock split?

27. If Best Co. had 10,000 shares of $20 par value common stock outstanding and declared a 5-for-1 stock split, how many shares would then be outstanding and what would be their par value after the split?

28. When a company appropriates retained earnings, does the company set aside cash for a specific use? Explain.

29. What is the largest source of financing for most U.S. businesses?

30. What is meant by *equity financing?* What is meant by *debt financing?*

31. What is a widely held corporation? What is a closely held corporation?

32. What are some reasons that a corporation might not pay dividends?

 ## MULTIPLE-CHOICE QUESTIONS

Multiple-choice questions are provided on the text website at www.mhhe.com/edmondssurvey3e

EXERCISES

All applicable Exercises are available with McGraw-Hill's *Connect Accounting.*

LO 1, 2

Exercise 8-1   *Effect of accounting events on the financial statements of a sole proprietorship*

A sole proprietorship was started on January 1, 2012, when it received $60,000 cash from Mark Pruitt, the owner. During 2012, the company earned $40,000 in cash revenues and paid $19,300 in cash expenses. Pruitt withdrew $5,000 cash from the business during 2012.

Required

Prepare the income statement, capital statement (statement of changes in equity), balance sheet, and statement of cash flows for Pruitt's 2012 fiscal year.

LO 1, 2

Exercise 8-2   *Effect of accounting events on the financial statements of a partnership*

Justin Harris and Paul Berryhill started the HB partnership on January 1, 2012. The business acquired $56,000 cash from Harris and $84,000 from Berryhill. During 2012, the partnership earned $65,000 in cash revenues and paid $32,000 for cash expenses. Harris withdrew $2,000 cash from the business, and Berryhill withdrew $3,000 cash. The net income was allocated to the capital accounts of the two partners in proportion to the amounts of their original investments in the business.

Required

Prepare the income statement, capital statement, balance sheet, and statement of cash flows for the HB partnership for the 2012 fiscal year.

LO 1, 2

Exercise 8-3   *Effect of accounting events on the financial statements of a corporation*

Morris Corporation was started with the issue of 5,000 shares of $10 par common stock for cash on January 1, 2012. The stock was issued at a market price of $18 per share. During 2012, the company earned $63,000 in cash revenues and paid $41,000 for cash expenses. Also, a $4,000 cash dividend was paid to the stockholders.

Required

Prepare the income statement, statement of changes in stockholders' equity, balance sheet, and statement of cash flows for Morris Corporation's 2012 fiscal year.

Exercise 8-4 *Effect of issuing common stock on the balance sheet*

Newly formed Home Medical Corporation has 100,000 shares of $5 par common stock authorized. On March 1, 2012, Home Medical issued 10,000 shares of the stock for $12 per share. On May 2 the company issued an additional 20,000 shares for $20 per share. Home Medical was not affected by other events during 2012.

Required

a. Record the transactions in a horizontal statements model like the following one. In the Cash Flow column, indicate whether the item is an operating activity (OA), investing activity (IA), or financing activity (FA). Use NA to indicate that an element was not affected by the event.

Assets	=	Liab.	+	Equity			Rev.	−	Exp.	=	Net Inc.	Cash Flow
Cash	=		+	Com. Stk.	+	Paid-in Excess						

b. Determine the amount Home Medical would report for common stock on the December 31, 2012, balance sheet.

c. Determine the amount Home Medical would report for paid-in capital in excess of par.

d. What is the total amount of capital contributed by the owners?

e. What amount of total assets would Home Medical report on the December 31, 2012, balance sheet?

Exercise 8-5 *Recording and reporting common and preferred stock transactions*

Rainoy, Inc., was organized on June 5, 2012. It was authorized to issue 400,000 shares of $10 par common stock and 50,000 shares of 4 percent cumulative class A preferred stock. The class A stock had a stated value of $25 per share. The following stock transactions pertain to Rainoy, Inc.

1. Issued 20,000 shares of common stock for $15 per share.
2. Issued 10,000 shares of the class A preferred stock for $30 per share.
3. Issued 50,000 shares of common stock for $18 per share.

Required

Prepare the stockholders' equity section of the balance sheet immediately after these transactions have been recognized.

Exercise 8-6 *Effect of no-par common and par preferred stock on the horizontal statements model*

Eaton Corporation issued 5,000 shares of no-par common stock for $20 per share. Eaton also issued 2,000 shares of $50 par, 6 percent noncumulative preferred stock at $60 per share.

Required

Record these events in a horizontal statements model like the following one. In the cash flow column, indicate whether the item is an operating activity (OA), investing activity (IA), or financing activity (FA). Use NA to indicate that an element was not affected by the event.

Assets	=	Equity					Rev.	−	Exp.	=	Net Inc.	Cash Flow
Cash	=	Pfd. Stk.	+	Com. Stk.	+	PIC in Excess						

Exercise 8-7 *Issuing stock for assets other than cash*

Kaylee Corporation was formed when it issued shares of common stock to two of its shareholders. Kaylee issued 5,000 shares of $10 par common stock to K. Breslin in exchange for $60,000 cash (the issue price was $12 per share). Kaylee also issued 2,500 shares of stock to T. Lindsay in exchange for a one-year-old delivery van on the same day. Lindsay had originally paid $35,000 for the van.

Required

a. What was the market value of the delivery van on the date of the stock issue?

b. Show the effect of the two stock issues on Kaylee's books in a horizontal statements model like the following one. In the Cash Flow column, indicate whether the item is an operating activity (OA), investing activity (IA), or financing activity (FA). Use NA to indicate that an element was not affected by the event.

Assets	=	Equity	Rev. − Exp. = Net Inc.	Cash Flow
Cash + Van =		Com. Stk. + PIC in Excess		

LO 5

Exercise 8-8   *Treasury stock transactions*

Graves Corporation repurchased 2,000 shares of its own stock for $40 per share. The stock has a par of $10 per share. A month later Graves resold 1,200 shares of the treasury stock for $48 per share.

Required

What is the balance of the treasury stock account after these transactions are recognized?

LO 5

Exercise 8-9   *Recording and reporting treasury stock transactions*

The following information pertains to Smoot Corp. at January 1, 2012.

Common stock, $10 par, 10,000 shares authorized,	
2,000 shares issued and outstanding	$20,000
Paid-in capital in excess of par, common stock	15,000
Retained earnings	65,000

Smoot Corp. completed the following transactions during 2012:

1. Issued 1,000 shares of $10 par common stock for $28 per share.
2. Repurchased 200 shares of its own common stock for $25 per share.
3. Resold 50 shares of treasury stock for $26 per share.

Required

a. How many shares of common stock were outstanding at the end of the period?

b. How many shares of common stock had been issued at the end of the period?

c. Organize the transactions data in accounts under the accounting equation.

d. Prepare the stockholders' equity section of the balance sheet reflecting these transactions. Include the number of shares authorized, issued, and outstanding in the description of the common stock.

LO 6

Exercise 8-10   *Effect of cash dividends on financial statements*

On October 1, 2012, Smart Corporation declared a $60,000 cash dividend to be paid on December 30 to shareholders of record on November 20.

Required

Record the events occurring on October 1, November 20, and December 30 in a horizontal statements model like the following one. In the Cash Flow column, indicate whether the item is an operating activity (OA), investing activity (IA), or financing activity (FA).

Date	Assets = Liab. + Com. Stock + Ret. Earn.	Rev. − Exp. = Net Inc.	Cash Flow

Exercise 8-11 *Accounting for cumulative preferred dividends*   **LO 6**

When Polledo Corporation was organized in January 2012, it immediately issued 5,000 shares of $50 par, 5 percent, cumulative preferred stock and 10,000 shares of $10 par common stock. The company's earnings history is as follows: 2012, net loss of $15,000; 2013, net income of $60,000; 2014, net income of $95,000. The corporation did not pay a dividend in 2012.

Required

a. How much is the dividend arrearage as of January 1, 2013?

b. Assume that the board of directors declares a $40,000 cash dividend at the end of 2013 (remember that the 2012 and 2013 preferred dividends are due). How will the dividend be divided between the preferred and common stockholders?

Exercise 8-12 *Cash dividends for preferred and common shareholders*

B&S Corporation had the following stock issued and outstanding at January 1, 2012:

1. 100,000 shares of $5 par common stock.
2. 5,000 shares of $100 par, 5 percent, noncumulative preferred stock.

On May 10, B&S Corporation declared the annual cash dividend on its 5,000 shares of preferred stock and a $1 per share dividend for the common shareholders. The dividends will be paid on June 15 to the shareholders of record on May 30.

Required

Determine the total amount of dividends to be paid to the preferred shareholders and common shareholders.

Exercise 8-13 *Cash dividends: common and preferred stock*   **LO 6**

Varsity Corp. had the following stock issued and outstanding at January 1, 2012.

1. 200,000 shares of no-par common stock.
2. 10,000 shares of $100 par, 8 percent, cumulative preferred stock. (Dividends are in arrears for one year, 2011.)

On February 1, 2012, Varsity declared a $200,000 cash dividend to be paid March 31 to shareholders of record on March 10.

Required

What amount of dividends will be paid to the preferred shareholders versus the common shareholders?

Exercise 8-14 *Accounting for stock dividends*   **LO 7**

Rollins Corporation issued a 5 percent stock dividend on 10,000 shares of its $10 par common stock. At the time of the dividend, the market value of the stock was $14 per share.

Required

a. Compute the amount of the stock dividend.

b. Show the effects of the stock dividend on the financial statements using a horizontal statements model like the following one.

Assets	=	Liab.	+	Com. Stk.	+	PIC in Excess	+	Ret. Earn.	Rev.	−	Exp.	=	Net Inc.	Cash Flow

Exercise 8-15 *Determining the effects of stock splits on the accounting records*   **LO 7**

The market value of Coe Corporation's common stock had become excessively high. The stock was currently selling for $180 per share. To reduce the market price of the common stock, Coe declared a 2-for-1 stock split for the 300,000 outstanding shares of its $10 par common stock.

Required

a. How will Coe Corporation's books be affected by the stock split?

b. Determine the number of common shares outstanding and the par value after the split.

c. Explain how the market value of the stock will be affected by the stock split.

LO 9

Exercise 8-16   *Corporate announcements*

Super Drugs (one of the three largest drug makers) just reported that its 2012 third-quarter profits had increased substantially over its 2011 third-quarter profits. In addition to this announcement, the same day, Super Drugs also announced that the Food and Drug Administration had just denied approval of a new drug used to treat high blood pressure that Super Drugs developed. The FDA was concerned about potential side effects of the drug.

Required

Using the above information, answer the following questions.

a. What do you think will happen to the stock price of Super Drugs on the day these two announcements are made? Explain your answer.

b. How will the balance sheet be affected on that day by the above announcements?

c. How will the income statement be affected on that day by the above announcements?

d. How will the statement of cash flows be affected on that day by the above announcements?

PROBLEMS

All applicable Problems are available with McGraw-Hill's
Connect Accounting.

LO 1, 2

e**X**cel

CHECK FIGURES
a. Net Income: $5,500
b. Macy Calloway Capital: $25,400

Problem 8-17   *Effect of business structure on financial statements*

Calloway Company was started on January 1, 2012, when the owners invested $40,000 cash in the business. During 2012, the company earned cash revenues of $18,000 and incurred cash expenses of $12,500. The company also paid cash distributions of $3,000.

Required

Prepare the 2012 income statement, capital statement (statement of changes in equity), balance sheet, and statement of cash flows using each of the following assumptions. (Consider each assumption separately.)

a. Calloway is a sole proprietorship owned by Macy Calloway.

b. Calloway is a partnership with two partners, Macy Calloway and Artie Calloway. Macy Calloway invested $25,000 and Artie Calloway invested $15,000 of the $40,000 cash that was used to start the business. A. Calloway was expected to assume the vast majority of the responsibility for operating the business. The partnership agreement called for A. Calloway to receive 60 percent of the profits and M. Calloway to get the remaining 40 percent. With regard to the $3,000 distribution, A. Calloway withdrew $1,200 from the business and M. Calloway withdrew $1,800.

c. Calloway is a corporation. It issued 5,000 shares of $5 par common stock for $40,000 cash to start the business.

LO 4–6

e**X**cel

CHECK FIGURES
b. Preferred Stock, 2012: $50,000
c. Common Shares Outstanding, 2013: 19,500

Problem 8-18   *Recording and reporting stock transactions and cash dividends across two accounting cycles*

Davis Corporation was authorized to issue 100,000 shares of $10 par common stock and 50,000 shares of $50 par, 6 percent, cumulative preferred stock. Davis Corporation completed the following transactions during its first two years of operation.

2012

Jan.   2   Issued 5,000 shares of $10 par common stock for $28 per share.

       15   Issued 1,000 shares of $50 par preferred stock for $70 per share.

Feb. 14   Issued 15,000 shares of $10 par common stock for $30 per share.

Dec. 31   During the year, earned $170,000 of cash service revenue and paid $110,000 of cash operating expenses.

     31   Declared the cash dividend on outstanding shares of preferred stock for 2012. The dividend will be paid on January 31 to stockholders of record on January 15, 2013.

2013

Jan. 31   Paid the cash dividend declared on December 31, 2012.

Mar. 1   Issued 2,000 shares of $50 par preferred stock for $58 per share.

June 1   Purchased 500 shares of common stock as treasury stock at $43 per share.

Dec. 31   During the year, earned $210,000 of cash service revenue and paid $175,000 of cash operating expenses.

     31   Declared the dividend on the preferred stock and a $0.60 per share dividend on the common stock.

Required

a. Organize the transaction data in accounts under an accounting equation.

b. Prepare the stockholders' equity section of the balance sheet at December 31, 2012.

c. Prepare the balance sheet at December 31, 2013.

Problem 8-19 *Recording and reporting treasury stock transactions*

Midwest Corp. completed the following transactions in 2012, the first year of operation.

1. Issued 20,000 shares of $10 par common stock at par.
2. Issued 2,000 shares of $30 stated value preferred stock at $32 per share.
3. Purchased 500 shares of common stock as treasury stock for $15 per share.
4. Declared a 5 percent dividend on preferred stock.
5. Sold 300 shares of treasury stock for $18 per share.
6. Paid the cash dividend on preferred stock that was declared in Event 4.
7. Earned cash service revenue of $75,000 and incurred cash operating expenses of $42,000.
8. Appropriated $6,000 of retained earnings.

Required

a. Organize the transaction in accounts under an accounting equation.

b. Prepare the stockholders' equity section of the balance sheet as of December 31, 2012.

Problem 8-20 *Recording and reporting treasury stock transactions*

Boley Corporation reports the following information in its January 1, 2012, balance sheet:

Stockholders' equity	
Common stock, $10 par value,	
50,000 shares authorized, 30,000 shares issued and outstanding	$300,000
Paid-in capital in excess of par value	150,000
Retained earnings	100,000
Total stockholders' equity	$550,000

During 2012, Boley was affected by the following accounting events.

1. Purchased 1,000 shares of treasury stock at $18 per share.
2. Reissued 600 shares of treasury stock at $20 per share.
3. Earned $64,000 of cash service revenues.
4. Paid $38,000 of cash operating expenses.

Required

Prepare the stockholders' equity section of the year-end balance sheet.

LO 5, 6, 8

 e**X**cel

CHECK FIGURE
b. Total Paid-In Capital: $264,900

LO 5

CHECK FIGURES
Total Paid-In Capital: $451,200
Total Stockholders' Equity:
$570,000

Problem 8-21   *Recording and reporting stock dividends*

Chan Corp. completed the following transactions in 2012, the first year of operation.

1. Issued 20,000 shares of $20 par common stock for $30 per share.
2. Issued 5,000 shares of $50 par, 5 percent, preferred stock at $51 per share.
3. Paid the annual cash dividend to preferred shareholders.
4. Issued a 5 percent stock dividend on the common stock. The market value at the dividend declaration date was $40 per share.
5. Later that year, issued a 2-for-1 split on the 21,000 shares of outstanding common stock.
6. Earned $210,000 of cash service revenues and paid $140,000 of cash operating expenses.

Required

a. Record each of these events in a horizontal statements model like the following one. In the Cash Flow column, indicate whether the item is an operating activity (OA), investing activity (IA), or financing activity (FA). Use NA to indicate that an element is not affected by the event.

Assets = Liab. +	Equity	Rev. − Exp. = Net Inc.	Cash Flow
	Pfd. Stk. + Com. Stk. + PIC in Excess PS + PIC in Excess CS + Ret. Earn.		

b. Prepare the stockholders' equity section of the balance sheet at the end of 2012.

Problem 8-22   *Analyzing the stockholders' equity section of the balance sheet*

The stockholders' equity section of the balance sheet for Brawner Company at December 31, 2012, is as follows:

Stockholders' Equity		
Paid-in capital		
Preferred stock, ? par value, 6% cumulative, 50,000 shares authorized, 30,000 shares issued and outstanding	$300,000	
Common stock, $10 stated value, 150,000 shares authorized, 50,000 shares issued and ? outstanding	500,000	
Paid-in capital in excess of par—Preferred	30,000	
Paid-in capital in excess of stated value—Common	200,000	
Total paid-in capital		$1,030,000
Retained earnings		250,000
Treasury stock, 1,000 shares		(100,000)
Total stockholders' equity		$1,180,000

Note: The market value per share of the common stock is $25, and the market value per share of the preferred stock is $12.

Required

a. What is the par value per share of the preferred stock?
b. What is the dividend per share on the preferred stock?
c. What is the number of common stock shares outstanding?
d. What was the average issue price per share (price for which the stock was issued) of the common stock?
e. Explain the difference between the average issue price and the market price of the common stock.
f. If Brawner declared a 2-for-1 stock split on the common stock, how many shares would be outstanding after the split? What amount would be transferred from the retained earnings account because of the stock split? Theoretically, what would be the market price of the common stock immediately after the stock split?

Problem 8-23   *Different forms of business organization*   **LO 1**

Shawn Bates was working to establish a business enterprise with four of his wealthy friends. Each of the five individuals would receive a 20 percent ownership interest in the company. A primary goal of establishing the enterprise was to minimize the amount of income taxes paid. Assume that the five investors are taxed at the rate of 15% on dividend income and 30% on all other income and that the corporate tax rate is 30 percent. Also assume that the new company is expected to earn $400,000 of cash income before taxes during its first year of operation. All earnings are expected to be immediately distributed to the owners.

Required

Calculate the amount of after-tax cash flow available to each investor if the business is established as a partnership versus a corporation. Write a memo explaining the advantages and disadvantages of these two forms of business organization. Explain why a limited liability company may be a better choice than either a partnership or a corporation.

Problem 8-24   *Effects of equity transactions on financial statements*   **LO 4–8**

The following events were experienced by Abbot Inc.:

1. Issued cumulative preferred stock for cash.
2. Issued common stock for cash.
3. Distributed a 2-for-1 stock split on the common stock.
4. Issued noncumulative preferred stock for cash.
5. Appropriated retained earnings.
6. Sold treasury stock for an amount of cash that was more than the cost of the treasury stock.
7. Distributed a stock dividend.
8. Paid cash to purchase treasury stock.
9. Declared a cash dividend.
10. Paid the cash dividend declared in Event 9.

Required

Show the effect of each event on the elements of the financial statements using a horizontal statements model like the following one. Use + for increase, − for decrease, and NA for not affected. In the Cash Flow column, indicate whether the item is an operating activity (OA), investing activity (IA), or financing activity (FA). The first transaction is entered as an example.

Event No.	Assets	=	Liab.	+	Equity	Rev.	−	Exp.	=	Net Inc.	Cash Flow
1	+		NA		+	NA		NA		NA	+ FA

ANALYZE, THINK, COMMUNICATE

ATC 8-1   Business Applications Case   *Understanding real-world annual reports*

Use the Target Corporation's annual report in Appendix B to answer the following questions.

Target Corporation

Required

a. What is the par value per share of Target's stock?

b. How many shares of Target's common stock were *outstanding* as of January 31, 2010?

c. Target's annual report provides some details about the company's executive officers. How many are identified? What is their minimum, maximum, and average age? How many are females?

d. Target's balance sheet does not show a balance for treasury stock. Does this mean the company has not repurchased any of its own stock? Explain.

ATC 8-2   Group Assignment   *Missing information*

Listed here are the stockholders' equity sections of three public companies for years ending in 2008 and 2007:

	2008	2007
Wendy's (in thousands) (merger with Triare in 2008)		
Stockholders' equity		
Common stock, ?? stated value per share, authorized:		
1,500,000; 470,424 in 2008 and 93,576 in		
2007 shares issued, respectively	$ 47,042	$ 9,357
Capital in excess of stated value	2,752,987	291,122
Retained earnings	(357,541)	167,267
Acc. other comp. income (loss)	(43,253)	(2,098)
Treasury stock, at cost: 1,220 in 2008 and 841 in 2007	(15,944)	(16,774)
Coca-Cola (in millions)		
Stockholders' equity		
Common stock, ?? par value per share, authorized:		
5,600; issued: 3,519 shares in 2008 and 3,519 shares in 2007	880	880
Capital surplus	7,966	7,378
Reinvested earnings	38,513	36,235
Acc. other comp. inc. (loss)	(2,674)	(626)
Treasury stock, at cost: (1,207 shares in 2008; 1,201 shares in 2007)	(24,213)	(23,375)
Harley-Davidson (dollar amounts are presented in thousands)		
Stockholders' equity		
Common stock, ?? par value per share, authorized: 800,000,000, issued:		
335,653,577 in 2008 and 335,211,201 shares in 2007	3,357	3,352
Additional paid-in capital	846,796	812,224
Retained earnings	6,458,778	6,117,567
Acc. other comp. inc. (loss)	(522,526)	(137,258)
Treasury stock, at cost: 102,889,370 for 2008 and 96,725,399 for 2007	(4,670,802)	(4,420,394)

Required

a. Divide the class in three sections and divide each section into groups of three to five students. Assign each section one of the companies.

Group Tasks

Based on the company assigned to your group, answer the following questions.

b. What is the per share par or stated value of the common stock in 2008?
c. What was the average issue price of the common stock for each year?
d. How many shares of stock are outstanding at the end of each year?
e. What is the average cost per share of the treasury stock for 2008?
f. Do the data suggest that your company was profitable in 2008?
g. Can you determine the amount of net income from the information given? What is missing?
h. What is the total stockholders' equity of your company for each year?

Class Discussion

i. Have each group select a representative to present the information about its company. Compare the share issue price and the par or stated value of the companies.
j. Compare the average issue price to the current market price for each of the companies. Speculate about what might cause the difference.

ATC 8-3   Research Assignment   *Analyzing PepsiCo's equity structure*

Using either Big Lots, Inc. most current Form 10-K or the company's annual report, answer the questions below. To obtain the Form 10-K use either the EDGAR system following the instructions in Appendix A or the company's website. The company's annual report is available on its website.

Required

a. What is the *book value* of Big Lots' stockholders' equity that is shown on the company's balance sheet?

b. What is the par value of Big Lots' common stock?

c. Does Big Lots have any treasury stock? If so, how many shares of treasury stock does the company hold?

d. Why does the stock of a company such as a Big Lots have a market value that is higher than its book value?

ATC 8-4 Writing Assignment *Comparison of organizational forms*

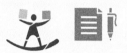

Jim Baku and Scott Hanson are thinking about opening a new restaurant. Baku has extensive marketing experience but does not know that much about food preparation. However, Hanson is an excellent chef. Both will work in the business, but Baku will provide most of the funds necessary to start the business. At this time, they cannot decide whether to operate the business as a partnership or a corporation.

Required

Prepare a written memo to Baku and Hanson describing the advantages and disadvantages of each organizational form. Also, from the limited information provided, recommend the organizational form you think they should use.

ATC 8-5 Ethical Dilemma *Bad news versus very bad news*

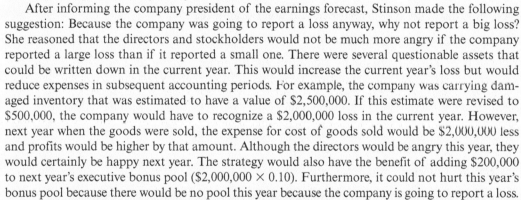

Louise Stinson, the chief financial officer of Bostonian Corporation, was on her way to the president's office. She was carrying the latest round of bad news. There would be no executive bonuses this year. Corporate profits were down. Indeed, if the latest projections held true, the company would report a small loss on the year-end income statement. Executive bonuses were tied to corporate profits. The executive compensation plan provided for 10 percent of net earnings to be set aside for bonuses. No profits meant no bonuses. While things looked bleak, Stinson had a plan that might help soften the blow.

After informing the company president of the earnings forecast, Stinson made the following suggestion: Because the company was going to report a loss anyway, why not report a big loss? She reasoned that the directors and stockholders would not be much more angry if the company reported a large loss than if it reported a small one. There were several questionable assets that could be written down in the current year. This would increase the current year's loss but would reduce expenses in subsequent accounting periods. For example, the company was carrying damaged inventory that was estimated to have a value of $2,500,000. If this estimate were revised to $500,000, the company would have to recognize a $2,000,000 loss in the current year. However, next year when the goods were sold, the expense for cost of goods sold would be $2,000,000 less and profits would be higher by that amount. Although the directors would be angry this year, they would certainly be happy next year. The strategy would also have the benefit of adding $200,000 to next year's executive bonus pool ($2,000,000 × 0.10). Furthermore, it could not hurt this year's bonus pool because there would be no pool this year because the company is going to report a loss.

Some of the other items that Stinson is considering include (1) converting from straight-line to accelerated depreciation, (2) increasing the percentage of receivables estimated to be uncollectible in the current year and lowering the percentage in the following year, and (3) raising the percentage of estimated warranty claims in the current period and lowering it in the following period. Finally, Stinson notes that two of the company's department stores have been experiencing losses. The company could sell these stores this year and thereby improve earnings next year. Stinson admits that the sale would result in significant losses this year, but she smiles as she thinks of next year's bonus check.

Required

a. Explain how each of the three numbered strategies for increasing the amount of the current year's loss would affect the stockholders' equity section of the balance sheet in the current year. How would the other elements of the balance sheet be affected?

b. If Stinson's strategy were effectively implemented, how would it affect the stockholders' equity in subsequent accounting periods?

c. Comment on the ethical implications of running the company for the sake of management (maximization of bonuses) versus the maximization of return to stockholders.

d. Formulate a bonus plan that will motivate managers to maximize the value of the firm instead of motivating them to manipulate the reporting process.

e. How would Stinson's strategy of overstating the amount of the reported loss in the current year affect the company's current P/E ratio?

CHAPTER 10

An Introduction to Managerial Accounting

LEARNING OBJECTIVES

After you have mastered the material in this chapter, you will be able to:

1 Distinguish between managerial and financial accounting.

2 Identify the cost components of a product made by a manufacturing company: the cost of materials, labor, and overhead.

3 Explain the effects on financial statements of product costs versus general, selling, and administrative costs.

4 Prepare a schedule of cost of goods manufactured and sold.

5 Distinguish product costs from upstream and downstream costs.

6 Explain how product costing differs in service, merchandising, and manufacturing companies.

7 Show how just-in-time inventory can increase profitability.

8 Identify and explain the standards contained in IMA's Statement of Ethical Professional Practice.

9 Identify emerging trends in accounting (Appendix A).

CHAPTER OPENING

Andy Grove, Senior Advisor to Executive Management of Intel Corporation, is credited with the motto "Only the paranoid survive." Mr. Grove describes a wide variety of concerns that make him paranoid. Specifically, he declares:

I worry about products getting screwed up, and I worry about products getting introduced prematurely. I worry about factories not performing well, and I worry about having too many factories. I worry about hiring the right people, and I worry about morale slacking off. And, of course, I worry about competitors. I worry about other people figuring out how to do what we do better or cheaper, and displacing us with our customers.

Do Intel's historically based financial statements contain the information Mr. Grove needs? No. **Financial accounting** is not designed to satisfy all the information needs of business managers. Its scope is limited to the needs of external users such as investors and creditors. The field of accounting designed to meet the needs of internal users is called **managerial accounting.**

The Curious Accountant

In the first course of accounting, you learned how retailers, such as Sears, account for the cost of equipment that lasts more than one year. Recall that the equipment was recorded as an asset when purchased, and then it was depreciated over its expected useful life. The depreciation charge reduced the company's assets and increased its expenses. This approach was justified under the matching principle, which seeks to recognize costs as expenses in the same period that the cost (resource) is used to generate revenue.

Is depreciation always shown as an expense on the income statement? The answer may surprise you. Consider the following scenario. Schwinn manufactures the bicycles that it sells to Sears. In order to produce the bicycles, Schwinn had to purchase a robotic machine that it expects can be used to produce 50,000 bicycles.

Do you think Schwinn should account for depreciation on its manufacturing equipment the same way Sears accounts for depreciation on its registers at the checkout counters? If not, how should Schwinn account for its depreciation? Remember the matching principle when thinking of your answer. (Answer on page 368.)

DIFFERENCES BETWEEN MANAGERIAL AND FINANCIAL ACCOUNTING

Distinguish between managerial and financial accounting.

While the information needs of internal and external users overlap, the needs of managers generally differ from those of investors or creditors. Some distinguishing characteristics are discussed in the following section.

Users and Types of Information

Financial accounting provides information used primarily by investors, creditors, and others *outside* a business. In contrast, managerial accounting focuses on information used by executives, managers, and employees who work *inside* the business. These two user groups need different types of information.

Internal users need information to *plan, direct,* and *control* business operations. The nature of information needed is related to an employee's job level. Lower level employees use nonfinancial information such as work schedules, store hours, and customer service policies. Moving up the organizational ladder, financial information becomes increasingly important. Middle managers use a blend of financial and nonfinancial information, while senior executives concentrate on financial data. To a lesser degree, senior executives also use general economic data and nonfinancial operating information. For example, an executive may consider the growth rate of the economy before deciding to expand the company's workforce.

External users (investors and creditors) have greater needs for general economic information than do internal users. For example, an investor debating whether to purchase stock versus bond securities might be more interested in government tax policy than financial statement data. Exhibit 10.1 summarizes the information needs of different user groups.

Level of Aggregation

External users generally desire *global information* that reflects the performance of a company as a whole. For example, an investor is not so much interested in the performance of a particular Sears store as she is in the performance of Sears Roebuck Company versus that of JC Penney Company. In contrast, internal users focus on detailed information about specific subunits of the company. To meet the needs of the different user groups, financial accounting data are more aggregated than managerial accounting data.

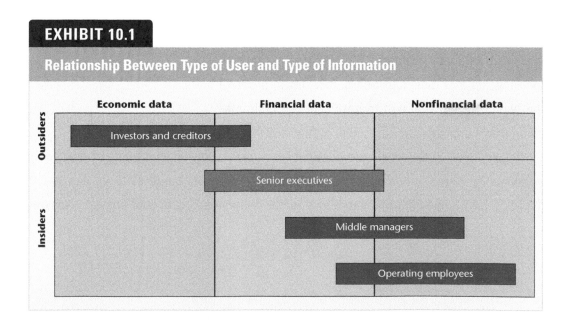

EXHIBIT 10.1

Relationship Between Type of User and Type of Information

Regulation

As previously discussed, the information in financial statements is highly regulated to protect the public interest.

Beyond financial statement data, much of the information generated by management accounting systems is proprietary information not available to the public. Because this information is not distributed to the public, it need not be regulated to protect the public interest. Management accounting is restricted only by the **value-added principle.** Management accountants are free to engage in any information gathering and reporting activity so long as the activity adds value in excess of its cost. For example, management accountants are free to provide forecasted information to internal users. In contrast, financial accounting as prescribed by GAAP does not permit forecasting.

Information Characteristics

While financial accounting is characterized by its objectivity, reliability, consistency, and historical nature, managerial accounting is more concerned with relevance and timeliness. Managerial accounting uses more estimates and fewer facts than financial accounting. Financial accounting reports what happened yesterday; managerial accounting reports what is expected to happen tomorrow.

Time Horizon and Reporting Frequency

Financial accounting information is reported periodically, normally at the end of a year. Management cannot wait until the end of the year to discover problems. Planning, controlling, and directing require immediate attention. Managerial accounting information is delivered on a continuous basis.

FOCUS ON INTERNATIONAL ISSUES

FINANCIAL ACCOUNTING VERSUS MANAGERIAL ACCOUNTING—AN INTERNATIONAL PERSPECTIVE

This chapter has already explained some of the conceptual differences between financial and managerial accounting, but these differences have implications for international businesses as well. With respect to financial accounting, publicly traded companies in most countries must follow the generally accepted accounting principles (GAAP) for their country, but these rules can vary from country to country. Generally, companies that are audited under the auditing standards of the United States follow the standards established by the Financial Accounting Standards Board. Most companies located outside of the United States follow the standards established by the International Accounting Standards Board. For example, the United States is one of very few countries whose GAAP allow the use of the LIFO inventory cost flow assumption.

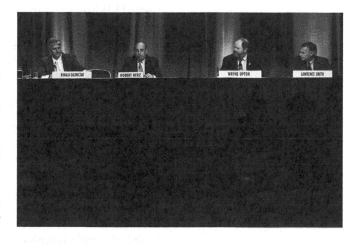

Conversely, most of the managerial accounting concepts introduced in this course can be used by businesses in any country. For example, *activity-based management (ABM)* is a topic addressed in the appendix to this chapter and is used by many companies in the United States. Meanwhile, a study published in *Accountancy Ireland** found that approximately one-third of the companies surveyed in Ireland, the United Kingdom, and New Zealand were also either using ABM, or were considering adopting it.

*Bernard Pierce, "Activity-Based Costing; the Irish Experience: True Innovation or Passing Fad?" *Accountancy Ireland,* October 2004, pp. 28–31.

EXHIBIT 10.2

Comparative Features of Managerial versus Financial Accounting Information

Features	Managerial Accounting	Financial Accounting
Users	Insiders including executives, managers, and operators	Outsiders including investors, creditors, government agencies, analysts, and reporters
Information type	Economic and physical data as well as financial data	Financial data
Level of aggregation	Local information on subunits of the organization	Global information on the company as a whole
Regulation	No regulation, limited only by the value-added principle	Regulation by SEC, FASB, and other determiners of GAAP
Information characteristics	Estimates that promote relevance and enable timeliness	Factual information that is characterized by objectivity, reliability, consistency, and accuracy
Time horizon	Past, present, and future	Past only, historically based
Reporting frequency	Continuous reporting	Delayed with emphasis on annual reports

Exhibit 10.2 summarizes significant differences between financial and managerial accounting.

PRODUCT COSTING IN MANUFACTURING COMPANIES

Identify the cost components of a product made by a manufacturing company: the cost of materials, labor, and overhead.

A major focus for managerial accountants is determining **product cost.**[1] Managers need to know the cost of their products for a variety of reasons. For example, **cost-plus pricing** is a common business practice.[2] **Product costing** is also used to control business operations. It is useful in answering questions such as: Are costs higher or lower than expected? Who is responsible for the variances between expected and actual costs? What actions can be taken to control the variances?

The cost of making products includes the cost of materials, labor, and other resources (usually called **overhead**). To understand how these costs affect financial statements, consider the example of Tabor Manufacturing Company.

Tabor Manufacturing Company

Tabor Manufacturing Company makes wooden tables. The company spent $1,000 cash to build four tables: $390 for materials, $470 for a carpenter's labor, and $140 for tools used in making the tables. How much is Tabor's expense? The answer is zero. The $1,000 cash has been converted into products (four tables). The cash payments for materials, labor, and tools (overhead) were *asset exchange* transactions. One asset (cash) decreased while another asset (tables) increased. Tabor will not recognize any expense until the tables are sold; in the meantime, the cost of the tables is held in an asset account called **Finished Goods Inventory.** Exhibit 10.3 illustrates how cash is transformed into inventory.

Average Cost per Unit

How much did each table made by Tabor cost? The *actual* cost of each of the four tables likely differs. The carpenter probably spent a little more time on some of the tables than

---

[1]This text uses the term *product* in a generic sense to mean both goods and services.
[2]Other pricing strategies will be introduced in subsequent chapters.

EXHIBIT 10.3

Transforming the Asset Cash Into the Asset Finished Goods Inventory

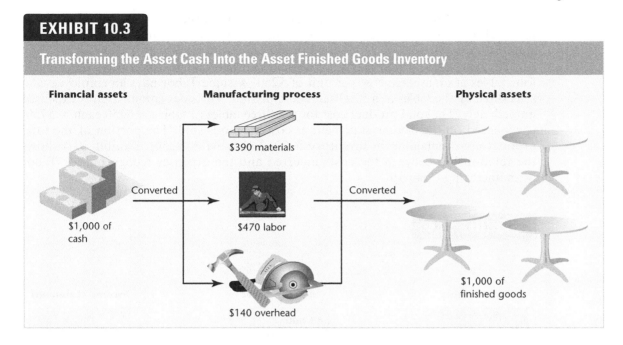

others. Material and tool usage probably varied from table to table. Determining the exact cost of each table is virtually impossible. Minute details such as a second of labor time cannot be effectively measured. Even if Tabor could determine the exact cost of each table, the information would be of little use. Minor differences in the cost per table would make no difference in pricing or other decisions management needs to make. Accountants therefore normally calculate cost per unit as an *average*. In the case of Tabor Manufacturing, the **average cost** per table is $250 ($1,000 ÷ 4 units). Unless otherwise stated, assume *cost per unit* means *average cost per unit*.

✓ CHECK YOURSELF 10.1

All boxes of General Mills' Total Raisin Bran cereal are priced at exactly the same amount in your local grocery store. Does this mean that the actual cost of making each box of cereal was exactly the same?

Answer No, making each box would not cost exactly the same amount. For example, some boxes contain slightly more or less cereal than other boxes. Accordingly, some boxes cost slightly more or less to make than others do. General Mills uses average cost rather than actual cost to develop its pricing strategy.

Costs Can Be Assets or Expenses

It might seem odd that wages earned by production workers are recorded as inventory instead of being expensed. Remember, however, that expenses are assets used in the process of *earning revenue*. The cash paid to production workers is not used to produce revenue. Instead, the cash is used to produce inventory. Revenue will be earned when the inventory is used (sold). So long as the inventory remains on hand, all product costs (materials, labor, and overhead) remain in an inventory account.

When a table is sold, the average cost of the table is transferred from the Inventory account to the Cost of Goods Sold (expense) account. If some tables remain unsold at the end of the accounting period, part of the *product costs* is reported as an asset (inventory) on the balance sheet while the other part is reported as an expense (cost of goods sold) on the income statement.

Costs that are not classified as product costs are normally expensed in the period in which they are incurred. These costs include *general operating costs, selling and administrative costs, interest costs,* and the *cost of income taxes.*

To illustrate, return to the Tabor Manufacturing example. Recall that Tabor made four tables at an average cost per unit of $250. Assume Tabor pays an employee who sells three of the tables at a $200 sales commission. The sales commission is expensed immediately. The total product cost for the three tables (3 tables × $250 each = $750) is expensed on the income statement as cost of goods sold. The portion of the total product cost remaining in inventory is $250 (1 table × $250). Exhibit 10.4 shows the relationship between the costs incurred and the expenses recognized for Tabor Manufacturing Company.

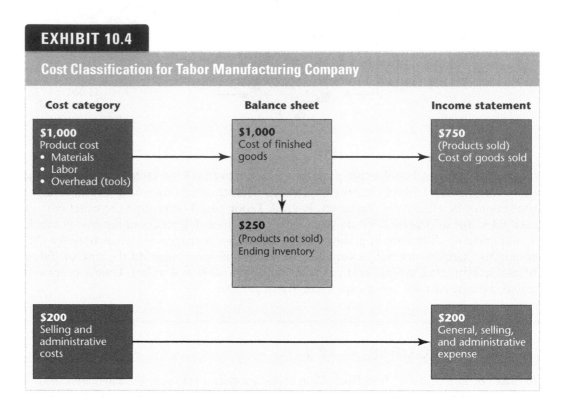

EXHIBIT 10.4

Cost Classification for Tabor Manufacturing Company

Cost category	Balance sheet	Income statement
$1,000 Product cost • Materials • Labor • Overhead (tools)	**$1,000** Cost of finished goods	**$750** (Products sold) Cost of goods sold
	$250 (Products not sold) Ending inventory	
$200 Selling and administrative costs		**$200** General, selling, and administrative expense

EFFECT OF PRODUCT COSTS ON FINANCIAL STATEMENTS

Explain the effects on financial statements of product costs versus general, selling, and administrative costs.

We illustrate accounting for product costs in manufacturing companies with Patillo Manufacturing Company, a producer of ceramic pottery. Patillo, started on January 1, 2012, experienced the following accounting events during its first year of operations.[3] *Assume that all transactions except 6, 8, and 10 are cash transactions.*

1. Acquired $15,000 cash by issuing common stock.
2. Paid $2,000 for materials that were used to make products. All products started were completed during the period.
3. Paid $1,200 for salaries of selling and administrative employees.
4. Paid $3,000 for wages of production workers.
5. Paid $2,800 for furniture used in selling and administrative offices.

---

[3]This illustration assumes that all inventory started during the period was completed during the period. Patillo therefore uses only one inventory account, Finished Goods Inventory. Many manufacturing companies normally have three categories of inventory on hand at the end of an accounting period: Raw Materials Inventory, Work in Process Inventory (inventory of partially completed units), and Finished Goods Inventory.

6. Recognized depreciation on the office furniture purchased in Event 5. The furniture was acquired on January 1, had a $400 estimated salvage value, and a four-year useful life. The annual depreciation charge is $600 [($2,800 − $400) ÷ 4].

7. Paid $4,500 for manufacturing equipment.

8. Recognized depreciation on the equipment purchased in Event 7. The equipment was acquired on January 1, had a $1,500 estimated salvage value, and a three-year useful life. The annual depreciation charge is $1,000 [($4,500 − $1,500) ÷ 3].

9. Sold inventory to customers for $7,500 cash.

10. The inventory sold in Event 9 cost $4,000 to make.

The effects of these transactions on the balance sheet, income statement, and statement of cash flows are shown in Exhibit 10.5. Study each row in this exhibit, paying particular attention to how similar costs such as salaries for selling and administrative personnel and wages for production workers have radically different effects on the financial statements. The example illustrates the three elements of product costs, materials (Event 2), labor (Event 4), and overhead (Event 8). These events are discussed in more detail below.

EXHIBIT 10.5

Effect of Product versus Selling and Administrative Costs on Financial Statements

Event No.		Assets					Equity							Cash Flow	
	Cash	+	Inventory	+	Office Furn.*	+	Manuf. Equip.*	=	Com. Stk.	+	Ret. Earn.	Rev.	− Exp.	= Net Inc.	Cash Flow	
1	15,000							=	15,000						15,000	FA
2	(2,000)	+	2,000												(2,000)	OA
3	(1,200)							=			(1,200)		− 1,200	= (1,200)	(1,200)	OA
4	(3,000)	+	3,000												(3,000)	OA
5	(2,800)	+			2,800										(2,800)	IA
6					(600)			=			(600)		− 600	= (600)		
7	(4,500)	+					4,500								(4,500)	IA
8			1,000	+			(1,000)									
9	7,500							=			7,500	7,500		= 7,500	7,500	OA
10			(4,000)					=			(4,000)		− 4,000	= (4,000)		
Totals	9,000	+	2,000	+	2,200	+	3,500	=	15,000	+	1,700	7,500	− 5,800	= 1,700	9,000	NC

*Negative amounts in these columns represent accumulated depreciation.

Materials Costs (Event 2)

Materials used to make products are usually called **raw materials.** The cost of raw materials is first recorded in an asset account (Inventory). The cost is then transferred from the Inventory account to the Cost of Goods Sold account at the time the goods are sold. Remember that materials cost is only one component of total manufacturing costs. When inventory is sold, the combined cost of materials, labor, and overhead is expensed as *cost of goods sold*. The costs of materials that can be easily and conveniently traced to products are called **direct raw materials** costs.

Labor Costs (Event 4)

The salaries paid to selling and administrative employees (Event 3) and the wages paid to production workers (Event 4) are accounted for differently. Salaries paid to selling and administrative employees are expensed immediately, but the cost of production wages is added to inventory. Production wages are expensed as part of cost of goods sold at the time the inventory is sold. Labor costs that can be easily and conveniently traced to products are called **direct labor** costs. The cost flow of wages for production employees versus salaries for selling and administrative personnel is shown in Exhibit 10.6.

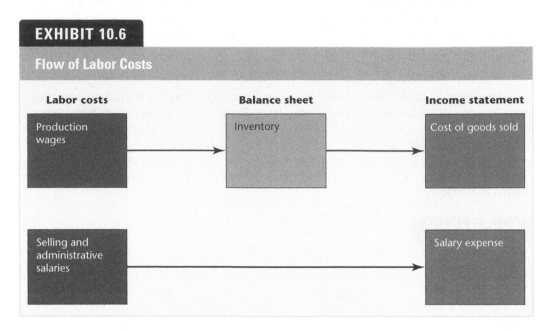

EXHIBIT 10.6

Flow of Labor Costs

Overhead Costs (Event 8)

Although depreciation cost totaled $1,600 ($600 on office furniture and $1,000 on manufacturing equipment), only the $600 of depreciation on the office furniture is expensed directly on the income statement. The depreciation on the manufacturing equipment is split between the income statement (cost of goods sold) and the balance sheet (inventory). The depreciation cost flow for the manufacturing equipment versus the office furniture is shown in Exhibit 10.7.

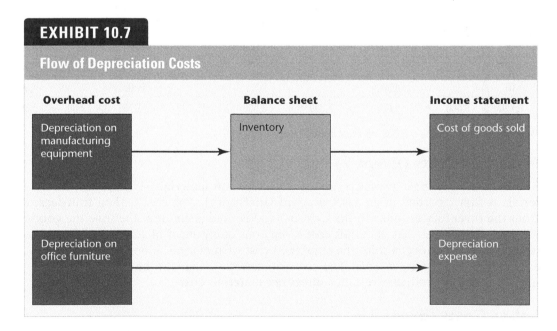

EXHIBIT 10.7

Flow of Depreciation Costs

Total Product Cost

A summary of Patillo Manufacturing's total product cost is shown in Exhibit 10.8.

EXHIBIT 10.8

Schedule of Inventory Costs

Materials	$2,000
Labor	3,000
Manufacturing overhead*	1,000
Total product costs	6,000
Less: Cost of goods sold	(4,000)
Ending inventory balance	$2,000

*Depreciation ([$4,500 − $1,500] ÷ 3)

General, Selling, and Administrative Costs

General, selling, and administrative costs (G,S,&A) are normally expensed *in the period* in which they are incurred. Because of this recognition pattern, nonproduct expenses are sometimes called **period costs.** In Patillo's case, the salaries expense for selling and administrative employees and the depreciation on office furniture are period costs reported directly on the income statement.

The income statement, balance sheet, and statement of cash flows for Patillo Manufacturing are displayed in Exhibit 10.9.

The $4,000 cost of goods sold reported on the income statement includes a portion of the materials, labor, and overhead costs incurred by Patillo during the year. Similarly, the $2,000 of finished goods inventory on the balance sheet includes materials, labor, and overhead costs. These product costs will be recognized as expense in the next accounting period when the goods are sold. Initially classifying a cost as a product cost delays, but does not eliminate, its recognition as an expense. All product costs are ultimately recognized as expense (cost of goods sold). Cost classification does not affect cash flow. Cash inflows and outflows are recognized in the period that cash is collected or paid regardless of whether the cost is recorded as an asset or expensed on the income statement.

EXHIBIT 10.9

PATILLO MANUFACTURING COMPANY
Financial Statements

Income Statement for 2012

Sales revenue	$ 7,500
Cost of goods sold	(4,000)
Gross margin	3,500
G, S, & A expenses	
Salaries expense	(1,200)
Depreciation expense—office furniture	(600)
Net income	$ 1,700

Balance Sheet as of December 31, 2012

Cash		$ 9,000
Finished goods inventory		2,000
Office furniture	$2,800	
Accumulated depreciation	(600)	
Book value		2,200
Manufacturing equipment	4,500	
Accumulated depreciation	(1,000)	
Book value		3,500
Total assets		$16,700
Stockholders' equity		
Common stock		$15,000
Retained earnings		1,700
Total stockholders' equity		$16,700

Statement of Cash Flows for 2012

Operating Activities	
Inflow from revenue	$ 7,500
Outflow for inventory	(5,000)
Outflow for S&A salaries	(1,200)
Net inflow from operating activities	1,300
Investing Activities	
Outflow for equipment and furniture	(7,300)
Financing Activities	
Inflow from stock issue	15,000
Net change in cash	9,000
Beginning cash balance	-0-
Ending cash balance	$ 9,000

Overhead Costs: A Closer Look

Costs such as depreciation on manufacturing equipment cannot be easily traced to products. Suppose that Patillo Manufacturing makes both tables and chairs. What part of the depreciation is caused by manufacturing tables versus manufacturing chairs? Similarly, suppose a production supervisor oversees employees who work on both tables and chairs. How much of the supervisor's salary relates to tables and how much to chairs? Likewise, the cost of glue used in the production department would be difficult to trace to tables versus chairs. You could count the drops of glue used on each product, but the information would not be useful enough to merit the time and money spent collecting the data.

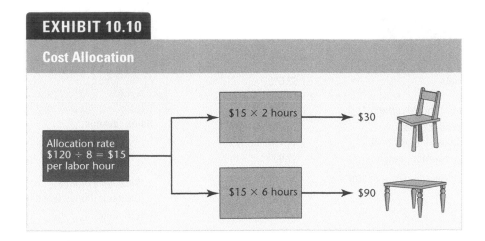

EXHIBIT 10.10

Cost Allocation

Costs that cannot be traced to products and services in a *cost-effective* manner are called **indirect costs.** The indirect costs incurred to make products are called **manufacturing overhead.** Some of the items commonly included in manufacturing overhead are indirect materials, indirect labor, factory utilities, rent of manufacturing facilities, and depreciation on manufacturing assets.

Because indirect costs cannot be effectively traced to products, they are normally assigned to products using **cost allocation,** a process of dividing a total cost into parts and assigning the parts to relevant cost objects. To illustrate, suppose that production workers spend an eight-hour day making a chair and a table. The chair requires two hours to complete and the table requires six hours. Now suppose that $120 of utilities cost is consumed during the day. How much of the $120 should be assigned to each piece of furniture? The utility cost cannot be directly traced to each specific piece of furniture, but the piece of furniture that required more labor also likely consumed more of the utility cost. Using this line of reasoning, it is rational to allocate the utility cost to the two pieces of furniture based on *direct labor hours* at a rate of $15 per hour ($120 ÷ 8 hours). The chair would be assigned $30 ($15 per hour × 2 hours) of the utility cost and the table would be assigned the remaining $90 ($15 × 6 hours) of utility cost. The allocation of the utility cost is shown in Exhibit 10.10.

We discuss the details of cost allocation in a later chapter. For now, recognize that overhead costs are normally allocated to products rather than traced directly to them.

Answers to The Curious Accountant

As you have seen, accounting for depreciation related to manufacturing assets is different from accounting for depreciation for nonmanufacturing assets. Depreciation on the checkout equipment at Sears is recorded as depreciation expense. Depreciation on manufacturing equipment at Schwinn is considered a product cost. It is included first as a part of the cost of inventory and eventually as a part of the expense, cost of goods sold. Recording depreciation on manufacturing equipment as an inventory cost is simply another example of the matching principle, because the cost does not become an expense until revenue from the product sale is recognized.

Manufacturing Product Cost Summary

As explained, the cost of a product made by a manufacturing company is normally composed of three categories: direct materials, direct labor, and manufacturing overhead. Relevant information about these three cost components is summarized in Exhibit 10.11.

EXHIBIT 10.11

Components of Manufacturing Product Cost

Component 1—Direct Materials
Sometimes called *raw materials*. In addition to basic resources such as wood or metals, it can include manufactured parts. For example, engines, glass, and car tires can be considered as raw materials for an automotive manufacturer. If the amount of a material in a product is known, it can usually be classified as a direct material. The cost of direct materials can be easily traced to specific products.

Component 2—Direct Labor
The cost of wages paid to factory workers involved in hands-on contact with the products being manufactured. If the amount of time employees worked on a product can be determined, this cost can usually be classified as direct labor. Like direct materials, labor costs must be easily traced to a specific product in order to be classified as a direct cost.

Component 3—Manufacturing Overhead
Costs that cannot be easily traced to specific products. Accordingly, these costs are called indirect costs. They can include but are not limited to the following:

1. Indirect materials such as glue, nails, paper, and oil. Indeed, note that indirect materials used in the production process may not appear in the finished product. An example is a chemical solvent used to clean products during the production process but not a component material found in the final product.

2. Indirect labor such as the cost of salaries paid to production supervisors, inspectors, and maintenance personnel.

3. Rental cost for manufacturing facilities and equipment.

4. Utility costs.

5. Depreciation.

6. Security.

7. The cost of preparing equipment for the manufacturing process (i.e., setup costs).

8. Maintenance cost for the manufacturing facility and equipment.

✓ CHECK YOURSELF 10.2

Lawson Manufacturing Company paid production workers wages of $100,000. It incurred materials costs of $120,000 and manufacturing overhead costs of $160,000. Selling and administrative salaries were $80,000. Lawson started and completed 1,000 units of product and sold 800 of these units. The company sets sales prices at $220 above the average per unit production cost. Based on this information alone, determine the amount of gross margin and net income. What is Lawson's pricing strategy called?

Answer   Total product cost is $380,000 ($100,000 labor + $120,000 materials + $160,000 overhead). Cost per unit is $380 ($380,000 ÷ 1,000 units). The sales price per unit is $600 ($380 + $220). Cost of goods sold is $304,000 ($380 × 800 units). Sales revenue is $480,000 ($600 × 800 units). Gross margin is $176,000 ($480,000 revenue − $304,000 cost of goods sold). Net income is $96,000 ($176,000 gross margin − $80,000 selling and administrative salaries). Lawson's pricing strategy is called *cost-plus* pricing.

SCHEDULE OF COST OF GOODS MANUFACTURED AND SOLD

To this point, we assumed all inventory started during an accounting period was also completed during that accounting period. All product costs (materials, labor, and manufacturing overhead) were either in inventory or expensed as cost of goods sold. At the end of an accounting period, however, most real-world companies have raw materials on hand, and manufacturing companies are likely to have in inventory items that have been started but are not completed. Most manufacturing companies accumulate product costs in three distinct inventory accounts: (1) **Raw Materials Inventory,** which includes lumber, metals, paints, and chemicals that will be used to make the company's products; (2) **Work in Process Inventory,** which includes partially completed products; and (3) **Finished Goods Inventory,** which includes completed products that are ready for sale.

The cost of materials is first recorded in the Raw Materials Inventory account. The cost of materials placed in production is then transferred from the Raw Materials Inventory account to the Work in Process Inventory account. The costs of labor and overhead are added to the Work in Process Inventory account. The cost of the goods completed during the period is transferred from the Work in Process Inventory account to the Finished Goods Inventory account. The cost of the goods that are sold during the accounting period is transferred from the Finished Goods Inventory account to the Cost of Goods Sold account. The balances that remain in the Raw Materials, Work in Process, and Finished Goods Inventory accounts are reported on the balance sheet. The amount of product cost transferred to the Cost of Goods Sold account is expensed on the income statement. Exhibit 10.12 shows the flow of manufacturing costs through the accounting records.

To help managers analyze manufacturing costs, companies frequently summarize product cost information is a report called a **schedule of cost of goods manufactured and sold.** To illustrate, assume that in 2013 Patillo Manufacturing Company purchased $37,950 of raw materials inventory. During 2013 Patillo used $37,000 of raw materials, incurred $34,600 of labor costs, and $26,700 of overhead costs in the process of making inventory. Also, during 2013 the company completed work on products that cost $94,600. Recall that Patillo had zero balances in its Raw Materials and Work in Process Inventory accounts at the end of 2012. It had a $2,000 balance in its Finished Goods Inventory account at the end of 2012. The 2012 ending balance becomes the

EXHIBIT 10.12

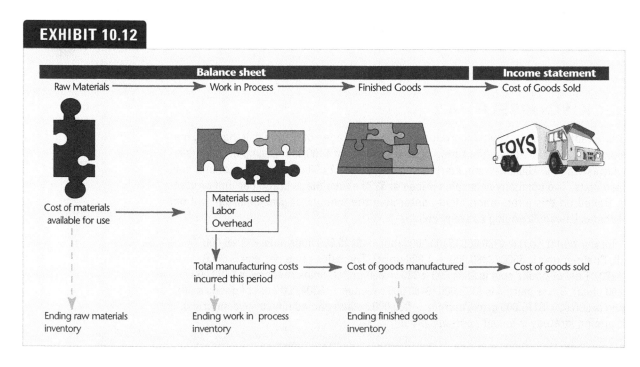

EXHIBIT 10.13

PATILLO MANUFACTURING COMPANY
Schedule of Cost of Goods Manufactured and Sold
For the Year Ended December 31, 2013

Beginning raw materials Inventory	$ 0
Plus: Raw materials purchases	37,950
Less: Ending raw materials inventory	(950)
Raw materials used	37,000
Labor	34,600
Overhead	26,700
Total manufacturing costs	98,300
Plus: Beginning work in process inventory	0
Total work in process inventory	98,300
Less: Ending work in process inventory	(3,700)
Cost of goods manufactured	94,600
Plus: Beginning finished goods inventory	2,000
Cost of goods available for sale	96,600
Less: Ending finished goods inventory	(3,200)
Cost of goods sold	$93,400

2013 beginning balance for finished goods. The 2013 ending balances for the inventory accounts were as follows: Raw Materials Inventory, $950; Work in Process Inventory, $3,700; Finished Goods Inventory, $3,200. Finally, during 2013 Patillo had sales revenue of $153,000. Patillo's schedule of cost of goods manufactured and sold for 2013 is shown in Exhibit 10.13

The $93,400 of cost of goods sold would appear on Patillo's 2013 income statement. A partial income statement for Patillo is shown in Exhibit 10.14

EXHIBIT 10.14

PATILLO MANUFACTURING COMPANY
Income Statement
For the Year Ended December 31, 2013

Sales revenue	$153,000
Cost of goods sold	(93,400)
Gross margin	$ 59,600

UPSTREAM AND DOWNSTREAM COSTS

Most companies incur product-related costs before and after, as well as during, the manufacturing process. For example, Ford Motor Company incurs significant research and development costs prior to mass producing a new car model. These **upstream costs** occur before the manufacturing process begins. Similarly, companies normally incur significant costs after the manufacturing process is complete. Examples of **downstream costs** include transportation, advertising, sales commissions, and bad debts. While upstream and downstream costs are not considered to be product costs for financial reporting purposes, profitability analysis requires that they be considered in cost-plus pricing decisions. To be profitable, a company must recover the total cost of developing, producing, and delivering its products to customers.

Distinguish product costs from upstream and downstream costs.

PRODUCT COSTING IN SERVICE AND MERCHANDISING COMPANIES

Companies are frequently classified as being service, merchandising, or manufacturing businesses. As the name implies, service organizations provide services, rather than physical products, to consumers. For example, St. Jude Children's Hospital provides treatment programs aimed at healing patient diseases. Other common service providers include

Explain how product costing differs in service, merchandising, and manufacturing companies.

public accountants, lawyers, restaurants, dry cleaning establishments, and lawn care companies. Merchandising businesses are sometimes called retail or wholesale companies; they sell goods other companies make. The Home Depot, Inc., Costco Wholesale Corporation, and Best Buy Co., Inc., are merchandising companies. Manufacturing companies make the goods they sell to their customers. Toyota Motor Corporation, Texaco, Inc., and American Standard Companies, Inc., are manufacturing businesses.

How do manufacturing companies differ from service and merchandising businesses? Do service and merchandising companies incur materials, labor, and overhead costs? Yes. For example, Ernst & Young, a large accounting firm, must pay employees (labor costs), use office supplies (material costs), and incur utilities, depreciation, and so on (overhead costs) in the process of conducting audits. *The primary difference between manufacturing entities and service companies is that the products provided by service companies are consumed immediately.* In contrast, products made by manufacturing companies can be held in the form of inventory until they are sold to consumers. Similarly, most labor and overhead costs incurred by merchandising companies result from providing assistance to customers. These costs are normally treated as general, selling, and administrative expenses rather than accumulated in inventory accounts. Indeed, merchandising companies are often viewed as service companies rather than considered a separate business category.

The important point to remember is that all business managers are expected to control costs, improve quality, and increase productivity. Like managers of manufacturing companies, managers of service and merchandising businesses can benefit from the analysis of the cost of satisfying their customers. For example, Wendy's, a service company, can benefit from knowing how much a hamburger costs in the same manner that Bayer Corporation, a manufacturing company, benefits from knowing the cost of a bottle of aspirin.

✓ CHECK YOURSELF 10.3

The cost of making a Burger King hamburger includes the cost of materials, labor, and overhead. Does this mean that Burger King is a manufacturing company?

Answer No, Burger King is not a manufacturing company. It is a service company because its products are consumed immediately. In contrast, there may be a considerable delay between the time the product of a manufacturing company is made and the time it is consumed. For example, it could be several months between the time Ford Motor Company makes an Explorer and the time the Explorer is ultimately sold to a customer. The primary difference between service and manufacturing companies is that manufacturing companies have inventories of products and service companies do not.

JUST-IN-TIME INVENTORY

LO 7

Show how just-in-time inventory can increase profitability.

Companies attempt to minimize the amount of inventory they maintain because of the high cost of holding it. Many **inventory holding costs** are obvious: financing, warehouse space, supervision, theft, damage, and obsolescence. Other costs are hidden: diminished motivation, sloppy work, inattentive attitudes, and increased production time.

Many businesses have been able to simultaneously reduce their inventory holding costs and increase customer satisfaction by making products available **just in time (JIT)** for customer consumption. For example, hamburgers that are cooked to order are fresher and more individualized than those that are prepared in advance and stored until a customer orders one. Many fast-food restaurants have discovered that JIT systems lead not only to greater customer satisfaction but also to lower costs through reduced waste.

Just-in-Time Illustration

To illustrate the benefits of a JIT system, consider Paula Elliot, a student at a large urban university. She helps support herself by selling flowers. Three days each week, Paula drives to a florist, purchases 25 single-stem roses, returns to the school, and sells the flowers to individuals from a location on a local street corner. She pays $2 per rose and sells each one for $3. Some days she does not have enough flowers to meet customer demand. Other days, she must discard one or two unsold flowers; she believes quality is important and refuses to sell flowers that are not fresh. During May, she purchased 300 roses and sold 280. She calculated her driving cost to be $45. Exhibit 10.15 displays Paula's May income statement.

After studying just-in-time inventory systems in her managerial accounting class, Paula decided to apply the concepts to her small business. She *reengineered* her distribution system by purchasing her flowers from a florist within walking distance of her sales location. She had considered purchasing from this florist earlier but had rejected the idea because the florist's regular selling price of $2.25 per rose was too high. After learning about *most-favored customer status,* she developed a strategy to get a price reduction. By guaranteeing that she would buy at least 30 roses per week, she was able to convince the local florist to match her current cost of $2.00 per rose. The local florist agreed that she could make purchases in batches of any size so long as the total amounted to at least 30 per week. Under this arrangement, Paula was able to buy roses *just in time* to meet customer demand. Each day she purchased a small number of flowers. When she ran out, she simply returned to the florist for additional ones.

The JIT system also enabled Paula to eliminate the cost of the *nonvalue-added activity* of driving to her former florist. Customer satisfaction actually improved because no one was ever turned away because of the lack of inventory. In June, Paula was able to buy and sell 310 roses with no waste and no driving expense. The June income statement is shown in Exhibit 10.16.

Paula was ecstatic about her $115 increase in profitability ($310 in June − $195 in May = $115 increase), but she was puzzled about the exact reasons for the change. She had saved $40 (20 flowers × $2 each) by avoiding waste and eliminated $45 of driving expenses. These two factors explained only $85 ($40 waste + $45 driving expense) of the $115 increase. What had caused the remaining $30 ($115 − $85) increase in profitability? Paula asked her accounting professor to help her identify the remaining $30 difference.

The professor explained that May sales had suffered from *lost opportunities.* Recall that under the earlier inventory system, Paula had to turn away some prospective customers because she sold out of flowers before all customers were served. Sales increased from 280 roses in May to 310 roses in June. A likely explanation for the 30 unit difference (310 − 280) is that customers who would have purchased flowers in May were unable to do so because of a lack of availability. May's sales suffered from the lost opportunity to earn a gross margin of $1 per flower on 30 roses, a $30 **opportunity cost.** This opportunity cost is the missing link in explaining the profitability difference between May and June. The total $115 difference consists of (1) $40 savings from waste elimination, (2) $45 savings from eliminating driving expense, and (3) opportunity cost of $30. The subject of opportunity cost has widespread application and is discussed in more depth in subsequent chapters of the text.

EXHIBIT 10.15

Income Statement for May

Sales revenue (280 units × $3 per unit)	$840
Cost of goods sold (280 units × $2 per unit)	(560)
Gross margin	280
Driving expense	(45)
Waste (20 units × $2 per unit)	(40)
Net income	$195

EXHIBIT 10.16

Income Statement for June

Sales revenue (310 units × $3 per unit)	$930
Cost of goods sold (310 units × $2 per unit)	(620)
Gross margin	310
Driving expense	0
Net income	$310

✓ CHECK YOURSELF 10.4

A strike at a General Motors brake plant caused an almost immediate shutdown of many of the company's assembly plants. What could have caused such a rapid and widespread shutdown?

Answer A rapid and widespread shutdown could have occurred because General Motors uses a just-in-time inventory system. With a just-in-time inventory system, there is no stockpile of inventory to draw on when strikes or other forces disrupt inventory deliveries. This illustrates a potential negative effect of using a just-in-time inventory system.

STATEMENT OF ETHICAL PROFESSIONAL PRACTICE

Identify and explain the standards contained in IMA's Statement of Ethical Professional Practice.

Management accountants must be prepared not only to make difficult choices between legitimate alternatives but also to face conflicts of a more troubling nature, such as pressure to

1. Undertake duties they have not been trained to perform competently.
2. Disclose confidential information.
3. Compromise their integrity through falsification, embezzlement, bribery, and so on.
4. Issue biased, misleading, or incomplete reports.

In Chapter 4 we explained how the American Institute of Certified Public Accountants' Code of Professional Conduct provides guidance for CPAs to avoid unethical behavior. To provide Certified Management Accountants (CMAs) with guidance for ethical conduct the Institute of Management Accountants (IMA) issued a *Statement of Ethical Professional Practice,* which is shown in Exhibit 10.17. Management accountants are also frequently required to abide by organizational codes of ethics. Failure to adhere to professional and organizational ethical standards can lead to personal disgrace, loss of employment, or imprisonment.

EXHIBIT 10.17

Statement of Ethical Professional Practice

Members of IMA shall behave ethically. A commitment to ethical professional practice includes overarching principles that express our values, and standards that guide our conduct. IMA's overarching ethical principles include: Honesty, Fairness, Objectivity, and Responsibility. Members shall act in accordance with these principles and shall encourage others within their organizations to adhere to them. A member's failure to comply with the following standards may result in disciplinary action.

Competence Each member has a responsibility to
- Maintain an appropriate level of professional expertise by continually developing knowledge and skills.
- Perform professional duties in accordance with relevant laws, regulations, and technical standards.
- Provide decision support information and recommendations that are accurate, clear, concise, and timely.
- Recognize and communicate professional limitations or other constraints that would preclude responsible judgment or successful performance of an activity.

Confidentiality Each member has a responsibility to
- Keep information confidential except when disclosure is authorized or legally required.
- Inform all relevant parties regarding appropriate use of confidential information. Monitor subordinates' activities to ensure compliance.
- Refrain from using confidential information for unethical or illegal advantage.

Integrity Each member has a responsibility to
- Mitigate actual conflicts of interest and avoid apparent conflicts of interest. Advise all parties of any potential conflicts.
- Refrain from engaging in any conduct that would prejudice carrying out duties ethically.
- Abstain from engaging in or supporting any activity that might discredit the profession.

Credibility Each member has a responsibility to
- Communicate information fairly and objectively.
- Disclose all relevant information that could reasonably be expected to influence an intended user's understanding of the reports, analyses, or recommendations.
- Disclose delays or deficiencies in information, timeliness, processing, or internal controls in conformance with organization policy and/or applicable law.

Resolution of Ethical Conflict In applying these standards, you may encounter problems identifying unethical behavior or resolving an ethical conflict. When faced with ethical issues, follow your organization's established policies on the resolution of such conflict. If these policies do not resolve the ethical conflict, consider the following courses of action.
- Discuss the issue with your immediate supervisor except when it appears that the supervisor is involved. In that case, present the issue to the next level. If you cannot achieve a satisfactory resolution, submit the issue to the next management level. Communication of such problems to authorities or individuals not employed or engaged by the organization is not considered appropriate, unless you believe there is a clear violation of the law.
- Clarify relevant ethical issues by initiating a confidential discussion with an IMA Ethics Counselor or other impartial advisor to obtain a better understanding of possible courses of action.
- Consult your own attorney as to legal obligations and rights concerning the ethical conflict.

REALITY BYTES

Unethical behavior occurs in all types of organizations. In its *2007 National Government Ethics Survey,* the Ethics Resource Center reported its findings on the occurrences and reporting of unethical behavior in local, state, and federal governments.

Fifty-seven percent of those surveyed reported having observed unethical conduct during the past year. Unethical conduct was reported most often by those in local governments (63%) and least often at the federal level (52%). The definition of ethical misconduct used in the study was quite broad, ranging from behavior such as an individual putting his or her personal interest ahead of the interest of the organization, to sexual harassment, to taking bribes. The more egregious offences, such as discrimination or taking bribes, were reported much less often than activities such as lying to customers, vendors, or the public.

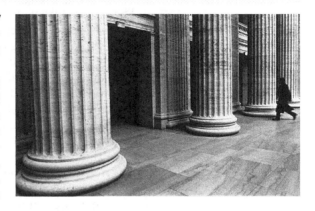

Once observed, unethical behavior often was not reported. For example, only 25 percent of observed incidents of the alteration of financial records were reported to supervisors or whistleblower hotlines, and only 54 percent of observed bribes were reported.

The survey also found that only 18 percent of government entities have ethics and compliance programs in place that could be considered well-implemented. However, where well-implemented programs do exist, observed unethical misconduct is less likely to occur and more likely to be reported. In these entities only 36 percent of respondents said they had observed misconduct (compared to 57 percent overall), and when they did observe misconduct, 75 percent said they reported it.

For the complete *2007 National Government Ethics Survey,* go to www.ethics.org.

A Look Back

Managerial accounting focuses on the information needs of *internal* users, while *financial accounting* focuses on the information needs of *external* users. Managerial accounting uses economic, operating, and nonfinancial, as well as financial, data. Managerial accounting information is local (pertains to the company's subunits), is limited by cost/benefit considerations, is more concerned with relevance and timeliness, and is future oriented. Financial accounting information, on the other hand, is more global than managerial accounting information. It supplies information that applies to the whole company. Financial accounting is regulated by numerous authorities, is characterized by objectivity, is focused on reliability and accuracy, and is historical in nature.

Both managerial and financial accounting are concerned with product costing. Financial accountants need product cost information to determine the amount of inventory reported on the balance sheet and the amount of cost of goods sold reported on the income statement. Managerial accountants need to know the cost of products for pricing decisions and for control and evaluation purposes. When determining unit product costs, managers use the average cost per unit. Determining the actual cost of each product requires an unreasonable amount of time and record keeping and it makes no difference in product pricing and product cost control decisions.

Product costs are the costs incurred to make products: the costs of direct materials, direct labor, and overhead. *Overhead costs* are product costs that cannot be cost effectively traced to a product; therefore, they are assigned to products using *cost allocation.* Overhead costs include indirect materials, indirect labor, depreciation, rent, and utilities for manufacturing facilities. Product costs are first accumulated in an asset account (Inventory). They are expensed as cost of goods sold in the period the inventory is sold. The difference between sales revenue and cost of goods sold is called *gross margin*.

General, selling, and administrative costs are classified separately from product costs. They are subtracted from gross margin to determine net income. General, selling, and administrative costs can be divided into two categories. Costs incurred before the manufacturing process begins (research and development costs) are *upstream costs*. Costs incurred after manufacturing is complete (transportation) are *downstream costs*. Service companies, like manufacturing companies, incur materials, labor, and overhead costs, but the products provided by service companies are consumed immediately. Therefore, service company product costs are not accumulated in an Inventory account.

A code of ethical conduct is needed in the accounting profession because accountants hold positions of trust and face conflicts of interest. In recognition of the temptations that accountants face, the IMA has issued a *Statement of Ethical Professional Practice,* which provides accountants guidance in resisting temptations and in making difficult decisions.

Emerging trends such as *just-in-time inventory* and *activity-based management* are methods that many companies have used to reengineer their production and delivery systems to eliminate waste, reduce errors, and minimize costs. Activity-based management seeks to eliminate or reduce *nonvalue-added activities* and to create new *value-added activities*. Just-in-time inventory seeks to reduce inventory holding costs and to lower prices for customers by making inventory available just in time for customer consumption.

>> A Look Forward

In addition to distinguishing costs by product versus G, S, & A classification, other classifications can be used to facilitate managerial decision making. In the next chapter, costs are classified according to the *behavior* they exhibit when the number of units of product increases or decreases (volume of activity changes). You will learn to distinguish between costs that vary with activity volume changes versus costs that remain fixed with activity volume changes. You will learn not only to recognize *cost behavior* but also how to use such recognition to evaluate business risk and opportunity.

APPENDIX A

Identify emerging trends in accounting.

Emerging Trends in Managerial Accounting

Global competition has forced many companies to reengineer their production and delivery systems to eliminate waste, reduce errors, and minimize costs. A key ingredient of successful **reengineering** is benchmarking. **Benchmarking** involves identifying the **best practices** used by world-class competitors. By studying and mimicking these practices, a company uses benchmarking to implement highly effective and efficient operating methods. Best practices employed by world-class companies include total quality management (TQM), activity-based management (ABM), and value-added assessment.

Total Quality Management

To promote effective and efficient operations, many companies practice **total quality management (TQM).** TQM is a two-dimensional management philosophy using (1) a systematic problem-solving philosophy that encourages frontline workers to achieve *zero defects* and (2) an organizational commitment to achieving *customer satisfaction*. A key component of TQM is **continuous improvement,** an ongoing process through which employees strive to eliminate waste, reduce response time, minimize defects, and simplify the design and delivery of products and services to customers.

Activity-Based Management

Simple changes in perspective can have dramatic results. For example, imagine how realizing the world is round instead of flat changed the nature of travel. A recent change in perspective developing in management accounting is the realization that an organization cannot manage *costs*. Instead, it manages the *activities* that cause costs to be incurred. **Activities** represent the measures an organization takes to accomplish its goals.

The primary goal of all organizations is to provide products (goods and services) their customers *value*. The sequence of activities used to provide products is called a **value chain**. **Activity-based management** assesses the value chain to create new or refine existing **value-added activities** and to eliminate or reduce *nonvalue-added activities*. A value-added activity is any unit of work that contributes to a product's ability to satisfy customer needs. For example, cooking is an activity that adds value to food served to a hungry customer. **Nonvalue-added activities** are tasks undertaken that do not contribute to a product's ability to satisfy customer needs. Waiting for the oven to preheat so that food can be cooked does not add value. Most customers value cooked food, but they do not value waiting for it.

To illustrate, consider the value-added activities undertaken by a pizza restaurant. Begin with a customer who is hungry for pizza; certain activities must occur to satisfy that hunger. These activities are pictured in Exhibit 10.18. At a minimum, the restaurant must conduct research and development (devise a recipe), obtain raw materials (acquire the ingredients), manufacture the product (combine and bake the ingredients), market the product (advertise its availability), and deliver the product (transfer the pizza to the customer).

EXHIBIT 10.18

Value Chain

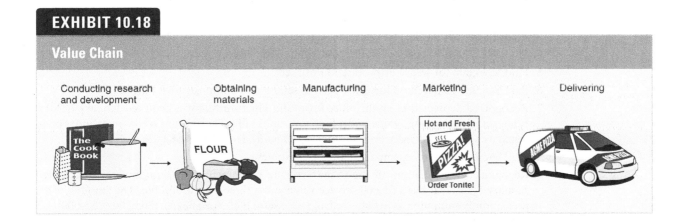

| Conducting research and development | Obtaining materials | Manufacturing | Marketing | Delivering |

Businesses gain competitive advantages by adding activities that satisfy customer needs. For example, Domino's Pizza grew briskly by recognizing the value customers placed on the convenience of home pizza delivery. Alternatively, Little Caesar's has been highly successful by satisfying customers who value low prices. Other restaurants capitalize on customer values pertaining to taste, ambience, or location. Businesses can also gain competitive advantages by identifying and eliminating nonvalue-added activities, providing products of comparable quality at lower cost than competitors.

Value Chain Analysis Across Companies

Comprehensive value chain analysis extends from obtaining raw materials to the ultimate disposition of finished products. It encompasses the activities performed not only by a particular organization but also by that organization's suppliers and those who service its finished products. For example, PepsiCo must be concerned with the activities of the company that supplies the containers for its soft drinks as well as the retail companies that sell its products. If cans of Pepsi fail to open properly, the customer is more likely to blame PepsiCo than the supplier of the cans. Comprehensive value chain analysis can lead to identifying and eliminating nonvalue-added activities that occur between companies. For example, container producers could be encouraged to build manufacturing facilities near Pepsi's bottling factories, eliminating the nonvalue-added activity of transporting empty containers from the manufacturer to the bottling facility. The resulting cost savings benefits customers by reducing costs without affecting quality.

A step-by-step audio-narrated series of slides is provided on the text website at www.mhhe.com/edmondssurvey3e.

SELF-STUDY REVIEW PROBLEM

Tuscan Manufacturing Company makes a unique headset for use with mobile phones. The company had the following amounts in its accounts at the beginning of 2012: Cash, $795,000; Raw Materials Inventory, $5,000; Work in process Inventory, $11,000; Finished Goods Inventory, $39,000; Common Stock, $650,000; and Retained Earnings, $200,000. Tuscan experienced the following accounting events during 2012. Other than the adjusting entries for depreciation, assume that all transactions are cash transactions.

1. Paid $50,000 of research and development costs to create the headset.
2. Paid $139,000 for raw materials will be used to make headsets.
3. Placed $141,000 of the raw materials cost into the process of manufacturing headsets.
4. Paid $82,200 for salaries of selling and administrative employees.
5. Paid $224,000 for wages of production workers.
6. Paid $48,000 to purchase furniture used in selling and administrative offices.
7. Recognized depreciation on the office furniture. The furniture was acquired January 1, 2012. It has an $8,000 salvage value and a four-year useful life. The amount of depreciation is computed as [(cost − salvage) ÷ useful life]. Specifically, ($48,000 − $8,000) ÷ 4 = $10,000.
8. Paid $65,000 to purchase manufacturing equipment.
9. Recognized depreciation on the manufacturing equipment. The equipment was acquired January 1, 2012. It has a $5,000 salvage value and a three-year useful life. The amount of depreciation is computed as [(cost − salvage) ÷ useful life]. Specifically, ($65,000 − $5,000) ÷ 3 = $20,000.
10. Paid $136,000 for rent and utility costs on the manufacturing facility.
11. Paid $41,000 for inventory holding expenses for completed headsets (rental of warehouse space, salaries of warehouse personnel, and other general storage costs.)
12. Completed and transferred headsets that had a total cost of $520,000 from work in process inventory to finished goods.
13. Sold headsets for $738,200.
14. It cost Tuscan $517,400 to make the headsets sold in Event 13.

Required

a. Show how these events affect the balance sheet, income statement, and statement of cash flows by recording them in a horizontal financial statement model.
b. Explain why Tuscan's recognition of cost of goods sold expense had no impact on cash flow.
c. Prepare a schedule of costs of goods manufactured and sold, an income statement, and a balance sheet.
d. Distinguish between the product costs and the upstream and downstream costs that Tuscan incurred.

Solution to Requirement *a*

Event No.	Cash	+	Raw Mat. Inv.	+	WIP Inv.	+	Finished Goods Inv.	+ Office Furn.*	+ Manuf. Equip.*	=	Com. Stk.	+ Ret. Earn.	Rev.	− Exp.	= Net Inc.	Cash Flow
	795,000		5,000		11,000		39,000			=	650,000	200,000			=	
1	(50,000)									=		(50,000)		− 50,000	= (50,000)	(50,000) OA
2	(139,000)		139,000							=					=	(139,000) OA
3			(141,000)		141,000					=					=	
4	(82,200)									=		(82,200)		− 82,200	= (82,200)	(82,200) OA
5	(224,000)				224,000					=					=	(224,000) OA
6	(48,000)						48,000			=					=	(48,000) IA
7								(10,000)		=		(10,000)		− 10,000	= (10,000)	
8	(65,000)								65,000	=					=	(65,000) IA
9					20,000				(20,000)	=					=	
10	(136,000)		136,000							=					=	(136,000) OA
11	(41,000)									=		(41,000)		− 41,000	= (41,000)	(41,000) OA
12					(520,000)		520,000			=					=	
13	738,200									=		738,200	738,200		= 738,200	738,200 OA
14							(517,400)			=		(517,400)		− 517,400	= (517,400)	
Totals	748,000	+	3,000	+	12,000	+	41,600 + 38,000	+ 45,000		=	650,000	+ 237,600	738,200	− 700,600	= 37,600	(47,000) NC

*Negative amounts in these columns represent accumulated depreciation.

Solution to Requirement *b*

Tuscan does not recognize a cash outflow at the time the goods are sold because the cash is paid when the materials, labor, and overhead are acquired.

Solution to Requirement *c*

TUSCAN MANUFACTURING COMPANY
Schedule of Cost of Goods Manufactured and Sold
For the Year Ended December 31, 2012

Beginning raw materials Inventory	$ 5,000
Plus: Raw materials purchases	139,000
Less: Ending raw materials inventory	(3,000)
Raw materials used	141,000
Labor	224,000
Overhead	156,000
Total manufacturing costs	521,000
Plus: Beginning work in process inventory	11,000
Total work in process inventory	532,000
Less: Ending work in process inventory	(12,000)
Cost of goods manufactured	520,000
Plus: Beginning finished goods inventory	39,000
Cost of goods available for sale	559,000
Less: Ending finished goods inventory	(41,600)
Cost of goods sold	$517,400

TUSCAN MANUFACTURING COMPANY
Income Statement
For the Year Ended December 31, 2012

Sales revenue	$738,200
Cost of goods sold	(517,400)
Gross margin	220,800
Research and development expenses	(50,000)
Selling and administrative salary expense	(82,200)
Selling and administrative depreciation expense	(10,000)
Inventory holding expenses	(41,000)
Net Income	$ 37,600

TUSCAN MANUFACTURING COMPANY
Balance Sheet
As of December 31, 2012

Assets	
Cash	$748,000
Raw materials inventory	3,000
Work in process inventory	12,000
Finished goods inventory	41,600
Manufacturing equipment less accumulated depreciation	45,000
Office furniture less accumulated depreciation	38,000
Total assets	$887,600
Equity	
Common stock	$650,000
Retained earnings	237,600
Total stockholders' equity	$887,600

Solution to Requirement *d*

Inventory product costs for manufacturing companies focus on the costs necessary to make the product. The cost of research and development (Event 1) occurs before the inventory is made and is therefore an upstream cost, not an inventory (product) cost. The inventory holding costs (Event 11) are incurred after the inventory has been made and are therefore downstream costs, not product costs. Selling costs (included in Events 4 and 7) are normally incurred after products have been made and are therefore usually classified as downstream costs. Administrative costs (also included in Events 4 and 7) are not related to making products and are therefore not classi-fied as product costs. Administrative costs may be incurred before, during, or after products are made, so they may be classified as either upstream or downstream costs. Only the costs of mate-rials, labor, and overhead that are actually incurred for the purpose of making goods (Events 3, 5, 9, and 10) are classified as product costs.

KEY TERMS

Activities 377

Activity-based management
(ABM) 377

Average cost 363

Benchmarking 376

Best practices 376

Continuous improvement 376

Cost allocation 368

Cost-plus pricing 362

Direct labor 366

Direct raw materials 365

Downstream costs 371

Financial accounting 359

Finished Goods Inventory 370

General, selling, and
administrative costs 367

Indirect costs 368

Inventory holding costs 372

Just in time (JIT) 372

Managerial accounting 359

Manufacturing overhead 368

Nonvalue-added activities 377   Raw Materials Inventory 370   Value-added activity 377
Opportunity cost 373   Reengineering 376   Value-added principle 361
Overhead 362   Schedule of cost of goods   Value chain 377
Period costs 367   manufactured and sold 370   Work in Process Inventory 370
Product costs 362   Total quality management
Product costing 362   (TQM) 376
Raw materials 365   Upstream costs 371

QUESTIONS

1. What are some differences between financial and managerial accounting?

2. What does the value-added principle mean as it applies to managerial accounting information? Give an example of value-added information that may be included in managerial accounting reports but is not shown in publicly reported financial statements.

3. How does product costing used in financial accounting differ from product costing used in managerial accounting?

4. What does the statement "costs can be assets or expenses" mean?

5. Why are the salaries of production workers accumulated in an inventory account instead of being directly expensed on the income statement?

6. How do product costs affect the financial statements? How does the classification of product cost (as an asset vs. an expense) affect net income?

7. What is an indirect cost? Provide examples of product costs that would be classified as indirect.

8. How does a product cost differ from a general, selling, and administrative cost? Give examples of each.

9. Why is cost classification important to managers?

10. What is cost allocation? Give an example of a cost that needs to be allocated.

11. What are some of the common ethical conflicts that accountants encounter?

12. What costs should be considered in determining the sales price of a product?

13. What is a just-in-time (JIT) inventory system? Name some inventory costs that can be eliminated or reduced by its use.

14. What are the two dimensions of a total quality management (TQM) program? Why is TQM being used in business practice? (Appendix)

15. What does the term *reengineering* mean? Name some reengineering practices. (Appendix)

16. How has the Institute of Management Accountants responded to the need for high standards of ethical conduct in the accounting profession? (Appendix)

17. What does the term *activity-based management* mean? (Appendix)

18. What is a value chain? (Appendix)

19. What do the terms *value-added activity* and *nonvalue-added activity* mean? Provide an example of each type of activity. (Appendix)

MULTIPLE-CHOICE QUESTIONS

Multiple-choice questions are provided on the text website at www.mhhe.com/edmondssurvey3e.

EXERCISES

All applicable Exercises are available with McGraw-Hill's *Connect Accounting*.

Exercise 10-1 *Identifying financial versus managerial accounting characteristics*   **LO 1**

Required

Indicate whether each of the following is representative of managerial or of financial accounting.

a. Information is factual and is characterized by objectivity, reliability, consistency, and accuracy.

b. Information is reported continuously and has a current or future orientation.

c. Information is provided to outsiders including investors, creditors, government agencies, analysts, and reporters.
d. Information is regulated by the SEC, FASB, and other sources of GAAP.
e. Information is based on estimates that are bounded by relevance and timeliness.
f. Information is historically based and usually reported annually.
g. Information is local and pertains to subunits of the organization.
h. Information includes economic and nonfinancial data as well as financial data.
i. Information is global and pertains to the company as a whole.
j. Information is provided to insiders including executives, managers, and operators.

LO 2

Exercise 10-2 *Identifying product versus general, selling, and administrative costs*

Required

Indicate whether each of the following costs should be classified as a product cost or as a general, selling, and administrative cost.

a. Direct materials used in a manufacturing company.
b. Indirect materials used in a manufacturing company.
c. Salaries of employees working in the accounting department.
d. Commissions paid to sales staff.
e. Interest on the mortgage for the company's corporate headquarters.
f. Indirect labor used to manufacture inventory.
g. Attorney's fees paid to protect the company from frivolous lawsuits.
h. Research and development costs incurred to create new drugs for a pharmaceutical company.
i. The cost of secretarial supplies used in a doctor's office.
j. Depreciation on the office furniture of the company president.

LO 2

Exercise 10-3 *Classifying costs: product or G, S, & A/asset or expense*

Required

Use the following format to classify each cost as a product cost or a general, selling, and administrative (G, S, & A) cost. Also indicate whether the cost would be recorded as an asset or an expense. The first item is shown as an example.

Cost Category	Product/ G, S, & A	Asset/ Expense
Research and development costs	G, S, & A	Expense
Cost to set up manufacturing facility		
Utilities used in factory		
Cars for sales staff		
Distributions to stockholders		
General office supplies		
Raw materials used in the manufacturing process		
Cost to rent office equipment		
Wages of production workers		
Advertising costs		
Promotion costs		
Production supplies		
Depreciation on administration building		
Depreciation on manufacturing equipment		

Exercise 10-4   *Identifying effect of product versus general, selling, and*   **LO 2, 3**
administrative costs on financial statements

Required

Nailry Industries recognized accrued compensation cost. Use the following model to show how this event would affect the company's financial statement under the following two assumptions: (1) the compensation is for office personnel and (2) the compensation is for production workers. Use pluses or minuses to show the effect on each element. If an element is not affected, indicate so by placing the letters NA under the appropriate heading.

	Assets	=	Liab.	+	Equity	Rev.	−	Exp.	=	Net Inc.	Cash Flow
1.											
2.											

Exercise 10-5   *Identify effect of product versus general, selling, and administrative*   **LO 2, 3**
costs on financial statements

Required

Milby Industries recognized the annual cost of depreciation on its December 31 financial statement. Using the following horizontal financial statements model, indicate how this event affected the company's financial statements under the following two assumptions: (1) the depreciation was on office furniture and (2) the depreciation was on manufacturing equipment. Indicate whether the event increases (I), decreases (D), or has no affect (NA) on each element of the financial statements. Also, in the Cash Flow column, indicate whether the cash flow is for operating activities (OA), investing activities (IA), or financing activities (FA). (Note: Show accumulated depreciation as a decrease in the book value of the appropriate asset account.)

Event No.		Assets						Equity			Rev.	−	Exp.	=	Net Inc.	Cash Flow
	Cash	+	Inventory	+	Manuf. Equip.	+	Office Furn.	=	Com. Stk.	+	Ret. Earn.					
1.																
2.																

Exercise 10-6   *Identifying product costs in a manufacturing company*   **LO 2**

Tiffany Crissler was talking to another accounting student, Bill Tyrone. Upon discovering that the accounting department offered an upper-level course in cost measurement, Tiffany remarked to Bill, "How difficult can it be? My parents own a toy store. All you have to do to figure out how much something costs is look at the invoice. Surely you don't need an entire course to teach you how to read an invoice."

Required

a. Identify the three main components of product cost for a manufacturing entity.

b. Explain why measuring product cost for a manufacturing entity is more complex than measuring product cost for a retail toy store.

c. Assume that Tiffany's parents rent a store for $7,500 per month. Different types of toys use different amounts of store space. For example, displaying a bicycle requires more store space than displaying a deck of cards. Also, some toys remain on the shelf longer than others. Fad toys sell quickly, but traditional toys sell more slowly. Under these circumstances, how would you determine the amount of rental cost required to display each type of toy? Identify two other costs incurred by a toy store that may be difficult to allocate to individual toys.

LO 2, 3

Exercise 10-7 *Identifying product versus general, selling, and administrative costs*

A review of the accounting records of Rayford Manufacturing indicated that the company incurred the following payroll costs during the month of August.

1. Salary of the company president—$32,000.
2. Salary of the vice president of manufacturing—$16,000.
3. Salary of the chief financial officer—$18,800.
4. Salary of the vice president of marketing—$15,600.
5. Salaries of middle managers (department heads, production supervisors) in manufacturing plant—$196,000.
6. Wages of production workers—$938,000.
7. Salaries of administrative secretaries—$112,000.
8. Salaries of engineers and other personnel responsible for maintaining production equipment—$178,000.
9. Commissions paid to sales staff—$252,000.

Required

a. What amount of payroll cost would be classified as general, selling, and administrative expense?
b. Assuming that Rayford made 4,000 units of product and sold 3,600 of them during the month of August, determine the amount of payroll cost that would be included in cost of goods sold.

LO 2, 3

Exercise 10-8 *Recording product versus general, selling, and administrative costs in a financial statements model*

Pappas Manufacturing experienced the following events during its first accounting period.

1. Recognized depreciation on manufacturing equipment.
2. Recognized depreciation on office furniture.
3. Recognized revenue from cash sale of products.
4. Recognized cost of goods sold from sale referenced in Event 3.
5. Acquired cash by issuing common stock.
6. Paid cash to purchase raw materials that were used to make products.
7. Paid wages to production workers.
8. Paid salaries to administrative staff.

Required

Use the following horizontal financial statements model to show how each event affects the balance sheet, income statement, and statement of cash flows. Indicate whether the event increases (I), decreases (D), or has no effect (NA) on each element of the financial statements. In the Cash Flow column, indicate whether the cash flow is for operating activities (OA), investing activities (IA), or financing activities (FA). The first transaction has been recorded as an example. (*Note:* Show accumulated depreciation as decrease in the book value of the appropriate asset account.)

Event No.	Assets				Equity					Cash Flow
	Cash +	Inventory +	Manuf. Equip. +	Office Furn. =	Com. Stk. +	Ret. Earn.	Rev. −	Exp. =	Net Inc.	
1.	NA	I	D	NA	NA	NA	NA	NA	NA	NA

LO 2, 3

Exercise 10-9 *Allocating product costs between ending inventory and cost of goods sold*

Howle Manufacturing Company began operations on January 1. During the year, it started and completed 1,700 units of product. The company incurred the following costs.

1. Raw materials purchased and used—$3,150.
2. Wages of production workers—$3,530.

3. Salaries of administrative and sales personnel—$1,995.
4. Depreciation on manufacturing equipment—$4,370.
5. Depreciation on administrative equipment—$1,835.

Howle sold 1,020 units of product.

Required

a. Determine the total product cost for the year.
b. Determine the total cost of the ending inventory.
c. Determine the total of cost of goods sold.

Exercise 10-10 *Financial statement effects for manufacturing versus service organizations*   **LO 6**

The following financial statements model shows the effects of recognizing depreciation in two different circumstances. One circumstance represents recognizing depreciation on a machine used in a factory. The other circumstance recognizes depreciation on computers used in a consulting firm. The effects of each event have been recorded using the letter (I) to represent increase, (D) for decrease, and (NA) for no effect.

| Event No. | Assets | | | | | Equity | | | | | | | |
	Cash	+	Inventory	+	Equip.	=	Com. Stk.	+	Ret. Earn.	Rev.	−	Exp.	=	Net Inc.	Cash Flow
1.	NA		NA		D		NA		D	NA		I		D	NA
2.	NA		I		D		NA		NA	NA		NA		NA	NA

Required

a. Identify the event that represents depreciation on the computers.
b. Explain why recognizing depreciation on equipment used in a manufacturing company affects financial statements differently from recognizing depreciation on equipment used in a service organization.

Exercise 10-11 *Identifying the effect of product versus general, selling, and administrative cost on the income statement and statement of cash flows*   **LO 3**

Each of the following events describes acquiring an asset that requires a year-end adjusting entry. December 31st is the end of year.

1. Paid $14,000 cash on January 1 to purchase printers to be used for administrative purposes. The printers had an estimated useful life of four years and a $2,000 salvage value.
2. Paid $14,000 cash on January 1 to purchase manufacturing equipment. The equipment had an estimated useful life of four years and a $2,000 salvage value.
3. Paid $12,000 cash in advance on May 1 for a one-year rental contract on administrative offices.
4. Paid $12,000 cash in advance on May 1 for a one-year rental contract on manufacturing facilities.
5. Paid $2,000 cash to purchase supplies to be used by the marketing department. At the end of the year, $400 of supplies were still on hand.
6. Paid $2,000 cash to purchase supplies to be used in the manufacturing process. At the end of the year, $400 of supplies were still on hand.

Required

Explain how acquiring the asset and making the adjusting entry affect the amount of net income and the cash flow reported on the year-end financial statements. Also, in the Cash Flow column, indicate whether the cash flow is for operating activities (OA), investing activities (IA), or financing activities (FA). Use (NA) for no effect. Assume a December 31 annual closing date.

The first event has been recorded as an example. Assume that any products that have been made have not been sold.

	Net Income	Cash Flow
Event No.	Amount of Change	Amount of Change
1. Purchase of printers	NA	(14,000) IA
1. Make adjusting entry	(3,000)	NA

LO 4

Exercise 10-12   *Missing information in a schedule of cost of goods manufactured*

Required

Supply the missing information on the following schedule of cost of goods manufactured.

DEWBERRY CORPORATION
Schedule of Cost of Goods Manufactured
For the Year Ended December 31, 2011

Raw materials		
Beginning inventory	$?	
Plus: Purchases	120,000	
Raw materials available for use	$148,000	
Minus: Ending raw materials inventory	?	
Cost of direct raw materials used		$124,000
Direct labor		?
Manufacturing overhead		24,000
Total manufacturing costs		310,000
Plus: Beginning work in process inventory		?
Total work in process		?
Minus: Ending work in process inventory		46,000
Cost of goods manufactured		$306,000

LO 4

Exercise 10-13   *Cost of goods manufactured and sold*

The following information pertains to Pandey Manufacturing Company for March 2012. Assume actual overhead equaled applied overhead.

March 1	
Inventory balances	
Raw materials	$125,000
Work in process	120,000
Finished goods	78,000
March 31	
Inventory balances	
Raw materials	$ 85,000
Work in process	145,000
Finished goods	80,000
During March	
Costs of raw materials purchased	$120,000
Costs of direct labor	100,000
Costs of manufacturing overhead	63,000
Sales revenues	350,000

Required

a. Prepare a schedule of cost of goods manufactured and sold.

b. Calculate the amount of gross margin on the income statement.

Exercise 10-14 *Upstream and downstream costs*

During 2011, Gallo Manufacturing Company incurred $90,000,000 of research and development (R&D) costs to create a long-life battery to use in computers. In accordance with FASB standards, the entire R&D cost was recognized as an expense in 2011. Manufacturing costs (direct materials, direct labor, and overhead) were expected to be $260 per unit. Packaging, shipping, and sales commissions were expected to be $50 per unit. Gallo expected to sell 2,000,000 batteries before new research renders the battery design technologically obsolete. During 2011, Gallo made 440,000 batteries and sold 400,000 of them.

Required

a. Identify the upstream and downstream costs.
b. Determine the 2011 amount of cost of goods sold and the ending inventory balance.
c. Determine the sales price assuming that Gallo desired to earn a profit margin equal to 25 percent of the *total cost* of developing, making, and distributing the batteries.
d. Prepare an income statement for 2011. Use the sales price determined in Requirement *c.*
e. Why would Gallo price the batteries at a level that would generate a loss for the 2011 accounting period?

Exercise 10-15 *Statement of Ethical Professional Practice*

In February 2006 former senator Warren Rudman of New Hampshire completed a 17-month investigation of an $11 billion accounting scandal at Fannie Mae (a major enterprise involved in home mortgage financing). The Rudman investigation concluded that Fannie Mae's CFO and controller used an accounting gimmick to manipulate financial statements in order to meet earnings-per-share (EPS) targets. Meeting the EPS targets triggered bonus payments for the executives. Fannie Mae's problems continued after 2006, and on September 8, 2008, it went into conservatorship under the control of the Federal Housing Financing Agency. The primary executives at the time of the Rudman investigation were replaced, and the enterprise reported a $59.8 billion loss in 2008.

Required

Review the principles of ethical professional practice shown in Exhibit 10.17. Identify and comment on which of the ethical principles the CFO and controller violated.

Exercise 10-16 *Using JIT to minimize waste and lost opportunity*

Ann Kyser, a teacher at Hewitt Middle School, is in charge of ordering the T-shirts to be sold for the school's annual fund-raising project. The T-shirts are printed with a special Hewitt School logo. In some years, the supply of T-shirts has been insufficient to satisfy the number of sales orders. In other years, T-shirts have been left over. Excess T-shirts are normally donated to some charitable organization. T-shirts cost the school $8 each and are normally sold for $14 each. Ms. Kyser has decided to order 800 shirts.

Required

a. If the school receives actual sales orders for 725 shirts, what amount of profit will the school earn? What is the cost of waste due to excess inventory?
b. If the school receives actual sales orders for 825 shirts, what amount of profit will the school earn? What amount of opportunity cost will the school incur?
c. Explain how a JIT inventory system could maximize profitability by eliminating waste and opportunity cost.

Exercise 10-17 *Using JIT to minimize holding costs*

Lee Pet Supplies purchases its inventory from a variety of suppliers, some of which require a six-week lead time before delivery. To ensure that she has a sufficient supply of goods on hand, Ms. Polk, the owner, must maintain a large supply of inventory. The cost of this inventory averages $21,000. She usually finances the purchase of inventory and pays a 9 percent annual finance charge. Ms. Polk's accountant has suggested that she should establish a relationship with a single large distributor who can satisfy all of her orders within a two-week time period. Given this quick turnaround time, she will be able to reduce her average inventory balance to $4,000.

Ms. Polk also believes that she could save $2,500 per year by reducing phone bills, insurance, and warehouse rental space costs associated with ordering and maintaining the larger level of inventory.

Required

a. Is the new inventory system available to Ms. Polk a pure or approximate just-in-time system?

b. Based on the information provided, how much of Ms. Polk's inventory holding cost could be eliminated by taking the accountant's advice?

LO 9

Exercise 10-18   *Value chain analysis (Appendix)*

Sonic Company manufactures and sells high-quality audio speakers. The speakers are encased in solid walnut cabinets supplied by Moore Cabinet Inc. Moore packages the speakers in durable moisture-proof boxes and ships them by truck to Sonic's manufacturing facility, which is located 50 miles from the cabinet factory.

Required

Identify the nonvalue-added activities that occur between the companies described in the above scenario. Explain how these nonvalue-added activities could be eliminated.

PROBLEMS

All applicable Problems are available with McGraw-Hill's *Connect Accounting.*

LO 2, 3

CHECK FIGURES
a. Average Cost per Unit: $8.40
f. $90,400

Problem 10-19   *Product versus general, selling, and administrative costs*

Jolly Manufacturing Company was started on January 1, 2011, when it acquired $90,000 cash by issuing common stock. Jolly immediately purchased office furniture and manufacturing equipment costing $10,000 and $28,000, respectively. The office furniture had a five-year useful life and a zero salvage value. The manufacturing equipment had a $4,000 salvage value and an expected useful life of three years. The company paid $12,000 for salaries of administrative personnel and $16,000 for wages to production personnel. Finally, the company paid $18,000 for raw materials that were used to make inventory. All inventory was started and completed during the year. Jolly completed production on 5,000 units of product and sold 4,000 units at a price of $12 each in 2011. (Assume all transactions are cash transactions.)

Required

a. Determine the total product cost and the average cost per unit of the inventory produced in 2011.

b. Determine the amount of cost of goods sold that would appear on the 2011 income statement.

c. Determine the amount of the ending inventory balance that would appear on the December 31, 2011, balance sheet.

d. Determine the amount of net income that would appear on the 2011 income statement.

e. Determine the amount of retained earnings that would appear on the December 31, 2011, balance sheet.

f. Determine the amount of total assets that would appear on the December 31, 2011, balance sheet.

g. Determine the amount of net cash flow from operating activities that would appear on the 2011 statement of cash flows.

h. Determine the amount of net cash flow from investing activities that would appear on the 2011 statement of cash flows.

LO 3

e**X**cel

CHECK FIGURES
Cash balance: $33,000
Net income: $4,600

Problem 10-20   *Effect of product versus period costs on financial statements*

Hoen Manufacturing Company experienced the following accounting events during its first year of operation. With the exception of the adjusting entries for depreciation, all transactions are cash transactions.

1. Acquired $50,000 cash by issuing common stock.

2. Paid $8,000 for the materials used to make products, all of which were started and completed during the year.

3. Paid salaries of $4,400 to selling and administrative employees.
4. Paid wages of $7,000 to production workers.
5. Paid $9,600 for furniture used in selling and administrative offices. The furniture was acquired on January 1. It had a $1,600 estimated salvage value and a four-year useful life.
6. Paid $13,000 for manufacturing equipment. The equipment was acquired on January 1. It had a $1,000 estimated salvage value and a three-year useful life.
7. Sold inventory to customers for $25,000 that had cost $14,000 to make.

Required

Explain how these events would affect the balance sheet, income statement, and statement of cash flows by recording them in a horizontal financial statements model as indicated here. The first event is recorded as an example. In the Cash Flow column, indicate whether the amounts represent financing activities (FA), investing activities (IA), or operating activities (OA).

Event No.	Assets					Equity							
	Cash	+	Inventory	+	Manuf. Equip.*	+	Office Furn.*	=	Com. Stk.	+	Ret. Earn.	Rev. − Exp. = Net Inc.	Cash Flow
1	50,000								50,000				50,000 FA

*Record accumulated depreciation as negative amounts in these columns.

Problem 10-21 *Product versus general, selling, and administrative costs*   **LO 3**

The following transactions pertain to 2012, the first year operations of Hall Company. All inventory was started and completed during 2012. Assume that all transactions are cash transactions.

CHECK FIGURES
Net income: $36
Total assets: $4,036

1. Acquired $4,000 cash by issuing common stock.
2. Paid $720 for materials used to produce inventory.
3. Paid $1,800 to production workers.
4. Paid $540 rental fee for production equipment.
5. Paid $180 to administrative employees
6. Paid $144 rental fee for administrative office equipment.
7. Produced 300 units of inventory of which 200 units were sold at a price of $12 each.

Required

Prepare an income statement, balance sheet, and statement of cash flows.

Problem 10-22 *Schedule of cost of goods manufactured and sold*   **LO 4**

Kirsoff Company makes eBook readers. The company had the following amounts at the beginning of 2011: Cash, $660,000; Raw Materials Inventory, $51,000; Work in Process Inventory, $18,000; Finished Goods Inventory, $43,000; Common Stock, $583,000; and Retained Earnings, $189,000. Kirsoff experienced the following accounting events during 2011. Other than the adjusting entries for depreciation, assume that all transactions are cash transactions.

1. Paid $23,000 of research and development costs.
2. Paid $47,000 for raw materials that will be used to make eBook readers.
3. Placed $83,000 of the raw materials cost into the process of manufacturing eBook readers.
4. Paid $60,000 for salaries of selling and administrative employees.
5. Paid $91,000 for wages of production workers.
6. Paid $90,000 to purchase equipment used in selling and administrative offices.
7. Recognized depreciation on the office equipment. The equipment was acquired on January, 1, 2011. It has a $10,000 salvage value and a five-year life. The amount of depreciation is computed as [(Cost − salvage) ÷ useful life]. Specifically, ($90,000 − $10,000) ÷ 5 = $16,000.

8. Paid $165,000 to purchase manufacturing equipment.

9. Recognized depreciation on the manufacturing equipment. The equipment was acquired on January 1, 2011. It has a $25,000 salvage value and a seven-year life. The amount of depreciation is computed as [(Cost − salvage) ÷ useful life]. Specifically, ($165,000 − $25,000) ÷ 7 = $20,000.

10. Paid $45,000 for rent and utility costs on the manufacturing facility.

11. Paid $70,000 for inventory holding expenses for completed eBook readers (rental of warehouse space, salaries of warehouse personnel, and other general storage cost).

12. Completed and transferred eBook readers that had total cost of $240,000 from work in process inventory to finished goods.

13. Sold 1,000 eBook readers for $420,000.

14. It cost Kirsoff $220,000 to make the eBook readers sold in Event 13.

Required

a. Show how these events affect the balance sheet, income statement, and statement of cash flows by recording them in a horizontal financial statements model.

b. Explain why Kirsoff's recognition of cost of goods sold had no impact on cash flow.

c. Prepare a schedule of cost of goods manufactured and sold, a formal income statement, and a balance sheet for the year.

d. Distinguish between the product costs and the upstream costs that Kirsoff incurred.

e. The company president believes that Kirsoff could save money by buying the inventory that it currently makes. The warehouse manager said that would not be a good idea because the purchase price of $230 per unit was above the $220 average cost per unit of making the product. Assuming the purchased inventory would be available on demand, explain how the company could be correct and why the production manager could be biased in his assessment of the option to buy the inventory.

LO 3, 6

CHECK FIGURES
a. Net loss: $20,000
b. Total assets: $55,000
c. Net income: $11,000

Problem 10-23 *Service versus manufacturing companies*

Goree Company began operations on January 1, 2011, by issuing common stock for $30,000 cash. During 2011, Goree received $40,000 cash from revenue and incurred costs that required $60,000 of cash payments.

Required

Prepare an income statement, balance sheet, and statement of cash flows for Goree Company for 2011, under each of the following independent scenarios.

a. Goree is a promoter of rock concerts. The $60,000 was paid to provide a rock concert that produced the revenue.

b. Goree is in the car rental business. The $60,000 was paid to purchase automobiles. The automobiles were purchased on January 1, 2011, had four-year useful lives and no expected salvage value. Goree uses straight-line depreciation. The revenue was generated by leasing the automobiles.

c. Goree is a manufacturing company. The $60,000 was paid to purchase the following items.

   (1) Paid $8,000 cash to purchase materials that were used to make products during the year.

   (2) Paid $20,000 cash for wages of factory workers who made products during the year.

   (3) Paid $2,000 cash for salaries of sales and administrative employees.

   (4) Paid $30,000 cash to purchase manufacturing equipment. The equipment was used solely to make products. It had a three-year life and a $6,000 salvage value. The company uses straight-line depreciation.

   (5) During 2011, Goree started and completed 2,000 units of product. The revenue was earned when Goree sold 1,500 units of product to its customers.

d. Refer to Requirement *c*. Could Goree determine the actual cost of making the 90th unit of product? How likely is it that the actual cost of the 90th unit of product was exactly the same as the cost of producing the 408th unit of product? Explain why management may be more interested in average cost than in actual cost.

Problem 10-24 *Importance of cost classification and ethics*

Cooke Manufacturing Company (CMC) was started when it acquired $40,000 by issuing common stock. During the first year of operations, the company incurred specifically identifiable product costs (materials, labor, and overhead) amounting to $24,000. CMC also incurred $16,000 of engineering design and planning costs. There was a debate regarding how the design and planning costs should be classified. Advocates of Option 1 believe that the costs should be classified as upstream general, selling, and administrative costs. Advocates of Option 2 believe it is more appropriate to classify the design and planning costs as product costs. During the year, CMC made 4,000 units of product and sold 3,000 units at a price of $24 each. All transactions were cash transactions.

Required

a. Prepare an income statement, balance sheet, and statement of cash flows under each of the two options.

b. Identify the option that results in financial statements that are more likely to leave a favorable impression on investors and creditors.

c. Assume that CMC provides an incentive bonus to the CFO who is a CMA. The bonus is equal to 13 percent of net income. Compute the amount of the bonus under each of the two options. Identify the option that provides the CFO with the higher bonus.

d. Assume the CFO knows that the design and planning costs are upstream costs that must be recognized as general, selling, and administrative expenses (Option 1). Even so, the CFO convinces management to classify the upstream costs as product cost in order to increase his bonus. Identify two principles in the Statement of Ethical Professional Practice that are violated by the CFO's behavior.

e. Comment on the conflict of interest between the company president as determined in Requirement *c* and owners of the company as indicated in Requirement *d*. Describe an incentive compensation plan that would avoid a conflict of interest between the president and the owners.

Problem 10-25 *Using JIT to reduce inventory holding costs*

Burt Manufacturing Company obtains its raw materials from a variety of suppliers. Burt's strategy is to obtain the best price by letting the suppliers know that it buys from the lowest bidder. Approximately four years ago, unexpected increase in demand resulted in materials shortages. Burt was unable to find the materials it needed even though it was willing to pay premium prices. Because of the lack of raw materials, Burt was forced to close its manufacturing facility for two weeks. Its president vowed that her company would never again be at the mercy of its suppliers. She immediately ordered her purchasing agent to perpetually maintain a one-month supply of raw materials. Compliance with the president's orders resulted in a raw materials inventory amounting to approximately $1,600,000. Warehouse rental and personnel costs to maintain the inventory amounted to $8,000 per month. Burt has a line of credit with a local bank that calls for a 12 percent annual rate of interest. Assume that Burt finances the raw materials inventory with the line of credit.

Required

a. Based on the information provided, determine the annual holding cost of the raw materials inventory.

b. Explain how a JIT system could reduce Burt's inventory holding cost.

c. Explain how most-favored customer status could enable Burt to establish a JIT inventory system without risking the raw materials shortages experienced in the past.

Problem 10-26 *Using JIT to minimize waste and lost opportunity*

CMA Review Inc. provides review courses for students studying to take the CMA exam. The cost of textbooks is included in the registration fee. Text material requires constant updating and is useful for only one course. To minimize printing costs and ensure availability of books on the first day of class, CMA Review has books printed and delivered to its offices two weeks in advance of the first class. To ensure that enough books are available, CMA Review normally orders 10 percent more than expected enrollment. Usually there is an oversupply of books that is thrown away. However, demand occasionally exceeds expectations by more than 10 percent and there are too few books available for student use. CMA Review had been forced to turn away students because of lack of textbooks. CMA Review expects to enroll approximately 100 students per course. The tuition fee is $800 per student. The cost of teachers is $25,000 per course, textbooks cost $60 each, and other operating expenses are estimated to be $35,000 per course.

Required

a. Prepare an income statement, assuming that 95 students enroll in a course. Determine the cost of waste associated with unused books.

b. Prepare an income statement, assuming that 115 students attempt to enroll in the course. Note that five students are turned away because of too few textbooks. Determine the amount of lost profit resulting from the inability to serve the five additional students.

c. Suppose that textbooks can be produced through a high-speed copying process that permits delivery *just in time* for class to start. The cost of books made using this process, however, is $65 each. Assume that all books must be made using the same production process. In other words, CMA Review cannot order some of the books using the regular copy process and the rest using the high-speed process. Prepare an income statement under the JIT system assuming that 95 students enroll in a course. Compare the income statement under JIT with the income statement prepared in Requirement *a*. Comment on how the JIT system would affect profitability.

d. Assume the same facts as in Requirement *c* with respect to a JIT system that enables immediate delivery of books at a cost of $65 each. Prepare an income statement under the JIT system, assuming that 115 students enroll in a course. Compare the income statement under JIT with the income statement prepared in Requirement *b*. Comment on how the JIT system would affect profitability.

e. Discuss the possible effect of the JIT system on the level of customer satisfaction.

LO 9

Problem 10-27 *Value chain analysis (Appendix)*

Jensen Company invented a new process for manufacturing ice cream. The ingredients are mixed in high-tech machinery that forms the product into small round beads. Like a bag of balls, the ice cream beads are surrounded by air pockets in packages. This design has numerous advantages. First, each bite of ice cream melts quickly in a person's mouth, creating a more flavorful sensation when compared to ordinary ice cream. Also, the air pockets mean that a typical serving includes a smaller amount of ice cream. This not only reduces materials cost but also provides the consumer with a low-calorie snack. A cup appears full of ice cream, but it is really half full of air. The consumer eats only half the ingredients that are contained in a typical cup of blended ice cream. Finally, the texture of the ice cream makes scooping it out of a large container easy. The frustration of trying to get a spoon into a rock-solid package of blended ice cream has been eliminated. Jensen Company named the new product Sonic Cream.

Like many other ice cream producers, Jensen Company purchases its raw materials from a food wholesaler. The ingredients are mixed in Jensen's manufacturing plant. The packages of finished product are distributed to privately owned franchise ice cream shops that sell Sonic Cream directly to the public.

Jensen provides national advertising and is responsible for all research and development costs associated with making new flavors of Sonic Cream.

Required

a. Based on the information provided, draw a comprehensive value chain for Jensen Company that includes its suppliers and customers.

b. Identify the place in the chain where Jensen Company is exercising its opportunity to create added value beyond that currently being provided by its competitors.

ANALYZE, THINK, COMMUNICATE

ATC 10-1   Business Applications Case   *Financial versus managerial accounting*

The following information was taken from the 2008 and 2009 Form 10-Ks for Dell, Inc.

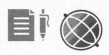

	Fiscal Year Ended	
	January 30, 2009	**February 1, 2008**
Number of regular employees	76,500	82,700
Number of temporary employees	2,400	5,500
Revenues (in millions)	$61,101	$61,133
Properties owned or leased in the U.S.	7.4 million square feet	8.2 million square feet
Properties owned or leased outside the U.S.	9.4 million square feet	9.7 million square feet
Total assets (in millions)	$26,500	$27,561
Gross margin (in millions)	$10,957	$11,671

Required

a. Explain whether each line of information in the table above would best be described as being primarily financial accounting or managerial accounting in nature.

b. Provide some additional examples of managerial and financial accounting information that could apply to Dell.

c. If you analyze only the data you identified as financial in nature, does it appear that Dell's 2009 fiscal year was better or worse than its 2008 fiscal year? Explain.

d. If you analyze only the data you identified as managerial in nature, does it appear that Dell's 2009 fiscal year was better or worse than its 2008 fiscal year? Explain.

ATC 10-2   Group Assignment   *Product versus upstream and downstream costs*

Victor Holt, the accounting manager of Sexton Inc., gathered the following information for 2011. Some of it can be used to construct an income statement for 2011. Ignore items that do not appear on an income statement. Some computations may be required. For example, the cost of manufacturing equipment would not appear on the income statement. However, the cost of manufacturing equipment is needed to compute the amount of depreciation. All units of product were started and completed in 2011.

1. Issued $864,000 of common stock.
2. Paid engineers in the product design department $10,000 for salaries that were accrued at the end of the previous year.
3. Incurred advertising expenses of $70,000.
4. Paid $720,000 for materials used to manufacture the company's product.
5. Incurred utility costs of $160,000. These costs were allocated to different departments on the basis of square footage of floor space. Mr. Holt identified three departments and determined the square footage of floor space for each department to be as shown in the table below.

Department	Square Footage
Research and development	10,000
Manufacturing	60,000
Selling and administrative	30,000
Total	100,000

6. Paid $880,000 for wages of production workers.
7. Paid cash of $658,000 for salaries of administrative personnel. There was $16,000 of accrued salaries owed to administrative personnel at the end of 2011. There was no beginning balance in the Salaries Payable account for administrative personnel.
8. Purchased manufacturing equipment two years ago at a cost of $10,000,000. The equipment had an eight-year useful life and a $2,000,000 salvage value.

9. Paid $390,000 cash to engineers in the product design department.
10. Paid a $258,000 cash dividend to owners.
11. Paid $80,000 to set up manufacturing equipment for production.
12. Paid a one-time $186,000 restructuring cost to redesign the production process to implement a just-in-time inventory system.
13. Prepaid the premium on a new insurance policy covering nonmanufacturing employees. The policy cost $72,000 and had a one-year term with an effective starting date of May 1. Four employees work in the research and development department and eight employees in the selling and administrative department. Assume a December 31 closing date.
14. Made 69,400 units of product and sold 60,000 units at a price of $70 each.

Required

a. Divide the class into groups of four or five students per group, and then organize the groups into three sections. Assign Task 1 to the first section of groups, Task 2 to the second section of groups, and Task 3 to the third section of groups.

Group Tasks

(1) Identify the items that are classified as product costs and determine the amount of cost of goods sold reported on the 2011 income statement.
(2) Identify the items that are classified as upstream costs and determine the amount of upstream cost expensed on the 2011 income statement.
(3) Identify the items that are classified as downstream costs and determine the amount of downstream cost expensed on the 2011 income statement.

b. Have the class construct an income statement in the following manner. Select a member of one of the groups assigned the first group task identifying the product costs. Have that person go to the board and list the costs included in the determination of cost of goods sold. Anyone in the other groups who disagrees with one of the classifications provided by the person at the board should voice an objection and explain why the item should be classified differently. The instructor should lead the class to a consensus on the disputed items. After the amount of cost of goods sold is determined, the student at the board constructs the part of the income statement showing the determination of gross margin. The exercise continues in a similar fashion with representatives from the other sections explaining the composition of the upstream and downstream costs. These items are added to the income statement started by the first group representative. The final result is a completed income statement.

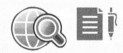

ATC 10-3   **Research Assignment**   *Identifying product costs at Snap-on, Inc.*

Use the 2008 Form 10-K for Snap-on, Inc., to complete the requirements below. To obtain the Form 10-K you can use the EDGAR system following the instructions in Appendix A, or it can be found under "Corporate Information" on the company's corporate website: www.snapon.com. Read carefully the following portions of the document.

■ "Products and Services" on page 5.
■ "Consolidated Statement of Earnings" on page 55.
■ The following parts of Note 1 on page 60:
   • "Shipping and handling"
   • "Advertising and promotion"
■ "Note 4: Inventories" on page 66.

Required

a. Does the level of detail that Snap-on provides regarding costs incurred to manufacture its products suggest the company's financial statements are designed primarily to meet the needs of external or internal users?
b. Does Snap-on treat shipping and handling costs as product or nonproduct costs?
c. Does Snap-on treat advertising and promotion costs as product or nonproduct costs?
d. In Chapter 3 you learned about a class of inventory called merchandise inventory. What categories of inventory does Snap-on report in its annual report?

ATC 10-4 Writing Assignment *Emerging practices in managerial accounting*

An annual report of the Maytag Corporation contained the following excerpt:

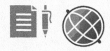

> *The Company announced the restructuring of its major appliance operations in an effort to strengthen its position in the industry and to deliver improved performance to both customers and shareowners. This included the consolidation of two separate organizational units into a single operation responsible for all activities associated with the manufacture and distribution of the Company's brands of major appliances and the closing of a cooking products plant in Indianapolis, Indiana, with transfer of that production to an existing plant in Cleveland, Tennessee.*

The restructuring cost Maytag $40 million and disrupted the lives of many of the company's employees.

Required

Assume that you are Maytag's vice president of human relations. Write a letter to the employees who are affected by the restructuring. The letter should explain why it was necessary for the company to undertake the restructuring. Your explanation should refer to the ideas discussed in the section "Emerging Trends in Managerial Accounting" of this chapter (see Appendix A).

ATC 10-5 Ethical Dilemma *Product cost versus selling and administrative expense*

Emma Emerson is a proud woman with a problem. Her daughter has been accepted into a prestigious law school. While Ms. Emerson beams with pride, she is worried sick about how to pay for the school; she is a single parent who has to support herself and her three children. She had to go heavily into debt to finance her own education. Even though she now has a good job, family needs have continued to outpace her income and her debt burden is staggering. She knows she will be unable to borrow the money needed for her daughter's law school.

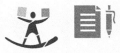

Ms. Emerson is the chief financial officer (CFO) of a small manufacturing company. She has just accepted a new job offer. She has not yet told her employer that she will be leaving in a month. She is concerned that her year-end incentive bonus may be affected if her boss learns of her plans to leave. She plans to inform the company immediately after receiving the bonus. She knows her behavior is less than honorable, but she believes that she has been underpaid for a long time. Her boss, a relative of the company's owner, makes twice what she makes and does half the work. Why should she care about leaving with a little extra cash? Indeed, she is considering an opportunity to boost the bonus.

Ms. Emerson's bonus is based on a percentage of net income. Her company recently introduced a new product line that required substantial production start-up costs. Ms. Emerson is fully aware that GAAP requires these costs to be expensed in the current accounting period, but no one else in the company has the technical expertise to know exactly how the costs should be treated. She is considering misclassifying the start-up costs as product costs. If the costs are misclassified, net income will be significantly higher, resulting in a nice boost in her incentive bonus. By the time the auditors discover the misclassification, Ms. Emerson will have moved on to her new job. If the matter is brought to the attention of her new employer, she will simply plead ignorance. Considering her daughter's needs, Ms. Emerson decides to classify the start-up costs as product costs.

Required

a. Based on this information, indicate whether Ms. Emerson believes the number of units of product sold will be equal to, less than, or greater than the number of units made. Write a brief paragraph explaining the logic that supports your answer.

b. Explain how the misclassification could mislead an investor or creditor regarding the company's financial condition.

c. Explain how the misclassification could affect income taxes.

d. Identify the specific components of the fraud triangle the were present in this case.

e. Review the Statement of Ethical Professional Practice shown in Exhibit 10.14 and identify at least two principles that Ms. Emerson's misclassification of the start-up costs violated.

f. Describe the maximum penalty that could be imposed under the Sarbanes-Oxley Act for the actions Ms. Emerson has taken.

CHAPTER 11

Cost Behavior, Operating Leverage, and Profitability Analysis

LEARNING OBJECTIVES

After you have mastered the material in this chapter, you will be able to:

1 Identify and describe fixed, variable, and mixed cost behavior.

2 Demonstrate the effects of operating leverage on profitability.

3 Prepare an income statement using the contribution margin approach.

4 Calculate the magnitude of operating leverage.

5 Demonstrate how the relevant range and decision context affect cost behavior.

6 Calculate the break-even point.

7 Calculate the sales volume required to attain a target profit.

8 Calculate the margin of safety in units, dollars, and percentage.

CHAPTER OPENING

Three college students are planning a vacation. One of them suggests inviting a fourth person along, remarking that four can travel for the same cost as three. Certainly, some costs will be the same whether three or four people go on the trip. For example, the hotel room costs $800 per week, regardless of whether three or four people stay in the room. In accounting terms the cost of the hotel room is a fixed cost. The total amount of a fixed cost does not change when volume changes. The total hotel room cost is $800 whether 1, 2, 3, or 4 people use the room. In contrast, some costs vary in direct proportion with changes in volume. When volume increases, total variable cost increases; when volume decreases, total variable cost decreases. For example, the cost of tickets to a theme park is a **variable cost**. The total cost of tickets increases proportionately with each vacationer who goes to the theme park. Cost behavior (fixed versus variable) can significantly impact profitability. This chapter explains cost behavior and ways it can be used to increase profitability.

The Curious Accountant

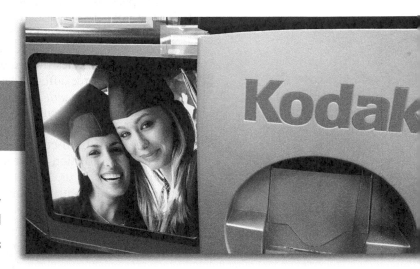

News flash! On April 29, 2009, Eastman Kodak, Inc., announced that its first quarter's revenues decreased 29 percent compared to the same quarter in 2008, yet its earnings had decreased by 213 percent. On May 4, 2009, Walt Disney announced that a decrease in revenue of 7 percent for the just-ended quarter would cause its earnings to decrease 46 percent compared to the same quarter in 2008. On April 12, 2009, Apple computer reported that its revenue for the quarter had increased by 9 percent compared to the previous year, but its earnings increased by 15 percent.

Can you explain why such relatively small changes in these companies' revenues resulted in such relatively large changes in their earnings or losses? In other words, if a company's sales increase 10 percent, why do its earnings not also increase 10 percent? (Answer on page 402.)

FIXED COST BEHAVIOR

LO 1

Identify and describe fixed, variable, and mixed cost behavior.

How much more will it cost to send one additional employee to a sales meeting? If more people buy our products, can we charge less? If sales increase by 10 percent, how will profits be affected? Managers seeking answers to such questions must consider **cost behavior.** Knowing how costs behave relative to the level of business activity enables managers to more effectively plan and control costs. To illustrate, consider the entertainment company Star Productions, Inc. (SPI).

SPI specializes in promoting rock concerts. It is considering paying a band $48,000 to play a concert. Obviously, SPI must sell enough tickets to cover this cost. In this example, the relevant activity base is the number of tickets sold. The cost of the band is a **fixed cost** because it does not change regardless of the number of tickets sold. Exhibit 11.1 illustrates the fixed cost behavior pattern, showing the *total cost* and the *cost per unit* at three different levels of activity.

Total versus *per-unit* fixed costs behave differently. The total cost for the band remains constant (fixed) at $48,000. In contrast, fixed cost per unit decreases as volume (number of tickets sold) increases. The term *fixed cost* is consistent with the behavior of *total cost.* Total fixed cost remains constant (fixed) when activity changes. However, there is a contradiction between the term *fixed cost per unit* and the *per-unit behavior pattern of a fixed cost.* Fixed cost per unit is *not* fixed. It changes with the number of tickets sold. This contradiction in terminology can cause untold confusion. Study carefully the fixed cost behavior patterns in Exhibit 11.2.

EXHIBIT 11.1

Fixed Cost Behavior

Number of tickets sold (a)	2,700	3,000	3,300
Total cost of band (b)	$48,000	$48,000	$48,000
Cost per ticket sold (b ÷ a)	$17.78	$16.00	$14.55

EXHIBIT 11.2

Fixed Cost Behavior

	When Activity Increases	When Activity Decreases
Total fixed cost	Remains constant	Remains constant
Fixed cost **per unit**	Decreases	Increases

The fixed cost data in Exhibit 11.1 help SPI's management decide whether to sponsor the concert. For example, the information influences potential pricing choices. The per-unit costs represent the minimum ticket prices required to cover the fixed cost at various levels of activity. SPI could compare these per-unit costs to the prices of competing entertainment events (such as the prices of movies, sporting events, or theater tickets). If the price is not competitive, tickets will not sell and the concert will lose money. Management must also consider the number of tickets to be sold. The volume data in Exhibit 11.1 can be compared to the band's track record of ticket sales at previous concerts. A proper analysis of these data can reduce the risk of undertaking an unprofitable venture.

OPERATING LEVERAGE

LO 2

Demonstrate the effects of operating leverage on profitability.

Heavy objects can be moved with little effort using *physical* leverage. Business managers apply **operating leverage** to magnify small changes in revenue into dramatic changes in profitability. The *lever* managers use to achieve disproportionate changes between revenue and profitability is fixed costs. The leverage relationships between revenue, fixed costs, and profitability are displayed in Exhibit 11.3.

When all costs are fixed, every sales dollar contributes one dollar toward the potential profitability of a project. Once sales dollars cover fixed costs, each

EXHIBIT 11.3

Operating Leverage

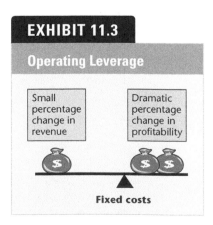

Small percentage change in revenue

Dramatic percentage change in profitability

Fixed costs

FOCUS ON INTERNATIONAL ISSUES

COST-VOLUME-PROFIT ANALYSIS AT A GERMAN CHEMICAL COMPANY

The greater the percentage of a company's total costs that are fixed, the more sensitive the company's earnings are to changes in revenue or volume. Operating leverage, the relationship between the changes in revenue and changes in earnings, introduced earlier, applies to companies throughout the world, large or small.

Large chemical manufacturers have significant fixed costs. It takes a lot of buildings and equipment to produce chemicals. BASF claims to be the largest chemical company in the world. It has its headquarters in Ludwigshafen, Germany. From 2004 through 2006 BASF's revenues increased 40.2 percent, but its earnings increased 60.4 percent. In other words, its earnings grew one and one-half times faster than its revenues.

Studying BASF offers insight into a true global enterprise. Though headquartered in Germany, it has manufacturing facilities at 150 locations throughout the world. Only 21 percent of its 2006 revenue came from sales within Germany, which was 1 percent less than the revenue it earned in the United States. Although its financial statements are presented in euros and prepared in accordance with international financial accounting standards, its stock is traded on the New York Stock Exchange as well as on the Frankfurt Stock Exchange.

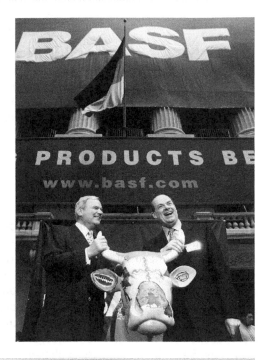

additional sales dollar represents pure profit. As a result, a small change in sales volume can significantly affect profitability. To illustrate, assume SPI estimates it will sell 3,000 tickets for $18 each. A 10 percent difference in actual sales volume will produce a 90 percent difference in profitability. Examine the data in Exhibit 11.4 to verify this result.[1]

EXHIBIT 11.4

Effect of Operating Leverage on Profitability

Number of tickets sold	2,700	⇐ −10% ⇐	3,000	⇒ +10% ⇒	3,300
Sales revenue ($18 per ticket)	$48,600		$54,000		$59,400
Cost of band (fixed cost)	(48,000)		(48,000)		(48,000)
Gross margin	$ 600	⇐ −90% ⇐	$ 6,000	⇒ +90% ⇒	$11,400

Calculating Percentage Change

The percentages in Exhibit 11.4 are computed as follows.

$$(\text{Alternative measure} - \text{Base measure}) \div \text{Base measure} = \% \text{ change}$$

The base measure is the starting point. To illustrate, compute the percentage change in gross margin when moving from 3,000 units (base measure) to 3,300 units (the alternative measure).

$$(\text{Alternative measure} - \text{Base measure}) \div \text{Base measure} = \% \text{ change}$$

$$(\$11,400 - \$6,000) \div \$6,000 = 90\%$$

---

[1]Do not confuse operating leverage with financial leverage. Companies employ *financial leverage* when they use debt to profit from investing money at a higher rate of return than the rate they pay on borrowed money. Companies employ *operating leverage* when they use proportionately more fixed costs than variable costs to magnify the effect on earnings of changes in revenues.

The percentage *decline* in profitability is similarly computed:

(Alternative measure − Base measure) ÷ Base measure = % change

($600 − $6,000) ÷ $6,000 = (90%)

Risk and Reward Assessment

Risk refers to the possibility that sacrifices may exceed benefits. A fixed cost represents a commitment to an economic sacrifice. It represents the ultimate risk of undertaking a particular business project. If SPI pays the band but nobody buys a ticket, the company will lose $48,000. SPI can avoid this risk by substituting *variable costs* for the *fixed cost*.

REALITY BYTES

The relationship among the costs to produce goods, the volume of goods produced, the price charged for those goods, and the profit earned is relevant to all industries, but perhaps no industry demonstrates the effects of these relationships more dramatically than automobile manufacturing. First, the automobile industry is characterized by having a lot of fixed production-costs for things such as buildings, equipment, research, and development, but also financing costs associated with borrowed funds, such as the interest expense on bonds. Second, the industry is globally competitive, and companies in the United States are often at a cost disadvantage. Some of this cost disadvantage comes from obvious sources, such as having to pay higher wages than do companies in countries such as South Korea. Finally, for many customers, price and quality are more important than brand loyalty.

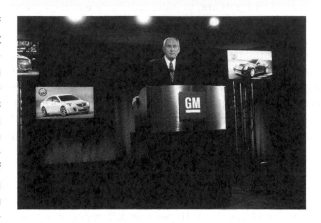

Over the past decades, domestic auto makers, and in particular General Motors (GM), have used different strategies to try to deal with the issues mentioned above. Early on, it had a dominant market share. As long as it produced more cars than its competitors, its fixed cost per car was lower, resulting in better profits. In the 1980s, however, foreign manufactures began increasing their market share and decreasing GM's. As its relative levels of production fell, its fixed cost per unit increased. In response, GM and others tried to regain market share by lowering prices, largely through rebates. Unfortunately this did not work, so the lower prices, combined with the higher relative fixed costs, seriously eroded profits.

These problems reached a crisis in 2008 and 2009 when GM and Chrysler sought financial help from the government and entered expedited bankruptcy proceedings.

What did GM and Chrysler hope to achieve? Primarily they needed to lower their costs, especially their fixed costs. As a result of bankruptcy proceedings, they were able to greatly reduce interest and principal payments on their outstanding bonds (fixed costs), reduce the number of brands (fixed costs), shut down some plants (fixed costs), reduce health care costs to retirees (fixed costs), and reduce the number of dealers. While reducing the number of dealers did reduce some cost to the companies, it also reduced price competition among the dealers, which had the potential of allowing the companies to charge more for their cars. All of these changes, it was hoped, would allow the companies to return to profitability.

However, before a company can be profitable, it must break even. At one time GM's break-even point was estimated at around 16 million vehicles per year. GM's CEO until 2000, Rick Wagoner, had implemented changes that reduced the company's break-even point to 12 million units. On March 29, 2009, as a condition of receiving government support, the administration of President Barack Obama asked Mr. Wagoner to resign as GM's CEO. Perhaps lost by many in the news coverage of Mr. Wagoner's resignation were reports by several news organizations that officials at the U.S. Treasury Department would ask the new leadership at GM to take steps to reduce the company's break-even point to 10 million units.

It would be a major achievement if GM can reduce its break even from 16 million units to 10 million units in the span of a few years. This may not be enough, however. In 2008 GM sold only 8.8 million units, and its sales in the first quarter of 2009 were even lower than the same quarter of 2008. Furthermore, it should be remembered that the objective of businesses is not simply to break even, but to make a profit.

VARIABLE COST BEHAVIOR

To illustrate variable cost behavior, assume SPI arranges to pay the band $16 per ticket sold instead of a fixed $48,000. Exhibit 11.5 shows the total cost of the band and the cost per ticket sold at three different levels of activity.

Identify and describe fixed, variable, and mixed cost behavior.

EXHIBIT 11.5

Variable Cost Behavior

Number of tickets sold (a)	2,700	3,000	3,300
Total cost of band (b)	$43,200	$48,000	$52,800
Cost per ticket sold (b ÷ a)	$16	$16	$16

Because SPI will pay the band $16 for each ticket sold, the *total* variable cost increases in direct proportion to the number of tickets sold. If SPI sells one ticket, total band cost will be $16 (1 × $16); if SPI sells two tickets, total band cost will be $32 (2 × $16); and so on. The total cost of the band increases proportionately as ticket sales move from 2,700 to 3,000 to 3,300. The variable cost *per ticket* remains $16, however, regardless of whether the number of tickets sold is 1, 2, 3, or 3,000. The behavior of variable cost *per unit* is contradictory to the word *variable.* Variable cost per unit remains *constant* regardless of how many tickets are sold. Study carefully the variable cost behavior patterns in Exhibit 11.6.

EXHIBIT 11.6

Variable Cost Behavior

	When Activity Increases	When Activity Decreases
Total variable cost	Increases proportionately	Decreases proportionately
Variable cost **per unit**	Remains constant	Remains constant

Risk and Reward Assessment

Shifting the cost structure from fixed to variable enables SPI to avoid the fixed cost risk. If no one buys a ticket, SPI loses nothing because it incurs no cost. If only one person buys a ticket at an $18 ticket price, SPI earns a $2 profit ($18 sales revenue − $16 cost of band). Should managers therefore avoid fixed costs whenever possible? Not necessarily.

Shifting the cost structure from fixed to variable reduces not only the level of risk but also the potential for profits. Managers cannot avoid the risk of fixed costs without also sacrificing the benefits. Variable costs do not offer operating leverage. Exhibit 11.7 shows that a variable cost structure produces a proportional relationship between sales and profitability. A 10 percent increase or decrease in sales results in a corresponding 10 percent increase or decrease in profitability.

Demonstrate the effects of operating leverage on profitability.

EXHIBIT 11.7

Variable Cost Eliminates Operating Leverage

Number of tickets sold	2,700	⇐ −10% ⇐	3,000	⇒ +10% ⇒	3,300
Sales revenue ($18 per ticket)	$48,600		$54,000		$59,400
Cost of band ($16 variable cost)	(43,200)		(48,000)		(52,800)
Gross margin	$ 5,400	⇐ −10% ⇐	$ 6,000	⇒ +10% ⇒	$ 6,600

✓ CHECK YOURSELF 11.1

Suppose that you are sponsoring a political rally at which Ralph Nader will speak. You estimate that approximately 2,000 people will buy tickets to hear Mr. Nader's speech. The tickets are expected to be priced at $12 each. Would you prefer a contract that agrees to pay Mr. Nader $10,000 or one that agrees to pay him $5 per ticket purchased?

Answer   Your answer would depend on how certain you are that 2,000 people will purchase tickets. If it were likely that many more than 2,000 tickets would be sold, you would be better off with a fixed cost structure, agreeing to pay Mr. Nader a flat fee of $10,000. If attendance numbers are highly uncertain, you would be better off with a variable cost structure thereby guaranteeing a lower cost if fewer people buy tickets.

Answers to The Curious Accountant

The explanation for how a company's earnings can rise faster, as a percentage, than its revenue rises is operating leverage, and operating leverage is due entirely to fixed costs. As the chapter explains, when a company's output goes up, its fixed cost per unit goes down. As long as it can keep prices about the same, this lower unit cost will result in higher profit per unit sold. In real-world companies, the relationship between changing sales levels and changing earnings levels can be very complex, but the existence of fixed costs helps to explain why a 9 percent rise in revenue can cause a 15 percent rise in net earnings.

✓ CHECK YOURSELF 11.2

If both Kroger Food Stores and Delta Airlines were to experience a 5 percent increase in revenues, which company would be more likely to experience a higher percentage increase in net income?

Answer   Delta would be more likely to experience a higher percentage increase in net income because a large portion of its cost (e.g., employee salaries and depreciation) is fixed, while a large portion of Kroger's cost is variable (e.g., cost of goods sold).

AN INCOME STATEMENT UNDER THE CONTRIBUTION MARGIN APPROACH

LO 3

Prepare an income statement using the contribution margin approach.

The impact of cost structure on profitability is so significant that managerial accountants frequently construct income statements that classify costs according to their behavior patterns. Such income statements first subtract variable costs from revenue; the resulting subtotal is called the **contribution margin.** The contribution margin represents the amount available to cover fixed expenses and thereafter to provide company profits. Net income is computed by subtracting the fixed costs from the contribution margin. A contribution margin style income statement cannot be used for public reporting (GAAP prohibits its use in external financial reports), but it is widely used for internal reporting purposes. Exhibit 11.8 illustrates income statements prepared using the contribution margin approach.

EXHIBIT 11.8

Income Statements

	Company Name	
	Bragg	Biltmore
Variable cost per unit (a)	$ 6	$ 12
Sales revenue (10 units × $20)	$200	$200
Variable cost (10 units × a)	(60)	(120)
Contribution margin	140	80
Fixed cost	(120)	(60)
Net income	$ 20	$ 20

MEASURING OPERATING LEVERAGE USING CONTRIBUTION MARGIN

A contribution margin income statement allows managers to easily measure operating leverage. The magnitude of operating leverage can be determined as follows.

$$\text{Magnitude of operating leverage} = \frac{\text{Contribution margin}}{\text{Net income}}$$

Calculate the magnitude of operating leverage.

Applying this formula to the income statement data reported for Bragg Company and Biltmore Company in Exhibit 11.8 produces the following measures.

Bragg Company:

$$\text{Magnitude of operating leverage} = \frac{140}{20} = 7$$

Biltmore Company:

$$\text{Magnitude of operating leverage} = \frac{80}{20} = 4$$

The computations show that Bragg is more highly leveraged than Biltmore. Bragg's change in profitability will be seven times greater than a given percentage change in revenue. In contrast, Biltmore's profits change by only four times the percentage change in revenue. For example, a 10 percent increase in revenue produces a 70 percent increase (10 percent × 7) in profitability for Bragg Company and a 40 percent increase (10 percent × 4) in profitability for Biltmore Company. The income statements in Exhibits 11.9 and 11.10 confirm these expectations.

EXHIBIT 11.9

Comparative Income Statements for Bragg Company

Units (a)	10		11
Sales revenue ($20 × a)	$200	⇒ +10% ⇒	$220
Variable cost ($6 × a)	(60)		(66)
Contribution margin	140		154
Fixed cost	(120)		(120)
Net income	$ 20	⇒ +70% ⇒	$ 34

EXHIBIT 11.10

Comparative Income Statements for Biltmore Company

Units (a)	10		11
Sales revenue ($20 × a)	$200	⇒ +10% ⇒	$220
Variable cost ($12 × a)	(120)		(132)
Contribution margin	80		88
Fixed cost	(60)		(60)
Net income	$ 20	⇒ +40% ⇒	$ 28

Operating leverage itself is neither good nor bad; it represents a strategy that can work to a company's advantage or disadvantage, depending on how it is used. The next section explains how managers can use operating leverage to create a competitive business advantage.

✓ CHECK YOURSELF 11.3

Boeing Company's 2001 10K annual report filed with the Securities and Exchange Commission refers to "higher commercial airlines segment margins." Is Boeing referring to gross margins or contribution margins?

Answer Because the data come from the company's external annual report, the reference must be to gross margins (revenue − cost of goods sold), a product cost measure. The contribution margin (revenue − variable cost) is a measure used in internal reporting.

COST BEHAVIOR SUMMARIZED

Identify and describe fixed, variable, and mixed cost behavior.

The term *fixed* refers to the behavior of *total* fixed cost. The cost *per unit* of a fixed cost *varies inversely* with changes in the level of activity. As activity increases, fixed cost per unit decreases. As activity decreases, fixed cost per unit increases. These relationships are graphed in Exhibit 11.11.

The term *variable* refers to the behavior of *total* variable cost. Total variable cost increases or decreases proportionately with changes in the volume of activity. In contrast, variable cost *per unit* remains *fixed* at all levels of activity. These relationships are graphed in Exhibit 11.12.

The relationships between fixed and variable costs are summarized in the chart in Exhibit 11.13. Study these relationships thoroughly.

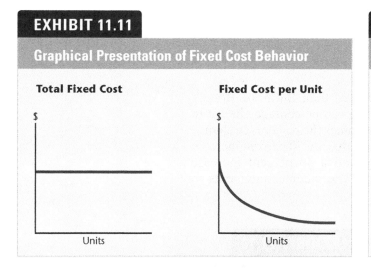

EXHIBIT 11.11

Graphical Presentation of Fixed Cost Behavior

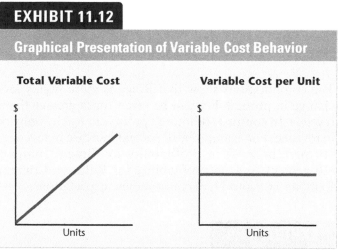

EXHIBIT 11.12

Graphical Presentation of Variable Cost Behavior

EXHIBIT 11.13

Fixed and Variable Cost Behavior

When Activity Level Changes	Total Cost	Cost per Unit
Fixed costs	Remains constant	Changes *inversely*
Variable costs	Changes in direct proportion	Remains constant

Mixed Costs (Semivariable Costs)

Mixed costs (semivariable costs) include both fixed and variable components. For example, Star Productions, Inc., frequently arranges backstage parties at which VIP guests meet members of the band. Party costs typically include a room rental fee and the costs of refreshments. The room rental fee is fixed; it remains unchanged regardless of the number of party guests. In contrast, the refreshments costs are variable; they depend on the number of people attending the party. The total party cost is a mixed cost.

Assuming a room rental fee of $1,000 and refreshments costs of $20 per person, the total mixed cost at any volume of activity can be computed as follows.

$$\text{Total cost} = \text{Fixed cost} + (\text{Variable cost per party guest} \times \text{Number of guests})$$

If 60 people attend the backstage party the total mixed cost is

$$\text{Total cost} = \$1,000 + (\$20 \times 60) = \$2,200$$

If 90 people attend the backstage party the total mixed cost is

$$\text{Total cost} = \$1,000 + (\$20 \times 90) = \$2,800$$

Exhibit 11.14 illustrates a variety of mixed costs businesses commonly encounter.

EXHIBIT 11.14

Examples of Mixed Costs

Type of Cost	Fixed Cost Component(s)	Variable Cost Component(s)
Cost of sales staff	Monthly salary	Bonus based on sales volume
Truck rental	Monthly rental fee	Cost of gas, tires, and maintenance
Legal fees	Monthly retainer	Reimbursements to attorney for out-of-pocket costs (copying, postage, travel, filing fees)
Outpatient service cost	Salaries of doctors and nurses, depreciation of facility, utilities	Medical supplies such as bandages, sterilization solution, and paper products
Phone services	Monthly connection fee	Per-minute usage fee
LP gas utility cost	Container rental fee	Cost of gas consumed
Cable TV services	Monthly fee	Pay-per-view charges
Training cost	Instructor salary, facility cost	Textbooks, supplies
Shipping and handling	Salaries of employees who process packages	Boxes, packing supplies, tape, and other shipping supplies, postage
Inventory holding cost	Depreciation on inventory warehouse, salaries of employees managing inventory	Delivery costs, interest on funds borrowed to finance inventory, cost of supplies

The Relevant Range

Suppose SPI, the rock concert promoter mentioned earlier, must pay $5,000 to rent a concert hall with a seating capacity of 4,000 people. Is the cost of the concert hall fixed or variable? Because total cost remains unchanged regardless of whether one ticket, 4,000 tickets, or any number in between is sold, the cost is fixed relative to ticket sales. However, what if demand for tickets is significantly more than 4,000? In that case, SPI might rent a larger concert hall at a higher cost. In other words, *the cost is fixed only for a designated range of activity (1 to 4,000).*

A similar circumstance affects many variable costs. For example, a supplier may offer a volume discount to buyers who purchase more than a specified number of products. The point is that descriptions of cost behavior pertain to a specified range of activity. The range of activity over which the definitions of fixed and variable costs are valid is commonly called the **relevant range.**

LO 5

Demonstrate how the relevant range and decision context affect cost behavior.

Context-Sensitive Definitions of Fixed and Variable

The behavior pattern of a particular cost may be either fixed or variable, depending on the context. For example, the cost of the band was fixed at $48,000 when SPI was considering hiring it to play a single concert. Regardless of how many tickets SPI sold, the total band cost was $48,000. However, the band cost becomes variable if SPI decides to hire it to perform at a series of concerts. The total cost and the cost per concert for one, two, three, four, or five concerts are shown in Exhibit 11.15.

In this context, the total cost of hiring the band increases proportionately with the number of concerts while cost per concert remains constant. The band cost is therefore variable. The same cost can behave as either a fixed cost or a variable cost, depending on the **activity base.** When identifying a cost as fixed or variable, first ask, fixed or variable *relative to what activity base?* The cost of the band is fixed relative to *the number of tickets sold for a specific concert;* it is variable relative to *the number of concerts produced.*

EXHIBIT 11.15

Cost Behavior Relative to Number of Concerts

Number of concerts (a)	1	2	3	4	5
Cost per concert (b)	$48,000	$48,000	$ 48,000	$ 48,000	$ 48,000
Total cost (a $\times$ b)	$48,000	$96,000	$144,000	$192,000	$240,000

✓ **CHECK YOURSELF 11.4**

Is the compensation cost for managers of Pizza Hut Restaurants a fixed cost or a variable cost?

Answer   The answer depends on the context. For example, because a store manager's salary remains unchanged regardless of how many customers enter a particular restaurant, it can be classified as a fixed cost relative to the number of customers at a particular restaurant. However, the more restaurants that Pizza Hut operates, the higher the total managers' compensation cost will be. Accordingly, managers' salary cost would be classified as a variable cost relative to the number of restaurants opened.

DETERMINING THE BREAK-EVEN POINT

Calculate the break-even point.

Bright Day Distributors sells nonprescription health food supplements including vitamins, herbs, and natural hormones in the northwestern United States. Bright Day recently obtained the rights to distribute the new herb mixture Delatine. Recent scientific research found that Delatine delayed aging in laboratory animals. The researchers hypothesized that the substance would have a similar effect on humans. Their theory could not be confirmed because of the relatively long human life span. The news media reported the research findings; as stories turned up on television and radio news, talk shows, and in magazines, demand for Delatine increased.

Bright Day plans to sell the Delatine at a price of $36 per bottle. Delatine costs $24 per bottle. Bright Day's management team suspects that enthusiasm for Delatine will abate quickly as the news media shift to other subjects. To attract customers immediately, the product managers consider television advertising. The marketing manager suggests running a campaign of several hundred cable channel ads at an estimated cost of $60,000.

Bright Day's first concern is whether it can sell enough units to cover its costs. The president made this position clear when he said, "We don't want to lose money on this product. We have to sell at least enough units to break even." In accounting terms, the **break-even point** is where profit (income) equals zero. So how many bottles of Delatine must be sold to produce a profit of zero? The break-even point is commonly computed using either the *equation method,* or the *contribution margin per unit method.* Both of these approaches produce the same result. They are merely different ways to arrive at the same conclusion.

Equation Method

The **equation method** begins by expressing the income statement as follows.

$$\text{Sales} - \text{Variable costs} - \text{Fixed costs} = \text{Profit (Net income)}$$

As previously stated, profit at the break-even point is zero. Therefore, the break-even point for Delatine is computed as follows.

$$\text{Sales} - \text{Variable costs} - \text{Fixed costs} = \text{Profit}$$

$$\$36N - \$24N - \$60,000 = \$0$$

$$\$12N = \$60,000$$

$$N = \$60,000 \div \$12$$

$$N = 5,000 \text{ Units}$$

Where:

N = Number of units

$36 = Sales price per unit

$24 = Variable cost per unit

$60,000 = Fixed costs

✓ CHECK YOURSELF 11.5

B-Shoc is an independent musician who is considering whether to independently produce and sell a CD. B-Shoc estimates fixed costs of $5,400 and variable costs of $2.00 per unit. The expected selling price is $8.00 per CD. Use the equation method to determine B-Shoc's break-even point.

Answer

$$\text{Sales} - \text{Variable costs} - \text{Fixed costs} = \text{Profit}$$

$$\$8N - \$2N - \$5,400 = \$0$$

$$\$6N = \$5,400$$

$$N = \$5,400 \div \$6$$

$$N = 900 \text{ Units (CDs)}$$

Where:

N = Number of units

$8 = Sales price per unit

$2 = Variable cost per unit

$5,400 = Fixed costs

Contribution Margin Per Unit Method

Recall that the *total contribution margin* is the amount of sales minus total variable cost. The **contribution margin per unit** is the sales price per unit minus the variable cost per unit. Therefore, the contribution margin per unit for Delatine is

Sales price per unit	$36
Less: Variable cost per unit	(24)
Contribution margin per unit	$12

For every bottle of Delatine it sells, Bright Day earns a $12 contribution margin. In other words, every time Bright Day sells a bottle of Delatine, it receives enough money to pay $24 to cover the variable cost of the bottle of Delatine and still has $12 left to go toward paying the fixed cost. Bright Day will reach the break-even point when it sells enough bottles of Delatine to cover its fixed costs. Therefore the break-even point can be determined as follows.

$$\text{Break-even point in units} = \frac{\text{Fixed costs}}{\text{Contribution margin per unit}}$$

$$\text{Break-even point in units} = \frac{\$60,000}{\$12}$$

$$\text{Break-even point in units} = 5,000 \text{ Units}$$

This result is the same as that determined under the equation method. Indeed, the contribution margin per unit method formula is an abbreviated version of the income statement formula used in the equation method. The proof is provided in the footnote below.[2]

Both the *equation method* and the *contribution margin per unit method* yield the amount of break-even sales measured *in units.* To determine the amount of break-even sales measured *in dollars,* multiply the number of units times the sales price per unit. For Delatine the break-even point measured in dollars is $180,000 (5,000 units × $36 per unit). The following income statement confirms this result.

Sales revenue (5,000 units × $36)	$180,000
Total variable expenses (5,000 units × $24)	(120,000)
Total contribution margin (5,000 units × $12)	60,000
Fixed expenses	(60,000)
Net income	$ 0

---

[2]The formula for the *contribution margin per unit method* is (where N is the number of units at the break-even point).

N = Fixed costs ÷ Contribution margin per unit

The income statement formula for the *equation method* produces the same result as shown below (where N is the number of units at the break-even point).

Sales − Variable costs − Fixed costs = Profit

Sales price per unit (N) − Variable cost per unit (N) − Fixed costs = Profit

Contribution margin per unit (N) − Fixed costs = Profit

Contribution margin per unit (N) − Fixed costs = 0

Contribution margin per unit (N) = Fixed costs

N = Fixed costs ÷ Contribution margin per unit

DETERMINING THE SALES VOLUME NECESSARY TO REACH A DESIRED PROFIT

Bright Day's president decides the ad campaign should produce a $40,000 profit. He asks the accountant to determine the sales volume that is required to achieve this level of profitability. Using the *equation method,* the sales volume in units required to attain the desired profit is computed as follows.

Calculate the sales volume required to attain a target profit.

$$\text{Sales} - \text{Variable costs} - \text{Fixed costs} = \text{Profit}$$
$$\$36N - \$24N - \$60,000 = \$40,000$$
$$\$12N = \$60,000 + \$40,000$$
$$N = \$100,000 \div \$12$$
$$N = 8,333 \text{ Units}$$

Where:

N = Number of units

$36 = Sales price per unit

$24 = Variable cost per unit

$60,000 = Fixed costs

$40,000 = Desired profit

The accountant used the *contribution margin per unit method* to confirm these computations as follows.

$$\text{Sales volume in units} = \frac{\text{Fixed costs} + \text{Desired profit}}{\text{Contribution margin per unit}}$$
$$= \frac{\$60,000 + \$40,000}{\$12} = 8,333.33 \text{ units}$$

The required volume in sales dollars is this number of units multiplied by the sales price per unit (8,333.33 units × $36 = $300,000). The following income statement confirms this result; all amounts are rounded to the nearest whole dollar.

Sales revenue (8,333.33 units × $36)	$300,000
Total variable expenses (8,333.33 units × $24)	(200,000)
Total contribution margin (8,333.33 units × $12)	100,000
Fixed expenses	(60,000)
Net income	$ 40,000

In practice, the company will not sell partial bottles of Delatine. The accountant rounds 8,333.33 bottles to whole units. For planning and decision making, managers frequently make decisions using approximate data. Accuracy is desirable, but it is not as important as relevance. Do not be concerned when computations do not produce whole numbers. Rounding and approximation are common characteristics of managerial accounting data.

✓ CHECK YOURSELF 11.6

VolTech Company manufactures small engines that it sells for $130 each. Variable costs are $70 per unit. Fixed costs are expected to be $100,000. The management team has established a target profit of $188,000. Use the contribution margin per unit method to determine how many engines VolTech must sell to attain the target profit.

Answer

$$\text{Sales volume in units} = \frac{\text{Fixed costs} + \text{Desired profit}}{\text{Contribution margin per unit}} = \frac{100,000 + 188,000}{\$130 - \$70} = 4,800 \text{ Units}$$

CALCULATING THE MARGIN OF SAFETY

Calculate the margin of safety in units, dollars, and percentage.

Based on the sales records of other products, Bright Day's marketing department believes that budgeted sales of 8,333 units is an attainable goal. Even so, the company president is concerned because Delatine is a new product and no one can be certain about how the public will react to it. He is willing to take the risk of introducing a new product that fails to produce a profit, but he does not want to take a loss on the product. He therefore focuses on the gap between the budgeted sales and the sales required to break even. The amount of this gap, called the *margin of safety,* can be measured in units or in sales dollars as shown here.

	In Units	In Dollars
Budgeted sales	8,333	$300,000
Break-even sales	(5,000)	(180,000)
Margin of safety	3,333	$120,000

The **margin of safety** measures the cushion between budgeted sales and the break-even point. It quantifies the amount by which actual sales can fall short of expectations before the company will begin to incur losses.

To help compare diverse products or companies of different sizes, the margin of safety can be expressed as a percentage. Divide the margin of safety by the budgeted sales volume[3] as shown here.

$$\text{Margin of safety} = \frac{\text{Budgeted sales} - \text{Break-even sales}}{\text{Budgeted sales}}$$

$$\text{Margin of safety} = \frac{\$300,000 - \$180,000}{\$300,000} \times 100 = 40\%$$

This analysis suggests actual sales would have to fall short of expected sales by 40 percent before Bright Day would experience a loss on Delatine. The large margin of safety suggests the proposed advertising program to market Delatine has minimal risk.

✓ CHECK YOURSELF 11.7

Suppose that Bright Day is considering the possibility of selling a protein supplement that will cost Bright Day $5 per bottle. Bright Day believes that it can sell 4,000 bottles of the supplement for $25 per bottle. Fixed costs associated with selling the supplement are expected to be $42,000. Does the supplement have a wider margin of safety than Delatine?

Answer Calculate the break-even point for the protein supplement.

$$\text{Break-even volume in units} = \frac{\text{Fixed costs}}{\text{Contribution margin per unit}} = \frac{\$42,000}{\$25 - \$5} = 2,100 \text{ Units}$$

Calculate the margin of safety. Note that the margin of safety expressed as a percentage can be calculated using the number of units or sales dollars. Using either units or dollars yields the same percentage.

$$\text{Margin of safety} = \frac{\text{Budgeted sales} - \text{Break-even sales}}{\text{Budgeted sales}} = \frac{4,000 - 2,100}{4,000} = 47.5\%$$

The margin of safety for Delatine (40.0 percent) is below that for the protein supplement (47.5 percent). This suggests that Bright Day is more likely to incur losses selling Delatine than selling the supplement.

---

[3]The margin of safety percentage can be based on actual as well as budgeted sales. For example, an analyst could compare the margins of safety of two companies under current operating conditions by substituting actual sales for budgeted sales in the computation, as follows: ([Actual sales − Break-even sales] ÷ Actual sales).

A Look Back

To plan and control business operations effectively, managers need to understand how different costs behave in relation to changes in the volume of activity. Total *fixed cost* remains constant when activity changes. Fixed cost per unit decreases with increases in activity and increases with decreases in activity. In contrast, total *variable cost* increases proportionately with increases in activity and decreases proportionately with decreases in activity. Variable cost per unit remains constant regardless of activity levels. The definitions of fixed and variable costs have meaning only within the context of a specified range of activity (the relevant range) for a defined period of time. In addition, cost behavior depends on the relevant volume measure (a store manager's salary is fixed relative to the number of customers visiting a particular store but is variable relative to the number of stores operated). A mixed cost has both fixed and variable cost components.

Fixed costs allow companies to take advantage of *operating leverage.* With operating leverage, each additional sale decreases the cost per unit. This principle allows a small percentage change in volume of revenue to cause a significantly larger percentage change in profits. The *magnitude of operating leverage* can be determined by dividing the contribution margin by net income. When all costs are fixed and revenues have covered fixed costs, each additional dollar of revenue represents pure profit. Having a fixed cost structure (employing operating leverage) offers a company both risks and rewards. If sales volume increases, fixed costs do not increase, allowing profits to soar. Alternatively, if sales volume decreases, fixed costs do not decrease and profits decline significantly more than revenues. Companies with high variable costs in relation to fixed costs do not experience as great a level of operating leverage. Their costs increase or decrease in proportion to changes in revenue. These companies face less risk but fail to reap disproportionately higher profits when volume soars.

Under the contribution margin approach, variable costs are subtracted from revenue to determine the *contribution margin.* Fixed costs are then subtracted from the contribution margin to determine net income. The contribution margin represents the amount available to pay fixed costs and provide a profit. Although not permitted by GAAP for external reporting, many companies use the contribution margin format for internal reporting purposes.

The *break-even point* (the point where total revenue equals total cost) in units can be determined by dividing fixed costs by the contribution margin per unit. The break-even point in sales dollars can be determined by multiplying the number of break-even units by the sales price per unit. To determine sales in units to obtain a designated profit, the sum of fixed costs and desired profit is divided by the contribution margin per unit.

The *margin of safety* is the number of units or the amount of sales dollars by which actual sales can fall below expected sales before a loss is incurred. The margin of safety can also be expressed as a percentage to permit comparing different size companies. The margin of safety can be computed as a percentage by dividing the difference between budgeted sales and break-even sales by the amount of budgeted sales.

A Look Forward

The next chapter begins investigating cost measurement. Accountants seek to determine the cost of certain objects. A cost object may be a product, a service, a department, a customer, or any other thing for which the cost is being determined. Some costs can be directly traced to a cost object, while others are difficult to trace. Costs that are difficult to trace to cost objects are called *indirect costs,* or *overhead.* Indirect costs are assigned to cost objects through *cost allocation.* The next chapter introduces the basic concepts and procedures of cost allocation.

A step-by-step audio-narrated series of slides is provided on the text website at www.mhhe.com/edmondssurvey3e.

SELF-STUDY REVIEW PROBLEM 1

Mensa Mountaineering Company (MMC) provides guided mountain climbing expeditions in the Rocky Mountains. Its only major expense is guide salaries; it pays each guide $4,800 per climbing expedition. MMC charges its customers $1,500 per expedition and expects to take five climbers on each expedition.

Part 1

Base your answers on the preceding information.

Required

a. Determine the total cost of guide salaries and the cost of guide salaries per climber assuming that four, five, or six climbers are included in a trip. Relative to the number of climbers in a single expedition, is the cost of guides a fixed or a variable cost?

b. Relative to the number of expeditions, is the cost of guides a fixed or a variable cost?

c. Determine the profit of an expedition assuming that five climbers are included in the trip.

d. Determine the profit assuming a 20 percent increase (six climbers total) in expedition revenue. What is the percentage change in profitability?

e. Determine the profit assuming a 20 percent decrease (four climbers total) in expedition revenue. What is the percentage change in profitability?

f. Explain why a 20 percent shift in revenue produces more than a 20 percent shift in profitability. What term describes this phenomenon?

Part 2

Assume that the guides offer to make the climbs for a percentage of expedition fees. Specifically, MMC will pay guides $960 per climber on the expedition. Assume also that the expedition fee charged to climbers remains at $1,500 per climber.

Required

g. Determine the total cost of guide salaries and the cost of guide salaries per climber assuming that four, five, or six climbers are included in a trip. Relative to the number of climbers in a single expedition, is the cost of guides a fixed or a variable cost?

h. Relative to the number of expeditions, is the cost of guides a fixed or a variable cost?

i. Determine the profit of an expedition assuming that five climbers are included in the trip.

j. Determine the profit assuming a 20 percent increase (six climbers total) in expedition revenue. What is the percentage change in profitability?

k. Determine the profit assuming a 20 percent decrease (four climbers total) in expedition revenue. What is the percentage change in profitability?

l. Explain why a 20 percent shift in revenue does not produce more than a 20 percent shift in profitability.

Solution to Part 1, Requirement *a*

Number of climbers (a)	4	5	6
Total cost of guide salaries (b)	$4,800	$4,800	$4,800
Cost per climber (b ÷ a)	1,200	960	800

Because the total cost remains constant (fixed) regardless of the number of climbers on a particular expedition, the cost is classified as fixed. Note that the cost per climber decreases as the number of climbers increases. This is the *per unit* behavior pattern of a fixed cost.

Solution to Part 1, Requirement *b*

Because the total cost of guide salaries changes proportionately each time the number of expeditions increases or decreases, the cost of salaries is variable relative to the number of expeditions.

Solution to Part 1, Requirements *c*, *d*, and *e*

Number of Climbers	4	Percentage Change	5	Percentage Change	6
Revenue ($1,500 per climber)	$6,000	⇐(20%)⇐	$7,500	⇒+20%⇒	$9,000
Cost of guide salaries (fixed)	4,800		4,800		4,800
Profit	$1,200	⇐(55.6%)⇐	$2,700	⇒+55.6%⇒	$4,200

Percentage change in revenue: ±$1,500 ÷ $7,500 = ±20%
Percentage change in profit: ±$1,500 ÷ $2,700 = ±55.6%

Solution to Part 1, Requirement *f*

Because the cost of guide salaries remains fixed while volume (number of climbers) changes, the change in profit, measured in absolute dollars, exactly matches the change in revenue. More specifically, each time MMC increases the number of climbers by one, revenue and profit increase by $1,500. Because the base figure for profit ($2,700) is lower than the base figure for revenue ($7,500), the percentage change in profit ($1,500 ÷ $2,700 = 55.6%) is higher than percentage change in revenue ($1,500 ÷ $7,500). This phenomenon is called *operating leverage*.

Solution for Part 2, Requirement *g*

Number of climbers (a)	4	5	6
Per climber cost of guide salaries (b)	$ 960	$ 960	$ 960
Cost per climber (b × a)	3,840	4,800	5,760

Because the total cost changes in proportion to changes in the number of climbers, the cost is classified as variable. Note that the cost per climber remains constant (stays the same) as the number of climbers increases or decreases. This is the *per unit* behavior pattern of a variable cost.

Solution for Part 2, Requirement *h*

Because the total cost of guide salaries changes proportionately with changes in the number of expeditions, the cost of salaries is also variable relative to the number of expeditions.

Solution for Part 2, Requirements *i*, *j*, and *k*

Number of Climbers	4	Percentage Change	5	Percentage Change	6
Revenue ($1,500 per climber)	$6,000	⇐(20%)⇐	$7,500	⇒+20%⇒	$9,000
Cost of guide salaries (variable)	3,840		4,800		5,760
Profit	$2,160	⇐(20%)⇐	$2,700	⇒+20%⇒	$3,240

Percentage change in revenue: ±$1,500 ÷ $7,500 = ±20%
Percentage change in profit: ±$540 ÷ $2,700 = ±20%

Solution for Part 2, Requirement *l*

Because the cost of guide salaries changes when volume (number of climbers) changes, the change in net income is proportionate to the change in revenue. More specifically, each time the number of climbers increases by one, revenue increases by $1,500 and net income increases by $540 ($1,500 − $960). Accordingly, the percentage change in net income will always equal the percentage change in revenue. This means that there is no operating leverage when all costs are variable.

A step-by-step audio-narrated series of slides is provided on the text website at www.mhhe.com/edmondssurvey3e.

SELF-STUDY REVIEW PROBLEM 2

Sharp Company makes and sells pencil sharpeners. The variable cost of each sharpener is $20. The sharpeners are sold for $30 each. Fixed operating expenses amount to $40,000.

Required

a. Determine the break-even point in units and sales dollars.

b. Determine the sales volume in units and dollars that is required to attain a profit of $12,000. Verify your answer by preparing an income statement using the contribution margin format.

c. Determine the margin of safety between sales required to attain a profit of $12,000 and break-even sales.

Solution to Requirement *a*

Formula for Computing Break-even Point in Units
Sales − Variable costs − Fixed costs = Profit
Sales price per unit (N) − Variable cost per unit (N) − Fixed costs = Profit
Contribution margin per unit (N) − Fixed costs = Profit
N = (Fixed costs + Profit) ÷ Contribution Margin per unit
N = ($40,000 + 0) ÷ ($30 − $20) = 4,000 Units

Break-even Point in Sales Dollars	
Sales price	$ 30
× Number of units	4,000
Sales volume in dollars	$120,000

Solution to Requirement *b*

Formula for Computing Unit Sales Required to Attain Desired Profit
Sales − Variable costs − Fixed costs = Profit
Sales price per unit (N) − Variable cost per unit (N) − Fixed costs = Profit
Contribution margin per unit (N) − Fixed costs = Profit
N = (Fixed costs + Profit) ÷ Contribution margin per unit
N = ($40,000 + 12,000) ÷ ($30 − $20) = 5,200 Units

Sales Dollars Required to Attain Desired Profit	
Sales price	$ 30
× Number of units	5,200
Sales volume in dollars	$156,000

Income Statement	
Sales volume in units (a)	5,200
Sales revenue (a × $30)	$156,000
Variable costs (a × $20)	(104,000)
Contribution margin	52,000
Fixed costs	(40,000)
Net income	$ 12,000

Solution to Requirement *c*

Margin of Safety Computations	Units	Dollars
Budgeted sales	5,200	$156,000
Break-even sales	(4,000)	(120,000)
Margin of safety	1,200	$ 36,000

Percentage Computation

$$\frac{\text{Margin of safety in \$}}{\text{Budgeted sales}} = \frac{\$36,000}{\$156,000} = 23.08\%$$

KEY TERMS

Activity base 406
Break-even point 407
Contribution margin 402
Contribution margin per
  unit 408

Cost behavior 398
Equation method 407
Fixed cost 398
Margin of
  safety 410

Mixed costs (semivariable
  costs) 405
Operating leverage 398
Relevant range 405
Variable cost 397

QUESTIONS

1. Define *fixed cost* and *variable cost* and give an example of each.

2. How can knowing cost behavior relative to volume fluctuations affect decision making?

3. Define the term *operating leverage* and explain how it affects profits.

4. How is operating leverage calculated?

5. Explain the limitations of using operating leverage to predict profitability.

6. If volume is increasing, would a company benefit more from a pure variable or a pure fixed cost structure? Which cost structure would be advantageous if volume is decreasing?

7. Explain the risk and rewards to a company that result from having fixed costs.

8. Are companies with predominately fixed cost structures likely to be most profitable?

9. How is the relevant range of activity related to fixed and variable cost? Give an example of how the definitions of these costs become invalid when volume is outside the relevant range.

10. Which cost structure has the greater risk? Explain.

11. The president of Bright Corporation tells you that he sees a dim future for his company. He feels that his hands are tied because fixed costs are too high. He says that fixed costs do not change and therefore the situation is hopeless. Do you agree? Explain.

12. All costs are variable because if a business ceases operations, its costs fall to zero. Do you agree with the statement? Explain.

13. Verna Salsbury tells you that she thinks the terms fixed cost and variable cost are confusing. She notes that fixed cost per unit changes when the number of units changes. Furthermore, variable cost per unit remains fixed regardless of how many units are produced. She concludes that the terminology seems to be backward. Explain why the terminology appears to be contradictory.

14. What does the term *break-even point* mean? Name the two ways it can be measured.

15. How does a contribution margin income statement differ from the income statement used in financial reporting?

16. If Company A has a projected margin of safety of 22 percent while Company B has a margin of safety of 52 percent, which company is at greater risk when actual sales are less than budgeted?

17. Mary Hartwell and Jane Jamail, college roommates, are considering the joint purchase of a computer that they can share to prepare class assignments. Ms. Hartwell wants a particular model that costs $2,000; Ms. Jamail prefers a more economical model that costs $1,500. In fact, Ms. Jamail is adamant about her position, refusing to contribute more than $750 toward the purchase. If Ms. Hartwell is also adamant about her position, should she accept Ms. Jamail's $750 offer and apply that amount toward the purchase of the more expensive computer?

MULTIPLE-CHOICE QUESTIONS

Multiple-choice questions are provided on the text website at
www.mhhe.com/edmondssurvey3e.

EXERCISES

connect
ACCOUNTING

All applicable Exercises are available with McGraw-Hill's
Connect Accounting.

LO 1, 5

Exercise 11-1 *Identifying cost behavior*

Deer Valley Kitchen, a fast-food restaurant company, operates a chain of restaurants across the nation. Each restaurant employs eight people; one is a manager who is paid a salary plus a bonus equal to 3 percent of sales. Other employees, two cooks, one dishwasher, and four waitresses, are paid salaries. Each manager is budgeted $3,000 per month for advertising cost.

Required

Classify each of the following costs incurred by Deer Valley Kitchen as fixed, variable, or mixed.

a. Cooks' salaries at a particular location relative to the number of customers.
b. Cost of supplies (cups, plates, spoons, etc.) relative to the number of customers.
c. Manager's compensation relative to the number of customers.
d. Waitresses' salaries relative to the number of restaurants.
e. Advertising costs relative to the number of customers for a particular restaurant.
f. Rental costs relative to the number of restaurants.

LO 1

Exercise 11-2 *Identifying cost behavior*

At the various activity levels shown, Amborse Company incurred the following costs.

	Units Sold	20	40	60	80	100
a.	Depreciation cost per unit	240.00	120.00	80.00	60.00	48.00
b.	Total rent cost	3,200.00	3,200.00	3,200.00	3,200.00	3,200.00
c.	Total cost of shopping bags	2.00	4.00	6.00	8.00	10.00
d.	Cost per unit of merchandise sold	90.00	90.00	90.00	90.00	90.00
e.	Rental cost per unit of merchandise sold	36.00	18.00	12.00	9.00	7.20
f.	Total phone expense	80.00	100.00	120.00	140.00	160.00
g.	Cost per unit of supplies	1.00	1.00	1.00	1.00	1.00
h.	Total insurance cost	480.00	480.00	480.00	480.00	480.00
i.	Total salary cost	$1,200.00	$1,600.00	$2,000.00	$2,400.00	$2,800.00
j.	Total cost of goods sold	1,800.00	3,600.00	5,400.00	7,200.00	9,000.00

Required

Identify each of these costs as fixed, variable, or mixed.

LO 1

Exercise 11-3 *Determining fixed cost per unit*

Henke Corporation incurs the following annual fixed costs.

Item	Cost
Depreciation	$ 50,000
Officers' salaries	120,000
Long-term lease	51,000
Property taxes	9,000

Required

Determine the total fixed cost per unit of production, assuming that Henke produces 4,000, 4,500, or 5,000 units.

Exercise 11-4   *Determining total variable cost*   **LO 1**

The following variable production costs apply to goods made by Watson Manufacturing Corporation.

Item	Cost per Unit
Materials	$5.00
Labor	2.50
Variable overhead	0.25
Total	$7.75

Required

Determine the total variable production cost, assuming that Watson makes 5,000, 15,000, or 25,000 units.

Exercise 11-5   *Fixed versus variable cost behavior*   **LO 1, 2**

Robbins Company's cost and production data for two recent months included the following.

	January	February
Production (units)	100	250
Rent	$1,500	$1,500
Utilities	$ 450	$1,125

Required

a. Separately calculate the rental cost per unit and the utilities cost per unit for both January and February.

b. Identify which cost is variable and which is fixed. Explain your answer.

Exercise 11-6   *Fixed versus variable cost behavior*   **LO 1**

Lovvern Trophies makes and sells trophies it distributes to little league ballplayers. The company normally produces and sells between 8,000 and 14,000 trophies per year. The following cost data apply to various activity levels.

Number of Trophies	8,000	10,000	12,000	14,000
Total costs incurred				
Fixed	$42,000			
Variable	42,000			
Total costs	$84,000			
Cost per unit				
Fixed	$ 5.25			
Variable	5.25			
Total cost per trophy	$10.50			

Required

a. Complete the preceding table by filling in the missing amounts for the levels of activity shown in the first row of the table. Round all cost per unit figures to the nearest whole penny.

b. Explain why the total cost per trophy decreases as the number of trophies increases.

LO 1, 5

Exercise 11-7   *Fixed versus variable cost behavior*

Harrel Entertainment sponsors rock concerts. The company is considering a contract to hire a band at a cost of $75,000 per concert.

Required

a. What are the total band cost and the cost per person if concert attendance is 2,000, 2,500, 3,000, 3,500, or 4,000?

b. Is the cost of hiring the band a fixed or a variable cost?

c. Draw a graph and plot total cost and cost per unit if attendance is 2,000, 2,500, 3,000, 3,500, or 4,000.

d. Identify Harrel's major business risks and explain how they can be minimized.

LO 1

Exercise 11-8   *Fixed versus variable cost behavior*

Harrel Entertainment sells souvenir T-shirts at each rock concert that it sponsors. The shirts cost $9 each. Any excess shirts can be returned to the manufacturer for a full refund of the purchase price. The sales price is $15 per shirt.

Required

a. What are the total cost of shirts and cost per shirt if sales amount to 2,000, 2,500, 3,000, 3,500, or 4,000?

b. Is the cost of T-shirts a fixed or a variable cost?

c. Draw a graph and plot total cost and cost per shirt if sales amount to 2,000, 2,500, 3,000, 3,500, or 4,000.

d. Comment on Harrel's likelihood of incurring a loss due to its operating activities.

LO 1

Exercise 11-9   *Graphing fixed cost behavior*

The following graphs depict the dollar amount of fixed cost on the vertical axes and the level of activity on the horizontal axes.

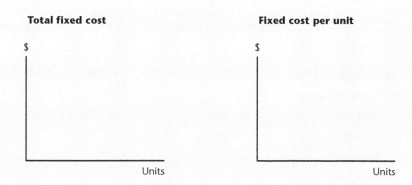

Required

a. Draw a line that depicts the relationship between total fixed cost and the level of activity.

b. Draw a line that depicts the relationship between fixed cost per unit and the level of activity.

Exercise 11-10   *Graphing variable cost behavior*   **LO 1**

The following graphs depict the dollar amount of variable cost on the vertical axes and the level of activity on the horizontal axes.

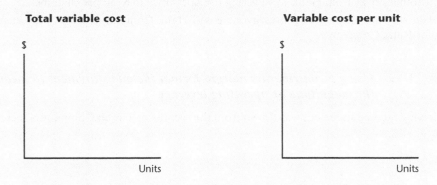

Total variable cost   **Variable cost per unit**

Required

a. Draw a line that depicts the relationship between total variable cost and the level of activity.

b. Draw a line that depicts the relationship between variable cost per unit and the level of activity.

Exercise 11-11   *Mixed cost at different levels of activity*   **LO 1**

Omar Corporation paid one of its sales representatives $4,300 during the month of March. The rep is paid a base salary plus $15 per unit of product sold. During March, the rep sold 200 units.

Required

Calculate the total monthly cost of the sales representative's salary for each of the following months.

Month	April	May	June	July
Number of units sold	240	150	250	100
Total variable cost				
Total fixed cost				
Total salary cost				

Exercise 11-12   *Using fixed cost as a competitive business strategy*   **LO 1, 2**

The following income statements illustrate different cost structures for two competing companies.

Income Statements		
	Company Name	
	Hank	**Rank**
Number of customers (a)	80	80
Sales revenue (a × $250)	$20,000	$20,000
Variable cost (a × $175)	N/A	(14,000)
Variable cost (a × $0)	0	N/A
Contribution margin	20,000	6,000
Fixed cost	(14,000)	0
Net income	$ 6,000	$ 6,000

Required

a. Reconstruct Hank's income statement, assuming that it serves 160 customers when it lures 80 customers away from Rank by lowering the sales price to $150 per customer.

b. Reconstruct Rank's income statement, assuming that it serves 160 customers when it lures 80 customers away from Hank by lowering the sales price to $150 per customer.

c. Explain why the price-cutting strategy increased Hank Company's profits but caused a net loss for Rank Company.

LO 3, 4

Exercise 11-13 *Using a contribution margin format income statement to measure the magnitude of operating leverage*

The following income statement was drawn from the records of Ulrich Company, a merchandising firm.

ULRICH COMPANY Income Statement For the Year Ended December 31, 2011	
Sales revenue (4,000 units × $150)	$600,000
Cost of goods sold (4,000 units × $80)	(320,000)
Gross margin	280,000
Sales commissions (10% of sales)	(60,000)
Administrative salaries expense	(90,000)
Advertising expense	(40,000)
Depreciation expense	(50,000)
Shipping and handling expenses (4,000 units × $1)	(4,000)
Net income	$ 36,000

Required

a. Reconstruct the income statement using the contribution margin format.

b. Calculate the magnitude of operating leverage.

c. Use the measure of operating leverage to determine the amount of net income Ulrich will earn if sales increase by 10 percent.

LO 4

Exercise 11-14 *Assessing the magnitude of operating leverage*

The following income statement applies to Stuart Company for the current year.

Income Statement	
Sales revenue (400 units × $25)	$10,000
Variable cost (400 units × $10)	(4,000)
Contribution margin	6,000
Fixed costs	(3,500)
Net income	$2,500

Required

a. Use the contribution margin approach to calculate the magnitude of operating leverage.

b. Use the operating leverage measure computed in Requirement *a* to determine the amount of net income that Stuart Company will earn if it experiences a 10 percent increase in revenue. The sales price per unit is not affected.

c. Verify your answer to Requirement *b* by constructing an income statement based on a 10 percent increase in sales revenue. The sales price is not affected. Calculate the percentage change in net income for the two income statements.

Exercise 11-15   *Break-even point*   LO 6

Connor Corporation sells products for $25 each that have variable costs of $13 per unit. Connor's annual fixed cost is $264,000.

Required

Determine the break-even point in units and dollars.

Exercise 11-16   *Desired profit*   LO 7

Garcia Company incurs annual fixed costs of $60,000. Variable costs for Garcia's product are $22.75 per unit, and the sales price is $35.00 per unit. Garcia desires to earn an annual profit of $45,000.

Required

Determine the sales volume in dollars and units required to earn the desired profit.

Exercise 11-17   *Determining fixed and variable cost per unit*   LO 1

Landry Corporation produced and sold 12,000 units of product during October. It earned a contribution margin of $96,000 on sales of $336,000 and determined that cost per unit of product was $25.

Required

Based on this information, determine the variable and fixed cost per unit of product.

Exercise 11-18   *Determining variable cost from incomplete cost data*   LO 1

Laya Corporation produced 200,000 watches that it sold for $16 each during 2012. The company determined that fixed manufacturing cost per unit was $7 per watch. The company reported a $800,000 gross margin on its 2011 financial statements.

Required

Determine the total variable cost, the variable cost per unit, and the total contribution margin.

Exercise 11-19   *Margin of safety*   LO 6, 7, 8

Information concerning a product produced by Askew Company appears here.

Sales price per unit	$145
Variable cost per unit	$55
Total annual fixed manufacturing and operating costs	$810,000

Required

Determine the following.

a. Contribution margin per unit.
b. Number of units that Askew must sell to break even.
c. Sales level in units that Askew must reach to earn a profit of $360,000.
d. Determine the margin of safety in units, sales dollars, and as a percentage.

Exercise 11-20   *Margin of safety*   LO 8

Jensen Company makes a product that sells for $38 per unit. The company pays $16 per unit for the variable costs of the product and incurs annual fixed costs of $176,000. Jensen expects to sell 21,000 units of product.

Required

Determine Jensen's margin of safety in units, sales dollars, and as a percentage.

PROBLEMS

All applicable Problems are available with McGraw-Hill's
Connect Accounting.

LO 1, 5

Problem 11-21 *Identifying cost behavior*

Required

Identify the following costs as fixed or variable.

Costs related to plane trips between Seattle, Washington, and Orlando, Florida, follow. Pilots are paid on a per trip basis.

a. Pilots' salaries relative to the number of trips flown.
b. Depreciation relative to the number of planes in service.
c. Cost of refreshments relative to the number of passengers.
d. Pilots' salaries relative to the number of passengers on a particular trip.
e. Cost of a maintenance check relative to the number of passengers on a particular trip.
f. Fuel costs relative to the number of trips.

First Federal Bank operates several branch offices in grocery stores. Each branch employs a supervisor and two tellers.

g. Tellers' salaries relative to the number of tellers in a particular district.
h. Supplies cost relative to the number of transactions processed in a particular branch.
i. Tellers' salaries relative to the number of customers served at a particular branch.
j. Supervisors' salaries relative to the number of branches operated.
k. Supervisors' salaries relative to the number of customers served in a particular branch.
l. Facility rental costs relative to the size of customer deposits.

Costs related to operating a fast-food restaurant follow.

m. Depreciation of equipment relative to the number of restaurants.
n. Building rental cost relative to the number of customers served in a particular restaurant.
o. Manager's salary of a particular restaurant relative to the number of employees.
p. Food cost relative to the number of customers.
q. Utility cost relative to the number of restaurants in operation.
r. Company president's salary relative to the number of restaurants in operation.
s. Land costs relative to the number of hamburgers sold at a particular restaurant.
t. Depreciation of equipment relative to the number of customers served at a particular restaurant.

LO 1, 6

e✗cel

CHECK FIGURES
c. Total supplies cost for cleaning 30 houses: $180
d. Total cost for 20 houses: $2,370

Problem 11-22 *Cost behavior and averaging*

Carlia Weaver has decided to start Carlia Cleaning, a residential house cleaning service company. She is able to rent cleaning equipment at a cost of $750 per month. Labor costs are expected to be $75 per house cleaned and supplies are expected to cost $6 per house.

Required

a. Determine the total expected cost of equipment rental and the expected cost of equipment rental per house cleaned, assuming that Carlia Cleaning cleans 10, 20, or 30 houses during one month. Is the cost of equipment a fixed or a variable cost?
b. Determine the total expected cost of labor and the expected cost of labor per house cleaned, assuming that Carlia Cleaning cleans 10, 20, or 30 houses during one month. Is the cost of labor a fixed or a variable cost?
c. Determine the total expected cost of supplies and the expected cost of supplies per house cleaned, assuming that Carlia Cleaning cleans 10, 20, or 30 houses during one month. Is the cost of supplies a fixed or a variable cost?
d. Determine the total expected cost of cleaning houses, assuming that Carlia Cleaning cleans 10, 20, or 30 houses during one month.

e. Determine the expected cost per house, assuming that Carlia Cleaning cleans 10, 20, or 30 houses during one month. Why does the cost per unit decrease as the number of houses increases?

f. If Ms. Weaver tells you that she prices her services at 25% above cost, would you assume that she means average or actual cost? Why?

Problem 11-23 *Context-sensitive nature of cost behavior classifications*

LO 5

CHECK FIGURE
b. Average teller cost for 60,000 transactions: $1.50

Pacific Bank's start-up division establishes new branch banks. Each branch opens with three tellers. Total teller cost per branch is $90,000 per year. The three tellers combined can process up to 90,000 customer transactions per year. If a branch does not attain a volume of at least 60,000 transactions during its first year of operations, it is closed. If the demand for services exceeds 90,000 transactions, an additional teller is hired, and the branch is transferred from the start-up division to regular operations.

Required

a. What is the relevant range of activity for new branch banks?

b. Determine the amount of teller cost in total and the teller cost per transaction for a branch that processes 60,000, 70,000, 80,000, or 90,000 transactions. In this case (the activity base is the number of transactions for a specific branch), is the teller cost a fixed or a variable cost?

c. Determine the amount of teller cost in total and the teller cost per branch for Pacific Bank, assuming that the start-up division operates 10, 15, 20, or 25 branches. In this case (the activity base is the number of branches), is the teller cost a fixed or a variable cost?

Problem 11-24 *Context-sensitive nature of cost behavior classifications*

LO 5

CHECK FIGURES
a. Average cost at 400 units: $200
b. Average price at 250 units: $265

Susan Hicks operates a sales booth in computer software trade shows, selling an accounting software package, *Dollar System*. She purchases the package from a software manufacturer for $175 each. Booth space at the convention hall costs $10,000 per show.

Required

a. Sales at past trade shows have ranged between 200 and 400 software packages per show. Determine the average cost of sales per unit if Ms. Hicks sells 200, 250, 300, 350, or 400 units of *Dollar System* at a trade show. Use the following chart to organize your answer. Is the cost of booth space fixed or variable?

	Sales Volume in Units (a)				
	200	**250**	**300**	**350**	**400**
Total cost of software (a × $175)	$35,000				
Total cost of booth rental	10,000				
Total cost of sales (b)	$45,000				
Average cost per unit (b ÷ a)	$ 225				

b. If Ms. Hicks wants to earn a $50 profit on each package of software she sells at a trade show, what price must she charge at sales volumes of 200, 250, 300, 350, or 400 units?

c. Record the total cost of booth space if Ms. Hicks attends one, two, three, four, or five trade shows. Record your answers in the following chart. Is the cost of booth space fixed or variable relative to the number of shows attended?

	Number of Trade Shows Attended				
	1	**2**	**3**	**4**	**5**
Total cost of booth rental	$10,000				

d. Ms. Hicks provides decorative shopping bags to customers who purchase software packages. Some customers take the bags; others do not. Some customers stuff more than one software package into a single bag. The number of bags varies in relation to the number of units sold, but the relationship is not proportional. Assume that Ms. Hicks uses $30 of bags for every 50 software packages sold. What is the additional cost per unit sold? Is the cost fixed or variable?

LO 1, 2

CHECK FIGURES
Part 1, b: $2,200
Part 2, h: $3,000 & 10%
Part 3, k: cost per student for 22 students: $25

Problem 11-25   *Effects of operating leverage on profitability*

Webster Training Services (WTS) provides instruction on the use of computer software for the employees of its corporate clients. It offers courses in the clients' offices on the clients' equipment. The only major expense WTS incurs is instructor salaries; it pays instructors $5,000 per course taught. WTS recently agreed to offer a course of instruction to the employees of Chambers Incorporated at a price of $400 per student. Chambers estimated that 20 students would attend the course.

Base your answer on the preceding information.

Part 1:

Required

a. Relative to the number of students in a single course, is the cost of instruction a fixed or a variable cost?

b. Determine the profit, assuming that 20 students attend the course.

c. Determine the profit, assuming a 10 percent increase in enrollment (i.e., enrollment increases to 22 students). What is the percentage change in profitability?

d. Determine the profit, assuming a 10 percent decrease in enrollment (i.e., enrollment decreases to 18 students). What is the percentage change in profitability?

e. Explain why a 10 percent shift in enrollment produces more than a 10 percent shift in profitability. Use the term that identifies this phenomenon.

Part 2:

The instructor has offered to teach the course for a percentage of tuition fees. Specifically, she wants $250 per person attending the class. Assume that the tuition fee remains at $400 per student.

Required

f. Is the cost of instruction a fixed or a variable cost?

g. Determine the profit, assuming that 20 students take the course.

h. Determine the profit, assuming a 10 percent increase in enrollment (i.e., enrollment increases to 22 students). What is the percentage change in profitability?

i. Determine the profit, assuming a 10 percent decrease in enrollment (i.e., enrollment decreases to 18 students). What is the percentage change in profitability?

j. Explain why a 10 percent shift in enrollment produces a proportional 10 percent shift in profitability.

Part 3:

WTS sells a workbook with printed material unique to each course to each student who attends the course. Any workbooks that are not sold must be destroyed. Prior to the first class, WTS printed 20 copies of the books based on the client's estimate of the number of people who would attend the course. Each workbook costs $25 and is sold to course participants for $40. This cost includes a royalty fee paid to the author and the cost of duplication.

Required

k. Calculate the workbook cost in total and per student, assuming that 18, 20, or 22 students attempt to attend the course.

l. Classify the cost of workbooks as fixed or variable relative to the number of students attending the course.

m. Discuss the risk of holding inventory as it applies to the workbooks.

n. Explain how a just-in-time inventory system can reduce the cost and risk of holding inventory.

Problem 11-26 *Effects of fixed and variable cost behavior on the risk and rewards*
of business opportunities

LO 1, 2

Eastern and Western Universities offer executive training courses to corporate clients. Eastern pays its instructors $5,310 per course taught. Western pays its instructors $295 per student enrolled in the class. Both universities charge executives a $340 tuition fee per course attended.

CHECK FIGURES
a. Western NI: $810
b. NI: $2,610

Required

a. Prepare income statements for Eastern and Western, assuming that 18 students attend a course.

b. Eastern University embarks on a strategy to entice students from Western University by lowering its tuition to $220 per course. Prepare an income statement for Eastern, assuming that the university is successful and enrolls 36 students in its course.

c. Western University embarks on a strategy to entice students from Eastern University by lowering its tuition to $220 per course. Prepare an income statement for Western, assuming that the university is successful and enrolls 36 students in its course.

d. Explain why the strategy described in Requirement *b* produced a profit but the same strategy described in Requirement *c* produced a loss.

e. Prepare income statements for Eastern and Western Universities, assuming that 15 students attend a course, assuming that both universities charge executives a $340 tuition fee per course attended.

f. It is always better to have fixed than variable cost. Explain why this statement is false.

g. It is always better to have variable than fixed cost. Explain why this statement is false.

Problem 11-27 *Analyzing operating leverage*

LO 3, 4

Justin Zinder is a venture capitalist facing two alternative investment opportunities. He intends to invest $1 million in a start-up firm. He is nervous, however, about future economic volatility. He asks you to analyze the following financial data for the past year's operations of the two firms he is considering and give him some business advice.

	Company Name	
	Ensley	**Kelley**
Variable cost per unit (a)	$21.00	$10.50
Sales revenue (8,000 units × $28)	$224,000	$224,000
Variable cost (8,000 units × a)	(168,000)	(84,000)
Contribution margin	56,000	140,000
Fixed cost	(25,000)	(109,000)
Net income	$ 31,000	$ 31,000

CHECK FIGURES
b. % of change for Kelley: 45.16
c. % of change for Ensley: (18.06)

Required

a. Use the contribution margin approach to compute the operating leverage for each firm.

b. If the economy expands in coming years, Ensley and Kelley will both enjoy a 10 percent per year increase in sales, assuming that the selling price remains unchanged. Compute the change in net income for each firm in dollar amount and in percentage. (*Note:* Because the number of units increases, both revenue and variable cost will increase.)

c. If the economy contracts in coming years, Ensley and Kelley will both suffer a 10 percent decrease in sales volume, assuming that the selling price remains unchanged. Compute the change in net income for each firm in dollar amount and in percentage. (*Note:* Because the number of units decreases, both total revenue and total variable cost will decrease.)

d. Write a memo to Justin Zinder with your analyses and advice.

Problem 11-28 *Determining the break-even point and preparing a contribution*
margin income statement

LO 3, 6

Inman Manufacturing Company makes a product that it sells for $60 per unit. The company incurs variable manufacturing costs of $24 per unit. Variable selling expenses are $12 per unit, annual fixed manufacturing costs are $189,000, and fixed selling and administrative costs are $141,000 per year.

CHECK FIGURE
a. 13,750 units

Required

Determine the break-even point in units and dollars using the following approaches.

a. Equation method.

b. Contribution margin per unit.

c. Contribution margin ratio.

d. Confirm your results by preparing a contribution margin income statement for the break-even sales volume.

LO 8

Problem 11-29 *Margin of safety and operating leverage*

Santiago Company is considering the addition of a new product to its cosmetics line. The company has three distinctly different options: a skin cream, a bath oil, or a hair coloring gel. Relevant information and budgeted annual income statements for each of the products follow.

	Relevant Information		
	Skin Cream	**Bath Oil**	**Color Gel**
Budgeted sales in units (a)	50,000	90,000	30,000
Expected sales price (b)	$7.00	$4.00	$13.00
Variable costs per unit (c)	$4.00	$1.50	$ 9.00
Income Statements			
Sales revenue (a × b)	$350,000	$360,000	$390,000
Variable costs (a × c)	(200,000)	(135,000)	(270,000)
Contribution margin	150,000	225,000	120,000
Fixed costs	(120,000)	(210,000)	(104,000)
Net income	$ 30,000	$ 15,000	$ 16,000

CHECK FIGURES
b. NI:
Skin Cream $60,000
Bath Oil $60,000
Color Gel $40,000

Required

a. Determine the margin of safety as a percentage for each product.

b. Prepare revised income statements for each product, assuming a 20 percent increase in the budgeted sales volume.

c. For each product, determine the percentage change in net income that results from the 20 percent increase in sales. Which product has the highest operating leverage?

d. Assuming that management is pessimistic and risk averse, which product should the company add to its cosmetic line? Explain your answer.

e. Assuming that management is optimistic and risk aggressive, which product should the company add to its cosmetics line? Explain your answer.

ANALYZE, THINK, COMMUNICATE

ATC 11-1 Business Applications *Operating leverage*

Description of Business for Amazon.com, Inc.

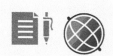

Amazon.com opened its virtual doors on the World Wide Web in July 1995 and we offer Earth's Biggest Selection. We seek to be Earth's most customer-centric company for three primary customer sets: consumer customers, seller customers and developer customers. In addition, we generate revenue through co-branded credit card agreements and other marketing and promotional services, such as online advertising.

Amazon.com	2008	2007
Operating revenue	$19,166	$14,835
Operating earnings	842	655

Description of Business for CSX, Inc.

CSX Corporations ("CSX") together with its subsidiaries (the "Company"), based in Jacksonville, Florida, is one of the nation's leading transportation suppliers. The Company's rail and inter-modal businesses provide rail-based transportation services including traditional rail service and the transport of intermodal containers and trailers.

CSX, Inc.	2008	2007
Operating revenue	$11,255	$10,030
Operating earnings	2,768	2,260

Required

a. Determine which company appears to have the higher operating leverage.

b. Write a paragraph or two explaining why the company you identified in Requirement *a* might be expected to have the higher operating leverage.

c. If revenues for both companies declined, which company do you think would likely experience the greater decline in operating earnings? Explain your answer.

ATC 11-2 Group Assignment *Operating leverage*

The Parent Teacher Association (PTA) of Meadow High School is planning a fund-raising campaign. The PTA is considering the possibility of hiring Eric Logan, a world-renowned investment counselor, to address the public. Tickets would sell for $28 each. The school has agreed to let the PTA use Harville Auditorium at no cost. Mr. Logan is willing to accept one of two compensation arrangements. He will sign an agreement to receive a fixed fee of $10,000 regardless of the number of tickets sold. Alternatively, he will accept payment of $20 per ticket sold. In communities similar to that in which Meadow is located, Mr. Logan has drawn an audience of approximately 500 people.

Required

a. In front of the class, present a statement showing the expected net income assuming 500 people buy tickets.

b. Divide the class into groups and then organize the groups into four sections. Assign one of the following tasks to each section of groups.

Group Tasks

(1) Assume the PTA pays Mr. Logan a fixed fee of $10,000. Determine the amount of net income that the PTA will earn if ticket sales are 10 percent higher than expected. Calculate the percentage change in net income.

(2) Assume that the PTA pays Mr. Logan a fixed fee of $10,000. Determine the amount of net income that the PTA will earn if ticket sales are 10 percent lower than expected. Calculate the percentage change in net income.

(3) Assume that the PTA pays Mr. Logan $20 per ticket sold. Determine the amount of net income that the PTA will earn if ticket sales are 10 percent higher than expected. Calculate the percentage change in net income.

(4) Assume that the PTA pays Mr. Logan $20 per ticket sold. Determine the amount of net income that the PTA will earn if ticket sales are 10 percent lower than expected. Calculate the percentage change in net income.

c. Have each group select a spokesperson. Have one of the spokespersons in each section of groups go to the board and present the results of the analysis conducted in Requirement *b*. Resolve any discrepancies in the computations presented at the board and those developed by the other groups.

d. Draw conclusions regarding the risks and rewards associated with operating leverage. At a minimum, answer the following questions.

(1) Which type of cost structure (fixed or variable) produces the higher growth potential in profitability for a company?

(2) Which type of cost structure (fixed or variable) produces the higher risk of declining profitability for a company?

(3) Under what circumstances should a company seek to establish a fixed cost structure?

(4) Under what circumstances should a company seek to establish a variable cost structure?

ATC 11-3   Research Assignment   *Fixed versus variable cost*

Use the 2008 Form 10-K for Black & Decker Corp. (B&D) to complete the requirements below. To obtain the Form 10-K you can use the EDGAR system following the instructions in Appendix A, or it can be found under "Investor Relations" on the company's corporate website: www.bdk.com. Be sure to read carefully the following portions of the document.

■ "General Development of the Business" on page 1.

■ "Consolidated Statement of Earnings" on page 36.

Required

a. Calculate the percentage decrease in B&D's sales and its "operating income" from 2007 to 2008.

b. Would fixed costs or variable costs be more likely to explain why B&D's operating earnings decreased by a bigger percentage than its sales?

c. On page 42 B&D reported that it incurred product development costs of $146 million in 2008. If this cost is thought of in the context of the number of units of products sold, should it be considered as primarily fixed or variable in nature?

d. If the product development costs are thought of in the context of the number of new products developed, should it be considered as primarily fixed or variable in nature?

ATC 11-4   Writing Assignment   *Operating leverage, margin of safety, and cost behavior*

In the early years of the 21st century the housing market in the United States was booming. Housing prices were increasing rapidly, new houses were being constructed at a record pace, and companies doing business in the construction and home improvement industry were enjoying rising profits. In 2006 the real estate market had slowed considerably, and the slump continued through 2007.

Home Depot was one major company in the building supplies industry that was adversely affected by the slowdown in the housing market. On August 14, 2007, it announced that its revenues for the first half of the year were 3 percent lower than revenues were for the first six months of 2006. Of even greater concern was the fact that its earnings for the first half of 2007 were 21 percent lower than for the same period in the prior year.

Required

Write a memorandum that explains how a 3 percent decline in sales could cause a 21 percent decline in profits. Your memo should address the following:

a. An identification of the accounting concept involved.

b. A discussion of how various major types of costs incurred by Home Depot were likely affected by the decline in its sales.

c. The effect of the decline in sales on Home Depot's margin of safety.

ATC 11-5   Ethical Dilemma   *Profitability versus social conscience (effects of cost behavior)*

Advances in biological technology have enabled two research companies, Bio Labs Inc. and Scientific Associates, to develop an insect-resistant corn seed. Neither company is financially strong enough to develop the distribution channels necessary to bring the product to world markets. World Agra Distributors Inc. has negotiated contracts with both companies for the exclusive right to market their seed. Bio Labs signed an agreement to receive an annual royalty of $1,000,000. In contrast, Scientific Associates chose an agreement that provides for a royalty of $0.50 per pound of seed sold. Both agreements have a 10-year term. During 2010, World Agra sold approximately 1,600,000 pounds of the Bio Labs Inc. seed and 2,400,000 pounds of the Scientific Associates seed. Both types of seed were sold for $1.25 per pound. By the end of 2010, it was apparent that the seed developed by Scientific Associates was superior. Although insect infestation was virtually nonexistent for both types of seed, the seed developed by Scientific Associates produced corn that was sweeter and had consistently higher yields.

World Agra Distributors' chief financial officer, Roger Weatherstone, recently retired. To the astonishment of the annual planning committee, Mr. Weatherstone's replacement, Ray Borrough, adamantly recommended that the marketing department develop a major advertising campaign to promote the seed developed by Bio Labs Inc. The planning committee reluctantly approved the recommendation. A $100,000 ad campaign was launched; the ads emphasized the ability of the Bio Labs seed to avoid insect infestation. The campaign was silent with respect to taste or crop yield. It did not mention the seed developed by Scientific Associates. World Agra's sales staff was instructed to push the Bio Labs seed and to sell the Scientific Associates seed only on customer demand. Although total sales remained relatively constant during 2011, sales of the Scientific Associates seed fell to approximately 1,300,000 pounds while sales of the Bio Labs Inc. seed rose to 2,700,000 pounds.

Required

a. Determine the amount of increase or decrease in profitability experienced by World Agra in 2011 as a result of promoting Bio Labs seed. Support your answer with appropriate commentary.

b. Did World Agra's customers in particular and society in general benefit or suffer from the decision to promote the Bio Labs seed?

c. Review the standards of ethical conduct in Exhibit 10.17 of Chapter 10 and comment on whether Mr. Borrough's recommendation violated any of the principles in the Statement of Ethical Professional Practice.

d. Comment on your belief regarding the adequacy of the Statement of Ethical Professional Practice for Managerial Accountants to direct the conduct of management accountants.